D1307851

CHEMISTRY AND BIOLOGY OF PTERIDINES

DEVELOPMENTS IN BIOCHEMISTRY

CHEMISTRY AND BIOLOGY OF PTERIDINES

Proceedings of The Sixth International Symposium on the Chemistry and Biology of Pteridines, La Jolla, California, September 25-28, 1978

Editors:

ROY L. KISLIUK
Department of Biochemistry, Tufts Medical School, Boston, Massachusetts, USA

and

GENE M. BROWN
Department of Biology, Massachusetts Institute of Technology, Cambridge, Massachusetts, USA

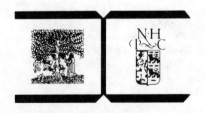

ELSEVIER/NORTH-HOLLAND
NEW YORK • AMSTERDAM • OXFORD

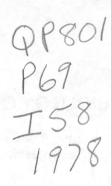

© 1979 by Elsevier North Holland, Inc.

with the exception of those articles authored by Descimon (pp. 93–98), Dorsett, Yim, and Jacobson (pp. 99–104), Kaufman (pp. 117–124), and Horne and Wagner (pp. 555–560) which are works of the United States Government.

Published by:

Elsevier North Holland, Inc.
52 Vanderbilt Avenue, New York, New York 10017

Sole distributors outside of the United States and Canada:

Elsevier/North-Holland Biomedical Press
335 Jan van Galenstraat, PO Box 211
Amsterdam, The Netherlands

ISSN: 0165-1714
ISBN: 0-444-00305-3 (volume 4)

Library of Congress Cataloging in Publication Data

International Symposium on Chemistry and Biology, 6th,
      La Jolla, Calif., 1978.
      Chemistry and biology of pteridines.

      (Developments in biochemistry; v. 4 ISSN 0165-1714)
      Bibliography: p.
      Includes index.
      1. Pteridines—Congresses. 2. Pteridines—Metabolism—
      Congresses. 3. Pterin—Metabolism—Congresses. 4. Vitamin M—
      Metabolism—Congresses. I. Kisliuk, Roy L. II. Brown, Gene M.
      III. Title. IV. Series.
QP801.P69I58 1978   574.1'924   78-26084
ISBN 0-444-00305-3

Manufactured in the United States of America

Contents

xiv

Preface

Research on pteridines has benefited greatly from several symposia since the first one held in Paris in 1952. Subsequent meetings were held in London in 1954, Stuttgart in 1962, Toba in 1969 and Konstanz in 1975. The present volume contains the proceedings of the Sixth International Symposium on the Chemistry and Biology of Pteridines held at LaJolla, California, from September 25 to September 28, 1978. It has been traditional at these meetings to bring together both chemists and bioligists to promote interactions and discussions that have been profitable for all, and in the past many cooperative efforts have grown out of contacts made at these meetings. The Organizing Committee for the Sixth Symposium strove to maintain the tradition of having a program balanced between chemistry and biology, although because of the recent increase in interest in the biological effects of unconjugated pteridines, folic acid and folic acid analogs the Committee felt justified in emphasizing the biological aspects to a somewhat greater extent than has been done in the previous symposia.

The Committee was pleasantly surprised at the large number of abstracts(140) that were submitted to the invitation to all interested investigators to participate in the Symposium. Since the number of submitted abstracts was too great to permit the scheduling of all of them for oral presentation, 80 were given as poster presentations. The Committee was particularly gratified at the success of the poster presentations; attendance was large, quality high, and the attendant discussions among individuals intense and productive.

The Organizing Committee consisted of J.J. Burchall, G.M. Brown, F.M. Huennekens, R.L. Kisliuk, S. Kaufman, J. Montgomery, T. Shiota, and J.M. Whiteley, all of whom enthusiastically contributed their time and talents to make the Symposium a success. Two preliminary meetings were graciously hosted by the Wellcome Research Laboratories, Research Triangle Park, North Carolina who also prepared the abstract book. We are grateful for the efficient manner with which Mrs. Nomi Feldman handled the details of arranging the meetings and the social activities. We are also grateful to Ms. Susan Koscielniak, representing **Elsevier** North-Holland, Inc., who attended the Symposium and took responsibility for collecting and processing the manuscripts. Finally, we wish to thank the participants for the quality of the presentations and for being so cooperative in the prompt submission of their manuscripts.

Cambridge and Boston, Massachusetts   G.M. Brown
October, 1978   R.L. Kisliuk

Acknowledgments

Financial support for this Symposium has been generously provided by:

Beckman Instruments, Inc.

Bristol Laboratories

Burroughs Wellcome Co.

Columbia Organic Chemicals Co.

Fisher Scientific Co.

FMC Corporation

Hoffmann-LaRoche, Inc.

Lederle Laboratories

Merck and Co., Inc.

Philip Morris, Inc.

Smith Kline and French Laboratories

Starks Associates, Inc.

The Upjohn Co.

VWR Scientific, Inc.

Wyeth Laboratories

and

by Grant CA22918 from the National Cancer Institute,

National Institutes of Health,

United States Public Health Service

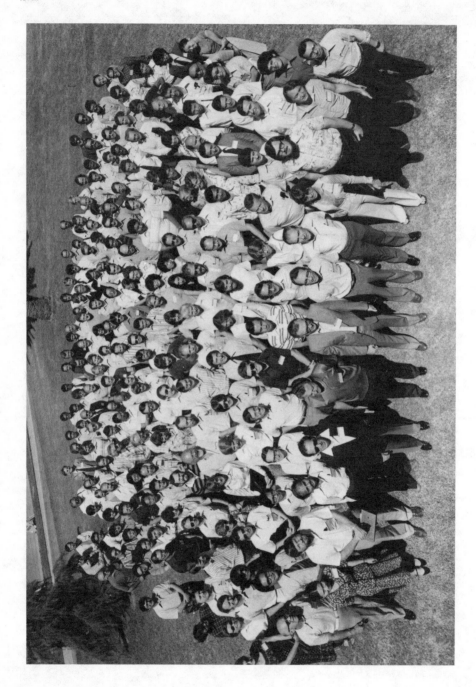

List of Participants

Akino, M.	Tokyo Metropolitan Univ., Tokyo, Japan
Albrecht, A.M.	Sloan-Kettering Institute, Rye, New York
Angier, R.B.	Lederle Laboratories, Pearl River, New York
Armarego, W.	Australian National Univ., Canberra
Ayling, J.E.	University of Texas, San Antonio
Baccanari, D.P.	Wellcome Research Labs., North Carolina
Baily, S.W.	University of Texas, San Antonio
Baugh, C.M.	University of South Alabama, Mobile
Baumgartner, K.T.	University of Zurich, Switzerland
Baur, R.	University of Konstanz, West Germany
Beck, W.S.	Massachusetts General Hospital, Boston
Bednarek, J.M.	University of South Carolina, Columbia
Benkovic, S.J.	Pennsylvania State Univ., University Park
Bertino, J.R.	Yale University, New Haven, Connecticut
Bieri, J.H.	University of Zurich, Switzerland
Blair, J.A.	University of Aston, Birmingham, England
Blakley, R.L.	University of Iowa, Iowa City
Blankenship, D.T.	University of Cincinnati, Ohio
Bowen, D.	Genesee Hospital, Rochester, New York
Boyle, P.H.	Trinity College, Dublin, Ireland
Braverman, E.B.	University of South Alabama, Mobile
Broadbent, H.S.	Brigham Young University, Provo, Utah
Brown, G.M.	Massachusetts Inst. Tech., Cambridge, Mass.
Bruck, P.	Cyclo Chemical, Los Angeles, California
Bruice, T.W.	University of California, San Francisco
Bullard, W.P.	University of California, San Diego
Burchall, J.J.	Wellcome Research Labs., North Carolina
Campbell, C.L.	University of Washington, Seattle
Caperelli, C.A.	Pennsylvania State Univ. University Park
Caston, J.D.	Case Western Reserve Univ., Cleveland, Ohio
Chan, K.	Hoffmann-LaRoche Inc., Nutley, New Jersey
Chanarin, I.	Northwick Park Hospital, Middlesex, England
Chello, P.L.	Sloan-Kettering Cancer Center, New York City
Cheng, Y.	Roswell Park Memorial Inst., Buffalo, N.Y.
Cocco, L.	University of Iowa, Iowa City
Colman, N.	Bronx VA Hospital, New York City
Colwell, W.T.	Stanford Research Inst., Menlo Park, Cal.
Connor, M.J.	University of Aston, Birmingham, England
Cook, R.J.	Vanderbilt University, Nashville, Tenn.
Cooper, B.A.	Royal Victoria Hospital, Montreal, Canada
Cossins, E.A.	University of Alberta, Edmonton, Canada
Cotton, R.G.H.	Royal Children's Hosp., Parkville, Australia
D'Ari, L.	University of California, Berkeley
daCosta, M.	New York Medical College, New York City
Dann, J.G.	Wellcome Research Labs., Beckenham, England
DeGraw, J.I.	Stanford Research Inst. Menlo Park, Cal.
Delk, A.S.	University of California, Berkeley
Descimon, H.A.	Ecole Normale Superieure, Paris, France
Diliberto,E., Jr.	Wellcome Research Labs, North Carolina
Doi, M.	University of Alabama, Birmingham
Dorsett, D.L.	Oak Ridge National Lab., Tennessee
Duch, D.S.	Wellcome Research Labs., North Carolina
Dunlap, R.B.	University of South Carolina, Columbia
Durrfeld, R.	University of South Florida, Tampa
Dwivedi, C.	Tufts University, Boston, Massachusetts
Eichner, E.R.	University of Oklahoma, Oklahoma City

Erbe, R.W.	Massachusetts General Hospital, Boston
Fan, C.	Scripps Clinic and Res. Found., La Jolla
Fan, C.L.	Beckman Instruments, Carlsbad, California
Fernandes, D.J.	Yale University, New Haven, Connecticut
Folsch, E.	Genessee Hospital, Rochester, New York
Foo, S.	University of Alberta, Edmonton, Canada
Forrest, H.S.	University of Texas, Austin
Freisheim, J.H.	University of Cincinnati, Ohio
Fry, D.W.	Medical College of Virginia, Richmond
Fujii, K.	Scripps Clinic and Res. Found., La Jolla
Fukushima, T.	Wellcome Research Labs., North Carolina
Furrer, H.	University of Zurich, Switzerland
Gal, E.M.	University of Iowa, Iowa City
Galivan, J.H.	New York State Dept. Health, Albany
Goldman, I.D.	Medical College of Virginia, Richmond
Goodford, P.J.	Wellcome Research Labs. Beckenham, England
Green, R.	Scripps Clinic and Res. Found., La Jolla
Groff, J.	University of Iowa, Iowa City
Grzelakowska-Sztabert, B.	Polish Academy of Sciences, Warsaw, Poland
Gupta, S.V.	Univ. of Saskatchewan, Saskatoon, Canada
Guynn, R.W.	University of Texas, Houston
Hagi, Y.	University of Alabama, Birmingham
Halsted, C.	University of California, Davis
Hansch, C.	Pomona College, Claremont, California
Hart, L.I.	Royal Cancer Hospital, Sutton, England
Harzer, G.	Scripps Clinic and Res. Found., La Jolla
Hasegawa, H.	National Inst. Mental Health, Bethesda, Md.
Henderson, G.B.	Scripps Clinic and Res. Found., La Jolla
Henkin, J.	University of Texas, Houston
Herbert, V.	Bronx VA Hospital, New York City
Himes, R.H.	University of Kansas, Lawrence
Hitchings, G.H.	Wellcome Research Labs., North Carolina
Horne, D.W.	VA Medical Center, Nashville, Tennessee
Howell, S.I.	University of California, San Diego
Huennekens, F.M.	Scripps Clinic and Res. Found., La Jolla
Hutchison, D.J.	Sloan-Kettering Institute, Rye, New York
Isacoff, W.H.	Harbor General Hospital, Torrance, Cal.
Iten, P.X.	University of Zurich, Switzerland
Iwai, K.	Kyoto University, Kyoto, Japan
Iwanami, Y.	Keio University, Yokohama, Japan
Jackson, R.	Indiana University, Indianapolis
Jacobsen, D.W.	Scripps Clinic and Res. Found., La Jolla
Jacobson, K.B.	Oak Ridge National Lab., Tennessee
Johns, D.G.	National Cancer Institute, Bethesda, Md.
Johnson, S.	Univ. of Saskatchewan, Saskatoon, Canada
Jongejan, J.A.	Technological Univ., Delft, Netherlands
Kalman, T.I.	State University of New York, Buffalo
Kamen, B.A.	Yale University, New Haven, Connecticut
Katoh, S.	Josai Dental Univ., Sakado-shi, Japan
Kaufman, S.	National Inst. Mental Health, Bethesda, Md.
Kaufman, E.	National Inst. Mental Health, Bethesda, Md.
Kaufman, B.T.	Nat. Inst. Arthr. Metab. Digest. Dis., Md.
Kim, D.H.	Wyeth Labs, Inc., Philadelphia, Pa.
Kiriasis, L.	University of Konstanz, West Germany
Kisliuk, R.L.	Tufts University, Boston, Massachusetts
Kompis, I.	Hoffmann-LaRoche, Inc., Nutley, New Jersey
Kozloff, L.M.	University of Colorado, Denver
Kraut, J.	University of California, San Diego
Krivi, G.G.	Massachusetts Inst. Tech., Cambridge, Mass.
Krumdieck, C.L.	University of Alabama, Birmingham

Kumar, A.A.	University of Cincinnati, Ohio
Kwee, S.	University of Aarhus, Aarhus, Denmark
Lai, P.	University of Iowa, Iowa City
Lee, C.	Wellcome Research Labs., North Carolina
Lewis, G.P.	Royal Alexandra Hosp.,Camperdown, Australia
Luthy, C.	Pennsylvania State Univ., University Park
MacKenzie, R.E.	McGill University, Montreal, Canada
Maley, F.	New York State Dept. Health, Albany
Maley, G.F.	New York State Dept. Health, Albany
Mandelbaum-Shavit, F.	Hadassah University, Jerusalem, Israel
Mangum, J.H.	Brigham Young University, Provo, Utah
Mathews, C.K.	Oregon State University, Corvallis
Matsuura, S.	Nagoya University, Nagoya, Japan
Matthews, D.A.	University of California, San Diego
Matthews, R.G.	University of Michigan, Ann Arbor
McCormick, J.I.	University of Cincinnati, Ohio
McDonald, C.	University of Oklahoma, Oklahoma City
McGuire, J.J.	Yale University, New Haven, Connecticut
Mehta, B.M.	Sloan-Kettering Institute, Rye, New York
Milstein, S.	National Inst. Mental Health, Bethesda, Md.
Moad, G.	Pennsylvania State Univ. University Park
Mogolesko, P.D.	American Cyanamid Co., Bound Brook, N.J.
Montgomery, J.A.	Southern Res. Inst., Birmingham, Alabama
Moran, R.G.	Children's Hospital of Los Angeles, Cal.
Morrison, R.W. Jr.	Wellcome Research Labs, North Carolina
Nadkarni, M.V.	National Cancer Institute, Bethesda, Md.
Nagasaki, T.	Scripps Clinic and Res. Found., La Jolla
Nakanishi, H.	Nippon Dental University, Tokyo, Japan
Nakanishi, N.	Josai Dental University, Sakado, Japan
Nagle, D.P., Jr.	University of California, Berkeley
Nair, M.G.	University of South Alabama, Mobile
Narisawa, K.	Tohoku University, Sendai, Japan
Nichol, C.A.	Wellcome Research Labs., North Carolina
Nixon, J.C.	Wellcome Research Labs., North Carolina
Noronha, J.M.	Bhabha Atomic Res. Centre, Bombay, India
O'Donnell J.M.	Carnegie-Mellon University, Pittsburgh, Pa.
Paris, G.Y.	Abbott Labs., Ltd., Montreal, Canada
Parish, W.W.	Parish Chemical, Provo, Utah
Pastore, E.J.	University of California, San Diego
Pendergast, W.	Wellcome Research Labs., North Carolina
Perry, J.R.	MRC Clinical Res. Centre, Harrow, England
Pfleiderer, W.	University of Konstanz, West Germany
Phillips, A.W.	Wellcome Research Labs., Beckenham, England
Piper, J.R.	Southern Res. Inst., Birmingham, Alabama
Piper, W.N.	University of California, San Francisco
Plante, L.T.	Tufts University, Boston, Massachusetts
Poe, M.	Merck Institute, Rahway, New Jersey
Priest, D.G.	University of South Carolina, Charleston
Rabinowitz, J.C.	University of California, Berkeley
Rode, W.K.	Yale University, New Haven, Connecticut
Rokos, H.	Henning Berlin GMBH, Berlin, West Germany
Roland, S.	Welcome Research Labs., North Carolina
Rosenberg, I.H.	University of Chicago, Chicago, Illinois
Rosenblatt, D.S.	Montreal Children's Hosp., Canada
Rosowsky, A.	Sidney Farber Cancer Inst. Boston, Mass.
Roth, B.	Wellcome Research Labs., North Carolina
Rothenberg, S.P.	New York Medical College, New York City
Rowe, P.B.	Royal Alexandra Hosp.,Camperdown,Australia
Santi, D.V.	University of California, San Francisco
Sauer, H.	Ludwig-Maximillian U., Munich, West Germany
Scanlon, K.J.	Yale University, New Haven, Connecticut

Schirch, L.G.	Medical College of Virginia, Richmond
Schmunk, G.A.	University of California, San Diego
Schrecker, A.W.	National Cancer Institute, Bethesda, Md.
Schwinck, I.	University of Connecticut, Storrs
Scott, J.M.	Trinity College, Dublin, Ireland
Scrimgeour, K.G.	University of Toronto, Toronto, Canada
Selhub, J.	University of Chicago, Chicago, Illinois
Shane, B.	Johns Hopkins Univ., Baltimore, Maryland
Shiota, T.	University of Alabama, Birmingham
Sirotnak, F.M.	Sloan-Kettering Cancer Center, New York
Smith, R.A.	University of California, Los Angeles
Smith, S.L.	Wellcome Research Labs., North Carolina
Spector, R.	University of Iowa, Iowa City
Steinberg, S.	University of Wasington, Seattle
Stephanson, L.G.	Scripps Clinic and Res. Found., La Jolla
Stokstad, E.L.R.	University of California, Berkeley
Stone, D.	Council for Tobacco Research, New York
Stone, D.	Wellcome Research Labs., Beckenham, England
Strum, W.	Scripps Clinic and Res. Found., La Jolla
Stuart, A.	Wellcome Foundation Ltd., Dartford, England
Shuresh, M.R.	Scripps Clinic and Res. Found., La Jolla
Suter, C.	Hoffmann-LaRoche, Basel, Switzerland
Szeto, D.W.	Roswell Park Memorial Inst., Buffalo, N.Y.
Tamura, T.	University of California, Davis
Tanaka, K.	Kobe-Gakuin University, Kobe, Japan
Taylor, E.C.	Princeton University, Princeton, New Jersey
Temple, C., Jr.	Southern Res. Inst., Birmingham, Alabama
Tisman, G.	Montebello, Calfornia
Tsusue, M.	Kitasato University, Sagamihara City, Japan
Turner, A.J.	University of Leeds, Leeds, England
Van der Plas, H.C.	Landbouwhogeschool, Wageningen, Netherlands
Viscontini, M.	University of Zurich, Switzerland
Vitols, K.S.	Scripps Clinic and Res. Found., La Jolla
Viveros, O.H.	Wellcome Research Labs., North Carolina
Wagner, C.	VA Hospital, Nashville, Tennessee
Walsh, C.T.	Massachusetts Inst. Tech., Cambridge, Mass.
Wang, E.A.	Massachusetts Inst. Tech., Cambridge, Mass.
Waxman, S.	Mount Sinai Hospital, New York City
Werbel, L.M.	Warner-Lambert/Parke-Davis, Ann Arbor, Mich.
Webber, S.	Scripps Clinic and Res. Found., La Jolla
Weinstock, J.	Smith Kline Corp., Philadelphia, Pa.
White, J.C.	Medical College of Virginia, Richmond
Whitehead, V.M.	Montreal Children's Hosp., Montreal, Canada
Whiteley, J.M.	Scripps Clinic and Res. Found., La Jolla
Wood, H.C.S.	University of Strathclyde, Glasgow, Scotland
Wu, S.	Montebello, California
Yellin, J.B.	Scripps Clinic and Res. Found., La Jolla
Ziegler, I.	Biochemical Institute, Munich, West Germany
Zielinska, Z.M.	Polish Academy of Sciences, Warsaw, Poland

THE STEREOSPECIFICITY OF 6-METHYL- AND 6,7-DIMETHYL-6,7(8H)-DIHYDROPTERIN COFACTORS TOWARDS DIHYDROPTERIDINE REDUCTASE

W. L. F. ARMAREGO

The Australian National University, Canberra, A.C.T. Australia

ABSTRACT

The effectiveness with which (+)-6-methyl, (-)-6-methyl, (±)-6-methyl, (±)-cis-6,7-dimethyl and a 1:1 mixture of (±)-cis and (±)-trans-6,7-dimethyl-6,7(8H)-dihydropterins oxidize NADH to NAD$^+$ in the presence of dihydropteridine reductase from sheep liver and human liver was compared under strictly similar conditions at 20°C and pH 7.2. The similarity of the K_m and $V_{max(app)}$ of the first three compounds and the differences in the K_m values of the last two compounds could be interpreted in terms of the conformation of the cofactors at the active site of the enzyme.

INTRODUCTION

The kinetic parameters (K_m and V_{max}) for the cofactor 6,7-dimethyl-6,7(8H)-dihydropterin and related pterins in the oxidation of NADH to NAD$^+$ using dihydropteridine reductase from various sources has been determined by several workers, notably Kaufman,[1] Scrimgeour,[2] Whiteley,[3] and Lind[4,5] and their coworkers. We were interested in the steric requirements of the enzyme dihydropteridine reductase towards pterin cofactors insofar as the alkyl groups at C-6 and C-7 can be accommodated at the active site of the enzyme. We have examined the kinetic parameters for the enantiomers of the 6-methyl derivative, the cis-isomer of the 6,7-dimethyl derivative and a 1:1 mixture of racemic cis- and trans-6,7-dimethyl derivatives,[6] together with racemic 6,7,7-trimethyl-6,7(8H)-dihydropterin, under strictly comparable conditions, and wish to discuss the data in terms of the conformation of the cofactors at the active site.

MATERIALS AND METHODS

Enzyme preparations. The enzyme from sheep liver was prepared essentially as before,[1,2] and purified up to the alkaline ammonium sulfate fractionation which gave a ca tenfold purification over the crude extract. The human liver enzyme was generously supplied by Dr. R. G. H. Cotton (Royal Children's Hospital, Melbourne, Australia). Two samples were used, the crude extract and the 250-fold purified enzyme which was prepared by Mr. F. Firgaira using a single step with the 1,2-naphthoquinone adsorbent of Cotton and Jenning.[7]

Cofactors. All cofactors were prepared *in situ* by oxidation of the respective 5,6,7,8-tetrahydropterins with peroxidase and hydrogen peroxide as described by Kaufman.[1] (+)-*cis*-6,7-Dimethyl-5,6,7,8-tetra-hydropterin hydrochloride was prepared by catalytic hydrogenation of 6,7-dimethylpterin.[6] It is important to point out that in all the previous literature where 6,7-dimethyl-5,6,7,8-tetrahydropterin was mentioned, the isomer used always had the *cis*-configuration. Reduction of 6,7-dimethylpterin with sodium in ethanol afforded a 1:1 mixture of (+)-*cis*- and (+)-*trans*-6,7-dimethyl-5,6,7,8-tetrahydropterin (clearly observable by p.m.r.).[6] The kinetic measurements were carried out with this mixture. Racemic 6-methyl-5,6,7,8-tetrahydropterin hydrochloride was resolved[8] by neutralizing the hydrochloride in ethanol with alcoholic KOH under dry nitrogen gas followed immediately by addition of an equimolar amount of 2S,3S(-)-di-*O*-benzoyl tartaric acid in the minimum volume of ethanol, and allowing to cool under nitrogen. The (+)base(-)-acid salt separated out almost quantitatively and was collected. The (-)base(-)acid salt was obtained from the mother liquors by addition of ether. Alternatively 2R,3R(+)-di-*O*-benzoyl tartaric acid can be used, in which case the solubilities of the diastereoisomeric salts were reversed. The hydrochlorides of the (+)- and (-)-6-methyl-5,6,7,8-tetra-hydropterins were recovered by dissolving the salts in aqueous 2N-hydrochloric acid, extracting exhaustively with chloroform to remove tartaric acid and freeze-drying the aqueous solution. The optical rotations were $[\alpha]_{435}^{20}$ + 25.8° and -25.0° in 2N-HCl, and displayed plain +ve and -ve ORD curves, respectively. Although we cannot as yet say that these enantiomers are optically pure, the magnitudes of the rotations with opposite signs are indicative of high optical purity. Also, the (+)-isomer gave a positive CD curve similar to that of unnatural optically pure tetrahydrobiopterin (HPLC) described recently by Bailey and Ayling.[9] The curve had a maximum at 263 nm with an ellipticity of 2.5 X 10^{-3} deg. cm.$^{-2}$ dmole^{-1} which compares favorably with the values[9] of pure natural and unnatural tetrahydrobiopterin considering that the latter have two more adjacent asymmetric centers which must affect the chromophore. Racemic 6,7,7-trimethyl-5,6,7,8-tetrahydropterin hydrochloride was prepared by catalytic hydrogenation of 6,7,7-trimethyl-7,8-dihydropterin.

Kinetic Runs. These were performed essentially as described by

Kaufman[1] using tris-chloride (100 μmoles), hydrogen peroxide (5 μmoles), peroxidase (20 μg), NADH (*ca* 0.07 μmoles), tetrahydropterin (0.01 to 0.07 μmoles) and enzyme (5 μl, 0.31 μg for pure human enzyme), all in 1 ml at 20°C, and giving a final pH of 7.2. The rate of change of optical density was followed at 340 nm. The NADH concentration was kept constant in all measurements and all determinations for comparisons (in duplicate) were made within a few days. The data were processed using an elaborate computer program supplied by Dr. J. F. Morrison (Australian National University) and *all* the runs were computed, hence the slightly larger s.e. values in some cases.

RESULTS AND DISCUSSION

6-Methyl-6,7(8*H*)-dihydropterins (6-MeDHP). The kinetic parameters for the racemate and the enantiomers with the human and sheep liver

TABLE

	(+)-6-MeDHP	(+)-6-MeDHP	(-)-6-MeDHP	
K_m	13.42 (se 0.99)μM	11.01 (se 0.8)μM	8.3 (se 0.33)μM	Human liver 250 fold purified
$V_{max.app}$	45.4 (se 1.3)	51.4 (se 1.3)	48.3 (se 0.6)	
K_m	35.9 (se 2.0)μM	33.7 (se 1.5)μM	32.7 (se 4.4)μM	Sheep liver 10 fold purified
$V_{max.app}$	2.74 (se 0.08)	2.74 (se 0.09)	3.29 (se 0.27)	

	cis-6,7-DiMeDHP	*cis+trans*-6,7-DiMeDHP(1:1)		
K_m	26.3 (se 3.3)μM	14.8 (se 1.4)μM	Crude	
$V_{max.app}$/5μl	0.0196 (se 0.001)	0.0154 (se 0.0003)		Human Liver
K_m	19.4 (se 1.9)μM	8.4 (se 0.5)μM	250 fold purified	
$V_{max.app}$	62.6 (se 2.5)	49.7 (se 0.9)		
K_m	38.4 (40.7) (se 1.1)μM	21.6 (se 1.5)μM	Sheep liver 10 fold purified	
$V_{max.app}$	2.78 (se 0.07)	3.0 (se 0.09)		

All these values were measured at 20°C, pH 7.2 and NADH conc. ∿ 70 μM.

	6,7,7-TriMeDHP	
K_m	47.7 (se 6.6)μM	Human liver 250 fold purified
$V_{max.app}$/mg	15.1 (se 1.1)	

At 20°C, pH 7.2 and NADH conc. ∿ 67 μM. $V_{max.app}$ are in μmoles NADH oxidized/min/mg.

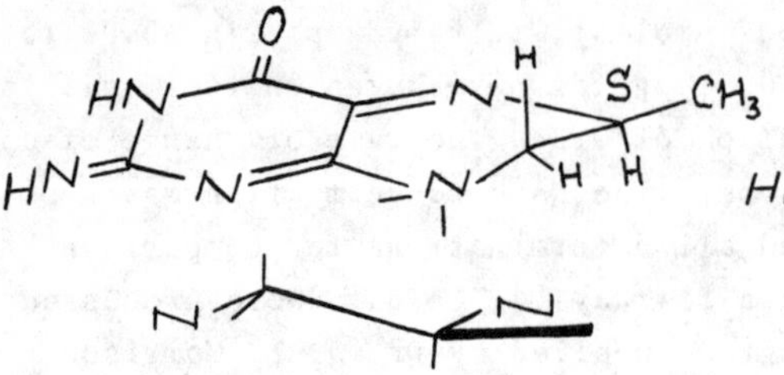

4

(1) 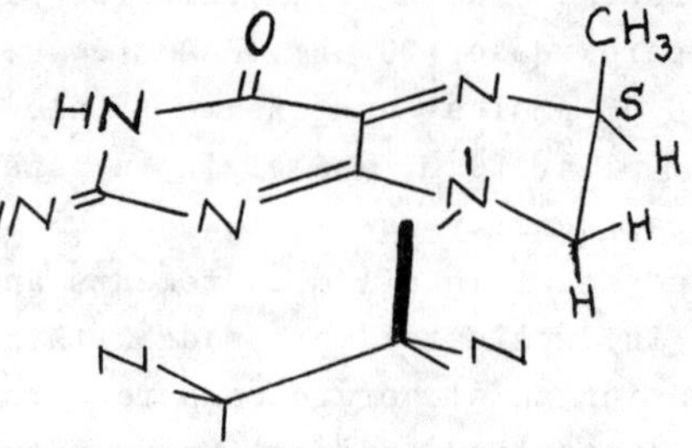   (2)

enzymes are in the Table. Although there is a trend in the K_m values
this is not significant enough, and it could be said that the compounds
have the same capabilities as cofactors. There can be two explanations
for this. In the first, if we fix the conformation of the S-isomer as
in (1) then the methyl group will be equatorial, and the molecule can
slot into the active site. The other conformer (2) will have the
methyl group in a pseudo-axial conformation and will need to undergo
a conformational change before it can be active. The R-isomer with
the hydropyrazine conformation (1), i.e. (3), will of necessity have a
pseudo-axial methyl group and will have to undergo a conformational
change to (4) in order to be active. Hence for both enantiomers to
have the same biological activity the S-isomer will have to function in
the conformation (1) and the R-isomer in the other conformation (4).
For the second explanation to hold there would need to be enough room
at the active site to accommodate either an axial or an equatorial 6-
methyl group. The test for this would be to find out if 6,6-dimethyl-
6,7(8H)-dihydropterin is active. In this case there will always be an
axial and equatorial methyl group in either conformation. The 5,6-
dimethyl compound has not yet been synthesized.

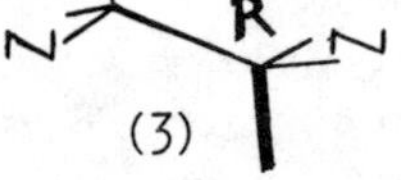

(3) 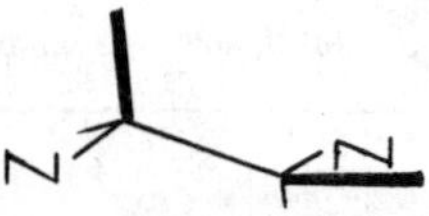   (5) 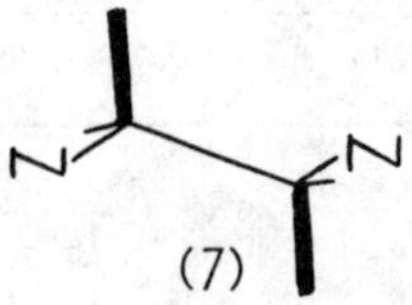   (7)

             CIS

                          TRANS

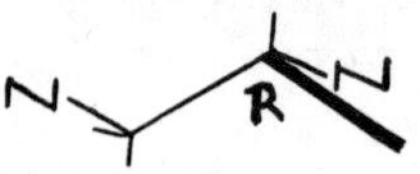

(4) 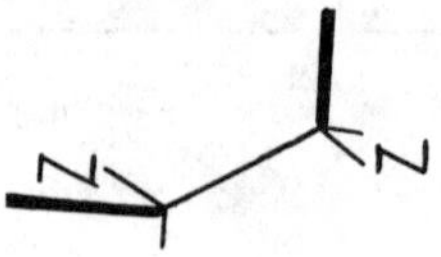   (6) 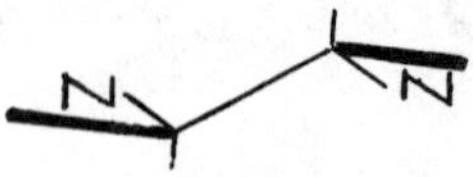   (8)

6,7-Dimethyl-6,7(8*H*)-dihydropterins (6,7-DiMeDHP). The data are in
the Table. The smaller K_m values of the *cis-trans*-mixture may be indicative of the fact that the *trans*-isomer binds more strongly to the
enzyme than the *cis*-isomer. This can be explained in conformational
terms. In the *cis*-isomer one methyl group is axial and the other
equatorial (5) and (6) irrespective of conformer. In the *trans*-isomer
one conformer (7, less favorable) has *trans*-diaxial methyl groups
whereas the favorable conformer has both methyl groups equatorial.
The latter conformer (8) would be more effective than any of the
conformers. Formulae (5) to (8) show only one of the two diastereomeric forms in each case. The double reciprocal plots for the *cis-
trans*-mixture, however, are slightly complicated because at low substrate concentrations (< ∿ 40 μM) the system is stimulated whereas
at higher concentrations it is inhibited compared with the *cis*-isomer
(see Fig.). This is an unusual case in which both *cis*- and *trans*-
isomers are effective substrates, and a clearer picture would be
obtained with the pure *trans*-isomer.

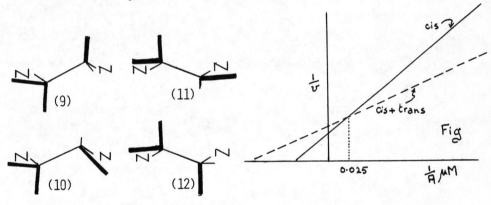

The 6,6-dimethyl derivative was not available for measurement, but
we have been able to study the effect of a gem-dimethyl group by
using 6,7,7-trimethyl-6,7(8*H*)-dihydropterin. This example has *cis*
and *trans* configurations of methyl groups in the same molecule (9)
to (12). The data (see Table) for 6,7,7-triMeDHP show that this compound not only has a comparatively low K_m value but also a lower
$V_{max(app)}$ compared with the other pterins, and is less effective as
a substrate than any of the above pterins in oxidizing NADH.

ACKNOWLEDGEMENTS
I thank Dr. R. G. H. Cotton for supplying the human liver enzyme
and Drs. Cotton, J. F. Morrison and E. Hyde for most helpful discussions.

6

REFERENCES

1. Craine, J.E., Hall, S.E. and Kaufman, S. (1972) J. Biol. Chem., 247, 6082.

2. Cheema, S., Soldin, S.J., Knapp, A., Hofmann, T. and Scrimgeour, K.G. (1973) Can. J. Biochem., 51, 1229.

3. Webber, S., Deits, T.L., Snyder, W.R. and Whiteley, J.M. (1978) Analyt. Biochem., 84, 491.

4. Lind, K.E. (1972) European J. Biochem., 25, 560.

5. Nielsen, K.H., Simsonsen, V. and Lind, K.E. (1969) European J. Biochem., 9, 497.

6. Armarego, W.L.F. and Schou, H. (1977) J. Chem. Soc., Perkin Trans. 1, 2529.

7. Cotton, R.G.H. and Jennings, J. (1978) European J. Biochem., 83, 319.

8. Schou, H., Ph.D. Thesis (1978) Australian National University.

9. Bailey, S. and Ayling, J. (1978) J. Biol. Chem., 253, 1598.

APPLICATION OF THE FRONTIER ORBITAL THEORY TO PTERINES

KONRAD BAUMGARTNER and JOST H. BIERI

Organisch-chemisches Institut, Universität Zürich-Irchel, Winterthurer-
str. 190, CH-8057 Zürich (Switzerland)

ABSTRACT

THE CNDO-CI calculation method[1] made it possible to make a contribution to the reaction mechanism and to the planning of the synthesis
of 7-aminoxanthopterin (V) from xanthopterin-7-carboxylic acid (IV)[2].

INTRODUCTION AND CALCULATION METHOD

According to the frontier orbital theory of Fukui, the orbital density of HOMO or LUMO predicts the position at which a molecule can be
attacked by an electrophilic or nucleophilic reagent[3]. This theory is
applied to reactions of xanthopterin (I)[4] and xanthopterin-7-carboxylic
acid (IV)[5]. The frontier electron densities were calculated according
to the CNDO-CI method (the most simple valence electron method with
explicit consideration of electron interaction). The calculation was
executed with a Fortran program by Kuhn using his set of parameters[6].
The atomic coordinates of the calculated compounds I and IV were determined with the X-ray diffraction data of xanthopterin monohydro--
chloride[7]. For additional partial structures, we used the customary
bond lengths and angles. The graphic representation of the molecule
orbitals was accomplished with the PLOT program by Haselbach and Schmelzer, where the diameters are proportional to the MO coefficients[8].

RESULTS

1. Nucleophilic reactions with xanthopterin (I)

In the literature, nucleophilic reactions at position 7 of xanthopterin (I) in acid, neutral, and basic solutions were described.
Xanthopterin-7-carboxylic amide (II)[9] and erythropterin (III)[10] are
formed as a result (diagram 1).

According to the frontier orbital theory applied to reactions with
a nucleophilic reagent, that position of the molecule is most likely
to react which has the greatest orbital density in the LUMO[3]. As
shown in figure 1, the frontier orbital density of I^{2-} is greatest

at position 7 (in the neutral and cationic molecules I and I⁺ the LUMO density is also greatest at position 7). The chemical experiments thus confirm the quantum chemistry calculations on I[9,10].

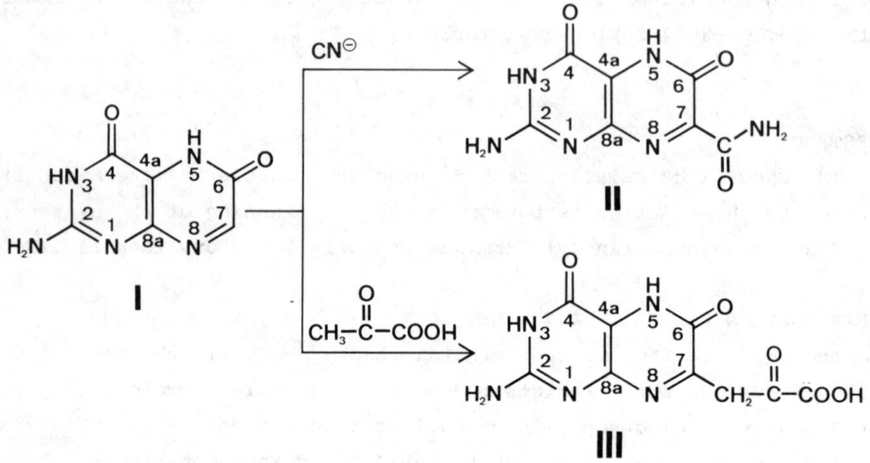

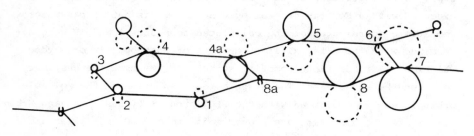

Diagram 1. Nucleophilic reactions with xanthopterin (I).

Fig. 1. LUMO of the xanthopterin dianion (I^{2-}) ($pK'_a = 6.59$; $pK''_a = 9.31$ [11]).

2. Nucleophilic reaction with xanthopterin-7-carboxylic acid (IV)

The chromatography of xanthopterin-7-carboxylic acid (IV) on cellulose with ammoniacal solvent unexpectedly yielded a product to which structure V was ascribed (diagram 2). Due to initial difficulties in the isolation and purification of 7-aminoxanthopterin (V), the postulated structure V could not be confirmed with standard spectroscopic methods. However, the quantum chemistry calculations (CNDO-CI) performed on IV justify the following statements: The calculated atomic charges of IV yield a -0.08 elementary charge on C(7)[4]. This indicates that a charge-controlled attack of the ammonia molecule at position 7 is impossible. However, the LUMO of IV (Fig. 2) shows that a nucleophilic, frontier-controlled attack of ammonia as a primary step seems quite probable[5].

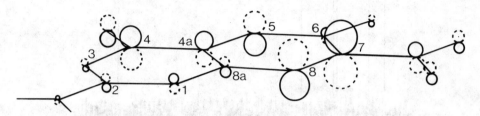

Fig. 2. LUMO of the xanthopterin-7-carboxylic acid trianion (IV^{3-}).

On the basis of these results, the reaction mechanism for the formation of V can be established (diagram 2) and the necessary consequences to optimize the preparation of V can be concluded (e.g. addition of MnO_2 in the oxidation step). It became thus possible after completion of the synthesis to confirm the structure of V with the help of ^{13}C-FT-NMR. (Fig. 3) and ^{15}N-FT-NMR. spectroscopy (Fig. 4).

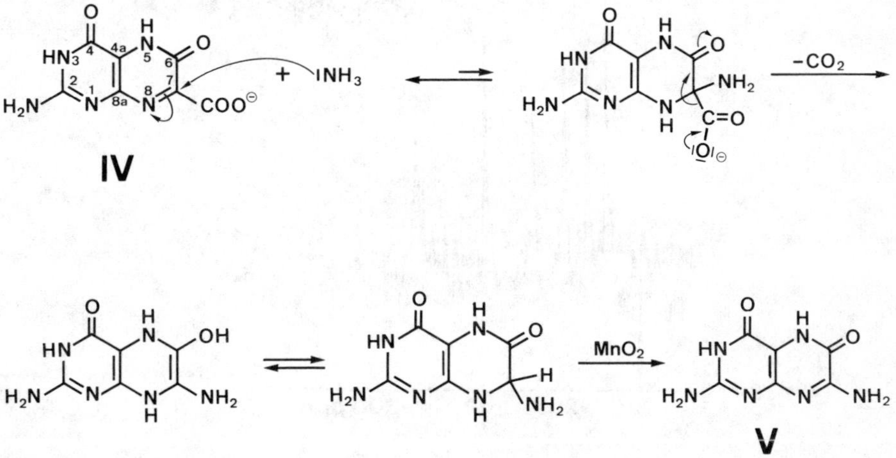

Diagram 2. Reaction mechanism of the formation of 7-aminoxanthopterin (V).

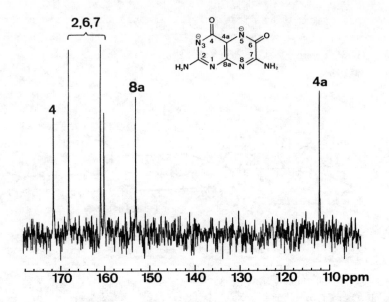

Fig. 3. ^{13}C-FT-NMR. spectrum of 7-aminoxanthopterin (V) in 1 N NaOD. (Assignment of signals according to ^{13}).

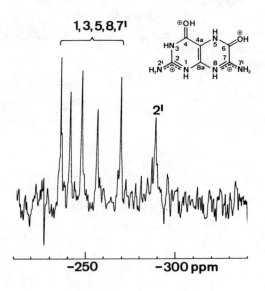

Fig. 4. ^{15}N-FT-NMR. spectrum of 7-aminoxanthopterin (V) in FSO$_3$H. (Assignment of signals only partially possible according to ^{14}).

ACKNOWLEDGMENTS

We should like to express our gratitude to Prof. Dr. M. Viscontini for helpful discussions, Mr. Dipl.-chem. W. Schwotzer (Department Prof. Dr. W. v.Philipsborn) for recording the ^{13}C-FT-NMR. and ^{15}N-FT-NMR. spectra and assisting with their interpretation, Dr. J. Kuhn for his CNDO-CI program, and the University of Zürich Data Processing Center for granting the necessary computer time.

REFERENCES

1. Pople, J.A. and Beveridge, D.L. (1970) Approximate Molecular Orbital Theory, McGraw-Hill, New York.

2. Purrmann, R. (1941) Annalen der Chemie, 548, 284.

3. Fukui, K. (1975) Theory of Orientation and Stereoselection, Springer, Berlin.

4. Baumgartner, K. (1977) Diplomarbeit, Universität Zürich.

5. Baumgartner, K. and Bieri, J.H. Helv. chim. Acta, to be published.

6. Kuhn, J. (1971) Dissertation, Universität Zürich.

7. Bieri, J.H. et al. (1976) Helv. chim. Acta, 59, 2374.

8. Haselbach, E. and Schmelzer, H. (1971) Helv. chim. Acta, 54, 1299.

9. Viscontini, M. and Piraux, M. (1962) Helv. chim. Acta, 45, 1000.

10. Viscontini M. and Stierlin, H. (1963) Helv. chim. Acta 46, 51.

11. Inoue, Y. and Perrin, D.O. (1962) J. chem. Soc., 2600.

12. Müller, G. and von Philipsborn, W. (1973) Helv. chim. Acta, 56, 2680.

13. Ewers, U. et al. (1973) Chem. Ber., 106, 3951; ibid. (1974) 107, 3275.

14. Schwotzer, W., Bieri, J.H. et al. (1978) Helv. chim. Acta, 61, in press.

PHOTOCHEMISTRY OF PTERIDINES

RALPH BAUR, MATTHIAS KAPPEL, RUDOLF MENGEL AND WOLFGANG PFLEIDERER
Fachbereich Chemie, Universität Konstanz
Postfach 7733, D-7750 Konstanz (West Germany)

ABSTRACT

Various new photochemical degradations are found in the lumazine
and pterin series. 8-Substituted lumazines (1) as well as 6- and 7-
polyhydroxyalkylpterins (3-5, 10) are degraded photochemically by a
Norrish type II cleavage reaction yielding lumazines (2) and the aut-
oxydizable 5,8-dihydropterin-6-(6,7) and 7-aldehydes (11) as interesting intermediates. Sepia-(13) and deoxysepiapterin (14) show a pH-dependent degradation on irradiation yielding pterin-6-carboxylic acid
at pH 5-12 and a simple photooxidation to 18 and 19 respectively at
pH 0. 7-Acyl-1,3-dimethyllumazines (21-24) are subject to a photochemical disproportionation reaction in acidic medium yielding the corresponding 5,8-dihydro (25-28) and N-1 dealkylated derivatives as well
as formaldehyde. 6-Acyl-1,3-dimethyllumazines (30-32) show also photo-
demethylation at N-1 to 34-36 of so far unknown mechanism. Photochemical decarboxylation takes place easily with 1,3-dimethyllumazine-7-
carboxylic acid (33) but not with the corresponding 6-isomer.

INTRODUCTION

Reports concerning the light sensitivity of naturally occurring
pteridine derivatives are frequently found in literature[1-4] but very
little is known about the photochemistry of this class of compounds.
In order to prevent the formation of artefacts during isolation and
work-up of such substances working in a dark-room usually is recommended. Since some of the reported photodegradations such as the conversion of biopterin into pterin-6-carboxylic acid[1,5] and of ichthio-
pterin into isoxanthopterin[3,4] are multistage reactions, we decided
to start some more systematic investigations in the lumazine and pterin
series in order to get detailed information about the complex mechanisms.

RESULTS

It was found with 8-substituted lumazines (1)[6] that especially
ß-hydroxy-, ß-alkoxy- and ß-aminoalkyl derivatives are subject to an
easy photodealkylation by a Norrish type II cleavage reaction converting the cross conjugated $\widetilde{\pi}$-system into a heteroaromatic configuration (2).

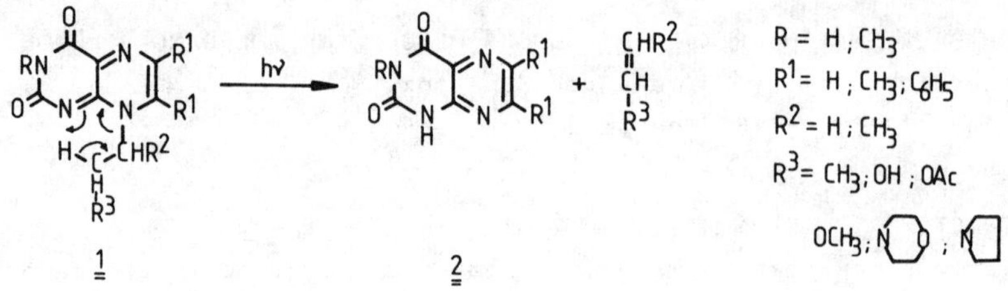

$$R = H; CH_3$$
$$R^1 = H; CH_3; C_6H_5$$
$$R^2 = H; CH_3$$
$$R^3 = CH_3; OH; OAc$$

Photolysis of biopterin (3) and neopterin (4) revealed an analogous photodegradation reaction forming under anaerobic conditions at
pH 10 via a Norrish type II mechanism a longwave absorbing substance
which is believed to be 5,8-dihydropterin-6-aldehyde (6) due to its
physical properties and due to the spontaneous dehydrogenation to
pterin-6-aldehyde (8) on admission of oxygen.

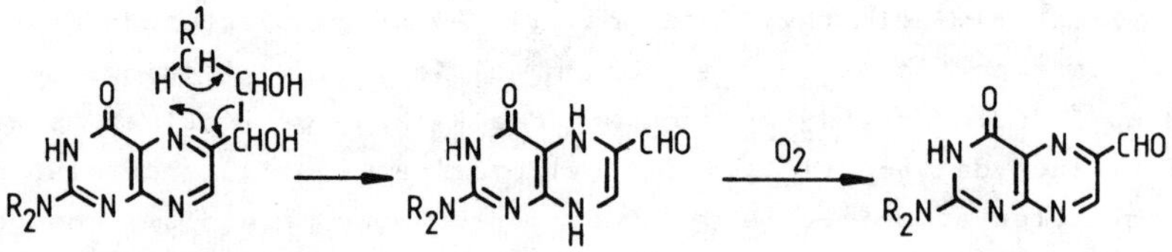

	R	R^1
3	H	H
4	H	OH
5	CH$_3$	H

	R
6	H
7	CH$_3$

	R
8	H
9	CH$_3$

The long wavelength absorption at 480-500 nm of low intensity
seems to be characteristic for 6- and 7-acyl-5,8-dihydrolumazines
and pterins respectively since the electrochemically prepared 6-
acetyl-1,3,7-trimethyl-5,8-dihydrolumazine[7] shows the same spectral
features and reactivities. 6 could also be obtained by photoreduction of 8 in the presence of 1,4-cyclohexadiene-1-carboxylic acid
indicating some thermodynamical stabilization of the formally antiaromatic dihydropyrazine moiety by the electron-attracting formyl
group. The Norrish type II cleavage of biopterin proceeds with a
quantum yield of 0.11 and is strongly pH-dependent. The anion reacts
most easily, in the neutral species the quantum yield is about one
half and the protonated form is relatively stable yielding on prolonged irradiation a complex mixture of compounds.

Neopterin (4) and 7-isobiopterin (10) are photochemically degraded in an analogous manner to 5,8-dihydropterin-6-(6) and 7-aldehyde

(11) respectively with a somewhat longer wavelength absorption band
of the latter at 500 nm.

A solvent dependence was also recognized showing a much faster
reaction in DMF than in buffer solution. The photodegradation of
2-N,N-dimethylbiopterin (5) proceeded again analogously in weakly
basic medium to 7, but at pH 1 another homogenous looking reaction
was observed contrary to 3. Irradiation effected the usual colour
change of the solution to red with an absorption band at 530 nm building up in 80 minutes to its highest extinction, but no 2-N,N-di-
methylpterin-6-aldehyde (9) could be detected after air oxidation.
Starting material 5 was found instead in 50 % yield after chromatographical separation from little byproducts. It is not yet clear where
the reduction equivalents come from to form the alleged 5,8-dihydro
structure and whether a simple 5,8-dihydropterin derivative without
a carbonyl function in 6- or 7-position respectively may give raise
to an absorption around 500 nm. It is, however, very much unlikely
that another chromophor will account for this fact.

There seems to be a general pH-dependence in the photochemistry
of pteridines since different degradations take place also with sepia-
(13) and deoxysepiapterin (14) (formerly called isosepiapterin) varying the pH. We could prove that sepiapterin is degraded at pH 5, 7
and 12 by light in presence of oxygen to pterin-6-carboxylic acid
(17)[5,8]. The mechanism is still unknown but may include in the first
step presumably also a photoelimination via the Norrish type II pathway yielding a ketene intermediate 15 which is the hydrated to 16
and oxidized to 17.

Photolysis of 13 and 14 respectively at pH 0 causes a much faster
spectral change which does, however, not include the side chain in
any elimination reaction according to the absence of pterin-6-carb-
oxylix acid (17) in tlc. We believe that a photooxidation to 6-lac-
toyl-(18) and 6-propionyl-pterin (19) takes place since the resulting
UV-spectrum resembles much more the model substance 6-acetyl-7-methyl-
pterin (20) than 17 especially if adjusted to pH 10 where the spectral
differences are more distinct.

These investigations have then been extended to 6- and 7-acyl-
1,3-dimethyllumazines respectively in order to establish possibly
a general reaction behaviour. It was found with 7-acetyl-(21), 7-
propionyl-(22), 7-butyroyl-(23) and 7-dihydrocinnamoyl-1,3-dimethyl-
lumazin (24) that on irradiation with a 250 Watt projector lamp again
a new absorption band in the visible region turned up under anaerobic
conditions with a maximum at 515 nm at pH 2.5 - 6 and 500 nm at pH
0 - 1. Obviously the 5,8-dihydro derivatives 25-28 have been formed
since air oxidation restored the UV-spectrum of the starting material
fast in neutral solution and much slower under acidic conditions.

	R
21	H
22	CH_3
23	C_2H_5
24	$CH_2C_6H_5$

	R
25	H
26	CH_3
27	C_2H_5
28	$CH_2C_6H_5$

The question then arose where the reduction equivalents come from
when having worked in aqueous solution and 0.1 N HCl respectively.
Chromatograms of the acidic case showed a second main spot which was

isolated in 20 % yield from a preparative scale (0.1 g 22) experiment
in an photoreactor and identified as 3-methyl-7-propionyllumazine
(29) by an NMR- mass spectrum as well as an elementary analysis.

We suggest that the photoreduction and photodealkytion are directly connected to each other revealing a special type of disproportionation reaction as seen from the 5,8-dihydro structure and the formation of formaldehyde which could be detected in the reaction solution[9]. Since the reaction rate increases with lowering the pH and
increase of concentration a bimolecular reaction is very much likely
involving the cation form as the acceptor molecule due to its substantially more basic properties in the excited state[10]. A radical
transfer by an H-atom followed by an electron is postulated since
no radical-cation could be found by ESR spectroscopy. A charge-trans-
fer situation analogous to findings in the pyrazine series[11] can be
ruled out by the spectral data. On these grounds we propose the following mechanism:

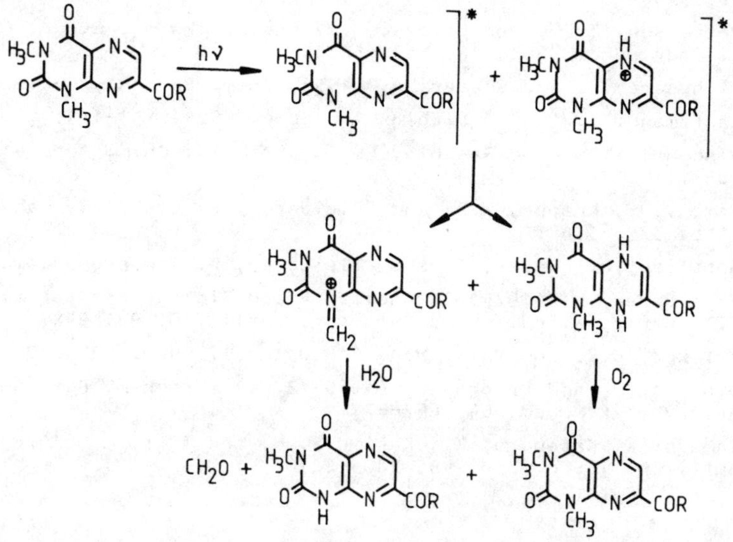

In order to prove the generality of the photochemical N-1 demethylation reaction in the lumazine series 1,3-dimethyllumazine (30),
its 6-propionyl-(31) and 7-methyl-6-propionyl derivatives (32) have
also been irradiated on 0.1 N HCl solution giving the dealkylated
products 34-36 in reasonable yields.

18

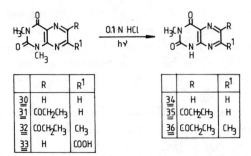

	R	R¹
30	H	H
31	COCH₂CH₃	H
32	COCH₂CH₃	CH₃
33	H	COOH

	R	R¹
34	H	H
35	COCH₂CH₃	H
36	COCH₂CH₃	CH₃

The mechanism of these photodegradations is not yet known and must be different from the above discussed 7-acyl isomers since the spectral changes do not show any absorption in the visible region.

REFERENCES

1. Forrest, H.S. and Mitchell, H.K. (1955) J. Amer. Chem. Soc. 77, 4865-4869.

2. Patterson, E.L., von Saltza, M.H. and Stockstad, E.L.R. (1956) J. Amer. Chem. Soc. 78, 5871-5873.

3. Tschesche, R. and Glaser, A. (1958) Chem. Ber. 91, 2081-2089.

4. Kauffmann, T. (1959) Liebigs Ann. Chem. 625, 133-139.

5. Viscontini, M. and Raschig, H. (1958) Helv. Chim. Acta 41, 108-113.

6. Ram, V.J., Knappe, W.R. and Pfleiderer, W. (1977) Tetrahedron Lett. 3795-3798.

7. Gottlieb, R., Geyer, I. and Pfleiderer, W., in preparation.

8. Pfleiderer, W. (1975) in Chemistry and Biology of Pteridines, Pfleiderer, W. ed., W. de Gruyter, Berlin, p. 941-948.

9. Bricker, C.E. and Vail, W.A. (1950) Anal. Chem. 22, 720-722.

10. Lippert, E. and Prigge, H. (1960) Z. Elektrochem. Ber. Bunsenges. Physik. Chem. 64, 662-671.

11. Yamada, K. Katsuura, K., Kasimura, H. and Iida, H. (1976) Bull. Chem. Soc. Jpn. 49, 2805-2810.

X-RAY ANALYSIS IN PTERIN CHEMISTRY

JOST H. BIERI

Organisch-chemisches Institut, Universität Zürich-Irchel, Winterthurer-
str. 190, CH-8057 Zürich (Switzerland)

ABSTRACT

The crystallographic structures of the following compounds are presented: xanthopterin-monohydrochloride (I)[1], 6-methyl-7,8-dihydro-
pterin-monohydrochloride-monohydrate (II)[2], 5-formyl-6,7-dimethyl-
5,6,7,8-tetrahydropterin (III)[3] and 5,6,7-trimethyl-5,6,7,8-tetra-
hydropterin-dihydrochloride-monohydrate (IV)[4].

CRYSTALLOGRAPHIC DETERMINATION

The crystallographic, diffractometric and structural data of I, II,
III and IV are given by [1,2,3,4].

RESULTS

1. Xanthopterin-monohydrochloride (I)

The molecule is protonated at N(1). This is identical to the protonation site postulated earlier on the basis of UV., ^{1}H-NMR. and [13]C-
NMR. spectroscopy in acidic solutions[5].

The chloride ion 18 exhibits its shortest distances with respect to
the atoms H(15) (2.198 Å) and H(12) (2.199 Å) but not as expected to
the latter and to one of the two hydrogen atoms at N(9). On the contrary, by the spatial arrangement of the chloride ion the N(9) grouping
with the atoms H(13) and H(14) is lifted out of the plane of the pyrimidine ring with concomitant distortion (fig. 2).

Based on these results the positive charge must be assumed to be de-
localised over the centers N(1), C(2), N(3) and N(9) (fig. 1).

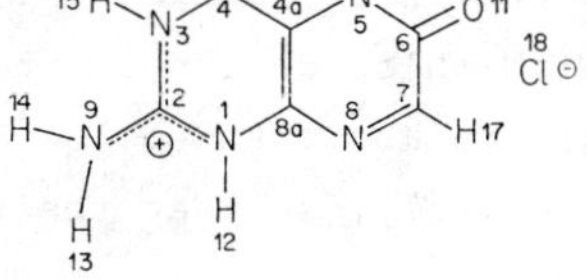

Fig. 1. Structure of xanthopterin-
monohydrochloride (I) with numbering
of atoms.

In contrast to planar pteridine[6] the planes 1 (pyrazine ring) and 2 (pyrimidine ring) present an angle of 2.02° with respect to each other.

The angles found at the carbonyl function C(4)=O(10) in I correspond to the usual values of these functional groups of 122.42°, 124,31° and 113.25°. They deviate markedly from those measured on guanine-hydro-chloride-monohydrate by X-ray diffraction (116°, 136° and 108°)[7].

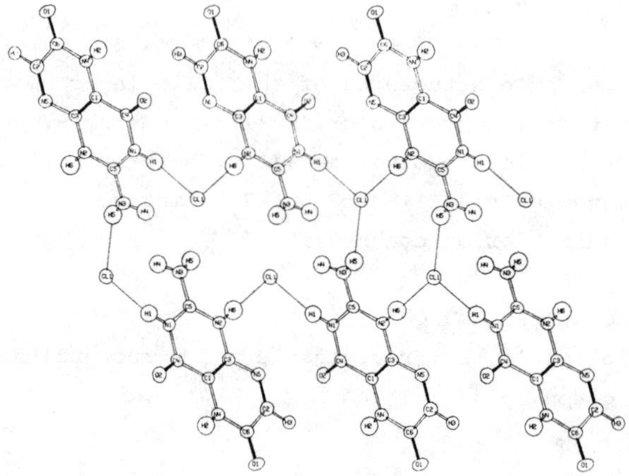

Fig. 2. Spatial representation of xanthopterin-monochloride (I).

2. 6-Methyl-7,8-dihydropterin-monohydrochloride-monohydrate (II)

The molecule is protonated at N(5). The chloride ion 22 has its shortest distances with respect to the atoms H(21) (2.339 Å) and H(25) (2.296 Å, hydrated) (fig. 4). The site of protonation and the short distance between chloride ion and H(21) indicate clearly the sequence of acid/base-strength in compound II.

Both the pyrimidine and pyrazine rings are planar with the amino group consisting of the atoms N(9), H(12) and H(13), and with the atoms H(14), O(10), H(15), C(11) and H(21) lying in the same respective planes. The angle between plane 1 (pyrimidine ring) and plane 2 (pyrazine ring) is 0.24° giving an overall planar molecular structure. Atom H(21) does not in this molecule stick out of the plane as has been observed previously in two 5,6,7,8-tetrahydropterin structures[3,4]. This may be explained by the strong interaction with chloride ion 22 which lies in the same plane. Atoms H(19) and H(20) are above and below the pyrazine plane by 0.818 Å and 0.705 Å, respectively, so that their environment will be symmetrical.

The N(8)-C(8a) bond (1.337 Å) of the vinylogous amide grouping displays distinct double bond characteristics. In view of the protonation site N(5) and of the bond lengths N(5)-C(6) (1.294 Å), C(6)-C(7) (1.491 Å) and C(6)-C(11) (1.483 Å) the acid-base catalysed exchange of the hydrogen atoms H(16), H(17), H(18) of the C(11)-methyl group and H(19) and H(20) of C(7) with deuterium can be readily explained.

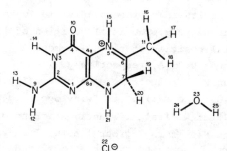

Fig. 3. Structure of 6-Methyl-7,8-dihydropterin-monohydrochloride-monohydrate (II) with numbering of atoms.

As indicated by the bond lengths of the pyrimidine ring there is a marked delocalisation of the π-electrons with the electron pair of N(9) contributing to the mesomeric system by means of the C(2)-N(9)-bond (1.329 Å). Fig. 4 shows furthermore that the pyrimidine rings of neighbouring molecules are arranged in a parallel manner. This is typical for aromatic molecules (or their substructures) where strong interactions between neighbouring π-electron systems occur.

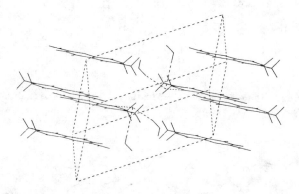

Fig. 4. ORTEP-presentation of the packing of molecules II in the unit cell.

3. 5-Formyl-6,7-dimethyl-5,6,7,8-tetrahydropterin (III)

The pyrimidine part of the molecule has a planar configuration with
the amino group (atoms N(9), H(15), H(16)) and the lactam function (including atoms H(17) and O(10)) lying in the same plane. Comparing the
positions of the atoms constituting the tetrahydropyrazine ring
with respect to the pyrimidine plane shows that N(5) (0.11 Å), C(7)
(0.12 Å) and N(8) (0.07 Å) lie almost in this plane whereas C(6) is
clearly above it by 0.84 Å. This results in a pronouncedly flattened
conformation for the tetrahydropyrazine ring. The axial position of the
C(13)-methyl group and the equatorial position of the C(14)-methyl group
is given by the values of 2.31 Å and 0.73 Å, respectively. The two
methyl groups have cis-configuration with respect to each other (fig.6).

The atoms O(10), C(4), C(4a), C(8a) and N(8) of the vinylogous amide
function lie in one plane with H(27) at N(8) significantly sticking out
(0.45 Å). The carbon atom 11 of the N(5)-formyl group lies well in the
planar system of the pyrimidine part whereas the oxygen atom 12 and the
hydrogen atom 18 protrude above (0.25 Å) and below (0.52 Å) the plane,
respectively. This must be assumed to be due to steric hindrance between the atoms O(10) and H(18) (interatomic distance: 2.59 Å). Thus,
the N(5)-formyl function possesses (E)-configuration (fig. 6).

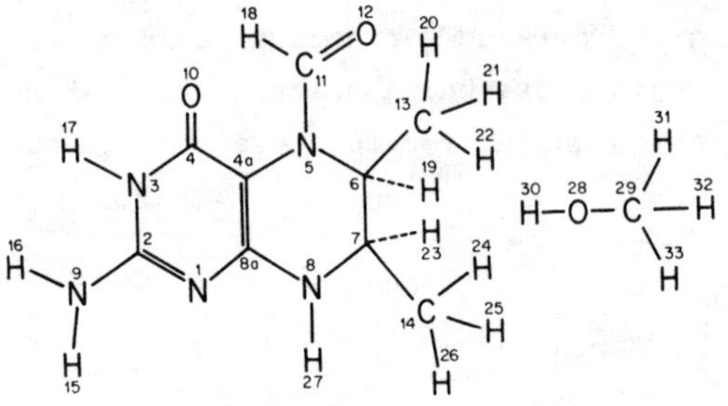

Fig. 5. Structure of 5-formyl-6,7-dimethyl-5,6,7,8-tetrahydropterin
(III) with numbering of atoms.

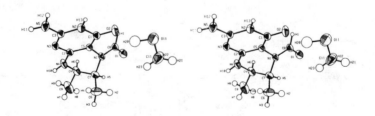

Fig. 6. ORTEP-stereoprojection of III.

4. 5,6,7-Trimethyl-5,6,7,8-tetrahydropterin-dihydrochloride-mono-hydrate (IV)

As expected this molecule is protonated at N(1) and N(5) (fig. 7).

The pyrimidine ring is planar with the atom H(14), the amino group consisting of the atoms N(9), H(15), H(16), the atom H(17) and the atoms O(10) and N(8) of the vinylogous amide function lying in the same plane. As previously demonstrated[3], the atom H(30) protrudes markedly from this plane by 0.20 Å. The chloride ion 31 also lies in the pyri-midine plane and has its shortest distances to the atoms H(14) (2.179 Å) and H(15) (2.503 Å). Cl(32), however, is situated above the plane with its shortest distances to the atoms H(16) (2.571 Å); H(17) (2.346 Å) and H(18) (2.198 Å). The N(8)-C(8a)-bond (1.318 Å) of the vinylogous amide grouping exhibits considerable double bond characteristics. Also the bonds N(1)-C(2) (1.326 Å), C(2)-N(3) (1.344 Å) and C(2)-N(9) (1.318 Å) are considerably shorter than single bonds indicating a strong delocalisation of the positive charge over the centers N(1), C(2), N(3) and N(9) as already discussed in [1].

The positional differences of the atoms constituting the tetrahydro-pyrazine ring with respect to the pyrimidine plane show N(5) (0.019 Å) and N(8) (0.011 Å) to be very close to the plane. C(6), however, is above by 0.600 Å and C(7) below 0.103 Å. The pseudoaxial and axial po-sitions, respectively, of the methyl groups C(11) and C(12) and the equatorial position of the C(13) methyl group are given by the values of 1.398 Å, 2.090 Å and 0.453 Å. The methyl groups C(11) and C(12) are trans to each other while the methyl groups C(12) and C(13) are in cis-configuration (fig. 8 and 9).

The calculated best planes of the pyrimidine and tetrahydropyrazine rings feature an angle of 7.39° between each other.

The protonation of the nitrogen atom N(5) determines the pseudo-axial arrangement of the C(11) methyl group. The trans-configuration of the methyl groups C(11) and C(12) corresponds to the conformation most favourable for the molecule.

In view of previous chemical and ^{1}H-NMR. spectroscopic investiga-tions of the molecule the formation of the cis-isomer upon N(5) proto-nation can be excluded[9].

24

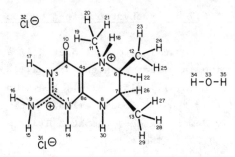

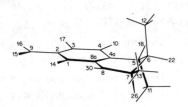

Fig. 7. Structure of 5,6,7-trimethyl-5,6,7,8-tetrahydropterin-dihydro-
chloride-monohydrate (IV) with numbering of atoms.

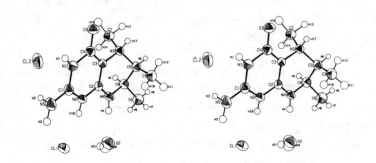

Fig. 8. Projection of the
molecular structure of IV.

Fig. 9. ORTEP stereoprojection of IV.

REFERENCES

1. Bieri, J.H. et al. (1976) Helv. chim. Acta 59, 2374.
2. Bieri, J.H. (1977) Helv. chim. Acta 60, 2303.
3. Bieri, J.H. and Viscontini, M. (1977) Helv. chim. Acta 60, 447.
4. Bieri, J.H. and Viscontini, M. (1977) Helv. chim. Acta 60, 1926.
5. Pfleiderer, W. et al. (1960) Chem. Ber. 93, 2015; Dieffenbacher, A.
   and v. Philipsborn, W. (1969) Helv. chim. Acta 52, 743; Müller, G.
   and v. Philipsborn, W. (1973) Helv. chim. Acta 56, 2680.
6. Hamor, T.A. and Robertson, M.J. (1956) J. chem. Soc., 3586; Shirell,
   C.D. and Williams, D.E. (1975) J. chem. Soc. Perkin II, 40.
7. Broomhead, J.M. (1951) Acta crystallogr. 4, 92.
8. Breitschmid, H.A. (1973) Dissertation, Universität Zürich; Weber, R.
   (1975) Dissertation, Universität Zürich.
9. Viscontini, M. and Bieri, J.H. (1972) Helv. chim. Acta 55, 21.

STRATEGY AND SYNTHESIS OF MIXED OLIGONUCLEOTIDES
CONTAINING LUMAZINES AND PURINES AS AGLYCONS

RAMAMURTHY CHARUBALA AND WOLFGANG PFLEIDERER
Fachbereich Chemie, Universität Konstanz
Postfach 7733, D-7750 Konstanz (West Germany)

ABSTRACT

The synthesis of tri-, penta- and nonameric mixed oligo-deoxy-nucleotides containing 6,7-diphenyllumazine and adenine as aglycons alternately via the phosphotriester method is described. The approach is based on 5'-O-monomethoxytrityl-3'-o-chlorophenyl-ß-cyanoethyl-phosphotriesters as universally feasible building blocks of selective reactivities at the 3'- and 5'-end. The condensation steps could be achieved by TPS in about 50 % yield and deblocking of the protecting groups proceeded smoothly without any side reactions yielding the trimer 11, pentamer 19 and nonamer 21 in HPLC pure form.

The oligomers show intra- and intermolecular interactions depending on the chain length as seen from the hypochromicities and CD-spectra.

INTRODUCTION

It is a well known fact that hydroxy- and amino-pteridines belong to the least soluble nitrogen-heterocycles due to very strong inter-molecular hydrogen bonds[1]. Some interesting effects may be expected from this property especially on base pairing interactions if the pteridine moiety functions as an aglycon in an oligonucleotidic chain. Since various pteridine nucleosides have been made easily available by our laboratory[2-7] in recent years we decided to approach the synthesis of mixed oligonucleotides consisting of deoxy-adenosine and 6,7-diphenyllumazine-1-ß-D-2'-deoxyriboside alternately as a first simple model with complementary base pairs.

The strategy of this synthesis was based on a "modified phospho-triester method"[8-11] using fully protected nucleotide triesters as universally feasible intermediates.

RESULTS

Starting from N^6-benzoyl-5'-O-monomethoxytrityl-2'-deoxy-adenosine
($\underline{1}$) and 6,7-diphenyl-5'-O-monomethoxytrityl-1-(2'-deoxy-ß-D-ribofurano-
syl)-1umazine ($\underline{4}$) respectively phosphorylation at 3'-position was
achieved in the first step of the synthesis by o-chlorophenylphosphoro-
ditriazolide in pyridine yielding phosphodiestermonotriazolides as
intermediates which on subsequent treatment with ß-cyanoethanol formed
the triesters $\underline{2}$ and $\underline{5}$. These building blocks are functionalized by an
acid labil group at the 5'-position and a base labil substituent at
the phosphotriester residue as a necessary presupposition for the formation of an internucleotidic linkage. Selective deblocking of $\underline{2}$ to
$\underline{3}$ by triethylamine and of $\underline{5}$ to $\underline{6}$ by 80 % acetic acid provided mono-
functional molecules which have been condensed by triisopropylbenzene-
sulfonylchloride (TPS) in pyridine to the dinucleosid diphosphate
triester $\underline{7}$ in 67 % yield. This compound can be regarded again as an
analogously substituted building block which possesses the same chemical characteristics at the 3'- and 5'-end of the molecule. ß-Elimination of the cyanoethyl group led to the diester $\underline{8}$ which was then
coupled with N^6-benzoyl-2'-deoxy-adenosine ($\underline{9}$) to the blocked trimer
$\underline{10}$ (yield 60 %).

Acid treatment of $\underline{7}$ offered the second component $\underline{12}$ deblocked at
the 5'-OH group ready for condensation with $\underline{8}$ by TPS to the fully protected tetramer $\underline{13}$ which was obtained in 55 % yield after separation
and purification by preparative tlc or column chromatography. Triethylamine in pyridine effected again ß-elimination of the cyanoethyl group
to $\underline{14}$ which on further condensation with N^6-benzoyl-2'-deoxyadenosine
($\underline{9}$) yielded the pentamer $\underline{16}$ (50 %). The chain elongation to the nonamer $\underline{20}$ was achieved in an analogous manner starting from $\underline{13}$ and forming the two components $\underline{14}$ and $\underline{15}$ respectively by selective deprotection of the privileged blocking groups for subsequent block conden-
sation to the octamer $\underline{17}$ (54 %). Its base treatment afforded $\underline{18}$ which
was again condensed with N^6-benzoyl-2'-deoxyadenosine to give the protected nonamer $\underline{20}$ in 47 % yield.

The cleavages of the various blocking groups to the unprotected
mixed oligonucleotides $\underline{11}$, $\underline{19}$ and $\underline{21}$ respectively was achieved first
by removal of the monomethoxytrityl group in 80 % acetic acid and se-
cond by reaction of conc. ammonia in dioxane for several days at room
temperature in the dark to hydrolyse the N-benzoyl group from the purine aglycon and the o-chlorophenyl group from the phosphotriester
functions.

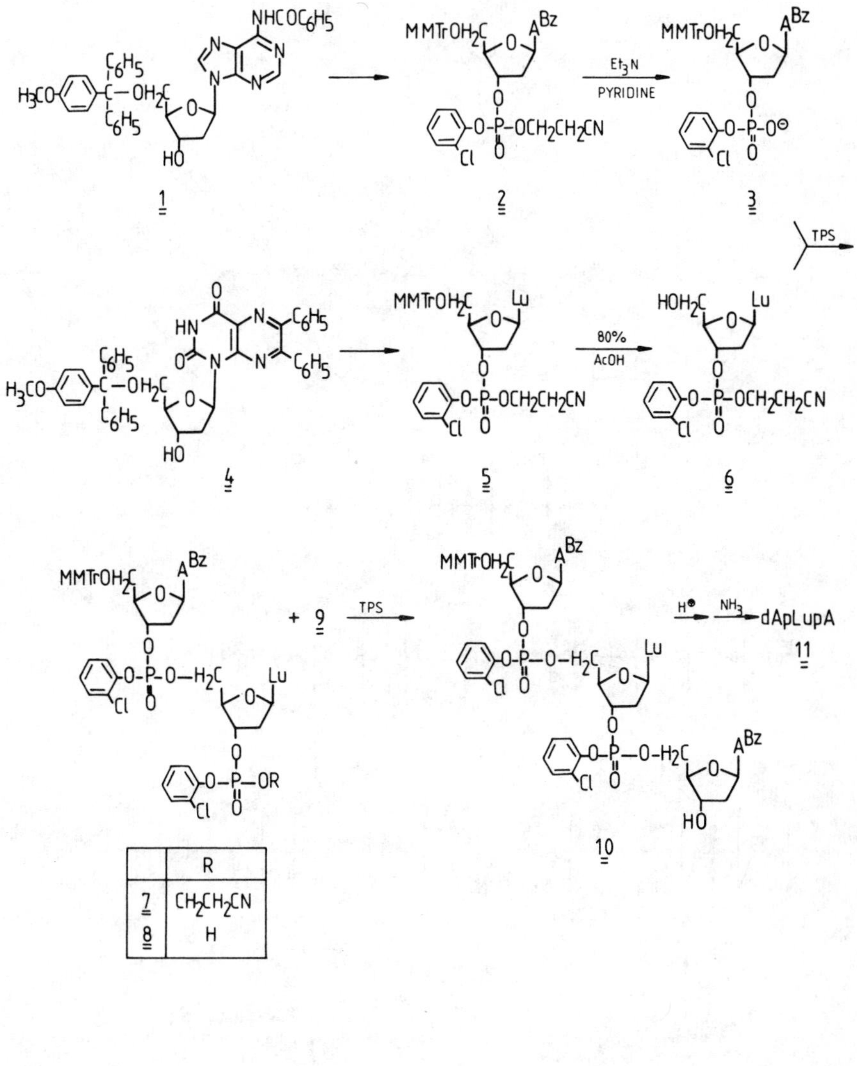

	R
7	CH_2CH_2CN
8	H

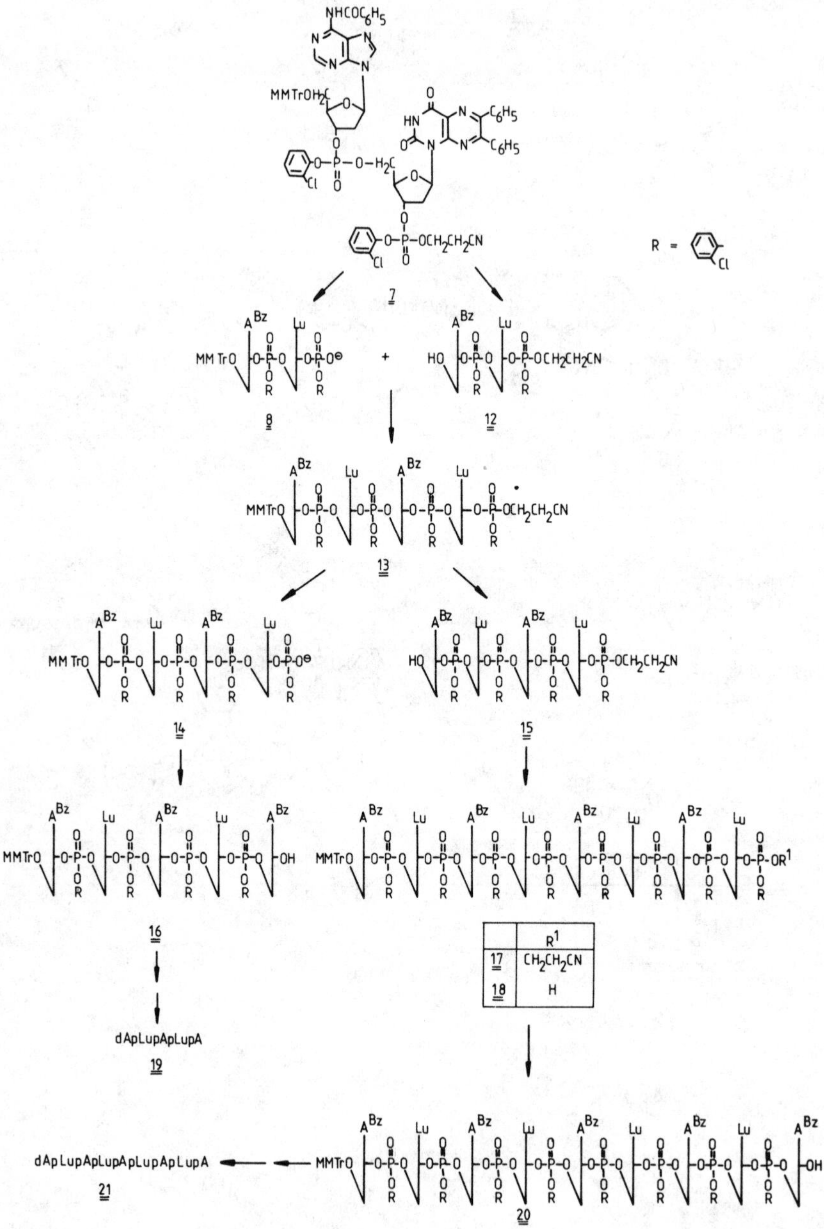

NHCOC6H5
MMTrOH2C
C6H5
C6H5
OCH2CH2CN
R =
7
8
12
13
14
15
16
R1
17 CH2CH2CN
18 H
dApLupApLupA
19
dApLupApLupApLupApLupA
21
20

These compounds were characterized by Rf-values, HPLC-determination, paper electrophoresis, UV- and CD-spectra. It was noticed hereby that strong intra- and intermolecular interactions are present in this type of molecules due to an increasing hypochromicity effect as well as dramatic changes in the CD curves depending on the chain length of the oligomer.

REFERENCES

1. Pfleiderer, W. (1963) in Physical Methods in Heterocyclic Chemistry, Katritzky, A.R. ed., Acad. Press, New York, p. 177-189.

2. Pfleiderer, W., Autenrieth, D. and Schranner, M. (1973) Chem. Ber. 106, 317-331.

3. Ritzmann, G. and Pfleiderer, W. (1973) Chem. Ber. 106, 1401-1417.

4. Schmid, H., Schranner, M. and Pfleiderer, W. (1973) Chem. Ber. 106, 1952-1975.

5. Ott, M. and Pfleiderer, W. (1974) Chem. Ber. 107, 339-361.

6. Itoh, T. and Pfleiderer, W., (1976) Chem. Ber. 109, 3228-3242.

7. Ritzmann, G., Ienaga, K. and Pfleiderer, W. (1977) Liebigs Ann. Chem. 1217-1234.

8. Amarnath, V. and Broom, A.D. (1977) Chem. Rev. 77, 183-217.

9. Letsinger, R.C. and Ogilvie, K.K. (1969) J. Amer. Chem. Soc. 91, 3350-3355.

10. Catlin, J.C. and Cramer, F. (1973) J. Org. Chem. 38, 245-250.

11. Itakura, K., Bahl, C.P., Katagiri, N., Michniewicz, J.J., Wightman, R.H. and Narang, S.A. (1973) Can. J. Chem. 51, 3649-3651.

OXIDATION AND CONVERSION OF REDUCED FORMS OF BIOPTERIN

TAKESHI FUKUSHIMA AND JON C. NIXON

The Wellcome Research Laboratories, Research Triangle Park, North Carolina   27709 (USA)

INTRODUCTION

Pfleiderer has reported the preparation of sepiapterin from BH_4* by air oxidation[1]. This conversion was assumed to occur through a key intermediate, BH_2. In this report, we present data which confirms that SP is a product of the oxidation of BH_2. By using reverse phase HPLC, we have examined the effects of temperature, pH and ionic conditions on the oxidative conversions of both BH_2 and BH_4.

MATERIALS AND METHODS

BH_4 was prepared by catalytic hydrogenation of biopterin. Methods previously reported were used for the preparation of BH_2[2], SP[2], DSP[3], and FDP[4].

HPLC[5]. For the analysis of yellow pterins (SP, DSP and FDP) a μBondapak C_{18} column (Waters) was used. Biopterin and pterin were analyzed by using a ODS column (Whatman). The yellow pterins were eluted isocratically with a methanol/water (1:4) solvent and monitored by absorbance at 420 nm. Biopterin and pterin were eluted isocratically with methanol/water (1:19) and monitored by using a fluorescence detector.

RESULTS

Air oxidation of BH_4 and BH_2 at room temperature. Ten to 30 μmoles of BH_4 or BH_2 were dissolved in 2-3 ml of various buffers. The reaction mixture was stirred in the dark for 2-3 days and the resulting pterins were analyzed.

When BH_4 was stirred in 0.025 M potassium succinate at pH 4, SP (9%) and DSP (3%) were obtained together with a large amount of biopterin. Almost the same results were obtained by the substitution of BH_2 for BH_4. If a potassium phosphate buffer (.1M, pH 6) was used for the oxidation, BH_4 was converted to SP (8%) and DSP (5%). When BH_2 was oxidized in this phosphate buffer, the yield of SP was slightly higher at 10% by which no DSP was detected. Autooxidation of BH_4 in 0.1 M sodium bicarbonate (pH 7.5) produced biopterin, xanthopterin and pterin, but the same treatment of BH_2 produced only biopterin and xanthopterin. These results are similar to those previously reported[1]. Small differences observed in the amount of SP recovered may be attributable to minor variation in reaction conditions. This experiment supports the assumption that BH_2 is an intermediate in the oxidative conversion of BH_4 to SP[1].

---

*Abbreviations used: BH_4, tetrahydrobiopterin; BH_2, 7,8 dihydrobiopterin; BQH_2, quinoid dihydrobiopterin; B, biopterin; SP, sepiapterin; DSP, deoxysepiapterin; FDP, 6-formyldihydropterin; HPLC, high performance liquid chromatography.

Air oxidation under high temperature. Since autooxidation of reduced biopterin proceeded slowly at room temperature, we examined the oxidative conversion at elevated temperatures. Two to 5 μmoles of BH_4 or BH_2 were dissolved in 2 ml of various buffers and incubated in hot water with gentle shaking.

As is shown in Table 1, BH_4 and BH_2 displayed quite different patterns in their oxidative conversion to yellow pterins. In most of the buffers, the recovery of SP is higher with the oxidation of BH_2 rather than BH_4. This may suggest that the conversion of BH_4 to BH_2 is not efficient under these conditions. The highest SP formation was observed when BH_2 was oxidized in .1M potassium phosphate buffer at pH 6.5.

Ionic composition is also important in the formation of SP. In potassium succinate buffer or Tris-HCl buffer the amount of SP recovered was much less than that observed when using phosphate buffer at a corresponding pH. The ratio of SP to DSP formed from the oxidative conversion of BH_4 is different from that observed using BH_2. This may indicate an additional pathway from BH_4 to DSP without BH_2 as an intermediate. The conversion of BH_2 to FDP was efficient in low ionic strength at high temperature in a pH range from neutral to slightly alkaline.

TABLE 1

OXIDATION OF REDUCED FORMS OF BIOPTERIN UNDER HIGH TEMPERATURE

		Starting Compound	BH_4			BH_2		
		Yellow Pterins Recovered(%)	SP	DSP	FDP	SP	DSP	FDP
	pH	Buffer						
	4	K succinate .025M	3	3	0.4	3	9	2
I	6.5	K succinate .025M	0	4	2	2	0	18
	6.5	K phosphate .1M	5	4	2	12	0.4	5
	7.5	K phosphate .1M	1	2	1	8	0	8
	--	H_2O	-	-	-	0.4	0	20
	6.5	K phosphate .1M	3	2	0	12	0.3	0.6
II	7.5	K phosphate .1M	1	2	0	9	0	1
	7.5	Tris-HCl .1M	2	3	0	2	0.2	1

I - Incubation at 80°C for 3 hrs.
II - Incubation at 60°C for 15 hrs.

Iodine oxidation of BH_4 and BH_2. It has been reported that when BH_4 is oxidized by iodine in .1N HCl, the resulting product shows *Crithidia* growth activity equal to that of biopterin. If iodine oxidation of BH_4 is conducted in .1N NaOH the resulting products show little *Crithidia* growth activity. In contrast, BH_2 oxidation by iodine in either HCl or NaOH results in products which have *Crithidia* growth activity comparable to that of biopterin[6]. We have confirmed these initial observations by direct analysis of the products of these reactions.

After iodine oxidation of BH_4 in .1N HCl and in .1N NaOH, reaction mixtures were separated by reverse phase HPLC. Approximately 90% of the BH_4 was recovered as B by the acid oxidation but only a few percent of BH_4 was recovered as B after alkaline oxidation. After alkaline oxidation, 80% of the BH_4 was recovered as 2-Amino-4-hydroxy-pteridine (pterin). Approximately 90% of BH_2 was recovered as B when oxidized in either HCl, NaOH or at neutral pH. However when BH_2 is oxidized with iodine at pH 4, the iodine consumption by BH_2 is approximately double that observed at .1N HCl or at neutral pH and the recovery of B decreases to 20-30%.

For further analysis, $[2-^{14}C]BH_2$ was treated with iodine at pH 4 and the reaction mixture was chromatographed on phospho-Sephadex. As shown in Fig. 1, radioactivity was eluted in three main peaks. Biopterin is eluted in fractions 11-15 under the second peak and the fluorescent compound in the first peak is probably 6-carboxy-pterin. Fractions 3,4,5 and 22 contained comparatively large amounts of radioactivity with little fluorescence. Therefore at pH 4, iodine oxidation appears to have converted BH_2 to non-pterin compound(s).

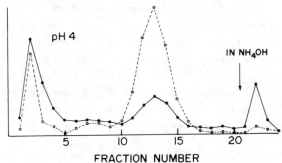

Fig. 1. Phospho-Sephadex column chromatography of iodine oxidation products from $[2-^{14}C]$ BH_2.

$[2-^{14}C]BH_2$ was oxidized by iodine in 0.1M potassium acetate, pH 4. Phospho-Sephadex was used in the H^+ form. The column was developed with water (fractions 1-20) and 1M NH_4OH (fractions 21-25). 0——0 Fluorescence; ●——● radioactivity (^{14}C)

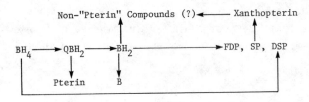

Fig. 2. Oxidative conversion of reduced forms of biopterin.

DISCUSSION

The oxidative conversion of BH_4 and BH_2 observed in the present work are summarized in Fig. 2. Throughout these experiments no 2-amino-4-hydroxy-pteridine (pterin) was formed from BH_2. Since pterin was observed in most reactions with BH_4 it would seem that the formation of a double bond between the 5 and 6 position on the pteridine ring of BH_4 or QBH_2 results in a loss of the dihydroxypropyl side chain. As indicated in the results, DSP may also be produced from a precursor other than BH_2. In this case, dihydro-DSP (6-propionyl tetrahydropterin) could be the precursor. Xanthopterin formed from BH_2 may be through SP or other yellow pterins. Nawa[7] observed the conversion of SP to dihydroxanthopterin in a borax buffer.

It is interesting that BH_2 was almost quantitatively oxidized by iodine at pH 1, but at pH 4 approximately 65% of BH_2 was oxidized to compounds other than biopterin (Fig. 1). Similarly, iodine oxidation of xanthopterin, although slower at pH 4, still results in products showing a loss of fluorescent properties. Since xanthopterin is covalently hydrated to a 7,8-dihydro form[8], this hydrated form may be susceptible to iodine oxidation. According to Rembold *et al.*[9], when $[2-^{14}C]BH_4$ was treated with iodine in 5% acetic acid and the products subsequently analyzed by phosphocellulose column chromatography, only 20% of the starting material was converted to ^{14}C-biopterin. Their data are similar to that presented in Fig. 1.

It has been generally accepted that most biopterin in mammals is present in its reduced forms. We have shown in this report that BH_4 and BH_2 are easily converted to other "pterins". Care should therefore be taken in the interpretation of analyses of biopterin and related "pterins" extracted by various techniques from tissues and fluids.

REFERENCES

1. Pfleiderer, W. (1975) in Chemistry and Biology of Pteridines, W. Pfleiderer ed., Walter de Gruter, Berlin, pp. 941-949.

2. Fukushima, T. and Akino, M. (1968) Arch. Biophys. Biochem., 128, 1-5.

3. Fukushima, T. and Shiota, T. (1972) J. Biol. Chem., 247, 4549-4556.

4. Chippel, D. and Scrimgeour, K.G. (1970) Can. J. Biochem., 48, 999-1009.

5. Fukushima, T. and Nixon, J.C. in preparation.

6. Fukushima, T. Kobayashi, K. Eto, I. and Shiota, T. (1978) Anal. Biochem., 89, 71-79.

7. Nawa, S. (1960) Bull. Chem. Soc. Japan 33, 1555-1560.

8. Inoue, Y. and Perrin, D.D. (1962) J. Chem. Soc. 2600-2606.

9. Rembold, H., Metzger, H., Sudershan, P. and Gutensohn, W. (1969) Biochim. Biophys. Acta 184, 386-396.

REVERSE-PHASE HIGH-PERFORMANCE LIQUID CHROMATOGRAPHIC SEPARATION OF UNCONJUGATED
PTERINS AND PTERIDINES

TAKESHI FUKUSHIMA AND JON C. NIXON

The Wellcome Research Laboratories, Research Triangle Park, North Carolina, 27709 (USA)

INTRODUCTION

Reverse-phase, high-performance liquid chromatography (HPLC) has been shown to be
useful for the separation of folates and diaminopteridines[1]. Pteridines have also
been separated by ion exchange methods utilizing HPLC[2]. We present in this report a
method for the extraction of various naturally occurring, unconjugated pterins
and pteridines and their separation and analysis by reverse phase HPLC.

MATERIALS AND METHODS

Instrumentation. A Model 6000A solvent delivery system, Model 440 absorbance
detector and Model U6K injector (all from Waters Associates, Inc., Milford, Mass.)
were used in all determinations. Additional detectors such as the SF 770 spectroflow
monitor and the FS 970 continuous flow fluorometer (Schoeffel Instrument Corp.,
Westwood, N.J.) were also used in routine analysis. Prepacked reverse-phase C_{18}
(octadecylsilane) columns were purchased from Waters Associates, Inc. and Whatman,
Inc., Clifton, N.J. Peak areas were determined by using an Autolab System IV
computing integrator (Spectra Physics, Schaumberg, IL).

HPLC solvent system. The HPLC separations described in this report were achieved
using an isocratic solvent system of methanol/H_2O (1:19).

Pterin extraction procedure. The biological sample (tissue or fluid) is homogenized in .1N HCl with iodine solution in excess to achieve oxidation of the pteridine
ring. Protein is removed by centrifugation 10,000 xg for 15 min. The supernatant is
applied directly to a Dowex 50 [H^+] column and washed with H_2O. Pterins are eluted
with .5N NH_4OH directly onto a Dowex 1 [OH^-] column and the Dowex 1 column is washed
with H_2O. Pterins are eluted from the Dowex 1 column with 1N acetic acid and the
eluate is analyzed directly by reverse-phase HPLC.

RESULTS AND DISCUSSION

The relative elution volume for various unconjugated pterins and pteridines is
presented in Table 1. The elution volumes for some pterins differ between the two
C_{18} columns used (Whatman ODS and Waters μBondapak). These differences can
probably be attributed to variation in compound interaction with both the nonpolar
C_{18} arm and the residual polar charge on the 10 micron particle.

Reduced pterins are generally labile to oxidation. Therefore for HPLC analysis,
pterins are oxidized to their more stable and more strongly fluorescent forms. Using
fluorescence monitoring, the minimal amount of biopterin detectable is 0.2 nanograms
with a good analytical range between 5→100 nanograms per injection. Analyses of

tissue total biopterin vary widely depending on the tissue type (Table 2). Pterin analyses of urine and other body fluids can be performed by procedures identical to those described for tissues.

TABLE 1

RELATIVE RETENTION TIME OF VARIOUS PTERIDINES SEPARATED BY REVERSE-PHASE HPLC

Compound	Whatman ODS	Waters μBondapak C_{18}
Biopterin	(100)	(100)
*Threo*biopterin	118	134
7,8-Dihydrobiopterin	123	100
Neopterin	63	62
*Threo*neopterin	72	75
7,8-Dihydroneopterin	76	62
6-Carboxypterin	23	23
6-Hydroxymethylpterin	124	115
Xanthopterin	86	83
*iso*Xanthopterin	115	115
Pterin	161	117
6-Formylpterin	151	179
Lumazine	102	102
6-Hydroxylumazine	42	48
7-Hydroxylumazine	23	23

Solvent system used in this study was Methanol:H_2O (1:19). Columns were of comparable size. At an elution flow rate of 0.5 ml/min., biopterin eluted in 8.5 ml from both columns.

TABLE 2

DISTRIBUTION OF BIOPTERIN IN RAT TISSUES

Tissue	Biopterin (μg/g wet weight)	Tissue	Biopterin (μg/g wet weight)
Pineal Body	12	Adrenal	0.7
Liver	1.3	Lung	0.35
Bone Marrow	1.2	Brain	0.11
Spleen	0.9	Pancreas	0.07

REFERENCES

1. Montgomery, J.A., Johnson, T.P., Thomas, H.J., Piper, J.R. and Temple Jr., C. (1977) Adv. Chromatog., 15, 169-195.

2. Bailey, S.W. and Ayling, J.E. (1975) in Chemistry and Biology of Pteridines, W. Pfleiderer ed. Walter de Gruter, Berlin, pp. 633-643.

LUMAZINES AS COENZYMES IN FLAVODOXIN:
EVIDENCE FOR THE OCCURRENCE OF LUMAZINE SEMIQUINONES

GERD HARZER and SANDRO GHISLA

Fachbereich Biologie der Universität Konstanz, Postfach 7733, D-775 Konstanz, W.
Germany

ABSTRACT

6,7-Dimethyl-N(8)-ribityllumazine-5'-phosphate 1, and 6,7-(2,3-dimethylbutano)-N
(8)-ribityllumazine-5'-phosphate 2, bind tightly to apoflavodoxin from *Megasphera
elsdenii*. The complexes are reduced by 0.5 equivalents of dithionite to form the
corresponding semiquinones (λ_{max} ∿ 460 - 475 nm). An enzyme bound dihydrolumazine
species cannot be obtained by direct reduction of the oxidized complexes; 7,8-
dihydrolumazine is modified upon binding to apoflavodoxin (λ_{max} ∿ 400 nm) suggesting
formation of a different tautomer, possibly the 5,8-dihydro form. The apoflavodoxin complexes of 1 and 2 show a catalytic activity, ∿ 30% and ∿ 90% that of the
native enzyme in the photosynthetic NADP reduction of spinach chloroplasts. This
allows the deduction that electron transfer in flavodoxins does not occur simply
via the flavin C(8) position.

INTRODUCTION

Pteridine cofactors play a well established role in enzymatic hydroxylations of
aromates[1] and methyl group transfer[2]. In addition to this, pteridine radicals
have been suggested to play a role in biological processes[3], e.g. they have been
implied to occur in photosynthesis[4]. The mechanism at molecular level of these
enzymatic reactions, however, has not been elucidated in detail so far. The
pteridine at its different oxidation levels, and pteridine radicals might be assumed
to exist in different tautomeric structures[3,5,6,7]. In order to obtain more information about these possible intermediates we addressed ourselves to the questions
of occurrence, stability and spectral characterization of pteridine related lumazines, at their 1 e$^-$ and 2 e$^-$ reduced states. In fact, ribityllumazine phosphate
is structurally related to the flavocoenzyme FMN, and as such is bound by several apo-
flavoproteins[8]. The latter in turn are known to stabilize specific flavine radical forms[9] as well as the 1,5-dihydroform of reduced flavins[10]. Thus a similar
stabilization of lumazine radicals and of specific dihydrolumazines bound to appropriate apoflavoenzymes might be expected which would then allow their spectral characterization. The similarity of the redox moiety of lumazines and flavins also
suggests that they might be interchangeable as cofactors in some enzymatic reactions;
specific steps in catalysis might thus become accessible to investigation, and allow
deductions about the mechanisms of both classes of coenzymes.

RESULTS AND DISCUSSION

6,7-Dimethyl-N(8)-ribityllumazine-5'-monophosphate (1) and 6,7-(2,3-dimethylbut-ano)-N(8)-ribityllumazine-5'-monophosphate (4H-FMN) (2) bind tightly to apoflavodoxin from *Megasphera elsdenii,* a strictly FMN specific flavoprotein[10,11].

Complex formation goes along with marked changes in the near UV portion of the luma-zine spectrum, and with a quenching of the fluorescence emission to <10% of the original value. The spectral changes parallel those observed upon binding of the native cofactor FMN to the same apoenzyme[12]. From fluorimetric titrations, K_d values of $\sim$ 1.5 X 10^{-8}M in the pH range 5-7 were estimated for 1, while 2 binds with a K_d of $\sim$ 5 X 10^{-9}M at pH 7. These values compare with a K_d of $\sim$ 4 X 10^{-10}M for the binding of FMN to the same apoflavodoxin[12]. These observations indicate that the lumazine coenzyme analogs and FMN must be bound at the same place on the apoprotein and in a very similar fashion. Furthermore, comparison of the binding constants in-dicate that the aromatic flavin benzene moiety does not play a major role in the binding of FMN to apoflavodoxin.

The reduction of lumazines 1 or 2 with dithionite under anaerobic conditions is very fast, the 7,8-dihydro form being formed isosbestically with 2 reducing equiva-lents. When the same titration is attempted with the apoflavodoxin complex of 1, however, the decrease in absorbance in the 400 nm region, which indicates reduction, proceeds very slowly and might require up to 1 hr (depending on the amount of $S_2O_4^{2-}$ added) until equilibration is obtained. Up to the addition of $\sim$ 0.5 molar equiva-lent of $S_2O_4^{2-}$ the reduction proceeds isosbestically and, in marked contrast to the reduction of free 1 or 2, goes along with the formation of a new species with λ_{max} at 470, 405 and 315 nm (Fig. 1). With the apoflavodoxin complex of 2 a similar species is formed with $S_2O_4^{2-}$. Admission of oxygen after the 1 e$^-$ reduction com-pletely and rapidly restores the oxidized lumazine spectra. Addition of further increments of $S_2O_4^{2-}$ causes only a very slow further reaction to occur which goes along with loss of the isosbestic points, but does not lead to complete disappear-ance of the long wave-length absorption. This indicates that the E_0' for the 2 e$^-$ reduction of the complex must be considerably lower than that of free lumazine (E_0' = -260 mV)[13] and comparable to that of dithionite[14]. The 1 e$^-$ reduced apoflavo-doxin complex of 2 shows an unresolved EPR signal with a line width comparable

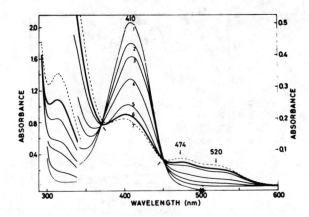

Fig. 1. Anaerobic reduction of the 6,7-dimethyl-N(8)-ribityllumazine phosphate (1)/ apoflavodoxin complex with dithionite. A solution of apoflavodoxin (1.5 X 10^{-4} M) in 0.01 M phosphate buffer pH 7.0 was incubated for 15 min at 0° with an excess of lumazine phosphate (1) and the complex was separated on a short G-25 Sephadex column. Curve 1 shows the spectrum of the complex, 6.2 X 10^{-5} M in 0.1 M phosphate buffer pH 7.0 at 25° and under anaerobic conditions. Curves 2-5 indicate the spectra obtained after addition of discrete amounts of a standardized solution of dithionite and after any time-dependent changes had gone to completion. Curves 6 and 7 represent the spectra obtained after addition of 0.50 and 0.575 equivalents respectively of reductant. The arrows indicate isosbestic points at 370 and 452 nm observed during the first phase of the reduction.

to that of native flavodoxin radicals. It should be pointed out that native flavodoxin radicals are formed analogously -- they have λ_{max} at 510 and 580 nm and are thermodynamically stabilized as compared to the free species[10].

From this we conclude that the long wavelength absorbing species indeed can be attributed to a (neutral ?) lumazine semiquinone. In good agreement with the radical spectra of Fig. 1 are the transient spectra obtained by Moorthy and Hayon in the microsecond range upon pulse radiolysis of pteridines[7].

Attempts to obtain complete reduction by photoirradiation in the presence of EDTA and catalytic amounts of deazaflavin[9] were unsuccessful as partial decomposition of the lumazine chromophore occurred. The complexes of the dihydrolumazines of 1 and 2 had thus to be obtained by a different approach, which relies on the expected kinetic lability of 7,8-dihydrolumzines towards tautomerism. Such experiments are outlined in Fig. 2. Lumazines 1 and 2 were first reduced with stoichiometric amounts of $S_2O_4^{2-}$, and then an excess of apoflavodoxin was added anaerobically. Marked spectral changes occurred immediately, and species with λ_{max} at ∿ 400 nm and a low intensity long wavelength absorption extending well over 500 nm were formed. Admission of air to these complexes lead to only very slow reappearance of the 410 nm absorbance, which is characteristic of oxidized lumazines. Similarly, aerobic

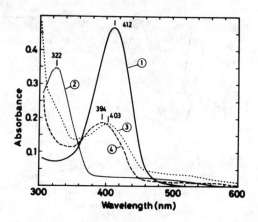

Fig. 2. Spectral changes accompanying binding of 7,8-dihydro-8-substituted "Luma-zines" to apoflavodoxin from *P. elsdenii*. A solution of 4H-FMN, 4 X 10^{-5} M in 0.05 M phosphate buffer pH 6.0 was made anaerobic (Curve 1) and then reduced with 1.05 equiv-alent dithionite to yield the 7,8-dihydro-form (Curve 2). From a side arm of the cuvet a 1.2 molar excess of apoflavodoxin, 5 X 10^{-4} M in the same buffer was then added anaerobically. The resulting spectrum is shown by Curve 3. When the same set of experiments was carried out starting from 6,7-dimethyl-8-ribityl-lumazine phosphate the spectrum of Curve 4 was obtained. The curves are corrected for dilution. 4H-FMN was obtained by catalytic reduction of FMN as described for riboflavin[19].

denaturation of the complex by heat treatment caused only partial recovery of the ab-sorption of 1 and 2. These spectral changes clearly indicate that the species bound by apoflavodoxin is not the 7,8-dihydro tautomer 3. That the 5,8-dihydro form is stabilized by apoflavodoxin is well conceivable, as in the native protein a hydrogen bond exists toward N(5), which stabilizes the blue radical[10]. This interaction could similarly induce a 7 → 5 tautomerism in the lumazine complexes. A dihydro pteridine with a long wave-length absorption, to which the 5,8-dihydro structure has been assigned, has been obtained by photodegradation of biopterin[16]. The lack of com-plete reoxidation of the complex might be attributed to the instability of inter-mediate reoxidation products either while bound to the protein, or upon release. However, alternative 5,6- or 6,7-dihydro tautomeric forms could exist as mesomeric structures, and could conceivably have absorptions in the 400 nm range, should also be considered as possible chromophores for the apoflavodoxin-bound species.

Nitrogen-(8)-substituted lumazines, and in particular 2, can be viewed as flavins lacking the benzene ring. This similarity might be expected within certain limits to result in an enzymatic activity when the flavocoenzyme is substituted by the lumazine analog. A case of particular interest, which would be accessible to experimental veri-fication by such an approach is the proposal put forward recently, that in the electron transfer enzyme flavodoxin, exchange of redox equivalents occurs through the flavin position C(8)[17]. In fact, from X-ray crystallography data it appears that this part of the flavin coenzyme is readily accessible and exposed to the solvent, while the actual redox moiety in the pyrazine/pyrimidine part is buried into the protein[10]. In flavodoxin reconstituted with 1 or 2 a conjugation to such a position is missing. Furthermore with 2 the hydrogenated xylene moiety should constitute a steric barrier for an approach leading to contact between redox partner and redox center.

For activity tests the photosynthetic NADP-reduction system of spinach chloroplasts, in which ferrodoxin can be replaced by flavodoxin, was employed[18]. The apoflavodoxin complex of 1 was found to have 30% of the activity of the native enzyme under standardized conditions. With the complex of 2, when the lumazine and flavodoxin were mixed immediately before assaying, an activity ∿ 90% that of the FMN enzyme was observed. However, as will be detailed later (Ghisla, S. and Harzer, G., to be published) complexes of 2 are not stable and decay with a half time of ∿ 4 hr at 25°C; the modified complex shows no electron transfer activity.

CONCLUSIONS

The results outlined above confirm the expectation that an apoflavodoxin can recognize a different redox system as a coenzyme when specific structural elements are maintained such as a 5'-phosphorylated ribityl side chain and an intact pyrimidine moiety. Binding to the protein induces a markedly different chemical reactivity into the pteridine system. Thus lumazine semiquinones show a remarkable stability when bound to apoflavodoxin, and could first be characterized spectrally. Similarly, a dihydrolumazine tautomer is being stabilized which is clearly not the usually stable 7,8-dihydro form, and which is tentatively suggested to be the 5,8-dihydro isomer. The reduction experiments carried out with dithionite indicate that the redox potentials of lumazines bound to apoflavodoxin are modified in a manner very much similar to those of the native coenzyme[10]; i.e., the radical form is markedly stabilized, while the potential for the second reduction step must be drastically lowered. This potential might be in the range of that of native enzyme (-420 mV[10]) as indicated by the relatively high activity found with the reconstituted enzymes as compared to native flavodoxin. With regard to the mechanism of electron transfer in flavodoxins, clearly the simple hypothesis that electron transfer between the redox partners requires involvement of the flavin C(8) position in catalysis[17] does not hold. Other mechanisms for electron transfer remain to be investigated. Possible alternatives include conformational changes occurring at the flavin side to allow in plane contact with the redox system or electron tunneling mechanisms.

ACKNOWLEDGEMENTS

Thanks are due to Prof. Dr. W. Pfleiderer for generous gifts of 8-ribityllumazine, and to Mr. M. Bartke for performing some of the experiments.

REFERENCES

1. Kaufman, S. and Fisher, D.B. (1974) in Molecular Mechanisms of Oxygen activation (Hayaishi, O., ed.) Academic Press, New York, London, pp. 285-369.

2. Blakley, R.L. (1969) The Biochemistry of Folic Acid and Related Pteridines (Neuberger, A. and Tatum, E.L., eds.) North-Holland, Amsterdam, London, pp. 332-358.

3. Ehrenberg, A., Hemmerich, P., Müller, F. and Pfleiderer, W. (1970) Eur. J. Biochem. 16, 584-591.

4. Fuller, R.C. and Nugent, N.A. (1969) Proc. Natl. Acad. Sci. USA, 63, 1311-1318.

5. Lund, H. (1975) in Chemistry and Biology of Pteridines (Pfleiderer, W., ed., W. de Gruyter, ed.) Berlin, New York, pp. 645-668.

6. Westerling, J., Mager, H.I. and Berends, W. (1977) Tetrahedron, 33, 2587-2594.

7. Moorthy, P.N. and Hayon, E. (1976) J. Org. Chem. 41, 1607-1613.

8. Harzer, G., Rokos, H., Otto, M.K., Bacher, A. and Ghisla, S. (1978) Biochim. Biophys. Acta 540, 48-54.

9. Massey, V. and Palmer, G. (1966) Biochemistry 5, 3181-3189.

10. Mayhew, S.G. and Ludwig, M.L. (1975) in The Enzymes (Boyer, P.D., ed.) Vol. XII 3rd ed. Academic Press, New York, London, pp. 57-118.

11. Mayhew, S.G. and Strating, M.J.J. (1975) Eur. J. Biochem., 59, 539-544.

12. Mayhew, S.G. (1971) Biochim. Biophys. Acta 235, 289-302.

13. Asahi, J. (1959)J. Pharm. Soc., Japan 79, 1574-1578.

14. Mayhew, S. G. (1978) Eur. J. Biochem. 85, 535-547.

15. Massey, V. and Hemmerich, P. (1978) Biochemistry, 17, 9-16.

16. Mengel, R., Pfleiderer, W. and Knappe, W.R. (1977) Tetrahedron Letters 32, 2817-2820.

17. Shiga, K. and Tollin, G. (1976) in Flavins and Flavoproteins (Singer, T.P., ed.) Elsevier, Amsterdam, pp. 422-433.

18. Böger, P. (1969) Z. Pflanzenphysiol. 61, 447-461.

19. Heizmann, C., Hemmerich, P., Mengel, R. and Pfleiderer, W. (1973) Helv. Chim. Acta 56, 1908-1920.

MASS SPECTRAL ASPECTS OF 7-(β-CARBONYL SUBSTITUTED)XANTHOPTERINS

YASUO IWANAMI

Department of Chemistry, Keio University, Hiyoshi 4-1, Yokohama
223 (Japan)

ABSTRACT

7-Acetonylxanthopterin and its derivatives have been characterized
by their mass spectra. The observed fragmentation pattern of these
compounds can be interpreted to mean that they exist in the enamine
form probably facilitated by an intramolecular hydrogen bonding even
in the gas phase. The main route of decomposition started with loss
of carbon monoxide from pyrazine rings without rupture of the chelated
side chain. In contrast, the un-chelated side chains of the 6-isomers
were not preserved and underwent scission via McLafferty rearrangement.

INTRODUCTION

It has been found that the hydrogen-bonded enamine form of some
xanthopterin and isoxanthopterin derivatives is an essential factor
to develop their growth-stimulating activity to Escherichia coli cells
in our laboratory[1,2]. Because the mass spectra of organic molecules
are markedly affected by structural changes, and mass spectral studies
are faster besides the conclusions are obtainable by the use of extremely small amounts of the samples, we have been using this technique
as part of our continuing program to examine the pteridine derivatives.
Thus, this also became a flexible tool to predict whether or not a
given pterin affect the microbial growth. This work concerns with the
application of mass spectroscopy to the xanthopterins having a β-carbo-
nyl side chain at 7-position with special attention being given to the
different fragmentations from those of the 6-isomers.

EXPERIMENTAL

Spectral measurement. The mass spectra were determined with a Hitachi RMS-4 and a JEOL 1SG-2 mass spectrometers, of which the latter
was used mainly for high resolution mass spectrometry by the courtesy
of JEOL Co. in their laboratory. Both spectrometers were operated at
an ionizing voltage of 70 eV and a sample temperature of about 175 -
250° C except for the intensity data for $\log(Z/Z_0)$ versus σ plots
which were measured at 40 eV.

Compounds. All samples were of analytical purity and were synthesized in a similar manner to that described previously[3].

RESULTS AND DISCUSSION

The mass spectra of 7-acetonylxanthopterin (I) and 6-acetonyliso-
xanthopterin (II) are shown in Fig. 1. The base peak of the former
spectrum (Fig. 1, above) is due to the molecular ion, which is likely
to be more stabilized as compared to that of II appearing as a lowerer
peak of 20% in the intensity. Between these two isomers I and II ,
many other differences are seen:

The latter 6-isomer (II) underwent side chain-scission with ketene
elimination as the result of a typical McLafferty rearrangement to
yield an ion a, m/e 193, which appears as the base peak in Fig.1
(below).

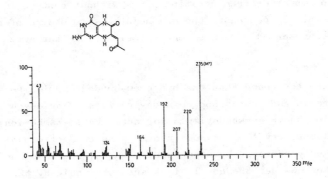

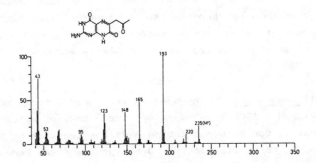

Fig. 1. Mass spectra (70 eV) of I and II.

This scission to ion <u>a</u> followed by expulsion of carbon monoxide to give ion <u>b</u>, m/e 165, was the main fragmentation process together with loss of a methyl radical from the molecular ion leading to ion <u>c</u>, m/e 220, which similarly lost carbon monoxide to afford ion <u>d</u>, m/e 192. These decompositions seem to proceed in a general manner with other heterocycles having a similar side chain[4]. Thus, it may fairly be presumed that II exists in the imine form of which acetonyl side chain is relatively free in its rotation.

M[+] 235   a   b
          m/e 193   m/e 165

In contrast, 7-isomer (I) decomposed by pyrazine ring cleavage with loss of carbon monoxide to yield an ion <u>f</u>, m/e 207. During the course, its side chain carbonyl remained intact even in the next step of demethylation to ion <u>g</u>, m/e 192. This ion <u>g</u> can also be formed in the reverse order. Further loss of another carbonyl from ion <u>g</u> resulted in an ion <u>h</u>, m/e 164. Special emphasis should be laid on that the acetonyl carbonyl in the side chain of I was being preserved at least in the initial steps of the fragmentation, and no indications of McLafferty rearrangement were given in the processes. It would, therefore, be reasonable to interpret these observations into that the acetonyl carbonyl is hydrogen-bonded with secondary amino group at 8-position which has been newly formed by migration of $C^7 = N^8$ double bond onto the side chain, i. e. the 7-isomer (I) exists in the enamine form with internal chelation. Although its existence in this form in the solution state (dimethyl sulfoxide-d_6) has been elucidated by the ^{1}H-NMR spectra, the mass spectral data give evidence anew in support of that the 7-isomer (I) was present in this chelated structure for duration of the gas phase reaction where the spectrum was measured.

Further investigation showed that some homologues of I and II, which are exemplified by 7-isobutyrylmethylxanthopterin (III) and 6-isobutyrylmethylisoxanthopterin (IV), respectively, fragmented by

M⁺ 235 → -CO → f m/e 207 → f m/e 207

$-\dot{C}H_3$

h m/e 164 ← -CO ← g m/e 192

parallel pathways. The homologues of II including IV initially lost part of the side chain yielding the same fragment ions a, b, c, and d, while those of I including III preserved their side chain carbonyl in the first steps of decomposition giving the identical ions f, g, and h. Moreover, this characteristic borne by the mass spectra of I, III, and their homologues are commonly found in those of 7-phenacyl-xanthopterin (V) and 7-(m- or p-substituted phenacyl)xanthopterins, which also lost carbon monoxide from their pyrazine ring initially[5]. Thus, all the enamine forms are probably fixed by the hydrogen bonding between respective phenacyl carbonyl and secondary amino group of the pyrazine ring.

More interestingly, however, the losses of m- or p-substituted benzoyl radicals are linearly related with the Hammett σ constants in spite of their carbonyl fixation in the chelated forms. In the order of electron-withdrawing tendency, the substituents facilitate splitting off substituted benzoyl radical.

It should be pointedly emphasized that no other pterins behave similarly in the fragmentations within our survey. Sepiapterin and biopterin display loss of a whole side chain[4]. Xanthopterin and 7-methylxanthopterin undergo rupture of pyrazine ring but in the opposite side with loss of hydrogen cyanide and methyl cyanide, respectively, resulting in the same ion. Some lumazines initiate their fragmentation pathways by cleavage of the pyrimidine rings[6].

The distinguishing feature of this series of compounds would thus be originated from their existence in the hydrogen-bonded enamine form.

ACKNOWLEDGEMENTS

Part of this work has been done in collaboration with Mr. Takeshi Inagaki, Central Research Laboratories, Nitto Chemical Industry Co. Ltd. We thank Mr. Tsutomu Kambe and Mr. Kazuyuki Tomiya for their assistance to make preparations of this paper.

REFERENCES

1. Iwanami, Y. (1976) in Chemistry and Biology of Pteridines, Proceedings of the Fifth International Pteridine Symposium, Pfleiderer, W. ed., Walter de Gruyter, Berlin, pp. 445-451.
2. Iwanami, Y. (1977) The 26th International Congress of Pure and Applied Chemistry, Abstracts, 1, 326.
3. Iwanami, Y. and Seki, T. (1972) Bull. Chem. Soc. Jpn., 45, 2829-2834.
4. Iwanami, Y. and Akino, M. (1972) Tetrahedron Lett., 31, 3219-3222.
5. Iwanami, Y., Inagaki, T. and Sakata, H. (1977) Org. Mass Spectrom. 12, 302-306.
6. Goto, M. (1968) Kagaku. Ryoiki, Zokan, 85, 141-180.

SYNTHESIS AND PROPERTIES OF NEW PTERIDINE NUCLEOSIDES

LEONIDAS KIRIASIS AND WOLFGANG PFLEIDERER
Fachbereich Chemie, Universität Konstanz
Postfach 7733, D-7750 Konstanz (West Germany)

ABSTRACT

The use of 4-amino-7-oxo-2-n-pentylthio-8(2,3,5-tri-O-benzoyl-ß-D-ribofuranosyl)-7,8-dihydropteridine (16) as starting material for further pteridine nucleoside syntheses is described. Peracid oxidation to the corresponding 2-n-pentylsulfonyl derivative 18 provides a reactive intermediate which is prone to various nucleophilic displacement reactions in position 2 forming new pteridine-N-8-ribosides (20-27). The structures of the newly synthesized compounds are proven by physical means and comparison with model substances.

INTRODUCTION

We have shown in a series of papers[1-7] that pteridine N-1 and N-8 nucleosides respectively could be synthesized from various hydroxypteridines by a modified Hilbert-Johnson procedure using the corresponding trimethylsilyloxy derivatives in the glycosidation step. It has been noticed during these investigations that ribosylation at N-8 encounters sometimes difficulties due to the chemical nature of the other substituents especially at C-2 and C-4 of the pyrimidine moiety of the molecule. Since 2-alkylthio-4-amino-7-oxo-7,8-dihydropteridine-N-8-ß-D-ribofuranosides[5] are easily obtained in good yields, we decided to study the displacement of the alkylthio group by various nucleophiles as an alternative approach to new types of 7-oxo-7,8-dihydropteridine-N-8-ribosides instead of a direct glycosidation reaction in the usual manner.

RESULTS

In order to get some information about the ease of displacing a 2-alkylthio group by various nucleophiles 4-amino-2-methylthio-7-phenylpteridine (1) and 4-amino-8-methyl-2-methylthio-7-oxo-7,8-dihydropteridine (5) have been treated by amines and hydrazine indicating that the displacement reactions afford severe conditions such as heating to 150°C or boiling in DMF as solvent. Since such reaction conditions are far too drastic for the nucleoside series conversion of the methylthio group to the methylsulfone was achieved by m-chloro-

perbenzoic acid oxidation in chloroform forming the highly reactive
4-amino-2-methylsulfonyl-7-phenyl-($\underline{2}$) and 4-amino-8-methyl-2-methyl-
sulfonyl-7-oxo-7,8-dihydropteridine ($\underline{6}$) respectively in good yields.

These compounds react very readily with nucleophiles even at room temperature, as seen from the hydrolysis of $\underline{2}$ and $\underline{6}$ respectively with
1 N KOH/dioxane (1/1) within 1 hour to $\underline{3}$ and $\underline{7}$. The analogous reaction with sodium methoxide in absol. methanol led after 1 hour stir-
ring at room temperature to $\underline{4}$ and $\underline{8}$ respectively.

Encouraged by these positive results 4-amino-7-oxo-2-n-pentyl-thio-
8-(2,3,5-tri-O-benzoyl-ß-D-ribofuranosyl)-7,8-dihydropteridine ($\underline{16}$)
was synthesized as starting material for similar displacement reactions in the pteridine nucleoside series. Hexamethyldisilazane treatment of 4-amino-7-oxo-2-n-pentylthio-7,8-dihydropteridine ($\underline{13}$), which
has been obtained by the sequence - alkylation of 4,6-diamino-2-thio-
pyrimidine ($\underline{9}$) with n-pentyliodide to $\underline{10}$, nitrosation at C-5 to $\underline{11}$,
reduction to the 5-amino derivative ($\underline{12}$) and cyclization with ethyl
glyoxylate hemiacetal - afforded the bis-trimethylsilyl derivative $\underline{14}$
as the reactive intermediate for the ribosylation reaction according
to a modified Hilbert-Johnson procedure[7]. It could be achieved best
with 1-O-acetyl-2,3,5-tri-O-benzoyl-ß-D-ribofuranose ($\underline{15}$) in dichloromethane and in presence of BF_3-etherate as Lewis acid catalyst. The
reaction was complete after 30 min. at room temperature yielding 64 %
of $\underline{16}$. The isolation and separation from minor byproducts was accomplished by silica gel column chromatography in chloroform.

The structure of 16 was characterized by an elementary analysis, an NMR-spectrum and UV-spectral comparison with 5 after deblocking to 17 by Zemplen's method[8].

Oxidation of 16 to the corresponding 4-amino-7-oxo-2-n-pentyl-sulfonyl-8-(2,3,5-tri-O-benzoyl-ß-D-ribofuranosyl)-7,8-dihydropteridine (18) has then been realized by m-chloroperbenzoic acid in absol. chloroform at room temperature yielding 77 % recrystallized material. Since a second component could be detected in the chromatogram the reaction was also achieved at -25°C with 1 equivalent of the oxidizing agent leading to the corresponding sulfoxide 19 in 76 % yield.

It is interesting to notice that the chemical and physical properties of 18 and 19 are very similar, as seen from almost identical UV-spectra and closely related NMR-spectra. The major spectral differences are observed already in the first oxidation step where the shape of the UV curve changes significantly. One absorption band is lost and the longwave maximum is shifted hypsochromically by about 10 nm. This influence is also seen in the NMR-spectra ($CDCl_3$), where the H-6 is shifted from δ = 7.92 ppm in 16 to 8.08 ppm in 19 and 8.2 ppm in 18 respectively according to the electron-attracting power of the sulfoxide and sulfone groups.

Furthermore the chemical reactivities of 18 and 19 respectively resemble each other very closely since treatment with dilute sodium

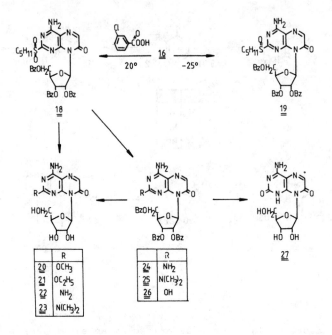

	R
20	OCH₃
21	OC₂H₅
22	NH₂
23	N(CH₃)₂

	R
24	NH₂
25	N(CH₃)₂
26	OH

methoxide solution at room temperature afforded not only deblocking of the sugar protecting groups but also displacement of the 2-substituents by the methoxy function giving 4-amino-2-methoxy-7-oxo-8-β-D-ribofuranosyl-7,8-dihydropteridine (20). Reaction with sodium ethoxide required a somewhat higher temperature (50°C) mainly due to steric reasons forming 21 in 70 % yield. Ammonia in dioxane and dimethylamine in chloroform respectively replace the n-pentylsulfonyl group selectively giving rise to 2,4-diamino-(24) and 4-amino-2-dimethylamino-7-oxo-8-(2,3,5-tri-O-benzoyl-β-D-ribofuranosyl)-7,8-dihydropteridine (25) respectively. Deblocking by sodium methoxide led again to the free nucleosides 22 and 23 in very good yields.

Difficulties, however, have been encountered during hydrolysis studies of the n-pentylsulfonyl group despite the high reactivity of this function towards nucleophiles. Treatment of 18 with aqueous base of different pH led to complex mixtures as seen from tlc and due to ring cleavage of the pyrazinone moiety. Acid hydrolysis turned out to be more successful if the acid strength was kept above pH 2 in order to avoid cleavage of the glycosidic linkage. Reflux of 18 in 5N acetic acid/acetone (1/1) for 5 days are so far the best conditions yielding 67 % of 26 in chromatographical pure form. Deprotection with methanolic ammonia gave 4-amino-2,7-dioxo-8-β-D-ribofuranosyl-tetrahydropteridine (27) in good yield.

Comparisons of physical data of 2Z with 4-amino-8-methyl-2,7-di-
oxotetrahydropteridine (Z) and 4-amino-2-methoxy-8-methyl-7-oxo-di-
hydropteridine (8) indicate that the ribosyl residue increases the
acid strength of Z as expected to a small extent of 0.2 pK units,
whereas the UV-spectra of the neutral molecular species reveal a
predominance in the tautomeric equilibrium of the lactam form 2Z.

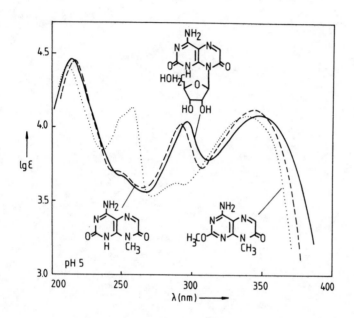

REFERENCES

1. Pfleiderer, W., Autenrieth, D. and Schranner, M. (1973)
    Chem. Ber. 106, 317-331.

2. Ritzmann, G. and Pfleiderer, W. (1973) Chem. Ber. 106, 1401-1417.

3. Harzer, K. and Pfleiderer, W. (1973) Helv. Chim. Acta 56,
    1225-1234.

4. Schmid, H., Schranner, M. and Pfleiderer, W. (1973)
    Chem. Ber. 106, 1952-1975.

5. Ott, M. and Pfleiderer, W. (1974) Chem. Ber. 107, 339-361.

6. Itoh, T. and Pfleiderer, W. (1976) Chem. Ber. 109, 3228-3242.

7. Ritzmann, G., Ienaga, K. and Pfleiderer, W. (1977)
    Liebigs Ann. Chem. 1217-1234.

8. Zemplén, G., Gerecs, A. and Hadacsy, I. (1936)
    Ber. Deut. Chem. Ges. 69, 1827-1829.

Kisliuk/Brown, eds. Chemistry and Biology of Pteridines

STUDIES ON 6-METHYL-5-DEAZATETRAHYDROPTERIN AND ITS OXIDATION PRODUCTS. EVIDENCE FOR THE INVOLVEMENT OF A 4a-ADDUCT IN THE OXIDATION OF TETRAHYDROPTERINS

GRAEME MOAD, CONNIE L. LUTHY AND STEPHEN J. BENKOVIC
Department of Chemistry, The Pennsylvania State University, University Park, PA 16802

INTRODUCTION

Although there have been many studies on the pterin-dependent amino acid hydroxylases, the precise mechanism of the hydroxylation they effect is not well understood. It is often assumed that the hydroxylation proceeds by way of a reactive intermediate derived from the interaction of oxygen with the tetrahydropterin cofactor. Various structures have been proposed for this intermediate;[1-3] most take the form of, or are derived from, a 4a- (or 8a-) adduct of the tetrahydropterin. However, since there is no reported isolation or synthesis of such adducts (presumably due to a predisposition of these compounds to undergo rearrangement and/or elimination) their properties are unknown and their intermediacy in the enzyme reaction remains unproved. Employing 6-methyl-5-deazatetrahydropterin (1)* we have been able to isolate and characterize various 4a-adducts and explore their chemistry and biochemistry.

PREPARATION

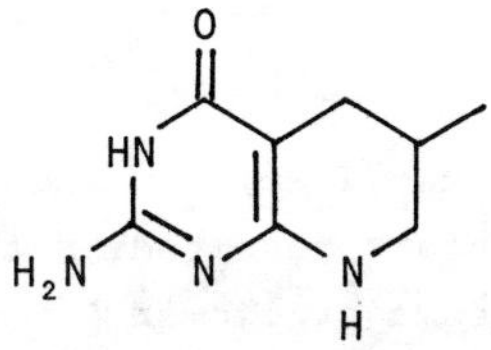

1

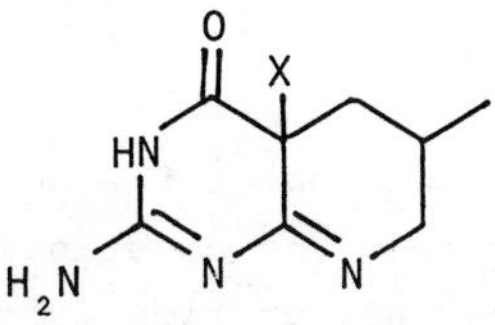

2

a X=Br
b X=Cl
c X=OH

The interaction of 1 with a variety of electrophilic reagents including bromine, N-chloro- and N-bromosuccinimide, and performic acid results in the initial formation of the respective 4a-adduct (2a-c).[4] These adducts have been isolated and characterized by their spectral properties and analytical data. The chloro- and hydroxy-adducts (2b and c) form as a mixture of isomers (isomer ratios ~9:1

*Prepared by catalytic hydrogenation of the fully aromatic precursor.[4]

for 2b and ~6:4 for 2c*). The major isomer of the hydroxy-adduct is obtained in >95% purity after fractional crystallization.

SPECTRAL DATA

Nuclear Magnetic Resonance

The ^{13}C NMR spectra of the major isomer of 2a-c are shown in Fig. 1. Peak assignments are based on a consideration of group additivity parameters[5] and the multiplicities observed in the fully coupled spectra. The ^{13}C NMR shielding of the 4a-carbon is characteristic of an aliphatic carbon bearing a bromo-, chloro- or hydroxy-substituent.[5] The shieldings of the remaining carbons are insensitive to the nature of the 4a-substituent and indicate the structural and stereochemical similarity of the adducts (2a-c). Additional support is derived from the spectral similarities of the minor isomer of 2b and c.

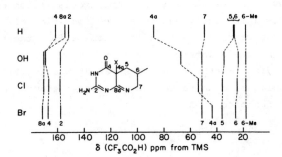

Fig. 1. ^{13}C NMR shieldings of 1 and 2a-c.

The 360 MHz ^{1}H NMR spectra of the adducts (2a-c) are shown in Fig. 2. An analysis of coupling constant data** resulted in the assignment of the trans-configuration to the major isomer formed during synthesis. This assignment concurs with the expected influence of steric factors on the electrophilic substitution reactions. The trans-isomer is free to assume the pseudo-chair conformation shown in Fig. 3 in which steric interactions are minimized, whereas the cis-isomer is forced into the distorted boat configuration

---

*The isomer ratio shows some dependence on the conditions used in the synthesis and isolation.

**For example, $J_{5,6}$=2.2 Hz (axial-equatorial) and 12.5 Hz (axial-axial) for the major isomer of 2b and $J_{5,6}$=8.3 Hz and 8.8 Hz for the minor isomer of 2b.

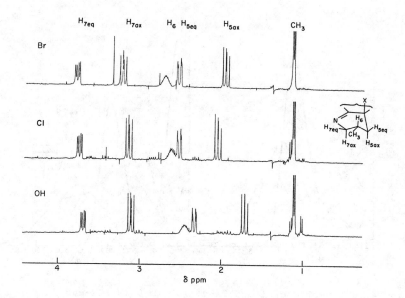

Fig. 2. 360 MHz ^{1}H NMR spectra of 2a-c.   δ(D$_2$O) ppm from TMS.

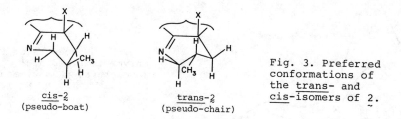

cis-2
(pseudo-boat)

trans-2
(pseudo-chair)

Fig. 3. Preferred
conformations of
the trans- and
cis-isomers of 2.

to avoid a severe 1,3-diaxial interaction between the 4a-substituent
and the 6-methyl group.

Ultraviolet Spectra

The UV spectra of 1 and 2a-c show a pronounced dependence on pH.
The spectra recorded at pH 1 and 8, attributed to the protonated and
neutral forms respectively, are shown in Fig. 4.   The pKa's associated
with this pH dependence are 3.5 for 6-methyl-5-deazatetrahydropterin
(1), 5.3 for the bromo- and chloro-adducts (2a,b), and 6.1 for the
hydroxy-adduct (2c).   The UV spectrum of the hydroxy-adduct (2c) bears
a striking resemblance to that determined by Kaufman[1] for a
tetrahydropterin-derived intermediate formed in the enzyme catalyzed
hydroxylation of phenylalanine (Fig. 5).

58

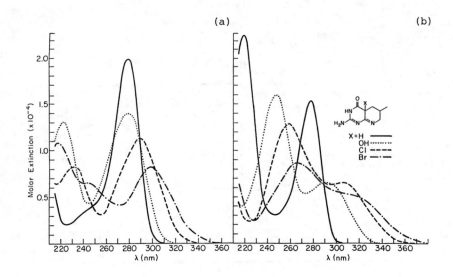

(a)   (b)

Fig. 4. UV spectra of 1 and 2a-c: (a) in 0.1N HCl and
(b) in 0.01M TRIS pH 8.0.

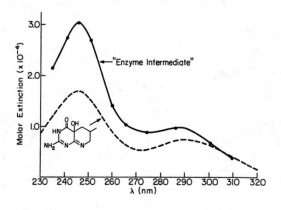

Fig. 5. UV spectra of the
enzyme intermediate[1]
(phosphate, pH 8.2) and
2c (0.1M TRIS, pH 8.2).

REACTIONS

The bromo-adduct (2a) is unstable in aqueous solution and reacts
with added nucleophiles or solvent to undergo an apparent substitution
reaction. For example, at pH>8, 2a is converted into the hydroxy-
adduct (2c). On the basis of HPLC data, this process proceeds
with >90% retention of configuration at the 4a-carbon. In the
presence of hydride reducing agents (NaBH$_4$, NADH) the bromo-adduct
(2a) is converted into 1 in high yield (90%). Second order kinetics
are obeyed (Rate=k[2a][H$^-$]). When 2a is reduced with sodium boro-
deuteride or with various reducing agents (NaBH$_4$, NaBD$_4$, NADH) in

deuterium oxide, no deuterium is incorporated into the product (1).
Therefore, a mechanism involving the intermediacy of a quinone
methide (3)--analogous in nature to the quinonoid intermediate
believed to be involved in the oxidation of tetrahydropterins--is
excluded.

In the absence of nucleophiles the bromo-adduct(2a) is observed
to undergo a slow conversion into 1. Plausible mechanisms for this
process include: (a) formation of the hydrate (4) and subsequent
elimination of hypobromous acid; or (b) the direct transfer of Br$^+$
to some acceptor molecule. These mechanisms also account for the
observation that in acidic media 2a effects para-bromination of
1,3-dimethoxybenzene (70% yield).

BIOLOGICAL ACTIVITY

The 6-methyl-5-deazatetrahydropterin (1) is a competitive
inhibitor of phenylalanine hydroxylase[6,7]--50% inhibition was obtained
with 14μM tetrahydrobiopterin and 50μM 1.[7] In addition, preliminary
results indicate that the bromo-* and hydroxy-adducts act as inhibitors. No cofactor activity has been observed with either 1 or the
adducts 2a and 2c. Compound 1 is also an inhibitor of brain tyrosine
hydroxylase.[7,8]

---

*The inhibition observed with 2a may be due to the formation of 1 or
2c during the assay (see Reactions).

60

Inhibition by 1 may stem, in part, from a significantly higher
oxidation potential relative to the natural cofactor. The peak
potential for the oxidation of 1 has been determined to be +0.75V vs.
Ag/AgCl on a carbon paste electrode at pH 9 relative to -0.08V for
6,7-dimethyltetrahydropterin under the same conditions.

SUMMARY

The results described above support the hypothesis that a 4a-
adduct derived from oxygen and a tetrahydropterin is involved in the
hydroxylation process.

ACKNOWLEDGEMENT

This work was supported in part by a grant from the National
Science Foundation.

REFERENCES
1. Kaufman, S. (1975) The Chemistry and Biology of Pteridines,
   Proc. 5th Int. Symp.,Pfleiderer, W. ed., de Gruyter, Berlin,
   pp. 291-304.
2. Kaufman, S. and Fisher, D.B. (1975) Molecular Mechanisms of
   Oxygen Activation, Hayaishi, O. ed., Academic Press, New York,
   pp. 285-369; Dmitrienko, G.I. Snieckus, V. and Viswanatha, T.
   (1977) Bioorganic Chem., 6, 421-429; Hamilton, G. (1975)
   Molecular Mechanisms of Oxygen Activation, Hayaishi, O. ed.,
   Academic Press, New York, pp. 405-451.
3. Mager, H.I.X. (1975) The Chemistry and Biology of Pteridines,
   Proc. 5th Int. Symp., Pfleiderer, W. ed., de Gruyter, Berlin,
   pp. 753-773; Viscontini, M. and Okada T. (1970) Helv. Chim.
   Acta. 50, 1492-1498; Gapski, G.R., Whitely, S.M. and
   Huennekens, F.M. (1971) Biochemistry, 10, 2930-2934; Blair, J.A.,
   Pearson, A.J. and Robb, A.J. (1975) J.C.S. Perkin II, 18-21.
4. Moad, G., Luthy, C.L., and Benkovic, S.J. (1978) Tetrahedron
   Lett., 2271-2274.
5. Clerk, P. and Simon, S. (1976) Tabellen zur Strukturaufklärung
   organischer Verbindungen mit speckroskopischen Methoden,
   Springer-Verlag, Berlin; Levy, G.C. and Nelson, G.L. (1972)
   Carbon-13 Nuclear Magnetic Resonance for Organic Chemists,
   Interscience, New York.
6. Ayling, J.E., personal communication.
7. Kaufman, S., personal communication.
8. Bullard, W.P., personal communication.

ROOM TEMPERATURE PHOSPHORESCENCE OF SELECTED PTERIDINES

R. T. PARKER, R. S. FREEDLANDER, E. M. SCHULMAN and R. B. DUNLAP
Department of Chemistry, University of South Carolina, Columbia, South Carolina 29208

Due to the nature of the phenomenon, phosphorescence analysis of organic compounds usually has been carried out only at very low temperatures (typically 77°K)[1]; however, the cumbersome techniques involved with these cryogenic methods have discouraged its application to routine analysis. Recently, phosphorescence analysis has gained considerable attention since the ability to make qualitative and quantitative measurements for a variety of organic and biomolecules at room temperature has been demonstrated[2]. Room temperature phosphorescence (RTP) can be observed from a number of polar organic compounds when solutions of these compounds are spotted on a suitable polar material (most commonly paper) and thoroughly dried. This method of analysis offers advantages of simplicity and selectivity over low temperature techniques and should compare favorably with or offer advantages over traditional procedures for clinical or biochemical analysis. Our interest in RTP and the biochemistry of various pteridines and folates has led us to investigate the phosphorescent properties of selected pteridines. Recent reports that elevated levels of 6-hydroxymethyl pterin may be indicative of neoplastic diseases has provided incentive for our development of analytical methods for pterins in tissues and body fluids[3].

Early in our studies, it was revealed that many pteridines exhibit intense phosphorescence at 77°K and that several of these compounds phosphoresce weakly at room temperature when adsorbed on Whatman 1 filter paper. The excitation maxima of the compounds studied were generally found to lie in the area of 370 nm and the emission maxima were typically around 500 nm. We further evaluated the phosphorescence properties of the pteridines on various supports.

When basic solutions of certain pterins were spotted on Whatman 1 filter paper which had previously been doped with sodium acetate, there was a very substantial increase in the RTP emission. In fact, those pteridines which displayed virtually no RTP when spotted on paper alone were observed to yield characteristic pteridine RTP spectra when subjected to the sodium acetate doping treatment. The RTP emission spectra for the pteridines also displayed an emission in the 450 nm region which coincides with the region of normal pteridine fluorescence. Our studies indicate that this emission is an E-type delayed fluorescence. The fact that we are observing delayed fluorescence is substantiated by the absence of this emission in the low temperature spectra together with other evidence to be presented in a future detailed report on the phosphorescent properties of selected pteridines.

The analytical utility of the RTP method for pteridine analysis was illustrated for pterin-6-carboxylic acid (PCA). By employing a special sample holder previously described by us[2], reproducible RTP intensity measurements could be made from samples spotted on 9/32" filter paper circles. Relative standard deviations for samples were generally around 3.5% for triplicate measurements, and a detection limit of 1 ng of material was possible. A calibration plot showed a linear range extending from the detection limit to slightly above 100 ng of PCA. It should be noted that the RTP emission from the pteridines is much more sensitive to quenching by moisture than many other compounds which show RTP; therefore, very thorough drying of the sample is necessary to observe reasonable RTP emission from the pteridines.

In conclusion, the RTP method presents a unique approach in the analysis of some of the pteridines, and our studies have demonstrated the extreme sensitivity and selectivity of this mode of analysis. RTP could readily be adapted to clinical analysis by use of an automated system which has been previously described[4]. Analysis by RTP may well hold advantages over many traditional techniques since the former method offers the potential of avoiding the complex separations often required in analyses of biological samples such as blood, urine and other body fluids.

ACKNOWLEDGEMENTS

This work was supported by funds awarded to R. T. Parker and R. S. Freedlander from an American Cancer Society Institutional Grant to the University of South Carolina. R. B. Dunlap is the recipient of an American Cancer Society Faculty Research Award (FRA-144).

REFERENCES

1. Zander, M. (1968) "Phosphorimetry," Academic Press, New York.

2. Schulman, E. M. and Parker, R. T. (1977) J. Phys. Chem., 81, 1932.

3. Stea, B., Backlund, P. S., Berkey, P. B., Cho, A. K., Halpern, B. C., Halpern, R. M. and Smith, R. A. (1978) Cancer Research, 38, 2378.

4. Vo-Dinh, T., Walden, G. L. and Winefordner, J. D. (1977) Anal. Chem., 49, 1126.

UNEXPECTED REACTIONS AND PROPERTIES OF PTERIDINES

WOLFGANG PFLEIDERER

Fachbereich Chemie, Universität Konstanz

Postfach 7733, D-7750 Konstanz (West Germany)

ABSTRACT

Electrochemical reductions of various pteridines provide an interesting tool for the synthesis of 5,8-, 5,6- and 7,8-dihydro derivatives depending on the reaction conditions. Radical anions as well
as pinacols starting from 6- and 7-acyllumazines could be achieved
by one electron reduction processes. Sterically crowded pinacols
cleave easily at the central long C-C bond.

1-(2'-Deoxy-ß-D-ribofuranosyl)-lumazine-5'-monophosphates show an
unexpected low stability of the glycosidic linkage at neutral pH presumably due to a neighbouring group participation effect of the phos-
phat function with intermediate pyrimidine ring opening.

The direct amination of 6- and 7-hydroxy-1,3-dimethyllumazine by
phenyl phosphodiamidates is described and some physical properties
of the corresponding amino derivatives discussed on the basis of
pK_a values and UV-spectra.

INTRODUCTION

Electrochemical studies of various 2,3-dioxotetrahydrochinoxa-
lines[1], 2,3-dioxotetrahydropyrido-[b]-pyrazines[2] and 6,7-dioxotetra-
hydropteridines[2,3] have shown that the electroactive part in these
di-amides are bounded by the adjacent carbonyl functions representing an 1,4-dioxadiene system. Extension of these findings to other
1,4-diheterodiene combinations in the pteridine field offers an interesting principle for a broad variety of potentially electrochemically active pteridine derivatives prone to cathodic reductions.

MATERIALS AND METHODS

The preparative electrolyses were carried out in electrolytic
cells[4] described elsewhere. The control and regulation of the electrochemical reduction processes were based on a commercially available potentiostat Jaissle, model 60T-B, and a coulometer built by
the electronic workshop of the University of Konstanz. A silver/sil-
ver chloride electrode was used as reference electrode. Nafion 125
of E.I. Dupont de Nemours and Co., Plastics Division, Wilmington,
Del./U.S.A., has been approved as excellent membrane material.

RESULTS

   The electroactive part in 1,3-dimethyllumazine (1) is localized
in the pyrazine moiety forming in a two electronic reduction step
the 5,8-dihydro derivative (2) which is thermodynamically unstable
due to the antiaromatic 8 $\widetilde{\pi}$-system and could therefore not be isolated. The formation of the 5,8-dihydro structure as an intermediate
was proven by trapping with acetic anhydride yielding 5,8-diacetyl-
1,3-dimethyl-5,8-dihydrolumazine (3). Its constitution has been elucidated by an X-ray analysis[5].

$$\underset{\underline{\underline{1}}}{} \qquad \underset{\underline{\underline{2}}}{} \qquad \underset{\underline{\underline{3}}}{}$$

   The initial step in such an electrochemical reduction may in general be an one-electron transfer giving rise to a radical anion which
could be detected by ESR during reduction in dry DMF in presence of
tetra-n-butylammonium iodide.

   The electrochemical reductive acylation process could be applied
to other 1,4-diazine systems such as chinoxalines, pyrido-pyrazines
and pyrazines forming stable 1,4-diacyl-1,4-dihydro derivatives in
high yields.

   A practical use of the potential controlled selective reduction
can be seen from the conversion of neopterin (4) to 7,8-dihydroneo-
pterin (5) in 55 % yield. The reaction proceeds in ammonium formiate
solution presumably via the 5,8-dihydro derivative which tautomerizes
to the thermodynamically more stable end product.

$$\underset{\underline{\underline{4}}}{} \qquad\qquad\qquad \underset{\underline{\underline{5}}}{}$$

An extension of the partial reductions to 6-acyl-lumazines offer
a series of new possibilities depending on reaction conditions and
structural features. 6-Acetyl-7-methyllumazines $\underline{7}$ - $\underline{9}$ were electrochemically reduced at pH 5 in n-propanol/0.3 M KCl-solution to the
corresponding 5,8-dihydro derivatives $\underline{10}$ - $\underline{12}$ which are stable to
some extent due to the electron-attracting power of the acetyl group.
The longwave absorption band of low extinction at 480-490 nm reveals
the 5,8-dihydro structure.

	R	R
$\underline{7}$	CH₃	CH₃
$\underline{8}$	CH₃	H
$\underline{9}$	H	CH₃

	R	R	λmax
$\underline{10}$	CH₃	CH₃	488
$\underline{11}$	CH₃	H	488
$\underline{12}$	H	CH₃	485

Reduction of $\underline{7}$ in acidic medium (0.5 N HCl/n-propanol) led to 6-
acetyl-1,3,7-trimethyl-7,8-dihydrolumazine ($\underline{6}$) whereas at pH 7 in
formamide and in presence of Robinson-Britton puffer a ring contrac-
tion to 8-acetonyl-coffein ($\underline{13}$) took place.

Another interesting substrate was found in 6-benzoyl-1,3-dimethyl-
7-phenyllumazine ($\underline{13}$) which reacts at pH 5 again to the 5,8-dihydro

form (14). At pH 8 in DMF/ammonium formiate solution a mixture of
the 5,6- (17) and 7,8-dihydro isomers (16) were formed, isolated and
characterized by physical means.

If the reduction was performed in n-propanol/0.3 M KCl solution
at pH 8 deacylation became the main reaction forming 73 % of 1,3-
dimethyl-7-phenyllumazine (15) besides 15 % of 16. This unusual deacylation may be a radical cleavage reaction since 6-benzoyl-1,3-
dimethyl-7-phenyl-5,6-dihydrolumazine (17) is easily converted by
base in presence of oxygen into 15.

An entirely different reaction was found with 6-acetyl-1,3,7-tri-
methyllumazine (7) during cathodic reduction in n-propanol/0.3 M KCl
at pH 8-10 forming the threo-pinacol 19 in an one-electron reduction
process in 84 % yield. 19 of which an X-ray analysis[6] has proven the
structure turned out to be a relatively labil compound presumably due
to its abnormal long central C-C bond of 1.589$\overset{\circ}{A}$. Treatment of 19
with oxygen in alcohols led to the starting material 7, which was
also obtained on attempted acetylation. Heating above the melting
point effected disproportionation to 7 and 6-(1-hydroxyethyl)-1,3,7-
trimethyllumazine.

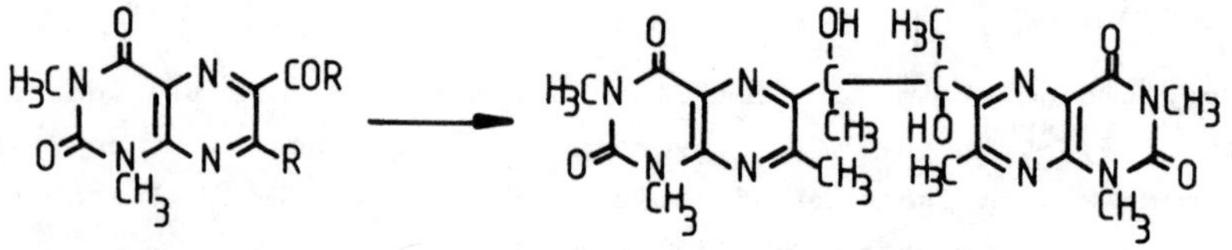

	R
7	CH₃
18	H

	R
19	CH₃
20	H

If 1,3-dimethyllumazine-6-aldehyde is reduced to the pinacol 20
the internal steric strain obviously is reduced drastically since 20
is a completely stable compound which could be acetylated to a diacetate and converted to its isopropylidene derivative by 2,2-di-
methoxypropane under acid catalysis.

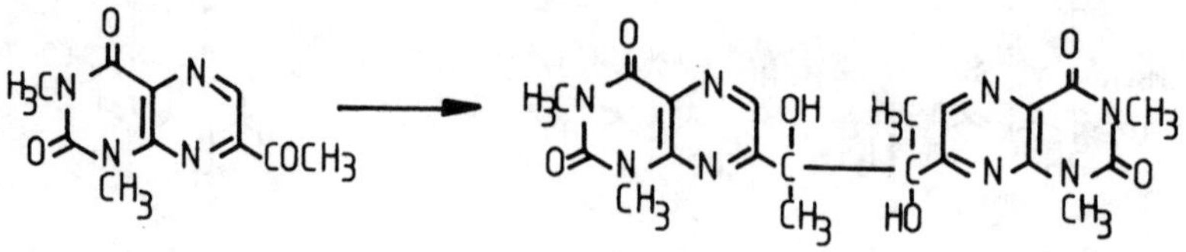

21

22

7-Acetyl-1,3-dimethyllumazine (21), however, formed another labil pinacol 22 indicating an unusual crowding effect at the alcoholic C-atoms.

Another interesting observation has been made during phosphoryla-tion studies of various pteridine nucleosides. We noticed that 1-(2'-deoxy-ß-D-ribofuranosyl)-lumazine-5'-monophosphates are very sensi-tive to cleavage of the glycosidic linkage especially at neutral pH in contrast to the corresponding pteridine N-1 ribonucleotides which behave analogously to the purine and pyrimidine nucleotides showing their maximum of stability exactly in physiological pH's. The reac-tion has been followed spectrophotometrically indicating a clean clea-vage to the lumazine aglycon with half-live-times of 15 to 20 hours depending on the various substituents.

	R
23	H
24	CH3

	R	50°C τ pH 9
25	H	20h
26	CH3	15h

27 28 29

We suggest that the cleavage of the glycosidic linkage does in-volve an intermediary ring opening of the pyrimidine ring facilitated by a neigbouring group participation effect of the phosphate function attacking nucleophilically the 2'-position to 27, conversion to 28 and hydrolysis of the Schiff's base to 29 which then cyclizes to the lumazines 25 and 26 respectively with loss of the sugar phosphate re-sidue. Since 2'-deoxy-ribonucleosides prefer in their sugar moiety an S-type conformation, the ribonucleosides, however, the N-type structure the phosphate group in the former is much closer located to the aglycon than in the latter. This may be an explanation of the large stability differences on molecular grounds.

6-(27) and 7-Hydroxy-1,3-dimethyllumazine (31) have been subject to direct aminations by phenyl phosphodiamidates yielding the corresponding 6-(28-30) and 7-amino-(32), 7-methylamino-(33) and 7-dimethylamino derivatives (34) respectively.

R	R^1
H	H
H	CH$_3$
CH$_3$	CH$_3$

	R	R^1	
28	H	H	32
29	H	CH$_3$	33
30	CH$_3$	CH$_3$	34

From the physical data such as pK$_a$ values and UV absorption spectra some features of the fine structure of these molecules could be recognized. The low basic pK$_a$ values of the 7-amino-1,3-dimethyllumazines indicate a strong vinylogous amide resonance in the neutral form and the bathochromic shift of the longwave absorption band on cation formation has to be explained by protonation at N-5. The basic strengths therefore increase in accordance to the electron-donating power of the amino substituent. In the 6-amino-1,3-dimethyllumazine series the basicities show a decrease in the same order indicating a protonation also at N-5 and some steric interferences due to the increasing bulkiness of the 6-substituent. Whereas 28 reveals a bathochromic shift on protonation the 6-dimethylamino-1,3-dimethyllumazine (30) is slightly hypsochromically shifted according to a less coplanar arrangement of the electron-donator with the heterocycle.

Finally we would like to emphasize that 7-acetonyl-xanthopterin (35), which prefer the more stable tautomeric vinylogous amide configuration[7], are valuable intermediates for the synthesis of leucopterins (36), 7-methylxanthopterins (37) and xanthopterin-7-carboxylic acids (38).

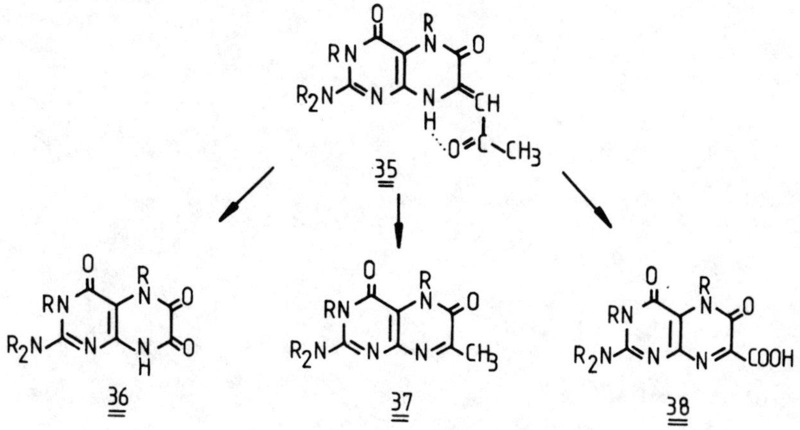

Treatment of 35 by sodium bicarbonate is initiated by nucleophilic attack of the hydroxide ion at C-7 giving leucopterins in hydrolyses, whereas 5N NaOH led to the 7-methylxanthopterins presumably via attack at the exocyclic carbonyl function of the anion form. Air oxidation in basic medium afforded oxidative degradation of the side-chain to xanthopterin-7-carboxylic acids (38).

ACKNOWLEDGEMENTS

Credits have to be given to Dr. R. Gottlieb, Dr. W. Bannwarth, I. Geyer and H. Steppan for their excellent work and cooperation leading to these results. The work has been sponsored by Deutsche Forschungsgemeinschaft.

REFERENCES

1. Gottlieb, R. and Pfleiderer, W. (1978) Chem.Ber. 111, 1753-1762.

2. Gottlieb, R. and Pfleiderer, W. (1975) in Chemistry and Biology of Pteridines, Pfleiderer, W. ed., W. de Gruyter, Berlin, pp. 681-685.

3. Gottlieb, R. and Pfleiderer, W. (1978) Chem.Ber. 111, 1763-1779.

4. Lund, H. (1970) in Advances in Heterocyclic Chemistry, Katritzky, A.R. and Boulton, A.J. eds., Academic Press, N.Y., Vol. 12, 233.

5. Kobayashi, Y., Iitaka, Y., Gottlieb, R. and Pfleiderer, W. (1977) Acta Cryst. B 33, 2911-2913.

6. Kobayashi, Y., Iitaka, Y., Gottlieb, R. and Pfleiderer, W. (1978) Acta Cryst., in press.

7. von Philipsborn, W., Stierlin, H. and Traber, W. (1963) Helv. Chim. Acta 46, 2592-2596.

SOME ISOMERS AND ANALOGS OF PTERIDINE NATURAL PRODUCTS
AND CHEMOTHERAPEUTIC AGENTS[1]

Edward C. Taylor,* Robert N. Henrie II and Donald J. Dumas

Department of Chemistry, Princeton University

Princeton, New Jersey 08540

Over the past several years we have developed a versatile synthetic approach to pteridines which permits the unequivocal placement
of substituents at either position 6 or 7.[2] This synthesis, which
employs as its key first (and unambiguous) step the cyclization of an
α-oximino carbonyl compound with an α-aminonitrile, leads to a 2-
amino-3-cyanopyrazine 1-oxide, which is then converted into pteridines
by deoxygenation and cyclization. This general approach has been
used, inter alia, for the unequivocal synthesis of xanthopterin,[3,4]
isoxanthopterin,[4] L-erythro-biopterin,[5] aminopterin,[6] methotrexate,[7]
folic acid,[8] asperopterin B,[9] and pterin-6-carboxaldehyde.[10]

Among the most versatile of the above pyrazine intermediates are
the chloromethyl derivatives 1 and 2, which are readily prepared by

$$\underline{1} \qquad\qquad\qquad \underline{2}$$

the reaction of aminomalononitrile tosylate with α-oximino-β-chloro-
propionaldehyde[11] and β-chloropyruvaldoxime[12] respectively. The
present paper describes the utilization of 1 for the preparation of
the pure 7-positional isomers of aminopterin and folic acid, and the
utilization of 2 for the synthesis of a novel group of biopterin
analogs in which both stereo- and regio-control over the introduction
of substituents into the C-6 sidechain have been achieved.

2-Amino-3-cyano-6-formylpyrazine (3) was prepared by two independent procedures. In the first, 2-amino-3-cyano-6-chloromethylpyrazine
(from PCl_3 deoxygenation of 1) was converted into its pyridinium salt,
which was condensed with p-dimethylaminonitrosobenzene, and the resulting nitrone hydrolyzed with dilute HCl (Kröhnke procedure).[13] In

the second, $\underline{1}$ was treated with n-propylamine, and the resulting imine
of $\underline{3}$ was hydrolyzed with dilute HCl. 7-Aminopterin (as its 10-acetyl
derivative $\underline{6}$) was then prepared from $\underline{3}$ by condensation with di-t-butyl
p-aminobenzoylglutamate, reduction of the resulting imine $\underline{4}$ with
sodium borohydride, protection of the fragile sidechain in $\underline{5}$ by acetylation of N-8, cyclization with guanidine, and hydrolysis. Attempts to
remove the 4-amino grouping of $\underline{6}$ (to give the 7-positional isomer of
folic acid) , or to remove the protecting acetyl grouping, were unsuccessful.[14]

Ar = –⟨ ⟩– CONHCHCH$_2$CH$_2$COO-t-Bu
                COO-t-Bu

Ar' = –⟨ ⟩– CONHCHCH$_2$CH$_2$COOH
                COOH

7-Folic acid, protected as its N-2'-acetyl derivative $\underline{11}$, was,
however, successfully prepared in the following unambiguous manner.
Pyruvaldehyde dimethylacetal was converted into its enamine $\underline{7}$ with
pyrrolidine and anhydrous magnesium sulfate in ether. Condensation of
$\underline{7}$ with the O-tosyl derivative of oximinomalononitrile gave the aza-
diene derivative $\underline{8}$, which was converted to 2-amino-3-cyano-6-dimethoxy-
methylpyrazine ($\underline{9}$) with ammonia.[15] The latter compound was condensed
with guanidine and the product hydrolyzed first with base (to remove
the 4-amino group) and then with acid to give pterin-7-carboxaldehyde
($\underline{10}$). Acetylation of $\underline{10}$, followed by condensation with di-t-butyl p-
aminobenzoylglutamate, reduction, and hydrolysis then gave $\underline{11}$. Both
$\underline{6}$ and $\underline{11}$ are thus available isomerically pure for biological evaluation.

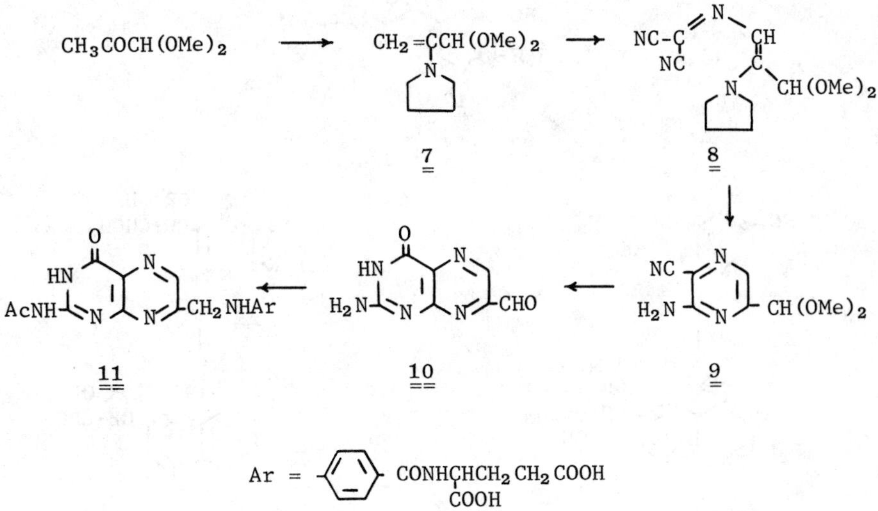

$$CH_3COCH(OMe)_2 \longrightarrow CH_2=\underset{\underset{N}{|}}{C}CH(OMe)_2 \longrightarrow$$

7

8

9

10

11

$$Ar = \underset{COOH}{\langle \ \rangle} CONHCHCH_2CH_2COOH$$

Some novel C-6 side chain analogs of biopterin have been prepared from the trans epoxide __12__ of 2-amino-3-cyano-5-(1-propenyl)pyrazine.[12] Hydrolysis of __12__ in aqueous acetonitrile containing Dowex 50W-X4 ion exchange resin gave the _threo_ glycol __13__ (R = H), which was converted to its acetonide and cyclized with guanidine. Aqueous acetic acid removed the acetonide protecting group to give 2,4-diamino-4-deoxy-d,l- _threo_-biopterin (__14__, R = H), which was hydrolyzed with base to d,l-_threo_-biopterin (__15__, R = H).

Reaction of __12__ with methanol containing a few drops of trifluoro-acetic acid gave the _threo_ glycol monomethyl ether __13__ (R = Me), in which both regio- and stereo-specificity of ring opening had been achieved. By contrast, utilization of anhydrous alumina doped with 4% methanol[16] gave exclusively the _erythro_ isomer __16__ (R = Me). Both __13__ (R = Me) and __16__ (R = Me) have been carried through to the corresponding 4-amino-4-deoxybiopterin and biopterin analogs __14__-__18__ (R = Me).

This would appear to be an exceptionally versatile route to biopterins and 4-amino-4-deoxybiopterins modified in the C-6 sidechain

threo series   erythro series

by replacement of the α-substituent by such groups as alkoxy, amino, substituted amino, alkylthio, mercapto, etc., both in the natural erythro and in the unnatural threo series.

REFERENCES

1. This work was supported by grants to Princeton University by the National Cancer Institute, National Institutes of Health (Grant # CA 12876), Eli Lilly & Co., and Hoffmann-La Roche & Co.

2. For a recent summary of this procedure, see E. C. Taylor in "Chemistry and Biology of Pteridines", W. Pfleiderer, ed., Walter de Gruyter, Berlin, 1975, pp. 543-573.

3. E. C. Taylor and P. A. Jacobi, J. Am. Chem. Soc., 95, 4455 (1973).

4. E. C. Taylor, R. F. Abdulla, K. Tanaka, and P. A. Jacobi, J. Org. Chem., 40, 2341 (1975).

5. E. C. Taylor and P. A. Jacobi, J. Am. Chem. Soc., 98, 2301 (1976).

6. E. C. Taylor and A. Nelson, unpublished results

7. (a) R. C. Portnoy, Ph.D. Thesis, Princeton University, 1975; (b) E. C. Taylor, R. C. Portnoy, and J. Wiecko, unpublished results.

8. (a) E. C. Taylor, R. N. Henrie II, and R. C. Portnoy, unpublished results; (b) E. C. Taylor, R. C. Portnoy, D. C. Hochstetler, and T. Kobayashi, J. Org. Chem., 40, 2347 (1975).

9. E. C. Taylor, P. A. Jacobi, and R. F. Abdulla, J. Org. Chem., 40, 2336 (1975).

10. E. C. Taylor, R. N. Henrie II, and R. C. Portnoy, J. Org. Chem., 43, 736 (1978).

11. E. C. Taylor and T. Kobayashi, J. Org. Chem., 41, 1299 (1976).

12. E. C. Taylor and T. Kobayashi, J. Org. Chem., 38, 2817 (1973).

13. This same sequence of reactions has recently been exploited for the conversion of 2-amino-3-cyano-5-chloromethylpyrazine to 2-amino-3-cyano-5-formylpyrazine, which was then converted to pterin-6-carboxaldehyde; see ref. 10.

14. (a) J. H. Boothe, J. H. Mowat, C. W. Waller, R. B. Angier, J. Semb, and A. L. Gazzola, J. Am. Chem.Soc., 74, 5407 (1952); (b) C. W. Waller, M. J. Fahrenbach, J. H. Boothe, R. B. Angier, B. L. Hutchings, J. H. Mowat, J. F. Poletto, and J. Semb, J. Am. Chem. Soc., 74, 5405 (1952).

15. This procedure for pyrazine synthesis was developed by J. Perchais and J-P. Fleury, Tetrahedron, 30, 99 (1974).

16. G. H. Posner and D. Z. Rogers, J. Am. Chem. Soc., 99, 8208, 8214 (1977).

STUDIES ON THE SYNTHESIS OF UROTHIONE AND DEOXYUROTHIONE

Edward C. Taylor* and Lawrence A. Reiter
Department of Chemistry, Princeton University
Princeton, New Jersey 08540

Urothione was first isolated from human urine nearly four

Urothione

decades ago.[1] Its concentration in urine is very low; only 20-80 mg
can be obtained from 1,000 liters. Since this early work, three
research groups undertook studies of this naturally occurring pteridine, and all three stated that at least part of their interest
arose from curiosity about its possible biological role.[1-3] However,
since significant quantities of urothione are clearly not conveniently
available from natural sources, a practical synthetic route would be
highly desirable. One synthesis of urothione has appeared,[4] but
the overall yield was extremely low and, judging from the lack of
further reports, this synthesis was apparently not capable of producing
amounts sufficient for biological studies. In light of current
increasing awareness of the biological importance of other naturally
occurring pteridines, we have undertaken a new total synthesis of
urothione.

The key distinction between the published synthesis and our
approach lies in the order of construction of the three rings of the
thieno(3,2-g)pteridine system. The published synthesis started with
a preformed pyrimidine, closed the pteridine ring, and then annulated
the thiophene ring. Our route involves the initial construction of
a multifunctional pyrazine intermediate which is first converted to
a thieno(2,3-b)pyrazine; formation of the fused pyrimidine ring to
generate the thieno(3,2-g)pteridine system is deferred until the
final stages of the synthesis.

Model experiments were directed towards the synthesis of deoxy-urothione (10), which we have successfully prepared as outlined in Scheme 1. Pyrazine 1, which was readily available[5] and contains functionality requisite for fusion of both the thiophene and pyrimidine rings, gave 2 (40%) with POCl$_3$ in DMF. Reaction of 2 with 1-mercapto-2-propanone gave 3 (90%), which was cyclized in quantitative yield to 4 with sodium ethoxide in ethanol.

Conversion of the 7-amino substituent in 4 to a methylthio grouping was accomplished in two steps by a Sandmeyer reaction to give the 7-bromo derivative 5 (50%), followed by treatment of 5 with sodium methyl mercaptide in THF at room temperature to give 6 (88%). Subsequent reduction of the carbonyl grouping in 6 with sodium borohydride in ethanol/THF gave 7 (70%) possessing the α-hydroxyethyl side chain required for deoxyurothione.

Considerable difficulties were encountered in the removal of the dimethylaminomethylene protecting group in 7, but this problem was eventually solved by treatment of 7 with p-toluenesulfonic acid in trimethyl orthoformate/methanol, which led not only to removal of the protecting group, but also to replacement of the α-hydroxyl group by a methoxy substituent. Cyclization of 8 with guanidine in refluxing methanol then gave the pteridine 9, which was converted directly to deoxyurothione with aqueous acid. We assume that loss of the methoxy group under these acidic conditions (as well as the reverse transformation observed in the conversion of 7 to 8) is assisted by the ortho-situated methylthio substituent. The overall yield of deoxyurothione (10) from the pyrazine 1 was 15%.

Scheme 1

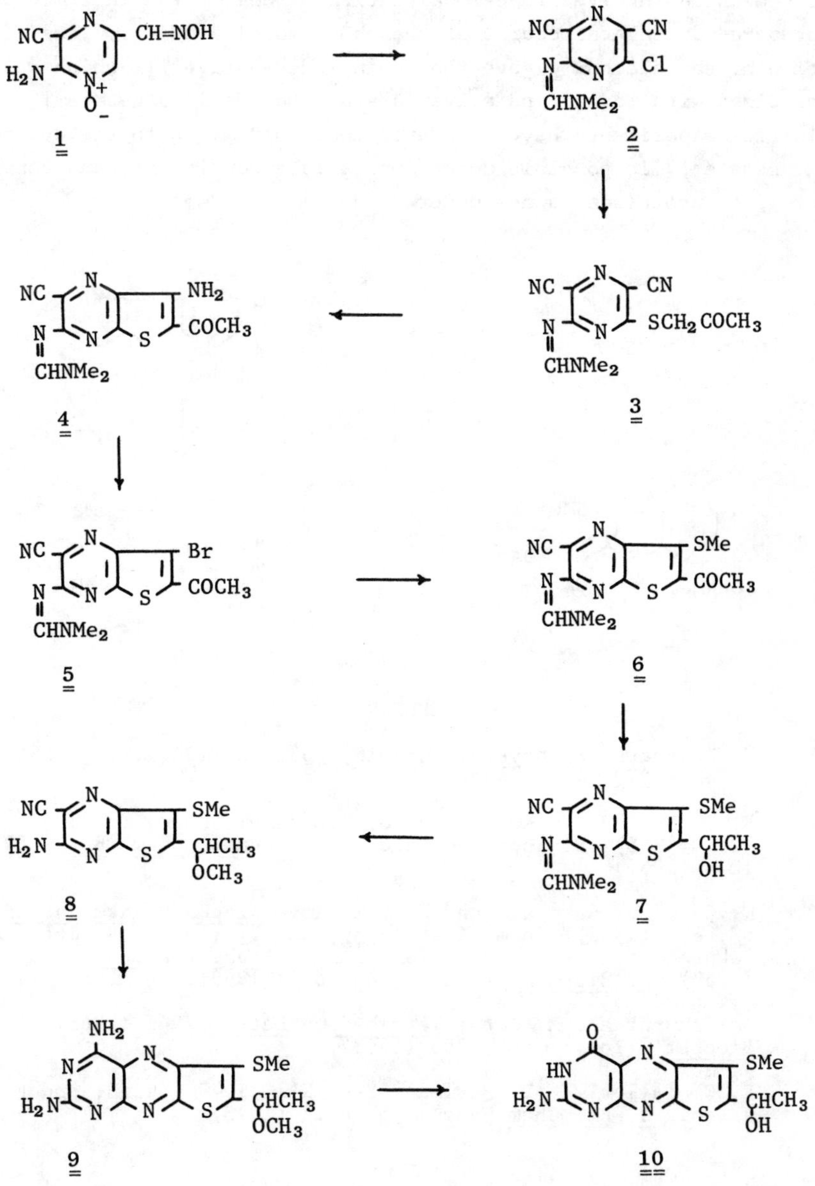

Attempts to apply the above synthesis to the preparation of urothione itself by utilizing intermediates possessing the additional primary hydroxyl group (in the thiophene side chain) have not been successful. As a consequence, we are currently exploring an alternate route which involves functionalization of one of the intermediates prepared during the course of the above model studies. Thus, dehydration of the alcohol 7 gave the 6-vinyl derivative 11, which was oxidized with iodine and silver acetate to the iodoacetate 12. Initial experiments have indicated that solvolysis to the desired diacetate 13 is possible under appropriate conditions, and conversion of 13 to urothione is now under study.

REFERENCES

1. W. Koschara, Z. physiol. Chemie, 263, 78 (1940); 277, 284 (1943); 279, 44 (1943).

2. R. Tschesche, F. Korte, and G. Heuschkel, Chem. Ber., 88, 1251 (1955); R. Tschesche and G. Heuschkel, Chem. Ber., 89, 1054 (1956).

3. M. Goto, A. Sakurai, and H. Yamakami, Nippon Kagaku Zasshi, 88, 897 (1967); Chem. Abstr., 69, 52107j (1968); M. Goto, A. Sakurai, K. Ohta, and H. Yamakami, Tetrahedron Lett., 4507 (1967); J. Biochem. (Tokyo), 65, 611 (1969).

4. A. Sakurai and M. Goto, Tetrahedron Lett., 2941 (1968); J. Biochem. (Tokyo), 65, 755 (1969).

5. E. C. Taylor, K. L. Perlman, Y-H. Kim, I. P. Sword, and P. A. Jacobi, J. Am. Chem. Soc., 95, 6413 (1973).

THE BIOSYNTHESIS OF PTERIDINES IN *DROSOPHILA MELANOGASTER*

GENE M. BROWN, GWEN G. KRIVI, CHING L. FAN AND THOMAS R. UNNASCH
Massachusetts Institute of Technology, Department of Biology, Building 56, Room 631,
Cambridge, Massachusetts 02139

ABSTRACT

The enzyme system that catalyzes the conversion of dihydroneopterin triphosphate to sepiapterin has been purified from extracts of *Drosophila melanogaster* and shown to consist of two Enzymes (A and B). Enzyme A catalyzes the removal of the three phosphate residues from the substrate to yield a product (not dihydroneopterin) which, in the presence of Enzyme B and NADPH, is converted to sepiapterin. During the latter conversion tritium from tritiated NADPH is incorporated into sepiapterin. Evidence concerning the identity of the intermediate produced by the action of Enzyme A is as follows: (a) it is capable of reacting to form a phenylhydrazone, (b) it can be reduced by sodium borohydride to a product identical with biopterin by paper chromatographic analyses, and (c) no oxidizing agent is needed during its enzymatic formation.

In the enzymatic conversion of sepiapterin to biopterin in the presence of NADPH and extracts of *Drosophila* we unexpectedly found that oxidized sepiapterin (K_m=10 μM) is preferred to sepiapterin (K_m=63 μM) as substrate. The products were identified as dihydrobiopterin (from sepiapterin) and biopterin (from oxidized sepiapterin).

We have found that *Drosophila* extracts contain an enzyme which catalyzes the oxidation of dihydropterins to pterins. The enzyme will utilize as substrate all dihydropterins that have been tested except for dihydroneopterin triphosphate. No NAD^+ or $NADP^+$ is required, but there is a requirement for O_2.

INTRODUCTION

The view that naturally-occurring pterins are made in animals from GTP with dihydroneopterin triphosphate (H_2-neopterin-P_3) as an intermediate has received support from reports that GTP cyclohydrolase I (the enzyme that catalyses the conversion of GTP to H_2-neopterin-P_3) occurs in animal tissues[1,2,3,4] and investigations on the enzymatic conversion of H_2-neopterin-P_3 to sepiapterin[5,6] and biopterin[4,7,8]. In the present report we present results of our investigations on the conversion of H_2-neopterin-P_3 to sepiapterin (formulas are shown in Fig. 1) and for the conversion of the latter compound to biopterin and H_2-biopterin in the presence of enzymes from *Drosophila melanogaster*. Since the details of the methodology used in these investigations are presented in other publications[5,6,8] they will not be repeated here.

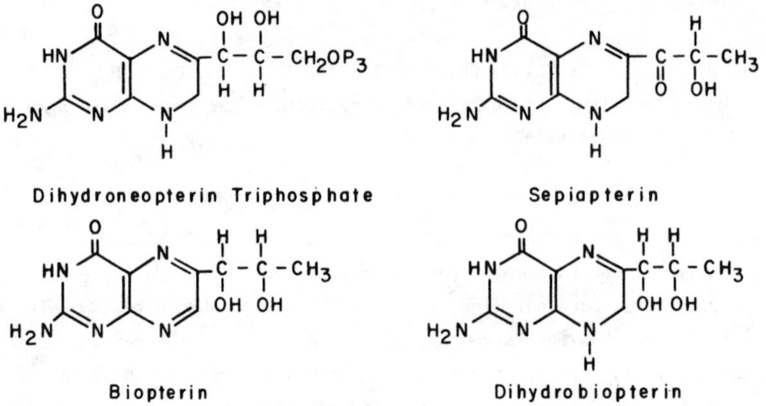

Fig. 1. Formulas of various pterins.

RESULTS

Enzymatic Synthesis of Sepiapterin - In preliminary experiments we found that ra-dioactive H_2-neopterin-P_3 could be converted to sepiapterin by incubation in the pre-sence of a crude extract of *Drosophila* heads[5]. Further work indicated that $MgCl_2$ and either $NADP^+$ or NADPH were required for maximal synthesis and that H_2-neopterin could not replace H_2-neopterin-P_3 as substrate[5].

Crude extracts have been subjected to fractionation successively: (a) with ammo-nium sulfate, (b) on a column of Blue Sepharose CL-6B, and finally (c) on a column of Ultrogel AcA44. The last step allowed the separation of the enzyme system into two fractions, both of which are required for the formation of sepiapterin from H_2-neo-pterin-P_3. The protein fraction which eluted first will be referred to as Enzyme A and the other fraction will be called Enzyme B. Other observations made with the use of the two purified enzymes, have indicated that (a) NADPH cannot be replaced by NADH, NAD^+, or $NADP^+$ (in contrast to the results obtained with the use of crude extracts), (b) the K_m for H_2-neopterin-P_3 is 10 μM; and (c) H_2-neopterin cannot replace H_2-neo-pterin-P_3 as substrate.

The need for two protein fractions for the conversion of H_2-neopterin-P_3 to sepia-pterin suggests that an intermediate may be produced. We conducted the experiments described below to obtain evidence bearing on this subject. H_2-neopterin-P_3 was in-cubated with either Enzyme A or Enzyme B and after the reaction mixture was heated at 100° (to inactivate the enzyme), the enzyme not present during the first incubation was added and the reaction mixture was reincubated. Although the yield of sepiapterin was relatively low (probably because of the instability of the intermediate during the heating) we were able to establish in a reproducible manner that incubation with Enzyme A followed by incubation with Enzyme B yielded sepiapterin whereas incubation in the reverse order yielded no sepiapterin. In similar experiments we established that Mg^{2+} is needed during the action of Enzyme A and that NADPH is needed only during the action of Enzyme B. These observations suggest that the reaction sequence involves a Mg^{2+}-dependent reaction catalyzed by Enzyme A to produce an intermediate which in the presence of NADPH and Enzyme B is converted to sepiapterin. Evidence for the formation of such an intermediate was obtained with the finding that when incubation is carried out in the presence of Enzymes A and B, but in the absence of NADPH, a compound is produced (detected by paper chromatography) which upon addition of NADPH and reincubation is converted to sepiapterin. We were also able to show that incubation of H_2-neopterin-P_3 with Enzyme A alone allowed the production of the same intermediate with the concomitant release of the 3 phosphate residues of the substrate. Since the release of at least the α-phosphate group of H_2-neopterin-P_3 cannot be hydrolytic (i.e., H_2-neopterin cannot be used as substrate for sepiapterin production), we conclude that the phosphate group is released as an elimination reaction, as shown in Fig. 2, to yield a substance which can exist either in the enol or keto form, shown in Fig. 2 as compounds II and III. We suggest that the intermediate is converted to sepiapterin in the presence of Enzyme B in a stepwise fashion through the utilization of NADPH to give perhaps an enzyme-bound intermediate (compound IV, Fig. 2) which can then be oxidized at the expense of the $NADP^+$ (produced in the first step) to yield sepiapterin.

If the reaction sequence of Fig. 2 is correct, tritium from NADPT should be incorporated into sepiapterin. We have done this experiment and observed that a substantial amount (0.63 moles ^3H per mole sepiapterin produced) of tritium is incorporated when the pro-R form of NADPT was supplied, but when the pro-S form was supplied a relatively insignificant amount (0.12 moles ^3H per mole sepiapterin) was incorporated. These observations strongly suggest that the pro-R form of NADPH is used in the enzymatic production of sepiapterin.

Unfortunately, the intermediate produced in the presence of Enzyme A is not stable enough to be produced and isolated in the amounts needed for chemical identification. We have therefore sought other ways to obtain evidence about its identity. If the intermediate is compound III, treatment with sodium borohydride should reduce it to biopterin. We have subjected the radioactive intermediate to this treatment and have found that the resulting radioactive product behaves as biopterin upon being subjected to paper chromatography in 3 different solvent systems. We also found that treatment of radioactive intermediate with dinitrophenylhydrazine yielded a radioactive derivative which behaved similarly to the dinitrophenylhydrazone of sepiapterin upon being subjected to analysis by paper chromatography. These results strongly suggest that the intermediate is a keto compound that can be reduced to biopterin. From

these observations compound III seems feasible since it can be reduced to biopterin and can react to form a phenylhydrazone. Another possibility would be a compound with a diketo side chain ($R-C-C-CH_3$), however if such a compound were produced en-
$$\overset{\parallel}{O}\,\overset{\parallel}{O}$$
zymatically, one would expect that an oxidizing agent should be needed during its production, since it is at a higher oxidation state than H_2-neopterin-P_3. However, during the enzymatic reaction (catalyzed by Enzyme A) there is no need for such an oxidant, including molecular oxygen (i.e., when the enzymatic reaction proceeds anaerobically the amount of intermediate produced is not diminished). Thus, the evidence summarized above is consistent with the intermediate being compound III (Fig. 2).

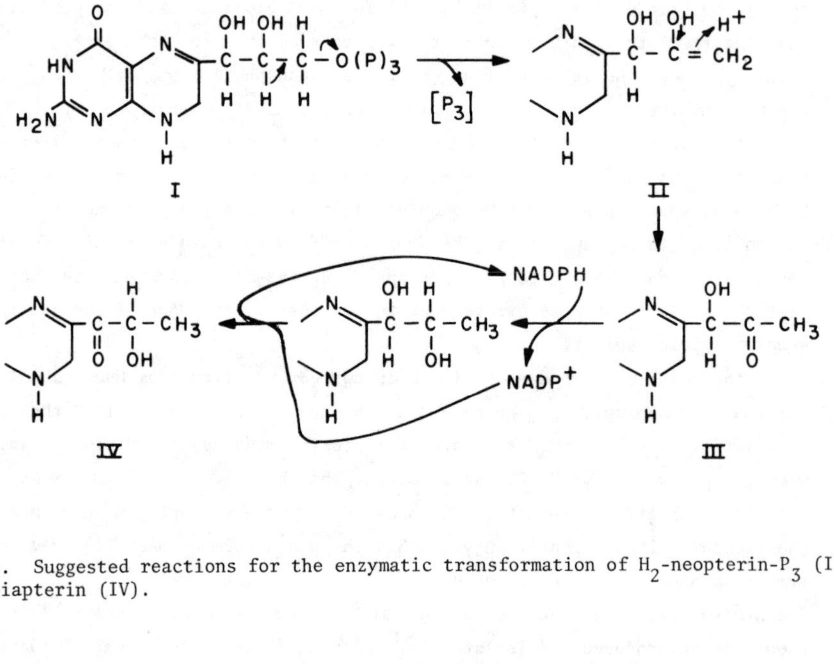

Fig. 2. Suggested reactions for the enzymatic transformation of H_2-neopterin-P_3 (I) to sepiapterin (IV).

Biopterin Synthase and H_2-Pterin Oxidase - Previous investigations in animal systems[9-14] have indicated that sepiapterin can be reduced enzymatically to H_2-biopterin. We initiated investigations to decide whether or not sepiapterin is a precursor of H_2-biopterin in *Drosophila*. In preliminary experiments, incubation of ^{14}C-labeled sepiapterin with a crude extract of *Drosophila* in the presence of NADPH resulted in the production of radioactive biopterin. In this experiment, biopterin was the product detected since we treated the incubated reaction mixture with I_2 to oxidize any H_2-biopterin that may have been produced to biopterin in order to simplify the analyses. When NADPH was deleted from the reaction mixture no biopterin (or H_2-biopterin) was produced, but all of the sepiapterin disappeared and a new blue-fluorescent compound appeared. It seemed reasonable that this substance might be oxidized sepiapterin since the treatment with I_2 would be expected to oxidize sepiapterin (a dihydropterin). Surprisingly, we found that when the treatment with I_2 was eliminated the blue-fluorescent compound was still produced in the absence of NADPH and, even more surprisingly, we found that when NADPH is included in the reaction mixture biopterin instead of H_2-biopterin was the enzymatic product, without the I_2 treatment. These observations indicate that an enzymatic oxidation occurs during the conversion of sepiapterin to biopterin. The consumption of sepiapterin in the absence of NADPH suggests that it is converted to oxidized sepiapterin and that the latter compound is converted, in the presence of NADPH, to biopterin. Conformation for this reaction sequence was obtained with the finding that the compound produced in the absence of NADPH disappears (and biopterin appears) when it is reincubated in the presence of NADPH. Finally, we were able to produce the blue-fluorescent compound in large enough amounts so that enough of it could be isolated for analysis. The UV spectra were exactly the same as standard oxidized sepiapterin. This evidence, along with the observations that the enzymatic product behaves as standard oxidized sepiapterin in paper chromatographic analyses with 7 different solvent systems, provides conclusive evidence that the enzymatic product is oxidized sepiapterin. For convenience, the enzyme will be called "H_2-pterin oxidase" in the remainder of this paper.

For the conversion of sepiapterin to oxidized sepiapterin an oxidizing agent must be present. Since there was no need to add such an agent to reaction mixtures, we considered the possibility that O_2 supplies oxidizing power. Confirmation of this possibility was obtained with the observation that under anaerobic conditions no oxidized sepiapterin was produced enzymatically from sepiapterin.

To obtain more information about the synthesis of biopterin from sepiapterin the enzymes were purified, with the primary goal of separating the oxidase from biopterin synthase. Extracts of a mixture of late larvae and early pupae were used as a source of enzymes. The purification scheme involved successively: fractionation with ammonium sulfate, chromatography on a column of DEAE-Sephadex, and chromatography on an Affi-gel Blue column. Each of these steps resulted in enrichment of the specific activities of the enzymes, but only the last step allowed the separation of H_2-pterin oxidase from biopterin synthase.

With the use of the purified biopterin synthase, (free from the oxidase), we have established that sepiapterin and oxidized sepiapterin can be converted to H_2-biopterin and biopterin, respectively, but oxidized sepiapterin is much the better substrate (the K_m is 10 μM whereas the K_m for sepiapterin is 63 μM). NADPH is needed and cannot be replaced by NADH.

The oxidase is not specific for sepiapterin as substrate; for example, H_2-pterin,

H_2-biopterin, and H_2-neopterin can also be used. In fact, the only H_2-pterin that has been tested and found not to be a substrate is H_2-neopterin-P_3.

Since, with the exception of sepiapterin, all of the pteridine pigments found in *Drosophila* apparently occur as the fully oxidized compounds (pterins), one can speculate that the physiological function of the oxidase is to catalyze the conversion of the biosynthetic dihydropterin compounds to the corresponding pterins which are the products normally found in the flies.

ACKNOWLEDGEMENTS

The work described in this paper was supported by research grants from the National Institutes of Health (AM03442) and the National Science Foundation (PCM-19513 A02).

REFERENCES

1. Fan, C.L. and Brown, G.M. (1976) Biochem. Genet., 14, 259.

2. Brown, G.M. and Fan, C.L. (1976) in Chemistry and Biology of Pteridines, Pfleiderer, W. ed., Walter de Gruyter, New York. pp. 265-272.

3. Fukushima, K., Richter, Jr., W.E., and Shiota, T. (1977) J. Biol. Chem., 252, 5750.

4. Gál, E.M., Nelson, J.M. and Sherman, A.D. (1978) Neurochem. Res., 1, 627.

5. Fan, C.L., Krivi, G.G., and Brown, G.M. (1975) Biochem. Biophys. Res. Commun. 67, 1047.

6. Krivi, G.G. and Brown, G.M. (1978) Biochem. Genet. (submitted for publication).

7. Eto, I., Fukushima, K., and Shiota, T. (1976) J. Biol. Chem., 251, 6505.

8. Fan, C.L. and Brown, G.M. (1978) Biochem. Genet. (submitted for publication).

9. Taira, T. (1961) Nature, 189, 231.

10. Matsubara, M., Tsusue, M., and Akino, M. (1963) Nature, 199, 908.

11. Matsubara, M. and Akino, M. (1964) Experientia, 20, 574.

12. Matsubara, M., Katoh, S., Akino, M., and Kaufman, S. (1966) Biochem. Biophys. Acta, 122, 202.

13. Nagai, M. (Matsubara) (1968) Arch. Biochem. Biophys. 126, 426.

14. Katoh, S., Nagai, M., Nagai, Y., Fukushima, T., and Akino, M. (1970) in Chemistry and Biology of Pteridines, Iwai, K., Akino, M., Goto, M. and Iwanami, Y., eds., International Academic Printing Co., Ltd., Tokyo, pp. 225-234.

THE PHARMACOLOGY OF STRIATAL PTERINS AND THE REGULATION OF DOPAMINERGIC FUNCTION

WILSON P. BULLARD, JOSEPH B. YELLIN, AND ARNOLD J. MANDELL
Department of Psychiatry, University of California at San Diego, La Jolla CA 92093

ABSTRACT

d-Amphetamine (d-AMP) decreases rat striatal reduced pterins (PH_4), and the change exhibits complex dose-time-effect relationships. Of 30 other drugs, none affects striatal PH_4, but some alter the d-AMP effect. Loss in PH_4 is due to oxidation yielding a non-quinoid dihydropterin (PH_2); and we have identified in the striatum a non-quinoid dihydropterin reductase (DPR) that is implicated in PH_4 restoration. Data are interpreted in terms of two PH_4 regenerating systems serving two dopamine (DA) synthetic pathways and suggest the primary d-AMP action involves DA release from one discrete system.

INTRODUCTION

We have previously established that the localization of PH_4 within the striatum reflects predominant, if not exclusive, association with dopaminergic systems[1]. As an essential coreactant in tyrosine hydroxylase (TYH)-catalyzed aromatic oxidation leading to DA, PH_4 is present primarily for the purpose of DA synthesis. The hydroxylation reaction exhibits adaptive regulatory mechanisms; in particular TYH is subject to feedback inhibition by DA in apparent competition with PH_4 and is conformationally flexible, its forms differing in the ratios of their affinities for DA and PH_4[2,3]. Further accumulation of evidence of pterin dynamics as a sensitive element in regulation of catecholaminergic function includes apparent CNS autoregulation of PH_4 supply via de novo synthesis from GTP within neuronal tissue[4-6]. We have taken a pharmacological approach in exploring the biochemistry of pterins in rat striatum and the integration of pterin dynamics with DA function.

MATERIALS AND METHODS

For measure of PH_4 and DPR activities a radioenzymatic assay based on PH_4-dependent phenylalanine hydroxylase (PAH)-catalyzed formation of L-tyrosine and ^3HOH from 4-^3H-phenylalanine was used. Total pterins (PH_x) were measured fluorimetrically after iodine oxidation. Quinoid and non-quinoid 7,8-dihydropterins (q.PH_2 and PH_2) were estimated by PH_4 measurement subsequent to attempted reduction using quinoid dihydropterin reductase (QDPR) or purified dihydrofolate reductase (DFR) in excess. 2,4-Diamino-5-(3,4-dichlorophenyl)-6-methylpyrimidine (DDMP) and the 6-ethyl homologue (DDEP) were gifts of C.A. Nichol, Burroughs Wellcome Research Laboratories.

In vivo drug trials. Using one or more groups of six experimental and six control animals and conducting two or more trials per drug, we tested more than 30 drugs for effect on striatal PH_4, including eight phenylethylamines, e.g. amphetamine, DOPA, and mescaline; the amphetamine analogue methylphenidate; three neuroleptics; apomorphine; the uptake inhibitors cocaine, benztropine, and imipramine; the monoamine oxidase inhibitor pargyline; the cholinergics physostigmine and scopolamine; reserpine (short time course); γ-butyrolactone; the DFR inhibitors methotrexate, DDMP, and DDEP. A series of drug combinations was also tested[7].

RESULTS AND DISCUSSION

Of the drugs tested, d-AMP only (and 1-amphetamine at higher doses)[*] reliably produced significant changes in PH_4. The d-AMP-induced decrease in striatal PH_4, observed in over 200 trials, is characterized by a "floor" effect. Above a threshold dose of 0.8 mg/kg a 25-30% decrease is observed at some point in the time course. The magnitude of decrease does not exceed 25-30% at any dose or time examined. A composite of time-dose-effect relationships (Fig. 1) is the product of two responses. A low-dose or "primary" event causes rapid loss of PH_4, approaching the 30% limit with increasing dose, the half-maximal effect occurring at 0.3 mg/kg. An antagonistic secondary effect is also seen; the initial <u>rate</u> of PH_4 loss decreases with increasing dose until at 5 mg/kg it takes about 120 min for PH_4 to reach the limiting value of 70% of control. The secondary component is half-maximal between 1 and 1.5 mg/kg. The biphasic or multiphasic effects of d-AMP on single unit discharge rates[8], locomotor and stereotypic behaviors[9], and DA synthesis or turnover in the striatum[10] have components that cluster similarly around doses of 0.3 and 1.3 mg/kg.

Comparison of d-AMP effects on PH_4 and on striatal DA synthesis velocities (Fig. 2) shows that increased DA synthesis mirrors PH_4 loss at low doses and decreased DA synthesis coincides with slower PH_4 loss at higher doses[10]. PH_4 utilization in DA synthesis provides an apparent basis for d-AMP-induced decrease in striatal PH_4 levels. However, the continued loss of PH_4 at higher d-AMP doses when DA synthesis velocities have fallen to below control values indicates a dissociation of PH_4 utilization and DA synthesis which is supported by the observation that a number of the drugs tested (Table 1) increase DA synthesis and are without effect on PH_4 levels[11]. The uniqueness of d-AMP in decreasing PH_4 levels and the uncoupling of PH_4 loss and DA synthesis suggest PH_4 changes reflect DA synthesis in only one of the two or more DA "pools" of the striatum[12] and that the PH_4 regeneration by the QDPR - $q.PH_2$ - NADH pathway is less efficient and supplemented or altogether supplanted by an alternate regenerating system in the pathway for synthesis of d-AMP-releasable DA.

Measurements of PH_4, PH_x, and $q.PH_2$ in striatal tissue of control and d-AMP-treated animals (Table 1), estimation of PH_2 by recovery with purified DFR in homogenates and following HPLC separation of striatal PH_4 and PH_2, and comparison of PH_4 recovery and reported synthesis rates, lead to the conclusions that 1) PH_2/PH_4 < 15% in control

---

[*] Changes observed with DDMP are discussed below.

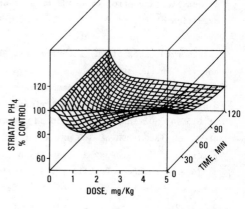

Fig. 1 Dose-time-effect surface
for d-AMP-induced changes in striatal
PH$_4$ levels.

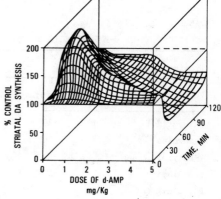

Fig. 2 Dose-time-effect surface
for d-AMP-induced changes in striatal
DA turnover[10].

TABLE 1

APPARENT DISTRIBUTION OF STRIATAL PTERINS AMONG REDOX AND TAUTOMERIC FORMS
IN CONTROL AND d-AMP TREATED ANIMALS

Treatment	(mg/kg)	(min)	Conditions of Tissue Preparation		
			Normal (PH_4)	Oxidizing (PH_x)	Reducing $(PH_4 + q.PH_2)$
Saline			100 ± 3	100 ± 4	100 ± 2
d-AMP	1	90	82 ± 2 *	109 ± 5	83 ± 3 *
d-AMP	5	120	73 ± 2 *	97 ± 4	--

* $p < 0.02$

animals, 2) PH_4 accounts for most of the total striatal pterins, 3) $q.PH_2$ is not detectable in control or d-AMP-treated animals, and 4) the PH_4 decrease reflects oxidation of PH_4 to PH_2 or a dihydropterin derivative and not a change in pterin synthesis or transport rates.

Observed rates of PH_4 recovery lead us to hypothesize a non-quinoid PH_2 reductase activity in the striatum. Using dihydrobiopterin (BH_2) as substrate and the PAH assay for PH_4 detection, we have demonstrated the enzyme activity in striatum and shown 1) a specific activity of 100 pmol/min/mg tissue, 2) a NADPH requirement, 3) pH optimum of 6.5, 4) 50% inhibition at 50 pM methotrexate, and 5) Michaelis constants for BH_2 of 30 µM, for NADPH of 3.0 µM, and for dihydrofolate of 11 µM. Two laboratories have reported a similar enzyme activity in rat and rabbit brain[13,14].

To explore the possibility that distinct PH_4 regenerating systems might be associated with discrete DA systems and underlie the effects on PH_4 elicited by d-AMP but not by other drugs that stimulate DA synthesis, we assessed the ability of several drugs to modify the d-AMP effect on striatal PH_4 (Table 2).

TABLE 2

MODIFICATION OF d-AMP EFFECTS ON STRIATAL PH_4

Treatments	Doses	Times			Modifications	
		min before d-AMP	min before sacrifice	min after d-AMP	% Change	
	mg/kg				Before	After
Haloperidol	1	30	90 *	45	+ 45	n.c.
Reserpine	2.5	30	90 *	45	− 77	− 100
γ-Butyrolactone	600	45	90 *	45	− 27	n.c.
Scopolamine	1	20	90 *		+ 32	
Physostigmine	1	40	45		− 41	
Pargyline	25	30	90 *	45		+ 32
Methylphenidate	10	40	45		− 92	
	10		90	60		− 75
	5	30	45		− 40	
	5	30	120		− 18	
Cocaine	10	30	45		− 119	
	10		75	45		n.c.

% Change in d-AMP effect = (combination − d-AMP)/(control − d-AMP).
+ = potentiation; − = antagonism; n.c. = no change. Changes are reported only if the effect of combined treatment differed from that of d-AMP alone and/or control groups at p < 0.05 in at least 2 trials. * d-AMP dose was 1 mg/kg; all others were 2 mg/kg.

The drug combination trials demonstrated that reserpine virtually blocks or reverses the d-AMP effect, which implies that excessive cytoplasmic DA prevents PH_4 utilization by inhibiting TYH. Modest alterations evoked by haloperidol and the cholinergics implicate the DA receptor and the striato-nigral descending pathway in the overall response.

Because methylphenidate (MPD) and d-AMP are thought to release DA from functionally discrete pools[15], we anticipated that MPD might, by release and reuptake, augment DA levels in the d-AMP-releasable pool, prolonging product inhibition of DA synthesis and delaying onset of PH_4 loss. MPD (5 mg/kg, Table 2) given 30 min before d-AMP significantly retards PH_4 loss measured 45 min after d-AMP; 75 min later PH_4 is significantly decreased, but less so than after d-AMP alone. The same dose of MPD given 60 min after d-AMP restores PH_4 to control levels. Cocaine (Table 2) at low doses blocks d-AMP-induced PH_4 loss, presumably by preventing primary d-AMP release of DA[16] in the pathway where PH_4 can be temporarily decreased because of its slow recovery. Cocaine administered after d-AMP is without effect, facilitation of DA release having been initiated.

The results are consistent with d-AMP facilitated release and stimulated synthesis of DA in a single pool as the primary event[17]. While DA synthesis in another pathway may be accompanied by nearly 100% efficient PH_4 regeneration via QDPR, in the PH_4 regeneration for the synthesis of d-AMP-releasable DA, tautomerization perhaps competes with reduction of $q.PH_2$, thus effecting a temporary loss to PH_2 which is recovered slowly by DPR.

We have observed that DDMP (5-10 mg/kg, s.c.) causes a 20% decrease in striatal PH_4 one to two hours after treatment, but have not demonstrated to our satisfaction that PH_2 recovery after d-AMP is substantially retarded by the DFR inhibitor. To complement the biochemical studies, we have begun a series of experiments observing and scoring stereotypic motor activities associated with d-AMP effects in rats. Preliminary results indicate that the lipid-soluble DPR inhibitor DDMP (5-15 mg/kg) elicits stereotyped behaviors. DDMP elicits 77% of the overall response observed with 2 mg/kg of d-AMP, and the effect endures 50% longer. The more potent inhibitor methotrexate does not readily enter the brain and at 2.5 mg/kg elicited no response that distinguished methotrexate-treated animals from saline-treated controls. The results are consonant with the pharmacodynamics of the compounds and with DPR involvement in DA function.

SUMMARY

The pharmacology of striatal PH_4 reveals a potential DA regulatory mechanism based on utilization and depletion of PH_4 and specifies some ideas of DA pool interactions and mechanisms of d-AMP action. The concept emerges of two distinct DA systems, one using about 70% of total PH_4 and a regenerating system involving $q.PH_2$, QDPR, and NADH; and the other, specifically responsive to d-AMP, using about

30% of total PH_4 and a less efficient regenerating system involving PH_2, DPR, and NADPH.

ACKNOWLEDGEMENTS

This work is supported by USPHS Grant DA-00265. We are grateful for the invaluable technical assistance of Patrick V. Russo.

REFERENCES

1. Bullard, W.P., Guthrie, P.B., Russo, P.V. and Mandell, A.J. (1978) J. Pharmacol. Exp. Ther., 206, 4-20.

2. Weiner, N. (1970) Ann. Rev. Pharmacol. 10, 273-290.

3. Mandell, A.J. (1978) Ann. Rev. Pharmacol. Toxicol. 18, 461-493.

4. Buff, K. and Dairman, W. (1975) in The Chemistry and Biology of Pteridines, Pfleiderer, W. ed., DeGruyter, New York, pp. 273-284.

5. Gal, E.M. and Sherman, A.D. (1976) Neurochem. Res., 1, 627-639.

6. Fukushima, K., Eto, I., Mayumi, T., Richter, W., Goodson, S. and Shiota, T. (1975) in The Chemistry and Biology of Pteridines, Pfleiderer, W. ed., DeGruyter, New York, pp. 247-264.

7. Bullard, W.P., Yellin, J.B., Russo, P.V. and Mandell, A.J. (1978) J. Pharmacol. Exp. Ther., in revision for publication.

8. Groves, P., Rebec, G. and Segal, D. (1974) Behav. Biol., 11, 33-47.

9. Segal, D.S. and Mandell, A.J. (1974) Pharmacol. Biochem. Behav., 2, 249-255.

10. Kuczenski, R. (1978) Neuropharmacology, in press.

11. Roth, R.H., Walters, J.R. and Aghajanian, G.K. (1973) in Frontiers in Catecholamine Research, Usdin, E. and Snyder, S. eds., Pergamon, New York, pp. 567-574.

12. Javoy, F. and Glowinski, J. (1971) J. Neurochem., 18, 1305-1311.

13. Abelson, H.T., Spector, R., Gorka, C. and Fosburg, M. (1978) Biochem. J., 171, 267-268.

14. Pollock, R.J. and Kaufman, S. (1978) J. Neurochem., 30, 253-256.

15. Moore, K.E., Chiueh, C.C. and Zeldes, G. (1976) in Cocaine and Other Stimulants, Ellinwood, E.H. and Kilbey, M.M. eds., Plenum, New York, pp. 143-157.

16. Heikkila, R.E., Orlansky, H., Mytilineou, C. and Cohen, G. (1975) J. Pharmacol. Exp. Ther., 194, 47-56.

17. Uretsky, N.J. and Snodgrass, S.R. (1977) J. Pharmacol. Exp. Ther., 202, 565-580.

18. Nichol, C.A., Cavallito, J.C., Wooley, J.L. and Sigel, C.W. (1977) Cancer Treat. Rep., 61, 559-564.

PTERIDINE BIOSYNTHESIS AND NITROGEN METABOLISM IN THE BUTTERFLY *COLIAS CROCEUS*
AND ITS *"ALBA"* MUTANT

HENRI DESCIMON

Ecole Normale Supérieure, Laboratoire de Zoologie, 46 rue d'Ulm, 75230 Paris cedex 05
France

ABSTRACT

The female mutant *Alba* of *Colias* synthesizes less pteridine wing pigments than the orange phenotype. ^{14}C-guanosine and ^{14}C-glycine have been injected into pupae of *C. croceus* at the beginning of pigment synthesis and their incorporation into various compounds has been studied. Males differ markedly from females; the orange morph excretes in meconium more guanosine derivatives than *Alba*. With glycine, no significant differences between both morphs are observed. The autoradiographic incorporation pattern in wings suggests that differential permeability plays a role with heavier precursors (guanosine, pterins) but not with glycine, where the uptake is more homogenous.

INTRODUCTION

The Pierid butterflies of the genus *Colias* are brightly coloured by pteridine pigments, which are mainly synthesized in the wing imaginal disks and deposited in the scales during the last third of metamorphosis[1,2]. In almost all species, the females are dimorphic: one morph is male-like coloured (yellow to red), the other one is whitish and named *Alba*. This latter character is determined by a single autosomal dominant gene[3]. Its expression may be influenced by modifier genes and environmental conditions[4,5].

It has been shown that *Alba* produces an overall reduction of pigment synthesis[6]. Watt[7] has suggested that this mutant devotes less GTP or guanosine to pteridine synthesis; the corresponding amount of guanosine might be used for other functions.

The ecological aspects of this polymorphism are beyond the scope of this article. It will be only mentionned that *Alba* is less resistant to diseases at high temperatures[8,9], which implies the presence of a metabolic difference already in the preimaginal stages. Since *Alba* remains present in natural populations, especially under cool conditions, a still unknown factor must counteract this disadvantage.

Some preliminary experiments have been undertaken to comparatively study the metabolism of two major pteridine precursors, glycine and guanosine, in males, orange (*"aa"*) and *Alba* (*"Aa"*) females of the european species *Colias croceus*.

MATERIALS AND METHODS

The *C. croceus* strain originates from South of France; the larvae are raised on

potted alfalfa in winter, in a cool greenhouse (5–15°C), under natural (short) photoperiod. After pupation, the insects are placed in a constant temperature room (20°C,
16h photoperiod). At the 8th day after pupation, $2-^{14}$C-guanosine and $1-^{14}$C-glycine
are injected into insects issued from *Aa* females mated by *aa* males, which give rise
to an 1:1 offspring of *aa* and *Aa* females. After hatching, the butterflies are killed
by freezing, the wings are cut off from the body, which is conserved in 2 ml of
absolute ethanol at –70°C. Meconium is cropped on Whatman n°1 chromatography paper.

The bodies are homogenized by lots of 5 or 10 in cold ethanol with Ultra-Turrax
and submitted to a sequence of differential extraction for small molecules, nucleic
acids and proteins by HClO4 and NaOH solutions, according to the method of Lafont et
al[10]. Aliquots of the extracts are counted by scintillation. Proteins and nucleic
acids are measured by classical methods[10].

The wing pteridines are analyzed by column chromatography on Ecteola-cellulose,
TLC and thin-layer electrophoresis[11].

Autoradiographs of the wings are made by application of the dried wings on Kodak
Kodirex film for 48h; the films are scanned with a Vernon densitometer.

RESULTS

General features of precursor incorporation

The methods used allow one to obtain data on the precursors incorporation into
i- small molecules present in the body; ii- meconium excretory compounds; iii- pigments and excreta deposited in the wings; iv- RNA; v- DNA; vi- proteins (table 1).
A slight contamination of DNA extracts by peptides does not allow the measurements of
their radioactivity to be significant in ^{14}C-glycine series.

Clearcut differences are observed between males and females. With guanosine, the
former show a lesser incorporation into nucleic acids, but a larger accumulation of
small molecules in the body and the wings. With glycine, the incorporation is less
in nucleic acids and in proteins; however, there is no compensatory incorporation into
other parts. Since there is a deficit in the total counts with respect to the amount
injected, it must be concluded that more than 40% of the glycine has been catabolized.
In females, the missing counts are approximately 25% only.

The differences observed between female phenotypes are slight: with guanosine, the
meconium contains clearly more radioactivity in *aa* than in *Aa*, which incorporates
slightly more into RNA, DNA, wing pigments and excreta. No differences at all are
observed with glycine.

Incorporation into wing pteridines

A typical elution diagram is represented in Fig. 1. In guanosine experiments, which
are the only ones to have been analyzed in detail, it appears that all the pterins are
labelled, with the exception of isoxanthopterin, which bears a very weak amount of
radioactivity. In all cases, the incorporation into xanthopterin is the largest, but

TABLE 1

INCORPORATION OF PTERIDINE PRECURSORS INTO VARIOUS TYPES OF COMPOUNDS DURING THE LAST THIRD OF METAMORPHOSIS IN *COLIAS CROCEUS* MALE, ORANGE AND *ALBA* FEMALES

A: after injection of 1.35 μCi (ca. 3×10^6 DPM) of 2-^{14}C-guanosine, B: after injection of 0.95 μCi (ca. 2×10^6 DPM° of 1-^{14}C-glycine into each pupa. Results for lots of 5 animals, in DPMx10^5. Specific activities (DPM/μg) in *italics*.

		Body compounds					*Wings*	*Meconium*
		Small molecules soluble in		RNA	DNA	Proteins	Pigments & excreta	Excreta
		EtOH	EtOH/EtO2 Water					
A	♂	0.8	0.2	21.4	26.0 *1195*	1.4 *590*	0	55.2	51.7
	aa ♀	1.0	0.1	11.6	31.9 *1205*	1.7 *650*	0	41.6	57.5
	Aa ♀	1.0	0.2	13.3	34.1 *1285*	1.8 *665*	0	48.3	44.8
B	♂	0.9	0.1	6.4	4.0 *206*	(3.7)[a]	18.9 *40*	14.0	11.7
	aa ♀	1.1	0.1	7.0	7.6 *280*	(7.0)[a]	26.7 *52*	16.4	8.0
	Aa ♀	1.6	0.1	8.8	7.2 *260*	(6.8)[a]	26.5 *51.5*	15.8	10.6

[a] Insignificant values, due to contamination by incipient hydrolysis of proteins

there is a very wide variation owing to the pteridines. Non-fluorescing compounds are also observed. One of them (peak 6 of the elution diagram) is especially abundant in males and is not yet identified. Quantitative results are given in Table 2.

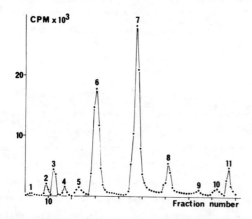

3=sepiapterin
7=xanthopterin
8=leucopterin
11=erythropterin

Fig. 1. Elution diagram of wing compounds of male *C. croceus* after injection of ^{14}C-guanosine on a 2x40 cm Ecteola-cellulose column. The pH of the elution buffer is decreased owing to a discontinuous gradient from 7 to 3. The fraction volume is 18 ml. Extract from the wings of 5 animals. Some peaks have been further purified by TLC. Isoxanthopterin is detected by its fluorescence, since it does not appear in the radioactivity diagram.

The most striking difference between the two kinds of females is the lesser incorporation into erythropterin in *Aa* which present, on the other hand, more radioactivity in leucopterin. The specific radioactivity (in mCi/mM) of erythropterin is 0.020 in males, 0.012 in *aa* 0.014 in *Aa* females. In glycine experiments, the specific radioactivity of the same pigment is 0.020 in males, 0.015 in *aa* and 0.018 in *Aa* females.

TABLE 2

RADIOACTIVITY OF PTERIDINES AFTER INJECTION OF GUANOSINE INTO PUPAE OF *COLIAS CROCEUS* MALE, ORANGE AND *ALBA* FEMALES

Same conditions as in Table 1. Radioactivity in $DPMx10^5$.

	Sepiapterin	Pterin	Xanthopterin	Isoxanthopterin	Leucopterin	Erythropterin
♂	1.2^a	0.1	12.1	< 0.01	2.2	3.7
aa♀	0.6^a	0.1	20.3	< 0.01	1.9	4.0
Aa♀	0.5^a	0.1	17.1	< 0.01	2.8	1.6

[a] Cumulated values of sepiapterin and 6-COOH-pterin, issued from the former by photolysis.

Incorporation and wing pattern

The amounts of the different pteridines vary according to the zones of the wing[6]. The autoradiographs of butterfly wings injected with ^{14}C-guanosine (as well as with [14]C- various pteridines[12]) show that the coloured wing-pattern is transferred with much fidelity (Fig. 2). Black areas incorporate very little, while the orange discoidal spot of the hindwings is strongly labelled. On the contrary, the pattern obtained with glycine is much less clearcut. Densitograms of these autoradiographs illustrate this phenomenon (Fig. 2). With both precursors, no significant differences have been observed between the two female phenotypes.

DISCUSSION AND CONCLUSIONS

It is well established today that the pteridines of the adult wing in *Pieridae* are not issued from a single source[12]. One minor part comes from fat body where breakdown products of coenzymes accumulate during larval life[13]. This is the case with leucopterin and isoxanthopterin, which are oserved in fat body during the first part of nymphosis[1]. In *Colias*, it is likely the only source for the latter, present in small amounts: its synthesis is negligible with guanosine[2] as well as with dihydroneopterin as a precursor[14] and the present experiments confirm these data. In *Colias*, on the contrary, isoxanthopterin synthesis is very important[15]; the difference lies probably at the level of the conversion dihydropterin→pterin or dihydroxanthopterin.

The simple hypothesis that *Alba* mutation operates at this level and that the pigments of this mutant are only issued from the former process, *in situ* synthesis being non-existent, is obviously ruled out by the experiments presented here.

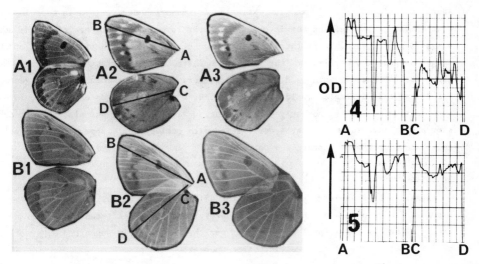

Fig. 2. Autoradiographs of *Colias croceus* wings after injection of ^{14}C-guanosine (A) and ^{14}C-glycine (B) into pupae at the 8th day of pupal stage. 1: male, 2: orange female, 3 *Alba* female. The original autoradiographs are used as a negative and so the prints reproduced here are inversed (labelled areas appear clear). 4: densitogram of A2, 5: densitogram of B2. The autoradiographs are scanned owing to A-B and C-D.

The major part of the wing pigments is synthesized *de novo* and *in situ*. But the question remain as to the major precursor, which must undergo a transport from fat body by haemolymph. GTP is excluded, because of its difficulty to pass through the cell membrane; thus guanosine and glycine remain the best candidates for this role. The former is released by the histolysis processes which characterize metamorphosis; it may also be synthesized in fat body and transported into the wings; however, it has not been observed in detectable amounts in *Pieris* haemolymph[16]. On the contrary, glycine is present in Insect haemolymph[17]. Autoradiographic results suggest that both play a role: guanosine, which penetrates differentially into the cells, produces the wing pattern; glycine, which is fixed homogenously, the overall coloration.

In the scheme issued from these data:

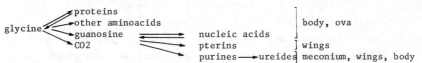

where lies the difference between orange and *Alba* females? The internal redistribution between pigments that appear in Table 2 is likely an ulterior effect of the primary factors, already quoted by Watt[7]. The available specific activities of nucleic acids, proteins and erythropterin fail to indicate any significant difference with glycine as well as with guanosine. This only means that a long-term single labelling is too coarse an experiment to unravel phenomena which are complex. The only datum which seems significant is that meconium excretion of guanosine derivatives is more important in orange females and the incorporation of this compound into nucleic acids and wings is higher in *Alba*. Further verification and study of the chemical nature of the compounds produced may lead to the conclusion that white females have a more parsimonious pool of nucleic acid (and pteridine) precursors. So, the metabolic divergence between *aa* and *Aa* females would be again earlier than Watt[7] suggested. This would have important consequences, not only on pigmentation and excretion, but also on reproduction physiology. In this case, a correlation with ecology would appear less chimerical. Future work must test this hypothesis.

AKNOWLEDGEMENTS

Thanks to R. Blanchard for providing the wild strain of *Colias croceus*, to J. Brulfert for help in breeding, To J.L. Pennetier for competent technical assistance and to R. Lafont for helpful advice. This work has been partly supported by grants of C.N.R.S., R.C.P. N° 317 "Polymorphisme-Spéciation-Mimétisme".

REFERENCES

1. Descimon, H. (1966) C.R. Soc. Biologie, 160, 928-933.
2. Watt, W.B. (1967) J. biol. Chem., 242, 565-572.
3. Remington, C.L. (1954) Adv. Genet., 6, 403-450.
4. Hoffmann, R.J. (1974) J. Insect Physiol., 20, 1913-1924.
5. Descimon, H., unpublished data.
6. Descimon, H. (1966) C. R. Acad. Sci. Paris, 262, 390-393.
7. Watt, W.B. (1973) Evolution, 27, 537-548.
8. Herman, C. and Lorkovic, Z. (1963) Bull. Sci. Cons. Acad. R.S.F. Yougosl., 8, 67.
9. Descimon, H., to be published.
10. Lafont, R. et al. (1975) Comp. Biochem. Physiol., 51B, 439-444.
11. Descimon, H. (1973) Bull. Soc. chim. France, 1973, 145-152.
12. Descimon, H. (1976) in Chemistry and Biology of Pteridines, Pfleiderer, W. ed., Walter de Gruyter, Berlin and New York, pp. 805-840.
13. Harmsen, R. (1966) J. Insect Physiol., 12, 9-22.
14. Descimon, H. (1976) in Chemistry and Biology of Pteridines, Pfleiderer, W. ed., Walter de Gruyter, Berlin and New York, pp. 841-847.
15. Lafont, R., (1972) Biochimie, 54, 73-81.
16. Lafont, R., personnal communication.
17. Gilmour, D. (1961) The Biochemistry of Insects, Academic Press, New York and London, p. 237.

BIOSYNTHESIS OF DROSOPTERINS IN THE HEAD OF <u>DROSOPHILA MELANOGASTER</u>

DALE L. DORSETT, JOHN J. YIM, AND K. BRUCE JACOBSON

University of Tennessee—Oak Ridge Graduate School of Biomedical Sciences and

Biology Division, Oak Ridge National Laboratory, Oak Ridge, Tennessee 37830 (U.S.A.)

ABSTRACT

Conditions are described that allow for the enzymatic conversion of dihydroneopterin triphosphate to neodrosopterin, isodrosopterin, fraction (e) [Schwinck and Mancini], aurodrosopterins, and sepiapterin. Synthesis of the "drosopterins" requires Mg^{2+} and either NADPH or NADH, whereas sepiapterin synthesis requires Mg^{2+} and NADPH. Drosopterin synthesis occurs enzymatically in three subcellular fractions, whereas the majority of sepiapterin synthesis occurs enzymatically in one subcellular fraction. Evidence presented suggests that sepiapterin is not a precursor to "drosopterins" but that they share a common precursor.

INTRODUCTION

The "drosopterin"[*] eye pigments of <u>Drosophila melanogaster</u> appear to be formed from two pteridine ring systems in which one of the pteridines has been altered.[1] During studies on sepiaterin synthase we found that radioactive dihydroneopterin triphosphate [H_2-neopterin-$(P)_3$] was converted not only to sepiapterin, but to six "drosopterins" as well. In this report the methods for preparation of enzyme fractions are described, as are some of the cofactor requirements for "drosopterin" biosynthesis.

The purple (<u>pr</u>) mutant is deficient in sepiapterin synthase,[2] an enzyme that requires both Mg^{2+} and NADPH to convert H_2-neopterin-$(P)_3$ to sepiapterin.[3] The level of enzyme activity in this mutant, 10–30% that of wild type, can be restored fully when the suppressor mutant <u>su(s)</u>[2] is also present in the genotype.[2] The amounts of "drosopterins" in the <u>pr</u> mutant are ~30% of normal and are also restored to normal by the <u>su(s)</u>[2] mutant.[4] To increase understanding of the mechanism of suppression, we wish to define the gene product of the <u>su(s)</u>[2] locus and how it affects the activity of the mutant sepiapterin synthase and the synthesis of "drosopterins."

THE ASSAY

The assay is an extension of the sepiapterin synthase assay used in a previous report.[2] [U-^{14}C]H_2-neopterin-$(P)_3$ prepared from [U-^{14}C]GTP by the action of purified <u>Escherichia coli</u>

---

[*] "Drosopterin" refers to the class of 6 dipteridine-derived red eye pigments of <u>Drosophila</u>; drosopterin refers to the individual compound.

GTP cyclohydrolase was incubated with Drosophila extracts in the presence of various cofactors and pteridines, depending upon the experiment. After the mixture was heated to stop the reaction, alkaline phosphatase was added to degrade the substrate; carrier sepiapterin and "drosopterins" were also added. The samples were centrifuged, sepiapterin and the "drosopterins" were separated by two-dimensional cellulose thin-layer chromatography, and their radioactivity was determined in a scintillation counter.

SUBSTRATE REQUIREMENTS

The conversion of $[U-^{14}C]H_2$-neopterin-$(P)_3$ into sepiapterin and the "drosopterins" depends on heat-labile factors present in extracts of fly heads (Figs. 1 and 2). $[3'-^3H]H_2$-neopterin-$(P)_3$ is not converted to radioactive "drosopterins," but $[^3H]$sepiapterin is readily formed (Fig. 2). If bacterial alkaline phosphatase is used to remove the phosphates from $[U-^{14}C]H_2$-neopterin-$(P)_3$ prior to its use as a substrate, conversion to "drosopterins" and sepiapterin is prevented (Fig. 2). The synthesis of sepiapterin and the "drosopterins" increases with extract concentration and time.

"DROSOPTERIN" BIOSYNTHESIS IN SUBCELLULAR ORGANELLES

Pigment granules containing "drosopterins" occur in the primary and secondary pigment cells of the ommatidia[5] and appear to sediment at 600g, forming a distinct red upper layer when a homogenate of Oregon-R heads is subjected to differential centrifugation. Pellets were also obtained after 15,000g and 100,000g centrifugations. Each pellet was washed twice, but these washings were not included in the 100,000g supernatant. "Drosopterin" biosynthesis was found in all fractions except the 15,000g pellet, whereas sepiapterin synthase was found mainly in the 100,000g supernatants (~12% is in the 100,000g pellet) (Fig. 3). The red pigmented upper layer of the 600g pellet is greatly enriched in "drosopterins," and it was routinely separated from the rest of the pellet and assayed alone. We shall refer to this as the red pellet. It is possible that the "drosopterin" biosynthesis is associated with the pigment granules in the red pellet.

As shown in Fig. 3, the red pellet had little sepiapterin synthase but was quite active in "drosopterin" biosynthesis. The red pellet was supplemented with sepiapterin synthase by addition of aliquots of the 100,000g supernatant. "Drosopterin" biosynthesis in this combination was additive, but sepiapterin synthase responded synergistically; the amount of sepiapterin produced by the combination of the red pellet and the 100,000g supernatant was nearly twice the amount each could produce alone (Fig. 4). When the red pellet was heated at 100°C for 5 min, the synergistic synthesis of sepiapterin did not occur (Fig. 4). When the wild-type red pellet was mixed with a pr[bw] mutant whole-fly 100,000g supernatant, a stimulation of sepiapterin synthase was also seen (Fig. 4). Krivi and Brown had communicated to us that they were able to separate sepiapterin synthase into two fractions, both fractions being required for sepiapterin synthesis. We propose that only the first is necessary for "drosopterin" biosynthesis and that this is the step lacking in the purple mutants. We suggest that the initial step of sepiapterin synthase is present in the red pellet and is limiting in the 100,000g supernatant. Mixing of the two fractions results in a synergistic synthesis of sepiapterin. Furthermore, if the enzymatic lesion in the purple mutant is in the first step of sepiapterin synthase, then the red pellet of wild-type flies should stimulate sepiapterin synthesis in a pr^{bw} 100,000g supernatant by providing a source of the enzyme for which this mutant is defective (Fig. 4).

Previously reported gene dosage data for pr^{+} revealed sepiapterin synthase activity ratios of 2.0 when flies with two gene doses were compared with those with one dose. But a ratio of only 1.2 instead of the expected 1.5 was found for flies with three doses as compared with those with two doses.[2] We suggest that the expected 1.5 ratio was not seen because flies with three doses of the initial enzymatic step of sepiapterin synthase may contain more activity for production of the sepiapterin precursor than the second enzyme which has to convert the precursor to sepiapterin. Further evidence for the hypothesis comes from cofactor and isotope-dilution studies with a soluble, pigment-free enzyme extract.

COFACTORS AND ISOTOPE DILUTION

Empirically it was found that buffers containing KCl could extract "drosopterin" synthesizing activity from the pellet fractions. A head homogenate was made in 50 mM Pipes (pH 7.0) containing 0.5 M KCl, then centrifuged at 15,000g for 10 min. Activity was extracted from the pellet once with 0.5 M KCl buffer, twice with 1.0 M KCl buffer, and twice with 1.5 M KCl buffer by homogenization and recentrifugation. The pellet extracts and original supernatant were pooled and fractionated with 40–60% saturated $(NH_4)_2SO_4$. This protein fraction was dissolved and chromatographed on a Sephadex G-25 column. The excluded, A_{280}-absorbing material was concentrated by vacuum dialysis to 10 mg protein per ml.

With this extract it was found that Mg^{2+} is required for both sepiapterin and "drosopterin" biosynthesis (Fig. 5). While NADPH was required for sepiapterin synthesis, "drosopterin" synthesis utilized either NADPH or NADH (Fig. 5). Apparently the production of the common precursor for sepiapterin and "drosopterins" requires Mg^{2+}; the conversion of the precursor to sepiapterin requires specifically NADPH, whereas the conversion to the "drosopterins" can be accommodated by either NADH or NADPH.

The presence of sepiapterin at a concentration 100 times that of H_2-neopterin-$(P)_3$ to a reaction in which "drosopterin" synthesis was occuring resulted in no decrease in the amount of radioactive drosopterins synthesized. While it is possible that sepiapterin may be converted to "drosopterins" by a first-order reaction or that the exogenously added sepiapterin does not equilibrate with the enzymatically produced sepiapterin, it is more likely that sepiapterin is not a precursor of "drosopterins," as the other evidence presented here suggests. A possible reaction sequence is illustrated in Fig. 2.

INTERCONVERSION OF "DROSOPTERINS"

The six "drosopterins" may not all be produced enzymatically. Pfleiderer has shown that neodrosopterin can rearrange in aqueous solutions to form drosopterin and isodrosopterin.[6] Schwinck and Mancini have demonstrated that fraction (e) and the aurodrosopterins behave as a group genetically.[7] Furthermore, aurodrosopterins consist of a pair of stereoisomers, analogous to the stereoisomeric pair of drosopterin and isodrosopterin.[6] Neodrosopterin and fraction (e) have similar visible color, fluorescent color, and R_f values. Thus there is a possibility that fraction (e) can give rise to the aurodrosopterins by means of a chemical conversion that is analogous to that by which neodrosopterin converts to drosopterin and isodrosopterin. From these considerations one might predict that the addition of unlabeled neodrosopterin or of a mixture of drosopterin and isodrosopterin would not dilute the amount of label incorporated into the "drosopterins" from $[U-^{14}C]H_2$-neopterin-$(P)_3$. Indeed, when these experiments were performed no isotope dilution was observed. A more critical experiment would be to prepare neodrosopterin and fraction (e) and see if they nonenzymatically convert to the other "drosopterins" under the reaction conditions used.

REACTION MECHANISM

In a possible scheme for the biosynthesis of "drosopterins" (Fig. 6) it is necessary to recognize that (1) the 3'-hydrogens of H_2-neopterin-$(P)_3$ do not appear in the final products and (2) there are three less carbons in drosopterin than there are in two molecules of H_2-neopterin-$(P)_3$. The removal of the 3'-hydrogens could be a consequence of (1) the loss of the 3' carbon, (2) the loss of two carbons or the entire side chain of H_2-neopterin-$(P)_3$, or (3) the oxidation of the 3'-carbon. Since the 3'-hydrogens do appear in sepiapterin, it is necessary to consider such alterations as occuring at some stage after the production of the common precursor. The mechanism by which the number of carbon atoms is reduced by three in the formation of drosopterin must also be sought. An enzyme activity that may be considered for this role was described recently;[8] this enzyme causes the cleavage of either two or three carbons from H_2-neopterin-$(P)_3$ and requires only Mg^{2+}.

Despite the coordinate control of the synthesis of sepiapterin and "drosopterins" by the pr mutant, it seems clear that sepiapterin is not a direct precursor of the "drosopterins." The identification of the common precursor of the "drosopterins" and sepiapterin is under way.

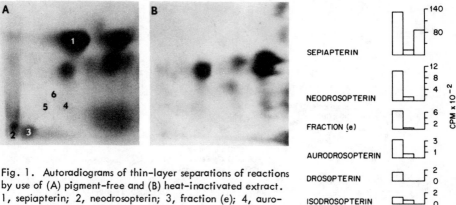

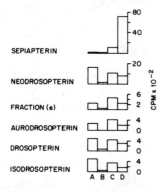

Fig. 1. Autoradiograms of thin-layer separations of reactions by use of (A) pigment-free and (B) heat-inactivated extract. 1, sepiapterin; 2, neodrosopterin; 3, fraction (e); 4, aurodrosopterin; 5, drosopterin; 6, isodrosopterin

Fig. 2. Substrate requirements for sepiapterin and "drosopterin" biosynthesis. A, $[U-^{14}C]H_2$-neopterin-$(P)_3$; B, phosphatase-treated A; C, $[3'-^3H]H_2$-neopterin-$(P)_3$.

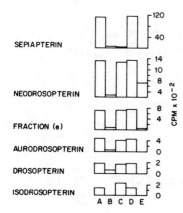

Fig. 3. Distribution of sepiapterin synthase and "drosopterin" biosynthesis among fractions from differential centrifugation of a head homogenate. A, 600g pellet; B, 15,000g pellet; C, 100,000g pellet; D, 100,000g supernatant.

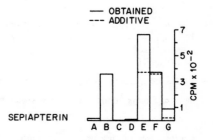

Fig. 4. Synergistic synthesis of sepiapterin by mixing 600g pellet of Oregon-R heads with a 100,000g supernatant of Oregon-R heads or pr^{bw} mutant whole flies. A, Oregon-R head 600g pellet; B, Oregon-R head 100,000g supernatant; C, heat-treated A; D, pr^{bw} whole-fly 100,000g supernatant; E, A + B; F, C + B; G, A + D.

Fig. 5. Cofactor requirements of sepiapterin and "drosopterin" biosynthesis in pigment-free extract. A, Mg^{2+} + NADPH + NADH; B, NADPH + NADH; C, Mg^{2+} + NADH; D, Mg^{2+} + NADPH; E, Mg^{2+}.

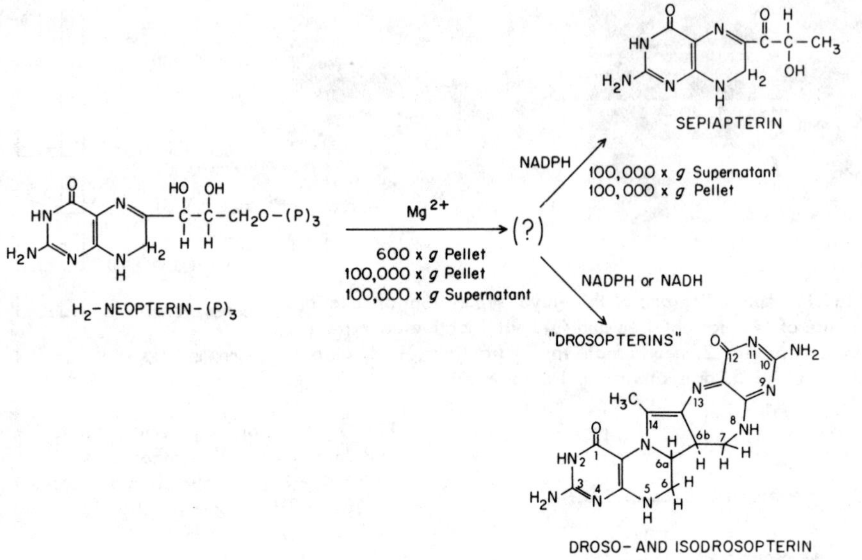

104

Fig. 6. Proposed reaction sequence and enzyme localization for sepiapterin and "drosopterin" biosynthesis.

ACKNOWLEDGEMENTS

Research sponsored by the Division of Biomedical and Environmental Research, U.S. Department of Energy, under contract W-7405-eng-26 with the Union Carbide Corporation. D.L.D. is supported by predoctoral training grant GM 1974 from the NIGMS, NIH. J.J.Y. was a postdoctoral investigator under subcontract 3322 from the Biology Division of ORNL to the University of Tennessee; present address: Dept. of Microbiology, Seoul National University, Seoul, Korea.

REFERENCES

1. Theobald, N. and Pfleiderer, W. (1977) Tetrahderon Lett., 10, 841.

2. Yim, J. J., Grell, E. H. and Jacobson, K. B. (1977) Science, 198, 1168.

3. Fan, C. L., Krivi, G. G. and Brown, G. M. (1975) Biochem. Biophys. Res. Commun., 67, 1047.

4. Wilson, T. G. and Jacobson, K. B. (1977) Biochem. Genet., 15, 321.

5. Shoup, J. R. (1966) J. Cell Biol., 29, 223.

6. Rokos, K. and Pfleiderer, W. (1975) Chem. Ber., 108, 2728.

7. Schwink, I. and Mancini, M. (1973) Arch. Genet., 46, 41.

8. Yim, J. J., Crummett, D. D. and Jacobson, K. B. (1978) Fed. Proc., 37, 1344.

RUSSUPTERIDINES: YELLOW LUMAZINES FROM RUSSULA SPECIES

PETER XAVER ITEN,[*] HANA MÄRKI-DANZIG AND CONRAD HANS EUGSTER
Organisch-chemisches Institut der Universität Zürich-Irchel,
Winterthurerstrasse 190, CH-8057 ZÜRICH, SWITZERLAND

ABSTRACT

Five yellow monomeric russupteridines have been isolated from
RUSSULA species. The structures of two of them are proposed; they
represent the first natural derivatives of 6,7-diamino-8-D-ribityl-
lumazine. A third is identified as riboflavine. Some chemical
properties of the remaining two are described.

INTRODUCTION

Fruiting bodies of the widespread genus RUSSULA (BASIDIOMYCETES)
are a unique and rich source of colorless, yellow, red and blue
compounds. All of them show a strong fluorescence under UV light and
those investigated so far have been found to be monomeric N(8)-D-
ribityl-lumazines [1,2] or dimeric compounds containing at least one
N(8)-D-ribityl-lumazine part and one D-ribosyl unit [1,3,4]. In this
paper we report on the yellow russupteridines (RP-yellow$_{I-V}$).

CHEMICAL PROPERTIES

We know from PC and TLC of at least seven yellow compounds from
different RUSSULA species. Five of them have been isolated in pure
form by repeated chromatography on cellulose and various sephadex
gels. For TLC data see Table 1.

RP-yellow$_{III}$ has been identified as riboflavine [2,5]. RP-yellow$_I$
and RP-yellow$_{II}$ both yield 6,7-dioxo-8-D-ribityl-5,6,7,8-tetrahydro-
lumazine on treatment with 2 percent degassed acetic acid in a sealed
tube at 150°C, whilst RP-yellow$_{IV}$ is even stable in boiling 0.1 N
HCl and 0.1 N NaOH. In contrast to this behaviour, RP-yellow$_I$ is
hydrolysed by the same reagents even at R.T. yielding formic acid and
an unstable intermediate, which from UV spectra is thought to be
6-amino-7-hydroxy-, 6-hydroxy-7-amino- or 6,7-diamino-8-D-ribityllumazine.

---

[*]New address: Kriminaltechnische Abteilung der Kantonspolizei Zürich,
Postfach 370, CH-8021 Zürich, Switzerland.

TABLE 1

R_f-VALUES AND FLUORESCENCES OF YELLOW RUSSUPTERIDINES

	4% Na Citrate		4% NH$_4$Cl		BAW (5:3:5)	
RP-yellow$_I$	0.40	lbl	0.48	gr-ye	0.31	bl
RP-yellow$_{II}$	0.31	ye	0.30	ye	0.22	ye
RP-yellow$_{III}$	0.37	dye	0.43	dye	0.79	dye
RP-yellow$_{IV}$	0.23	lbl	0.27	lbl	0.23	lbl
RP-yellow$_V$	0.24	gr-ye	0.44	gr-ye	0.45	gr-ye

Cellulose layer Polygram CEL 300-UV$_{254}$; color of fluorescence (UV$_{350}$):
bl = blue; lbl = light blue; ye = yellow; dye = dark yellow;
gr-ye = green yellow.

Final identification by comparison has not yet been possible because
these compounds are still unknown. Treatment of this intermediate with
acetic acid as described above again gave 6,7-dioxo-8-D-ribityl-
5,6,7,8-tetrahydrolumazine.

RP-yellow$_V$ has been hitherto isolated from several RUSSULA species
only in very small amounts. The best source seems to be RUSSULA
OCHROLEUCA, a yellow earth mushroom. Little is known about its
chemistry and structure.

STRUCTURE OF RUSSUPTERIDINE-YELLOW$_{IV}$

RP-yellow$_{IV}$* is present in very small amounts in RUSSULA SARDONIA.
From 300 kg we isolated only 25 mg of pure compound. The UV/VIS
spectra (see Figure 1) show a new type of chromophore, similar to
that of 6,7,8-substituted lumazines. From the ^{1}H-NMR spectrum (see
Figure 2) and ^{13}C-NMR spectrum (48.52; 63.31; 68.05; 72.21; 72.91
ppm) the presence of a ribityl group is proved. Furthermore there
are two protons exchangeable with D$_2$O (singlett 11.5 ppm). Of the
twelve carbon atoms in the ^{13}C-NMR spectrum [1], six belong to the
lumazine nucleus, five to the ribityl group and the remaining one,
on the basis of its chemical shift (163.93 ppm), is adjacent to an
amide or lactam group. Combined evidence from the microanalysis,
the electrophoretic behaviour, the IR- and mass-spectra give us every

*In earlier papers [1,6,7] RP-yellow$_{IV}$ was called Russupteridine-
colorless$_{III}$ because of its very pale yellow color.

reason to propose for russupteridine-yellow$_{IV}$ the following structure:

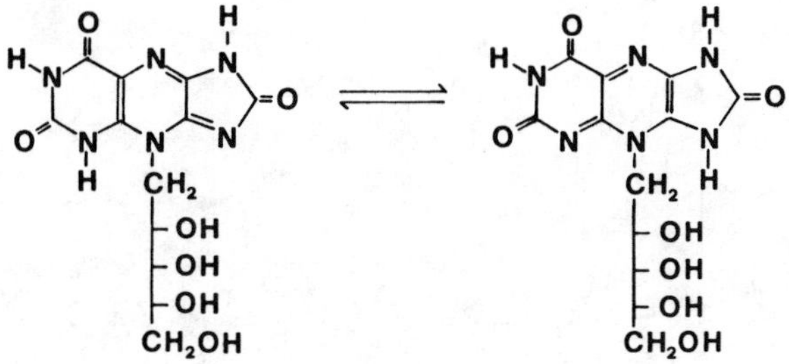

Russupteridine-yellow$_{IV}$;
4-(D-Ribityl)-imidazolo[4,5-g]pteridine-2,6,8(1H,4H,5H,7H)-trione.

The structure of RP-yellow$_{IV}$ has been confirmed by synthesis. Condensation of 4-D-ribitylamino-5-amino-uracil with parabanic acid in ethylene glycol with a catalytic amount of p-toluenesulfonic acid (see Scheme 1) yielded RP-yellow$_{IV}$ in low yield, which was identical in TLC with several solvents and in spectral and chiroptical data with the natural product.

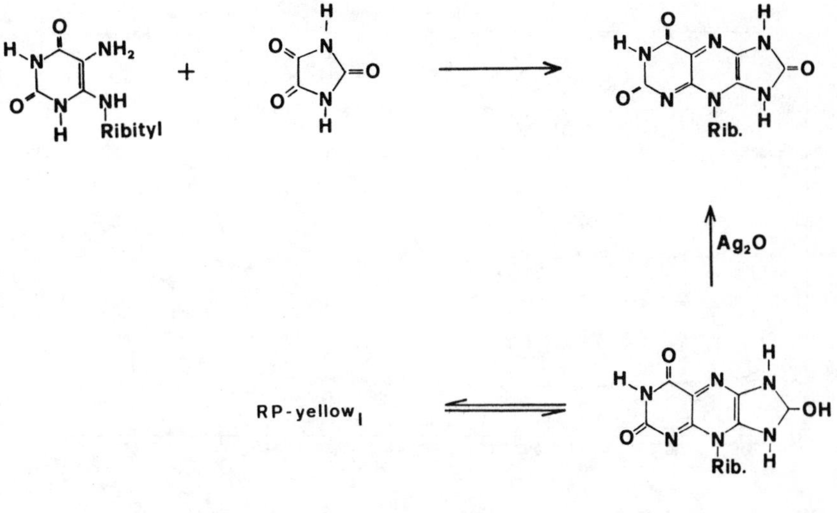

Scheme 1. Synthesis of Russupteridine-yellow$_{IV}$ and transformation of Russupteridine-yellow$_I$ into Russupteridine-yellow$_{IV}$ by silver oxide oxidation.

108

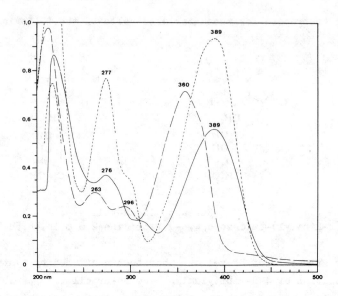

Fig. 1.   UV/VIS absorption spectra of Russupteridine-yellow$_{IV}$.
────── in 0.1 N NaOH;   ------ in 0.1 N HCl;
•••••• in H$_2$O; concentration of all spectra 16 mg/l.

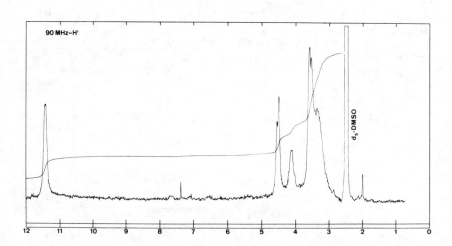

Fig. 2. ^{1}H-NMR spectrum of Russupteridine-yellow$_{IV}$
in d$_6$-DMSO, relative to TMS (= 0 ppm).

We were also able to transform RP-yellow$_I$ into RP-yellow$_{IV}$ by oxidation with silver oxide in sodium hydroxide solution (see Scheme 1). Therefore we now (c.f. [1]) propose the two following isomeric structures for RP-yellow$_I$:

Russupteridine-yellow$_I$;
The two isomers and some of their tautomeric forms.

RP-yellow$_I$, RP-yellow$_{IV}$ and probably also RP-yellow$_{II}$ represent the first naturally occurring 6,7-diamino-lumazine derivatives ever found.

ACKNOWLEDGEMENTS

This work was supported by the Swiss National Foundation for Scientific Research.

REFERENCES

[1] Eugster, C.H. and Iten, P.X. (1976) Chemistry and Biology of Pteridines, Walter de Gruyter, Berlin and New York, p 881.

[2] Eugster, C.H. (1973) Zeitschrift für Pilzkunde, 39, 45.

[3] Eugster, C.H., Frauenfelder, E.F. and Koch, H. (1970) Helvetica chimica acta 53, 131.

[4] Iten, P.X., Arihara, S. and Eugster, C.H. (1973) Helvetica chimica acta 56, 303.

[5] Koch, H. (1975) Dissertation Universität Zürich.

[6] Märki-Danzig, H. (1976), Diplomarbeit Universität Zürich.

[7] Eugster, C.H. (1977) Abstract of a lecture presented at the Second International Mycological Congress, University of South Florida, Tampa, USA.

ISOLATION AND CHARACTERIZATION OF 6-HYDROXYMETHYLPTERIN FROM SPINACH
CHLOROPLASTS AND ITS FUNCTION IN PHOTOSYNTHETIC ELECTRON TRANSPORT

KAZUO IWAI, MASAHIRO KOBASHI, TETSUYA SUZUKI AND MASAYASU BUNNO
Research Institute for Food Science, Kyoto University, Uji, Kyoto,
611 (Japan)

ABSTRACT

6-Hydroxymethylpterin was isolated from spinach chloroplasts by
chromatography on DEAE-Sephadex A-50, DEAE-cellulose and Sephadex G-25
columns and by preparative thin-layer chromatography. A fluorimetric
method and biological assay procedure were used to quantify the pterin.
To identify the pterin, gas chromatography-mass spectrometry was used.
Sonicated lamellar preparations of spinach chloroplasts catalyzed the
light reduction of 6-hydroxymethyldihydropterin. The reduced component
was active in cytochrome c dark reduction in the presence of FMN, or Pi
and ADP. 6-Hydroxymethylpterin was also reduced by light in the
presence of the chloroplasts.

INTRODUCTION

6-Alkylpterin compounds promote the growth of the trypanosomid flagellate Crithidia fasciculata when grown on a chemically defined medium
limited in folic acid.[1] Some compounds promoting the growth of C. fasciculata, but differing from biopterin, exist in spinach leaves as well
as in other vegetables.[2,3] No pterin compounds have ever been isolated
from green leaves, whereas three derivatives of lumazine have been isolated from spinach leaves.[4,5]

Pterin and lumazine compounds promote photophosphorylation in the
presence of a reducing agent and stimulate cytochrome c photooxidation
in sonicated spinach chloroplasts.[6] Tetrahydropterin compounds also
promote photophosphorylation in broken spinach chloroplasts,[6] and their
protein complex also stimulates photophosphorylation[7] and photoreduction of pea ferredoxin, ferricyanide and NADP in sonicated pea chloroplasts.[8] Tetrahydropterin compounds are produced by light reduction of
the dihydropterin compounds in a bacterial chromatophore fraction.[9]

This work deals with the isolation and chracterization of the naturally occurring pterin in spinach chloroplasts and its function in
photosynthetic electron transport.

MATERIALS AND METHODS

Chemicals. Synthetic 6-hydroxymethylpterin was a gift of Dr. S. Matsuura, Nagoya University. Its dihydro form was prepared by the method of Kaufman[13] and its tetrahydro form was prepared by catalytic reduction with hydrogen over PtO_2 in 0.1N HCl. Cytochrome c from horse heart was obtained from Sigma Chemical Co., and other chemicals were obtained from Nakarai Chemicals Ltd.

Fluorimetric method for pterin compounds. A fluorimetric method using excitation at 360 nm and emission at 440 nm was used.[11]

Biological assay procedure for pterin compounds. The assay procedure[3] with Crithidia fasciculata ATCC 12857 as the test organism was used in isolating the pterin compound from spinach chloroplasts.

Preparation of sonicated chloroplasts. Spinach leaves were sliced and homogenized with 20 mM Tris-HCl buffer (pH 7.8) containing 0.35 M NaCl for 30 sec. The homogenate was centrifuged at 10,000 x g for 30 min. Before being used, the precipitate was stored in 10 mM Tris-HCl buffer (pH 7.6) containing 0.4 M sucrose, 10 mM NaCl and 50 % glycerol at -20°C. The suspension was diluted 30-fold with cold water, stirred for 20 min, and centrifuged at 12,000 x g for 15 min. The precipitate was suspended in water and the suspension was sonicated for 1 min and centrifuged at 14,000 x g for 30 min. The green supernatant was used for sonicated chloroplasts.

Reduction of cytochrome c by the reduced pterin compound formed by light exposure. To cuvettes were added 0.1 M Tricin-KOH buffer (pH 7.5), sonicated chloroplasts (7.5 µg of chlorophyll) and 178 nmoles of 6-hydroxymethyldihydropterin for a total volume of 0.97 ml. The cuvettes were bubbled with argon at 30°C for 5 min and exposed to light (light intensity, 400 W/m^2) for 3 min under argon bubbling. After turning light off, 25 nmoles of FMN and 20 nmoles of cytochrome c were added to make a final volume of 1.00 ml. The absorbance difference (Δ552-536 nm) between dark and exposed samples was monitored by a JASCO UVIDEC -1 MS spectrophotometer (Japan Spectroscopic Co. Ltd.). For a coupling reaction of pterin reduction with photophosphorylation, $MgCl_2$ (1 µmole), K_2HPO_4 (0.25 µmole) and ADP (50 nmoles) were added to the cuvettes and exposed to light for 3 min. After turning light off, only cytochrome c was added.

RESULTS AND DISCUSSIONS

Isolation of 6-hydroxymethylpterin from chloroplasts[12]. Spinach chloroplasts were obtained from 207 kg of market spinach according to the method of Black et al.[14] Pterin compounds were purified from extract of chloroplasts by chromatography on DEAE-Sephadex A-50 (10 x 80

cm), DEAE-cellulose (10 x 60 cm) and Sephadex G-25 (3 x 81 cm) columns
and by preparative thin-layer chromatography using MN-cellulose 300 G,
developed with n-propanol/1% ammonia (2:1). A fluorescent band (Rf
0.38) with the growth-promoting activity for C. fasciculata was scraped
off and eluted with ethanol/3% ammonia (1:1). The eluate was lyophilized (yield 23.5 mg).

Characterization of the isolated compound. The isolated compound
was chromatographically pure, the Rf values were the same as those of
6-hydroxymethylpterin in the four solvent systems (Table I) and the
infrared spectrum was indistinguishable from that of the latter.

TABLE I. Rf VALUES OF THE ISOLATED COMPOUND AND ITS OXIDATION PRODUCT

Compound	Rf values in solvent system*			
	A	B	C	D
Isolated compound	0.45	0.30	0.38	0.20
6-Hydroxymethylpterin	0.45	0.30	0.38	0.19
Permanganate oxidation product of isolated compound	0.25	0.12	0.47	0.12
6-Carboxypterin	0.25	0.12	0.47	0.11
Biopterin	0.55	0.42	0.55	0.27

*Solvents: A,Ethanol/Acetic acid/Water(15:1:34); B,n-Propanol/1%
Ammonia(2:1); C,50mM Phosphate buffer, pH 7.0; D,n-Butanol/Acetic
acid/Water(4:1:1).

The corrected excitation and emission spectra of the compound were
measured with a Hitachi MPF-4 fluorescence spectrophotometer; Excitation; λ_{max}, 269 and 345 nm; emission; λ_{max}, 445 nm at pH 6.5. The Rf
values of the permanganate oxidation product was indistinguishable from
those of authentic 6-carboxypterin (Table I). Finally, the structure
of the isolated compound was determined by gas-liquid chromatography-
mass spectrometry after silylation of the compound. For the silylation
an excess amount of fresh N,O-bis(trimethylsilyl) acetamide in acetonitrile was added to a dry powder of the sample, and heated at 60°C for
10 min. After silylation of the sample, 2 µl of the solution was subjected to a Shimadzu-LKB 9000 gas chromatograph-mass spectrometer
equipped with a column (2m x 3 mm i.d.) of 3 % silicone gum SE-52 on
60-80 mesh Chromosorb W (acid-washed and silanized) with helium as the
carrier gas at 30 ml/min. For the chemical ionization method, a separation column (1m x 3 mm i.d.) packed with 3 % JXR silicone on 80-100
mesh GAS-CHROM-Q was used. Figure 1 shows the gas chromatogram and
mass spectra of the trimethylsilyl derivative of the isolated compound.

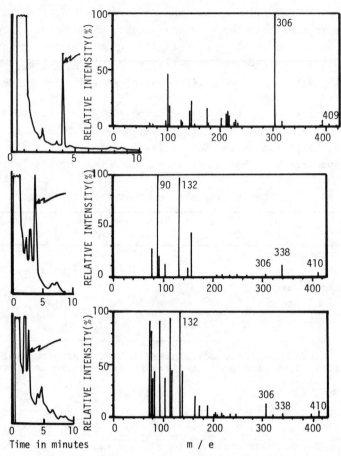

Fig. 1. Gas chromatogram and mass spectra of trimethylsilylated derivative of the isolated compound obtained with the electron impact method
(upper panel), and with the chemical ionization method using ammonia
(middle panel) and isobutane(lower panel) as the reactant gas[12].

From the parent ion peak of m/e=409 (upper panel in Fig. 1), and a
quasi molecular ion peak of m/e=410 which corresponds to $(M + 1)^+$
(middle and lower panels), the molecular weight of the compound was
estimated to be 193. From this value and the fragmentation patterns of
the trimethylsilyl compound, the isolated compound was identified as 6-
hydroxymethylpterin. This is the first case as far as we know that the
pterin compound has been isolated and identified from green leaves.
Since 6-hydroxymethylpterin in a 7,8-dihydro form has been known to be
an intermediate in the biosynthesis of folic acid,[15-17] the dihydro

form would be a functional form existing in chloroplasts.

Reduction of 6-hydroxymethyldihydropterin by light exposure in the presence of sonicated chloroplasts. Authentic 6-hydroxymethyltetrahydropterin had the λ_{max} at 302 nm in Tricin buffer at pH 7.5. Figure 2 shows that Δ optical density at 302 nm increases with light-exposure time. This suggests that the reduced pterin compound formed by light exposure in the presence of sonicated chloroplasts is a tetrahydro form.

Reduction of cytochrome c by 6-hydroxymethyltetrahydropterin. 6-Hydroxymethyltetrahydropterin formed from its dihydro form by light exposure in the presence of sonicated chloroplasts catalyzed the dark reduction of cytochrome c as shown in Fig. 3. The reduction of cyto-

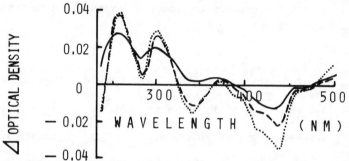

Fig. 2. Effect of light on the reduction of 6-hydroxymethyldihydropterin in the presence of sonicated chloroplasts. ——,1 min;— — —,3 min; ·······,5 min. Each spectra is a subtraction of each difference spectra between exposed and unexposed samples. 6-Hydroxymethyldihydropterin (71 nmoles) and chloroplasts(4.7 μg of chlorophyll) were used.

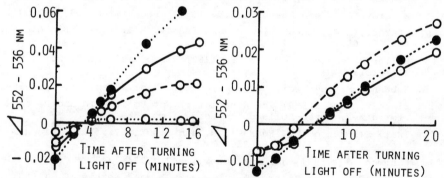

Fig. 3. Effect of 6-hydroxymethyltetrahydropterin produced from its dihydro form by light exposure on cytochrome c reduction in the presence of sonicated chloroplasts as a function of time after turning light off. O····O, 0; O— —O,71; O——O,178; ●····●, 355 nmoles of 6-hydroxymethyldihydropterin.

Fig. 4. Effect of additions of ADP and Pi (O—O) or FMN (●···●) on cytochrome c reduction catalyzed by the reduced pterin compound in the presence of sonicated chloroplasts. O——O, no addition. Experimental conditions are given in the test.

chrome c was increased with additions of concentrations of the dihydropterin compound. The formation of the tetrahydropterin compound and
the cytochrome c reduction were stimulated by the addition of ADP and
Pi, or FMN as shown in Fig. 4. This suggests that the pterin reduction
may couple with photophosphorylation and photosynthetic electron transport.

6-Hydroxymethylpterin was also reduced by light exposure under the
same conditions as in the above experiment.

These results indicate that 6-hydroxymethylpterin and its dihydro
form existing in chloroplasts are reduced to the tetrahydro form by
light exposure and that the tetrahydropterin compound may actually play
a key role in photophosphorylation and photosynthetic electron transport in spinach chloroplast.

REFERENCES

1. Guttman, H.N. and Wallace, F.G. (1964) in Biochemistry and
   Physiology of Protozoa, Vol.3, Hutner, S.H. ed., Academic Press,
   New York, pp. 459-494.

2. Wacker, A., Lochmann, E.-R. and Kirshfeld, S. (1959) Z. Naturforsch.
   14 b, 150-151.

3. Iwai, K., Kobashi, M. and Fujisawa, H. (1970) J. Bacteriol. 104,
   197-201.

4. Sugiura, K. and Goto, M. (1966) J. Biochem. 60, 335-337

5. Kobayashi, K., Forrest, H.S. and El -Emary, M. (1967) Arch. Biochem.
   Biophys. 121, 220-223.

6. Maclean, F.I., Fujita, Y., Forrest, H.S. and Myers, J. (1976)
   Plant Physiol. 41, 774-779.

7. Makarov, A.D. and Stakhov, L.F. (1974) Biokhimiya, 39, 499-503.

8. Stakhov, L.F., Makarov, A.D. and Ivanov, B.I. (1976) Biokhimiya,
   41, 655-659.

9. Fuller R.C. and Nugent, M.A. (1969) Proc. Natl. Acad. Sci., 63,
   1311-1318.

10. Kobashi, M. and Iwai, K. (1972) Agric. Biol. Chem. 36, 1685-1693.

11. Blakely, R.L. (1969) The Biochemistry of Folic Acid and Related
    Pteridines, North-Holland, Amsterdam, pp. 58-105.

12. Iwai, K., Bunno, M., Kobashi, M. and Suzuki, T. (1976) Biochim.
    Biophys. Acta, 444, 618-622.

13. Kaufman, S. (1967) J. Biol. Chem., 242, 3934-3943.

14. Black, C.C., San Pietro, A., Limback, D. and Norris, G. (1963)
    Proc. Natl. Acad. Sci., U. S., 50, 37-43.

15. Brown, G.M., Weisman, R.A. and Lolnar, D.A. (1961) J. Biol. Chem.,
    236, 2534-2543.

16. Mitsuda, H., Suzuki, Y., Tadera, K. and Kawai, F. (1965)
    J. Vitaminol., 11, 122-138.

17. Iwai, K., Okinaka, O. and Suzuki, N. (1968) J. Vitaminol., 14,
    160-169.

BIOPTERIN AND METABOLIC DISEASE

SEYMOUR KAUFMAN
Laboratory of Neurochemistry, National Institute of Mental Health,
Bethesda, Maryland 20014

ABSTRACT

The molecular defects in several newly recognized inborn errors
of metabolism have been shown to involve, either directly or indirectly,
the biosynthesis of tetrahydrobiopterin. In one of these diseases,
the defect has been identified as a deficiency of dihydropteridine
reductase. In the second one, the defect is in a step in the biosynthesis of biopterin. These conditions appear to lead to functional
deficiencies of the 3 pterin-dependent aromatic amino acid hydroxylases,
phenylalanine, tyrosine, and tryptophan hydroxylases. As a result
of these multiple effects, patients with a deficiency of tetrahydrobiopterin show neurological symptoms that are not manifest in the
form of phenylketonuria (PKU) that is caused by a lack of phenylalanine
hydroxylase; i.e., classical PKU.

Biochemistry has contributed enormously to our understanding
of the genetic disease, phenylketonuria (PKU).[1] More recently,
the situation has changed and studies on patients with various
forms of PKU have contributed to our understanding of certain aspects
of biopterin biochemistry.

Before discussing some of these recent findings, it may be useful
to review briefly the reactions involved in the hydroxylation of
phenylalanine. The hepatic phenylalanine hydroxylating system
is a complex one consisting of at least two essential enzymes,
phenylalanine hydroxylase and dihydropteridine reductase (DHPR),
and a new, unique coenzyme, tetrahydrobiopterin.[2] Phenylalanine
hydroxylase catalyzes the reaction shown in equation 1, in which
both phenylalanine and tetrahydrobiopterin are oxidized to tyrosine
and quinonoid dihydrobiopterin, respectively.

$$\text{Tetrahydrobiopterin} + O_2 + \text{phenylalanine} \rightarrow$$
$$\text{quinonoid dihydrobiopterin} + \text{tyrosine} + H_2O \quad (1)$$

The second essential enzyme in the hydroxylating system is dihydropteridine reductase. It catalyzes the NADH or NADPH-mediated reduction
of the quinonoid dihydrobiopterin back to the tetrahydro level

according to equation 2, thus allowing the biopterin to function catalytically in the hydroxylation system.[2]

$$NADH(NADPH) + H^+ + \text{quinonoid dihydrobiopterin} \rightarrow$$

$$NAD^+(NADP^+) + \text{tetrahydrobiopterin} \qquad (2)$$

Quinonoid dihydrobiopterin is an extremely unstable compound that undergoes tautomerization to 7,8-dihydrobiopterin.[3] The 7,8-dihydrobiopterin is not a substrate for dihydropteridine reductase, but is a substrate for dihydrofolate reductase,[4] which catalyzes reaction 3.

$$NADPH + H^+ + \text{7,8-dihydrobiopterin} \rightarrow$$

$$\text{tetrahydrobiopterin} + TPN^+ \qquad (3)$$

In addition to serving a role in the reduction to the tetrahydro level of any quinonoid dihydrobiopterin that may undergo tautomerization before it could be reduced by dihydropteridine reductase, dihydrofolate reductase may be involved in the de novo biosynthesis of tetrahydrobiopterin.[5]

As soon as we had established that the phenylalanine hydroxylating system consisted of these 3 essential components, the hydroxylase, DHPR, and the pterin cofactor, it was evident that PKU might, in theory, be caused by the lack of any of these 3 components, i.e., that there might be 3 distinct forms of the disease. Indeed, in all of our early biochemical studies on liver biopsy samples obtained from PKU patients, we always measured the levels of these 3 components. Without exception, we found that phenylalanine hydroxylase was the only one that was deficient.[6,7] These studies helped to establish that the classic form of PKU is caused by the lack of phenylalanine hydroxylase.

In spite of these findings, the expectation remained that two other variant forms of PKU - caused by deficiency of DHPR or biopterin - might be encountered. Furthermore, because it had been established that DHPR and tetrahydrobiopterin are essential components of the tyrosine[8] and tryptophan[9] hydroxylating systems, and therefore should be required for the synthesis of the neurotransmitters, dopamine, norepinephrine and serotonin, it was expected that a deficiency of either the reductase or of biopterin would lead to clinical problems even if dietary restriction of phenylalanine were used to prevent the increased levels of phenylalanine in the blood and brain.

In 1975, the first case of PKU or hyperphenylalaninemia caused by a deficiency of DHPR was reported.[10] This child showed neurological deterioration despite early and excellent dietary control of his hyperphenylalaninemia. We measured all of the known components of the phenylalanine hydroxylating system in a biopsy liver sample and found them all to be present at adequate levels except for DHPR which was not detectable. With the use of a specific antiserum to sheep liver DHPR, which we showed to be capable of reacting with the normal human liver enzyme, no precipitin line was obtained with extracts of the patient's liver.[11] Furthermore, reductase could not be detected in a biopsy sample of brain tissue or in fibroblasts cultured from the patient's skin, although comparable tissue samples from control patients had readily detectable levels of the enzyme.

Results of biochemical analysis carried out on a liver biopsy sample from a second child who appeared to have the same disease were essentially the same: adequate hepatic levels of all of the known components of the phenylalanine hydroxylating system but with no detectable DHPR activity activity.[12]

The first, and most obvious lesson to be learned from this patient is that DHPR is indeed an essential component of the phenylalanine hydroxylating system in the intact organism. Although this is precisely the conclusion that we had reached from our earlier analysis of the isolated enzyme system, and there was never any reason to doubt that it played the same role in vivo, there are those who harbor the secret belief that once the enzymologist gets his hands on a tissue he creates a world full of artifacts. Perhaps our results with reductase-deficient patients will convince them about its assigned role.

A second conclusion, related to the first, is that not only does DHPR play this role in vivo, but that in humans, at least, there is no other system that is capable of substituting for it. This conclusion follows directly from the finding that DHPR deficiency leads to hyperphenylalaninemia. These results are of interest because there are at least two other potential candidates for regeneration in vivo of tetrahydrobiopterin from the dihydro level: naturally occurring reducing agents, such as glutathione and ascorbate, can reduce quinonoid dihydropterins to the tetrahydro level in vitro,[13] and dihydrofolate reductase, which catalyzes the reduction of 7,8-dihydrobiopterin to tetrahydrobiopterin (see equation 3). It is clear that in liver, the tissue in which most phenylalanine hydroxylation occurs, neither of these reactions occurs at a rate that is adequate for normal phenylalanine metabolism. It must be emphasized, on the other hand, that either of these alternative reactions might be responsible for supporting some phenylalanine hydroxylation.

It is also clear from our results with these patients that DHPR also must be playing its role in the tyrosine and tryptophan hydroxylating systems in brain. This conclusion is based on the evidence that the turnover of dopamine, and serotonin in the cnetral nervous system of these reductase-deficient patients is low.[14].

The last point that I want to discuss about DHPR-deficiency is one that is provocative. Based on the assumption that the neurological deterioration that characterized patients with this disease is due to a deficiency of the tyrosine and tryptophan-derived neurotransmitters, we proposed that the condition could be treated by a combination of dietary restriction of phenylalanine to control the hyperphenylalaninemia, and administration of 3,4-dihydroxyphenylalanine (DOPA) and 5-hydroxy-tryptophan, the precursors of dopamine, norepinephrine and serotonin, to supply the products beyond the metabolic blocks caused by the lack of fully functional tyrosine and tryptophan hydroxylases.[10] Although there is evidence that this treatment is beneficial,[12,14,15] at least one patient has died, presumably while still on this therapy.

If DHPR deficiency proves to be a lethal disease even when it is treated early with DOPA and 5-hydroxytryptophan, the possibility would be raised that DHPR may play a role in metabolism other than its known role in the 3 aromatic amino acid hydroxylating systems. In this regard, we have shown that DHPR can function in brain homogenates to keep folate in the tetrahydro form[16] and have proposed that, especially in a tissue like brain, with low dihydrofolate reductase levels, another role for DHPR may be to help keep folate in the tetrahydro form.[16]

Recently, the first case of hyperphenylalaninemia caused by a severe hepatic deficiency of biopterin was described.[17,18] This child also showed signs of neurological deterioration despite early dietary control of his elevated blood phenylalanine levels. Analysis of the components of the phenylalanine hydroxylating system in a liver biopsy sample showed that phenylalanine hydroxylase and DHPR levels were in the normal range but the level of hydroxylation cofactor, as measured with purified rat liver phenylalanine hydroxylase, was less than 10% of normal. Serum and urine levels of biopterin-like compounds, determined microbiologically with the organism, Crithidia fasiculata, were lower than levels in control children.

Since this was the first patient with a documented hepatic deficiency of pterin cofactor, it was difficult to predict precisely how much of a decrease in overall phenylalanine hydroxylase activity to expect from a 90-95% decrease in hepatic cofactor levels. To determine phenylalanine hydroxylase activity in vivo in this patient, we measured the rate of release into body fluids of tritiated water after the oral administration of ring-tritiated phenylalanine.[19] From the rate of release of tritiated water into the blood, which was fairly linear between 1 and 6 hours, we calculated that this child has about 2.3% of the normal level of phenylalanine hydroxylase.*

There are several possible explanations for the low biopterin in the patient's liver including a) a defect in biosynthesis; b) excessive catabolism; c) excessive urinary loss. The last explanation can be ruled out by the finding that urinary levels of biopterin-like compounds are low rather than high.

To distinguish between defective synthesis and excessive catabolism, we measured the blood levels of biopterin-related compounds in this patient during a phenylalanine challenge. We thought that this study would be informative because Leeming et al. had reported that patients with classical PKU have higher plasma levels of biopterin

---

* Although we had shown previously that the rate of release of deuterated or tritiated water into body fluids after administration of ring-deuterated or tritiated phenylalanine is a valid measure of normal in vivo phenylalanine hydroxylase activity[19], the possibility remained that small amounts of release might take place through a non-phenylalanine hydroxylase catalyzed reaction. Whereas the error introduced into the estimate of normal phenylalanine hydroxylase activity by such a minor pathway would be expected to be trivial, it could significantly affect the estimates of extremely low levels of phenylalanine hydroxylase activity. The only other known metabolic route that might lead to the liberation of readily measurable amounts of the ring tritium or hydrogen atoms from phenylalanine is the conversion of phenylalanine to o-hydroxyphenylacetic acid (OHPAA) via phenylpyruvate, a pathway in which one mole of hydrogen is released for each mole of OHPAA formed. To assess the contribution of this pathway to the total tritiated water released, we measured the amount of OHPAA excreted in the urine of this patient during the phenylalanine challenge. From this value, we calculated that only 1% of the observed tritium released could have been due to the formation of OHPAA. These results demonstrate, therefore, that contrary to the assertion of Curtius et al.,[20] there appear to be no alternative pathways in which the ring-hydrogen atoms of phenylalanine are liberated at a rate that can complicate the accurate measurement of even extremely low levels of phenylalanine hydroxylase activity by our method.

than do normals.[21] Furthermore, they found that an oral load of phenylalanine given to normal subjects led to a 4 to 5-fold increase in biopterin-related compounds. They also observed that a non-classical PKU patient with mild hyperphenylalaninemia of uncertain origin showed only a small rise in biopterin compounds in response to a phenylalanine load.

To have a basis for comparison, we studied this phenylalanine response in the biopterin-deficient patient as well as in classical PKU patients and their siblings. As can be seen in Fig. 1, patients with classical PKU and their normal and heterozygous siblings show an increase in serum levels of biopterin when challenged with an oral load of phenylalanine. We have also found that a DHPR-deficient patient shows an increase in serum levels of biopterin-like pterins in response to an oral phenylalanine challenge (data not shown). By contrast, the serum level of biopterin-related pterins in our biopterin-deficient patient did not increase in response to an oral load of phenylalanine. It should be noted, in confirmation of the finding of Leeming et al.,[21] that the initial serum levels of biopterin is elevated in classical PKU patients.

The observation that phenylalanine increases blood levels of biopterin in normals could have been due to release into the blood of the dihydro form of the pterin from liver (and kidney) in response to an increased rate of phenylalanine hydroxylation in these tissues. Our finding (Fig. 1) that classical PKU patients also show this response indicates that phenylalanine hdroxylase is not required for the phenylalanine-induced increase in blood levels of biopterin and therefore makes this explanation unlikely.

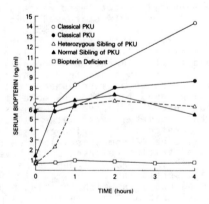

Fig. 1. Serum biopterin levels in patients after a phenylalanine load.

Other explanations for the effect are that phenylalanine either stimulates biosynthesis or inhibits catabolism of biopterin. If the latter explanation were correct, and the patient's low level of biopterin prior to the phenylalanine load were due to excessive catabolism, phenylalanine should have increased his blood levels of biopterin. On the other hand, if phenylalanine works by stimulating biosynthesis and the patient is defective in biosynthesis, then it can be predicted that this patient would be unable to increase his blood levels of biopterin in response to a phenylalanine load. The failure to show this response, therefore, strongly supports the conclusion that phenylalanine normally acts by stimulating a step in the biosynthesis of biopterin and that this patient has a defect in biopterin biosynthesis. From this analysis, it is likely that the hyperphenylalaninemic patient described by Rey et al.[15], whose plasma levels of biopterin also failed to increase in response to a phenylalanine load, was deficient in biopterin because of a defect in synthesis.

In collaboration with Dr. Jon Nixon of the Wellcome Research Laboratories, we have been examining the pattern of pterins in the urine of the biopterin-deficient. The results show that the ratio of neopterin derivatives to biopterin derivatives in the patient's urine is much higher than this ratio in urine from control subjects. These results indicate that the biopterin-deficient patient is blocked in the step in the biopterin biosynthetic pathway between neopterin and biopterin. Furthermore, these results provide strong evidence that a neopterin derivative is a normal intermediate in the biosynthesis of biopterin.

REFERENCES

1. Kaufman, S. (1976) in Advances in Neurochemistry, Vol. 2, Agranoff, B.W. and Aprison, M.H. eds., Plenum Press, New York, pp. 1-132.

2. Kaufman, S. (1971) Adv. Enzymol., 35, 245-319.

3. Kaufman, S. (1964) J. Biol. Chem., 239, 332-338.

4. Kaufman, S. (1967) J. Biol. Chem., 242, 3934-3943.

5. Kaufman, S. (1967) Ann. Rev. Biochem., 36, 171-184.

6. Kaufman, S. (1958) Science, 128, 1506-1508.

7. Friedman, P.A., Fisher, D.B., Kang, E.S. and Kaufman, S. (1973) Proc. Nat. Acad. Sci. USA, 70, 552-556.

8. Shiman, R., Akino, M. and Kaufman, S. (1971) J. Biol. Chem. 246, 1330-1340.

9. Friedman, P.A., Kappelman, A.H., and Kaufman, S. (1972) J. Biol. Chem., 247, 4165-4173.

10. Kaufman, S., Holtzman, N.A., Milstien, S., Butler, I.J. and Krumholz, A. (1975) New Eng. J. Med., 293, 785-790.

11. Milstien, S. and Kaufman, S. (1975) Biochem. Biophys. Res. Commun., 66, 475-481.

12. Brewster, T.G., Abroms, I.F., Kaufman, S., Breslow, J.L., Moskowitz, M.A., Villee, D.B. and Snodgrass, R.S. (1976) Ped. Res., 10, 446.

13. Kaufman, S. (1959) J. Biol. Chem., 234, 2677-2682.

14. Butler, I.J., Koslow, S.H., Krumholz, A., Holtzman, N.A. and Kaufman, S. (1978) Ann. Neurol., 3, 224-230.

15. Rey, F., Harpey, J.P., Leeming, R., Blair, J.A., Aicardi, J. and Rey, J. (1977) Arch. Franc. Ped., 34, 109-120.

16. Pollock, R.J. and Kaufman, S. (1978) J. Neurochem., 31, 115-123.

17. Kaufman, S., Berlow, S., Summer, G.K., Milstien, S., Schulman, J., Orloff, S., Spielberg, S. and Pueschel, S. (in press) New Eng. J. Med.

18. Milstien, S., Orloff, S., Spielberg, S., Berlow, S., Schulman, J.D. and Kaufman, S. (1977) Ped. Res., 11, 460.

19. Milstien, S. and Kaufman, S. (1975) J. Biol. Chem., 250, 4782-4785.

20. Curtius, H.-Ch., Zagalak, M.J., Baerlocher, K., Schaub, J., Leimbacher, W. and Redweik, U. (1977) Helv. paediat. Acta, 32, 461-469.

21. Leeming, R.J., Blair, J.A., Green, A. and Raine, D.N. (1976) Arch. Dis. Child., 51, 771.

BIOSYNTHESIS OF BIOPTERIN IN RAT BRAIN

CHING-LUN LEE, TAKESHI FUKUSHIMA AND JON C. NIXON

The Wellcome Research Laboratories, Research Triangle Park, North Carolina, 27709 (USA)

INTRODUCTION

Tetrahydrobiopterin probably serves as a natural cofactor mediating several mixed function oxygenases including tyrosine hydroxylase[1] and trytophan hydroxylase[2], the initial rate limiting enzymes in the biosynthesis of catecholamines and serotonin, respectively[3,4]. Regulation of tyrosine hydroxylase is accomplished, in part, by end product, feedback inhibition[3,4] in which catecholamines inhibit the enzyme by competitive binding at the tetrahydropterin binding site[5]. The relatively low concentration of tetrahydrobiopterin reported in brain would indicate that it may be present at less than a saturation level for optimum tyrosine hydroxylase activity. This would imply that the maintainance of an available pool of tetrahydrobiopterin may be a direct control on the regulation of catecholamine biosynthesis.

The biosynthesis of pterins by *Escherichia coli* has been extensively studied by Brown *et al.*[6]. GTP cyclohydrolase I, the initial enzyme in bacterial pterin synthesis, catalyzes the conversion of GTP to D-*erythro*dihydroneopterin triphosphate[7,8]. A similar enzymatic conversion of purines to pterins has been demonstrated in mammalian tissues[9,10]. Eto *et al.*[11] have also demonstrated biopterin biosynthesis in a soluble tissue extract from the kidney of the Syrian golden hamster. We have been successful in demonstrating biopterin biosynthesis in brain and the results presented below describe some of the requirements for this enzymatic pathway.

MATERIALS AND METHODS

GTP was purchased from P-L Biochemicals and [U-^{14}C]-GTP (ammonium salt, 52.8 mCi/mmole) was secured from Amersham/Searle. L-biopterin was secured from Dr. M. Viscontini, Zurich, Switzerland. ECTEOLA-Sephadex was prepared from G-25 Sephadex (fine) by the method of Peterson and Sober[12] and titrated to a final pH of 6.8 with 1N HCl[13]. The quantitation of authentic biopterin, solubilized in 0.1N NaOH, was based on ε_m = 8300 at λ = 362nm[14]. *Escherichia coli* GTP cyclohydrolase I was purified by the method of Yim and Brown[8]. With GTP as a substrate, a unit of activity for this enzyme is defined as that amount which generates 1 nmole/min of product at 42°C.

Thin layer chromatography. Precoated TLC cellulose plates (EM Laboratories, Inc.) were used for pterin separation and developed in the dark with the following solvent systems: A. 3% NH_4Cl; B. 1-propanol-ethylacetate-H_2O (7:1:2); C. ethanol-ammonium-borate (pH 8, 5% as boric acid)-3% NH_4Cl (2:1:1); D. 1-propanol-1% NH_3 (2:1); E. 1-butanol-acetic acid-H_2O (20:3:7). Radioactivity scanning of TLC plates was accomplished using a Berthold Model LB 2760 radioscanning unit. Fluorescence scanning of TLC plates was performed using a Schoeffel SD 3000 spectrodensitometer.

High-Performance Liquid Chromatography (HPLC). A ODS-2 reverse phase C_{18} column
(Whatman Inc.) was used for analytical determinations of pterins. Pterins were eluted
from this column using an isocratic solvent system of methanol/water (1:19). Pterins
separated by this procedure were quantitated using a Schoeffel FS-970 continuous
flow fluorescence monitor. A precolumn purification of reaction samples was done
using Dowex-50 and Dowex-1.

Male Sprague-Dawley rats (180-200 g) were used in this study. A crude soluble rat
brain extract was prepared by homogenization of the whole brain in buffer containing
10 mM Tris-HCl, pH 8.0 and 40 mM KCl. The crude homogenate was then centrifuged at
17,000 x g for 60 min. and the resulting supernatant was used in the following
in vitro studies.

RESULTS

A reaction with a total volume of 1.0 ml typically contained 0.2 µmoles of GTP with
1.25 µCi [U-^{14}C]-GTP, soluble rat brain fraction (2.8 mg protein), 0.46 units of pure
E. coli GTP cyclohydrolase I, 50 µmoles $MgCl_2$, 1 µmole of NADPH and was buffered with
0.1 M Tris-HCl at pH 7.2. This coupled enzyme reaction with *E. coli* GTP cyclohydrolase I was protected from light and incubated at 37°C for 4 hours. After incubation,
the products were oxidized with iodine, isolated using separate Dowex 50 and Dowex 1
columns and subsequently analyzed by HPLC. After repeated (3 x) rechromatography
by HPLC (Fig. 1), the purified fluorescent product had an identical retention volume
to that of authentic biopterin was purified. The recovered biopterin (74 ng) had a
specific activity 0.86 x that of the initial substrate [U-^{14}C]-GTP. Control reactions run without GTP, GTP cyclohydrolase I or rat brain soluble fraction failed
to generate biopterin or other fluorescent products.

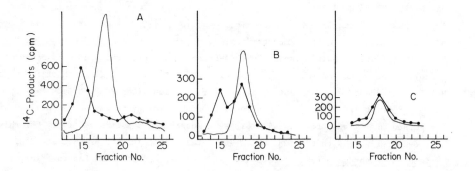

Fig. 1. HPLC purification of [U-^{14}C]-biopterin synthesized in a soluble brain extract.
A. Elution profile of products isolated from Dowex 1.
B. Rechromatography of A, pooled fractions 16-20.
C. Rechromatography of B, pooled fractions 16-20.
●—● ^{14}C-Reaction products; ——— Relative fluorescence.

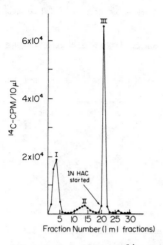

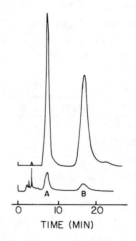

Fig. 2. Chromatography of ^{14}C-reaction
products on ECTEOLA-Sephadex (pH 6.8).
Products were eluted with H$_2$O through
fraction 20, then eluted with 1N acetic
acid.

Fig. 3. HPLC separation of Peak II from
ECTEOLA-Sephadex.
Upper tracing = Relative fluorescence
Lower tracing = UV [λ = 254 (.1 OD-FS)]
A = Neopterin, B = Biopterin

A separation of the ^{14}C-reaction products was also accomplished using ECTEOLA-
Sephadex (Fig. 2). Peak II contained all of the fluorescent products but only 9.8% of
the total eluted radioactivity. Peak II was collected, lyophilized and analyzed by
HPLC. The results presented in Fig. 3 show that fluorescent compounds with identical
elution volumes to those of biopterin and neopterin were present in the peak II fraction isolated from ECTEOLA-Sephadex. The biopterin peak was collected from the HPLC
separation and was found to have a specific activity of 0.91 that of the initial substrate [U-^{14}C]-GTP. The collected peak B, Fig. 3, was then analyzed by thin layer
chromatography using the various solvent systems described in the Methods section.
The results presented in Table 1 demonstrate that in each of the 5 different TLC solvent systems used, the ^{14}C-product measured by radiometric scanning had an identical
R$_f$ value to authentic biopterin measured by TLC fluorometric scanning.
TABLE 1

THIN LAYER CHROMATOGRAPHY OF ISOLATED ^{14}C-PRODUCT

Solvent*	R$_f$ of Authentic Biopterin TLC fluorometric Scan	R$_f$ of ^{14}C-Product TLC Radiometric Scan
A	0.49	0.49
B	0.19	0.18
C	0.55	0.55
D	0.37	0.34
E	0.26	0.26

*Solvents are described in Materials and Methods.

The effects of Mg^{++} and NADPH on biopterin synthesis is shown in Table 2. There is a one hundred fold increase in biopterin synthesis when both NADPH and Mg^{++} are present. A significant decrease in activity is observed when either of these cofactors is omitted from the reaction.

TABLE II

EFFECTS OF NADPH AND Mg^{++} ON BIOPTERIN SYNTHESIS

Reaction	NADPH (0.8 mM)	Mg^{++} (40 mM)	Relative Activity
I	+	+	103
II	+	−	20
III	−	+	4
IV	−	−	1

CONCLUSION

The results presented here indicate that the enzymatic pathway necessary for the conversion of D-*erythro*dihydroneopterin triphosphate to biopterin is present in brain. This enzymatic conversion is stimulated by Mg^{++} and NADPH. Neither neopterin nor dihydroneopterin appear to be substrates of preference for this pathway. Sepiapterin reductase requires the cofactor NADPH and has been previously reported in rat brain[14]. The Mg^{++} is probably involved in the conversion of neopterin triphosphate to sepiapterin, a step which may also require NADPH. Therefore the biopterin biosynthetic pathway in brain appears to be similar to that previously described in the kidney[11].

REFERENCES

1. Lloyd, T. and Weiner, N. (1971) Mol. Pharmacol., 7, 569-580.
2. Friedman, P.A., Kappelman, A.H. and Kaufman, S. (1972) J. Biol. Chem., 247, 4165-4173.
3. Levitt, M., Spector, S., Sjoerdsma, A., and Udenfriend, S. (1965) J. Pharmacol. Exptl. Therap., 148, 1-8.
4. Nagatsu, T., Levitt, M. and Udenfriend, S. (1964) J. Biol. Chem., 239, 2910-2917.
5. Nagatsu, T., Mizutani, K., Nagatsu, I., Matsuura, S. and Sugimoto, T. (1972) Biochem. Pharmacol., 21, 1945-1953.
6. Brown, G.M., Yim, J., Suzuki, Y., Heine, M.C. and Foor, F. (1975) in Chemistry and Biology of Pteridines, W. Pfleiderer ed., Walter deGruter, Berlin, pp. 219-245.
7. Burg, A.W. and Brown, G.M. (1968) J. Biol. Chem., 243, 2349-2358.
8. Yim, J. and Brown, G.M. (1976) J. Biol. Chem., 251, 5087-5098.
9. Fukushima, T., and Shiota, T. (1974) J. Biol. Chem., 249, 4445-4451.
10. Fukushima, K., Eto, I., Mayumi, T., Richter, W., Goodson, S. and Shiota, T. (1975) in Chemistry and Biology of Pteridines, W. Pfleiderer ed., pp. 247-263.
11. Eto, I., Fukushima, K. and Shiota, T. (1976) J. Biol. Chem., 251, 6505-6512.
12. Peterson, E.A. and Sober, H.A. (1956) J. Am. Chem. Soc., 78, 751-755.
13. Fukushima, T. and Shiota, T. (1972) J. Biol. Chem., 247, 4549-4556.
14. Rembold, H. and Metzger, H. (1963) Chem. Ber., 96, 1395-1405.
15. Katoh, S. (1971) Arch. Biochem. Biophys., 146, 202-214.

OCCURRENCE OF β-HYDROXY-α-KETOBUTYRIC ACID IN DROSOPHILA MELANOGASTER, WITH REFERENCE
TO DROSOPTERINS

M. MASADA, S. WATABE AND M. AKINO
Department of Biology, Tokyo Metropolitan University, Tokyo 158, Japan

ABSTRACT

A substance, designated as compound D, which reacts spontaneously with reduced
pterin to give drosopterins, is found in Drosophila melanogaster. The compound was
partially purified from the extract of flies by column chromatography and identified
as β-hydroxy-α-ketobutyric acid by analysis of its 2,4-dinitrophenylhydrazone, by mass
spectrometry and by reactivity with reduced pterin. Highly significant correlation
($r=0.95$, $p<0.001$) was found between amounts of the compound and drosopterins in the
wild type and eye-pigment mutants of D. melanogaster. Changes of the compound during
development of the wild type flies were also closely related to those of drosopterins.
These observations suggest a possibility that the compound participates in drosopterin biosynthesis in Drosophila.

INTRODUCTION

Concerning biosynthesis of drosopterins, some radioisotope-trace experiments
showed incorporation of glycine, formate, glucose[1,2] and reduced pterin $(AHPH_2)$[3]
into drosopterins in D. melanogaster. Recently, we have reported incorporation of
radioactivity of $[^{14}C(U)]GTP$ into drosopterins in the swordtail fish, Xiphophorus
helleri and noticed occurrence in the swordtail extract of a substance, which reacts
spontaneously with $AHPH_2$ to give drosopterins[4]. A compound with similar property
was also found in the extract of D. melanogaster and designated as compound D.

In the present paper, we wish to describe a fractionation method of compound D
from the fly extract and characterization of the compound. Relative quantities of
compound D and drosopterins in several eye-pigment mutants of D. melanogaster and
changes of these substances during developmental stages of flies are also reported.

MATERIALS AND METHODS

Adult flies within 24 h after eclosion were used. A method of $(7-^{14}C)AHPH_2$
synthesis and fractionation procedures of pterins from the acid alcohol extract of
flies were essentially the same as described previously[4]. For determination of
compound D, flies were extracted with acid alcohol, and the extract was heated with
$^{14}C-AHPH_2$ (160,000 cpm) at 85° for 15 min. Radioactivity of drosopterins (drosopterin plus isodrosopterin) purified from the reaction mixture was determined.
During the purification steps of compound D, each fraction was treated with $^{14}C-AHPH_2$
as described above, and after being neutralyzed with HCl, the reaction mixture was

130

supplemented with authentic drosopterins. Radioactivity of the purified drosopterin
fraction was counted. One unit of compound D was defined as an amount which produces
1,000 cpm of drosopterins under the conditions.

Keto acid 2,4-dinitrophenylhydrazones were analyzed by high performance liquid
chromatography (HPLC : Hitachi 635) using a Lichrosorb RP-18 column (Merck, 4 x 500
mm) with a solvent system : water-acetonitrile-10% H_3PO_4-methanol (52:30:10:8, v/v).
Amino acids were analyzed by an automatic analyzer (Hitachi, KLA-5) and by thin
layer chromatography (TLC) using three solvent systems : phenol-water (4:1, v/v) ;
n-butanol-acetic acid-water (4:1:2, v/v) ; 77% aqueous ethanol.

RESULTS AND DISCUSSION

Fractionation and characterization of compound D   Flies (5-10 g) were extracted
with 10 vol. of 80% aqueous ethanol. The compound in the extract was purified by
successive column chromatography on Dowex 50W, DEAE-Sephadex A-25, and Dowex 1. The
final column was eluted with a linear gradient composed of 25-300 mM NaCl containing
1 mM HCl. The fractions collected from the final column were analyzed with respect
to compound D, carboxyl[5] and carbonyl[6] groups (α-Ketobutyric acid was used as a
standard). Elution pattern is shown in Fig. 1. The peak fraction of compound D

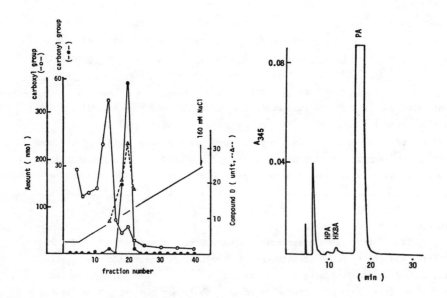

Fig. 1.(left) Column chromatography of the compound D fraction on Dowex 1.

Fig. 2.(right) HPLC analysis of 2,4-dinitrophenylhydrazones prepared from the
compound D fraction. HPA : β-hydroxypyruvic acid. HKBA : β-hydroxy-α-ketobutyric
acid. PA : pyruvic acid

coincided with that of carbonyl groups and a minor peak of carboxyl groups. Since the molar ratio of carboxyl groups to carbonyl groups in the compound D fraction was about 1:1, the fraction seemed to contain keto acid(s). Then, the fraction was treated with 2,4-dinitrophenylhydrazine to give dinitrophenylhydrazones. When the hydrazone sample was analyzed by HPLC, several absorption peaks (at 345 nm) appeared (Fig. 2). Of these, three peaks were assigned to hydrazones of pyruvic, β-hydroxy-pyruvic and β-hydroxy-α-ketobutyric acid, respectively, by comparing with authentic materials. Among these, pyruvic acid hydrazone was exceedingly predominant. To confirm the presence of these keto acid hydrazones, the hydrazone sample was reduced with aluminum amalgam to a corresponding amino acid mixture[7]. Analysis with TLC revealed that the reduced product contained alanine, serine and threonine as principal amino acids. The result was also confirmed by analysis with an automatic amino acid analyzer. Relative amounts of the amino acids are shown in Table 1.

TABLE 1

AMINO ACID ANALYSIS IN THE REDUCED PRODUCT OF 2,4-DINITROPHENYLHYDRAZONES PREPARED FROM THE COMPOUND D FRACTION

Amino acid	Relative amount (nmol)/10 g of flies	
alanine	620	(100)
serine	12.0	(1.93)
threonine	22.4	(3.61)
glycine	trace	

It can be concluded from above results that main keto acids in the compound D fraction are pyruvic, β-hydroxypyruvic and β-hydroxy-α-ketobutyric acid. The presence of the last keto acid was also confirmed by mass spectrometry of the compound D fraction (molecular ion peak, m/e=118). Although β-hydroxy-α-ketobutyric acid is known to react spontaneously with AHPH$_2$ to give drosopterins[8], drosopterin-forming ability of the main keto acids contained in the compound D fraction was re-examined under the conditions adopted in the present work. As shown in Table 2, radioactivity is efficiently incorporated into drosopterins from ^{14}C-AHPH$_2$ only when β-hydroxy-α-ketobutyric acid was used, whereas radioactivity of the drosopterin fraction was negligible in the cases of other keto acids. It could be concluded from the result that compound D is identical with β-hydroxy-α-ketobutyric acid.

Relative amounts of compound D together with those of pterins in the wild type and several eye-pigment mutants of D. melanogaster were surveyed. Since presently direct determination of compound D in the fly extract was impossible, the amount was tentatively expressed as units based on reactivity with ^{14}C-AHPH$_2$ as described in

TABLE 2

REACTIVITY OF KETO ACIDS WITH ^{14}C-AHPH$_2$ IN THE FORMATION OF DROSOPTERINS

The mixture of keto acid with ^{14}C-AHPH$_2$ (160,000 cpm), pH 6.0, was heated at 85° for 15 min. After supplement of authentic drosopterins, the drosopterin fraction was purified by column chromatography.

Keto acid	Amount (nmol)	Radioactivity of the drosopterin fraction (cpm)
Pyruvic acid	70	20
	550	18
β-Hydroxypyruvic acid	70	18
	550	10
β-Hydroxy-α-ketobutyric acid	70	2,700
	550	21,300
α-Ketobutyric acid (for comparison)	70	38
	550	24

TABLE 3

AMOUNTS OF COMPOUND D AND PTERINS IN THE EYE-PIGMENT MUTANTS OF D. MELANOGASTER

Starting material : 100 mg of flies

Strain	Compound D (unit)	Amount (nmol)				
		Drosopterin + Isodrosopterin	AHP	Sepiapterin	Biopterin	Isoxanthopterin
wild	12.7	100.0	10.6	-	11.2	31.4
	15.0	93.0	9.7	1.2	8.3	49.9
bar	1.96	31.2	-	-	5.8	77.6
rosy	0.23	18.1	22.5	8.1	11.8	4.2
claret	0.26	12.9	-	15.0	28.2	72.7
sepia	0.05	-	42.3	112.5	4.3	35.2
white	0.15	-	-	-	-	5.7
brown	0	-	-	-	8.0	24.9

- : undetectable

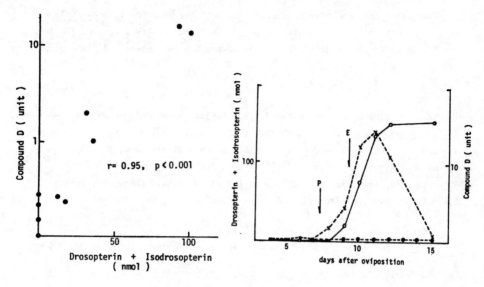

Fig. 3.(left) Correlation between amounts of compound D and drosopterins.

Fig. 4.(right) Changes of amounts of compound D and drosopterins in the wild type and mutant brown of D. melanogaster during development. -o- : Drosopterins (wild). -•- : Compound D (brown). -x- : Compound D (wild). Arrows in the figure indicate time of pupariation (P) and eclosion (E), respectively.

MATERIALS AND METHODS. One of the analytical results is summarized in Table 3.
In Fig. 3, the amounts of compound D in Drosophila mutants are plotted against those of drosopterins. Both values were taken from Table 3. The correlation coefficient (r) was calculated to be 0.95 (p<0.001), indicating highly significant correlation of both compounds. By contrast, no significant correlation was found between amounts of compound D and other pterins analyzed (AHP, sepiapterin, biopterin and isoxantho-pterin). There was also no correlation between amounts of drosopterins and other pterins. Neither drosopterins nor compound D were detectable in the mutant brown of D. melanogaster.

     In order to find further evidence indicating correlation between compound D and drosopterins, changes of these substances during development were analyzed using the wild type and mutant brown of D. melanogaster. Results are depicted in Fig. 4.
In the wild type flies, compound D appeared after pupariation, reached maximum at about 2 days after eclosion and decreased rapidly thereafter. Appearance of droso-pterins was somewhat later, and the amount rose with increase of compound D and reached almost plateau at about 3 days after eclosion. These changes of drosopterins during development of the wild flies are very similar to those reported by Fan et al[9]. In the mutant brown, neither compound D nor drosopterins were detectable throughout the developmental stages.

134

Although we have no evidence showing the presence of AHPH$_2$ in <u>Drosophila</u> and origin of compound D also remains to be studied, the results presented in Figs. 3 and 4 seem to suggest a definite role of compound D in biosynthesis of drosopterins in <u>Drosophila</u>.

REFERENCES

1. Brenner-Holzach, O. and Leuthardt, F. (1961) Helv. Chim. Acta, 44, 1480-1495.

2. Brenner-Holzach, O. and Leuthardt, F. (1965) Helv. Chim. Acta, 48, 1569-1578.

3. Goto, M., Okada, T. and Forrest, H.S. (1964) J. Biochem., 56, 379.

4. Watabe, S. and Akino, M. (1977) Annot. Zool. Japon., 50, 1-11.

5. Kasai, Y., Tanimura, T. and Tamura, Z. (1975) Anal. Chem., 47, 34-37.

6. Kalckar, H.M., Kjeldgaard, N.O. and Klenow, H. (1950) Biochim. Biophys. Acta, 5, 586-594.

7. Sprinson, D.B. and Chargaff, E. (1946) J. Biol. Chem., 146, 417-432.

8. Sugiura, K., Goto, M. and Nawa, S. (1969) Tetrahedron Letters, 34, 2963-2965.

9. Fan, C.L., Hall, L.M., Skrinska, A.J. and Brown, G.M. (1976) Biochem. Genet., 14, 271-280.

SEPIAPTERIN AND ITS CATABOLIC CONVERSION TO 6-(1-CARBOXYETHOXY)PTERIN

BY *Bacillus subtilis*

SADAO MATSUURA, TAKASHI SUGIMOTO, CHIZUKO KITAYAM YOKOKAWA*, and MOTOO TSUSUE*
Department of Chemistry, College of General Education, Nagoya University, Chikusa-ku,
Nagoya 464, Japan. * Biological Laboratory, Kitasato University, Sagamihara-City,
Kanagawa 228, Japan

ABSTRACT

The absolute strucures of sepiapterin and its catabolite by *B. subtilis* are
described. The former was determined to be 2-amino-7,8-dihydro-6-(s)-lactoyl-4(3H)-
pteridinone by analysis of the L-lactic acid produced from sepiapterin by oxidative
cleavage in aqueous sodium borate solution. The catabolite was estimated to be
2-amino-6-(1-carboxyethoxy)-4(3H)-pteridinone (from spectroscopic and degradation
studies), which was confirmed by an unambiguous synthesis. The absolute configuration of the 6-side chain was determined to be the (s)-configuration, by analysis of
the lactic acid produced by acid hydrolysis of the catabolite. These results suggest that the side chain of sepiapterin is rearranged intact during the catabolic
conversion. A possible mechanism for the conversion is presented.

INTRODUCTION

Sepiapterin, first isolated as an eye pigment from *sepia* mutant of *Drosophila
melanogaster*[1,2], has attracted much interest from both chemical and biological point
of view. The planar structure of sepiapterin was revealed to be 2-amino-7,8-dihy-
dro-6-lactoyl-4(3H)-pteridinone by Nawa in 1960[3]. Sepiapterin is optically active[2,4]
owing to the chiral carbon at the 2-position of the side chain. However, its absolute configuration had not been determined till the work of Pfleiderer[5], who synthesized natural type sepiapterin by oxidation of 5,6,7,8-tetrahydrobiopterin and determined the absolute configuration of the chiral carbon to be the (s)-configuration.

The biological role of sepiapterin has also been a center of interests, since this
compound is thought to be a key intermediate in the biosynthesis of tetrahydrobiopterin[6]. Three enzymes have been found which catalyze the conversion of sepiapterin:
these are sepiapterin reductase[7,8], a dihydrofolate reductase[9], and a deaminase[10].

Recently we found that various bacteria, including *Bacillus subtilis*, catabolize
sepiapterin into an intensely blue fluorescent compound A[11]. In the present work,
we describe the determination of the absolute structure of the catabolite A, and an
alternative approach for determining the absolute structure of sepiapterin. A tentative reaction mechanism for conversions of sepiapterin into 7,8-dihydroxanthopterin
(chemical) and into the catabolite A (biological) is presented to explain the two
types of the conversion by an essentially same mechanism.

THE ABSOLUTE CONFIGURATION OF SEPIAPTERIN[12]

It is known that sepiapterin (1) undergoes degradation into 7,8-dihydroxanthopte-rin (2) and lactic acid in a 4% sodium borate solution under aerobic conditions[3]. Since the chiral 2-position of the lactoyl group is not involved in the degradation, the configuration of the chiral carbon comes into the lactic acid unchanged. Hence, it is possible to determine the absolute configuration of sepiapterin by examining the configuration of the lactic acid produced.

We carried out the oxidative degradation of sepiapterin in a 4% sodium borate solution as described in the literature[3]. After completion of the reaction, we ana-lysed the lactic acid by an enzymatic method using L- and D-lactic acid dehydrogenases (LDH and DLDH)[13]. It turned out that the standard method[13] could not be applied directly to this case, since the LDH activities were hindered by borate ions pre-sent in the solution. However, the hindrance effects disappeared upon the addition of D-ribose to the assay solution prior to the addition of NAD and the enzyme. By the present slightly modified method, a 1.03 ± 0.01 molar amound of L-lactic acid and no D-lactic acid were detected from the degradation solution of sepiapterin. From these data, it is clear that the configuration at the chiral 2-position of the side chain of sepiapterin is the (s)-configuration as shown in the formula (1). Our present conclusion is consistent with that of Pfleiderer[5].

THE ABSOLUTE STRUCTURE OF THE CATABOLITE A

Isolation. B. subtilis IAM 1069 was incubated in a 0.74% brain-heart infusion (1000 ml) containing sepiapterin (24 mg) by shaking in 10 ml volume L-shaped tubes at 37°C under aerobic conditions in a dark room for several days untill the initial yellow fluorescence changed to blue. The combined medium, after centrifugation and concentration in vacuo, was submitted for column chromatography successively in the following manner: on ECTEOLA-cellulose (eluted by 0.3M acetic acid), on P-cellulose (eluted by water, repeated twice), on ECTEOLA-cellulose (eluted by 0.2M acetic acid), and finally on Sephadex G-25 (eluted by water). These procedures afforded 0.94 mg of the pure catabolite A, estimated from the UV absorbance.

The planar structure of A. The compound A was methylated by diazomethane to give a compound with a molecular formula of $C_{11}H_{13}N_5O_4$ ditermined by high-resolution mass spectrometry (M^+: 279.0999. Calcd for $C_{11}H_{13}N_5O_4$: 279.0965). The mass spectrum of A itself showed M^+ at m/e 251. These results indicated that two methyl groups were introduced on methylation, and hence a molecular formula of $C_9H_9N_5O_4$ was given for $\underline{A}$. The pK_a values and UV spectra of $\underline{A}$ were very similar to those of 6-methoxypterin[14] (Table 1). From these results and the finding that $\underline{A}$ yielded xantho-pterin (3) on hydrolysis in 5M HCl, we assumed $\underline{A}$ to be 2-amino-4(3H)-pteridinone with a $-O-C_3H_5O_2$ side cahin at the 6-position. Among the several possible structures ^{1}HNMR spectrum of $\underline{A}$ allowed to choose two structures (6) and (7), as more probable ones, both of which fitted well to the signals of a doublet (J=7 Hz) at $\delta 1.36$ (a methyl group), a quartet (J=7 Hz) at $\delta 5.05$ (methin pro-

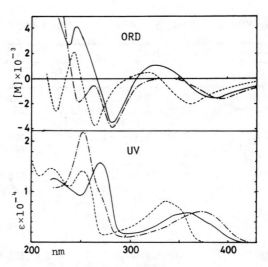

Fig. 1. ORD and UV spectra of $\underline{A}$.
----- , at pH 0.0 (cation),
——— , at pH 5.5 (neutral molecule),
—·— , at pH 11.0 (anion).

ton adjacent to the methyl group), and a singlet at $\delta 8.22$ (an aromatic proton at the 7-position of the pteridine ring). We designated $\underline{A}$ as the ether (6) rather than the ester (7), since $\underline{A}$ was stable in alkaline solution. This conclusion was confirmed by an unambiguous synthesis of (6) as illustrated in the Scheme 1. Condensation of (3) with propylene glycol in the presence of hydrogen chloride gave two ethers, (4) and (5). Permanganate oxidation of (4) in an alkaline solution gave (6), whose R_f values, pK_a values, UV spectra, ^{1}HNMR spectrum, and mass spectrum were all in complete agreement with those of $\underline{A}$ (Table 1).

Scheme 1

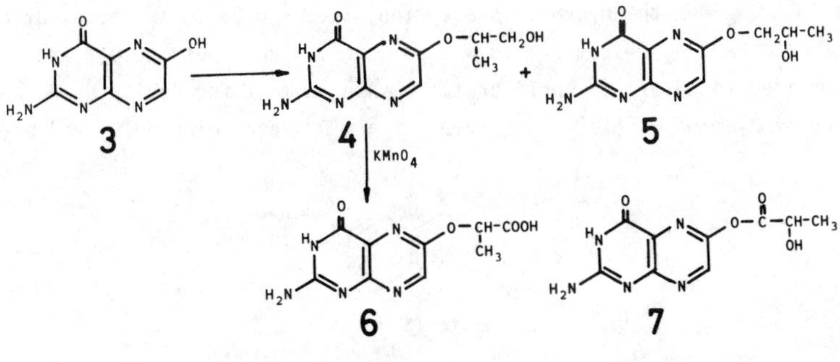

TABLE 1.

R_f VALUES, pK_a VALUES, AND UV SPECTRA OF 6-ALKOXYPTERINS

6-Substituted pterins	R_f values		pK_a	UV spectra	
	a	b		pH	λ_{max} (log ε)
-O-CH$_3$ *	0.36	0.51	2.37	0.0	222(4.10), 255(4.12), 340(3.85)
			8.15	5.0	231(4.01), 270(4.16), 360(3.73)
				12.0	253(4.32), 373(3.80
(4) -O-CH-CH$_2$OH CH$_3$	0.47	0.52	2.67	0.0	224(4.15), 257(4.18), 344(3.90)
			8.38	6.0	228(4.09), 273(4.20), 364(3.78)
				11.0	255(4.35), 376(3.82)
(5) -O-CH$_2$CH-CH$_3$ OH	0.38	0.43	2.68	0.0	224(4.13), 256(4.15), 343(3.87)
			8.28	6.0	228(4.03), 273(4.18), 363(3.76)
				11.0	255(4.33), 377(3.81)
(6) -O-CH-COOH CH$_3$	0.66	0.35	2.65	0.0	222(4.15), 255(4.14), 340(3.88)
			8.53	6.0	225(4.09), 273(4.19), 363(3.75)
				11.0	255(4.33), 374(3.77)
(A)**	0.66	0.35	2.65	0.0	222(4.19), 255(4.15), 340(3.87)
			8.53	6.0	224(4.13), 272(4.19), 363(3.75)
				11.0	255(4.34), 374(3.80)

a: 4% sodium citrate, b: n-butanol, acetic acid, water; 4:1:1. * The pK_a values and UV spectra are taken from reference 14. ** Since A could not be weighed, the extinctions were calculated by estimating the absorbance of the neutral molecule (at pH 6.0) at 363 nm as log ε = 3.75 by analogy to (6).

The stereochemical structure of A. Compound A is optically active, as shown by its ORD curves (Fig. 1.), due to the chiral carbon in the side chain. In order to determine the absolute structure of A, we carried out hydrolysis of A, and examined the configuration of the lactic acid thus formed by means of the above mentioned enzymatic method[13]. The hydrolysis became complete when A was heated in 5M HCl at 80°C for 5 hr. From the hydrolysis solution, 1.02 ± 0.01 molar amount of L-lactic acid was detected; no D-lactic acid was detected. From these result the side chain was determined to be of (s)-configuration, same as that for sepiapterin, and the structure of 2-amino-6-[(1s)-1-carboxyethoxy]-4(3H)-pteridinone (8) was given for A.

A POSSIBLE MECHANISM FOR THE CONVERSION OF SEPIAPTERIN TO A AND TO 7,8-DIHYDRO-XANTHOPTERIN

The present study revealed that both sepiapterin and its catabolite A possesse the same (s)-configuration. This indicates that sepiapterin might have been converted to A by the following intramolecular rearrangement, retaining the configuration of the side chain (Scheme 2). The rearrangement is initiated by addition of the 2'-OH group to the 5,6-double bond, followed by oxidation of the resulting tetrahydropterin (9) into a quinonoid dihydropterin (10). The quinonoid dihydropterin might be expected to undergo cleavage of the C_6-C_1, bond to give (11), the 7,8-dihydro derivative of A, which should be easily oxidized to the aromatic compound A. Throughout the rearrangement, the configuration at the chiral 2'-carbon is retained.

An indirect support for the present intramolecular rearrangement mechanism was obtained from an experiment using radio active lactic acid: *B. subtilis* was incubated exactly in the same way as above described except the addition of $[U-^{14}C]$-lactic acid. From the compound A thus formed, no radio activity was detected, indicating that the side chain of A came from sepiapterin by the above mechanism and not from other sourses.

Scheme 2.

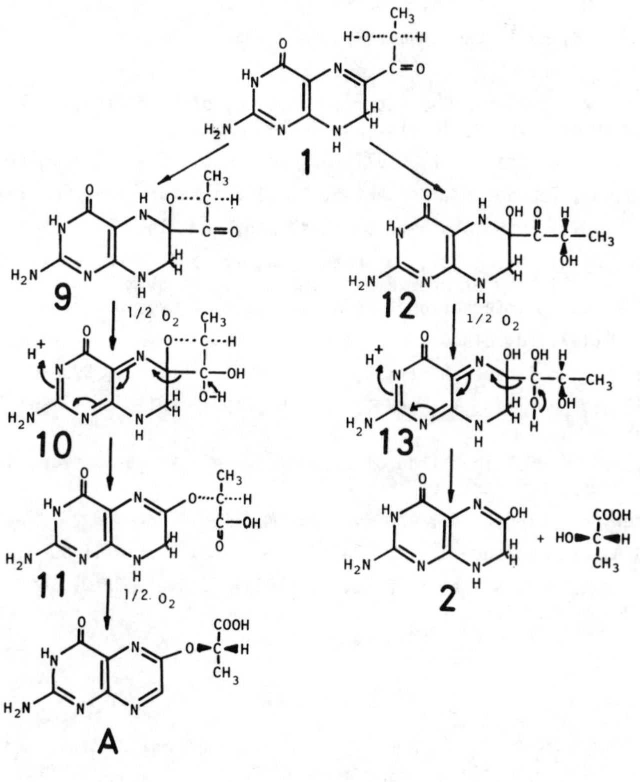

A similar reaction mechanism is applicable to the oxidative degradation of sepia-pterin into 7,8-dihydroxanthopterin (2) and L-lactic acid; where the reaction is initiated by the addition of water to the 5,6-double bond, again giving a tetra-hydropterin (12). Oxidation of (12) to a quinonoid dihydro pterin (13) by air and subsequent cleavage of the C_6-C_1, bond would give 7,8-dihydroxanthopterin (2) and L-lactic acid.

Other examples to support the present mechanism are available. Several 5,6,7,8-tetrahydropterins with a -C-X side chain (where X is an amino or hydroxy group) at the 6-position, such as tetrahydrobiopterin or tetrahydrofolic acid, are known to undergo cleavage of the C_6-C_1, bond during oxidation[2,5,15]. Also several isoxantho-pterin derivatives having a COOH, CH_2NH_2, or $CH(OH)CH_3$ group at the 6-position undergo cleavage of the C_6-C_1, bond to give isoxanthopterin, when they are reduced (presumably to a 5,6-dihydro derivative) by aluminium amalgam[16]. All of these cleavage reactions can be reasonably explained by the above mechanism proceeding through a quinonoid dihydropteridine.

REFERENCES

1. Forrest, H.S. and Mitchell, H.K. (1954) J. Amer. Chem. Soc. 76, 5656-5658.

2. Viscontini, M. and Möhlmann, E. (1959) Helv. chim. Acta 42, 836-841.

3. Nawa, S. (1960) Bull. Chem. Soc. Jpn. 33, 1555-1560.

4. Tsusue, M. and Akino, M. (1965) Zool. Mag. 74, 91-94.

5. Pfleiderer, W. (1975) in Chemistry and Biology of Pteridines, Pfleiderer, W. ed., Walter de Gruyter, Berlin, pp. 941-949.

6. Fukushima, T. and Shiota, T. (1974) J. Biol. Chem. 249, 4445-4451.

7. Matsubara, M., Tsusue, M., and Akino, M. (1963) Nature 199, 908-909.

8. Katoh, S. (1971) Arch. Biochem. Biophys. 146, 202-214.

9. Katoh, S., Nagai, M., Nagai, Y., Fukushima, T., and Akino, M. (1970) in Chemistry and Biology of Pteridines, Iwai, K., Akino, M., Goto, M., and Iwanami, Y. eds., International Academic Press, Tokyo, pp. 225-234.

10. Tsusue, M. (1971) J. Biochem. Tokyo 69, 781-788.

11. Kitayama, C. and Tsusue, M. (1975) Agric. Biol. Chem. 39, 905-906.

12. Matsuura, S., Sugimoto, T., and Tsusue, M. (1977) Bull. Chem. Soc. Jpn. 50, 2168-2169.

13. Hohorst, H.J. (1963) in Method of Enzymatic Analysis, Bergmeyer, H.U. ed., Academic Press, New York, pp. 266-270.

14. Pfleiderer, W., Liedek, E., and Rukwied, M. (1962) Chem. Ber. 95, 755-762.

15. Blair, J.A. and Pearson, A.J. (1974) J.Chem. Soc. Perkin II 80-88.

16. Nawa, S., Matsuura, S., and Hirata, Y. (1953) J. Amer. Chem. Soc. 75, 4450-4451.

141

DROSOPTERINS AND THE IN VIVO MODULATION OF THEIR SYNTHESIS BY IMPLANTATION OF
METABOLITES IN EYE COLOR MUTANTS OF DROSOPHILA MELANOGASTER

ILSE SCHWINCK

Biological Sciences Group, University of Connecticut, Box U-42
Storrs, Connecticut, 06268   (U.S.A.)

ABSTRACT

In the Drosophila melanogaster mutants ruby and orange[66k], which permit partial
synthesis of the red drosopterins, the upward modulation of the drosopterin synthesis by phenylalanine implants is not effected by the presence or absence of the biosynthesis of the brown ommochrome pigment xanthommatin, nor by the presence or absence of metabolites of the three ommochrome pathway blocks, the vermilion, the
cinnabar, and the scarlet mutant.

INTRODUCTION

The ontogenetic development in holometabolic insects and its regulation by well
coordinated sequences of épigenetic events mediated by low molecular metabolites is
a challenge to experimental biologists, especially if cell-cell interactions, diffu-
sible metabolites, and experimental modulation in the differentiation system permit
an in vivo analysis. During metamorphosis, the eye pigment synthesis in the pharate
pupae and young Drosophila fly presents such an experimental tool. The rather stable
Drosophila eye pigments, the brown ommochromes and the red drosopterins, permit quantitative studies of these biosynthetic endproducts. Two days before eclosion, the
melanin synthesis in the cuticle and the ommochrome synthesis in the adult eyes begin; one day later, the red drosopterins first appear in the adult eyes, and drosopterins continue to increase for several days after eclosion. Several dozen mutants
are known to effect the synthesis of drosopterins. The post-eclosion synthesis is
extensive in some of these mutants and can add as much as 100%. Furthermore, mutants
controlling the synthesis of drosopterins show a different quantitative distribution
of the five major drosopterin pigments[1,2]; for several mutants, this "fingerprint
pattern" of drosopterins changes during the post-eclosion synthesis.

In my earlier studies, I demonstrated that the pre-eclosion and post-eclosion
synthesis of drosopterins can be augmented by supplemental phenylalanine, either entering dissected pupae osmotically, or by implantation of phenylalanine crystals into pharate pupae or newly eclosed flies[3,4]. The implanted phenylalanine also causes
a shift in the fingerprint pattern, specifically an augmentation of the aurodrosopterins[1,5,6]. I postulated a mechanism involving the cofactor of phenylalanine
hydroxylase -- a biopterin derivative -- that may cause the upward modulation of the
biosynthesis of drosopterins[3,4,6].

A dipteridyl structure for four of these red pigments has been suggested by W. Pfleiderer's group[7,8,9]; however, they recently revised it[10] and details are under further investigation. Until more information on the molecular structure is available, these red pigments as a group will be called "drosopterin pigments" or "drosopterins", and the single pigments "drosopterin"[2], "isodrosopterin", "neodrosopterin"[11], and "aurodrosopterin"[6,8,9] and "fraction e"[2].

In our first transplantation study of the non-autonomous red pigment synthesis in the rosy mutant (for symbols and description of mutants see [12]), we observed lower amounts of red pigments in double mutant flies, with rosy and the two ommochrome blocking mutants vermilion and cinnabar; and we stated in 1956 that the pleiotropic side effect of these ommochrome mutants has an influence on the red pigment synthesis[13,14]. Recently, Parisi et al, in their quantitative study with various mutants of the ommochrome and drosopterin pathway suggested several indirect interactions of metabolites of both pathways; they propose a model where the brown ommochrome pigment xanthommatin has a cofactor function in the biosynthesis of the red drosopterins[15]. Furthermore, they demonstrate the involvement of xanthine dehydrogenase in the xanthommatin biosynthesis[16], and they also report an increase of xanthommatin and of drosopterins in a maroonlike phenocopy with a vermilion-maroon-like genotype, caused by feeding the missing metabolite of the xanthommatin pathway[17]. Another indication for some kind of an ommochrome-drosopterin pathway interaction is reported from Howells' laboratory in a study of partially purified particulate phenoxazinone synthase from fly heads[18]. This enzyme is assumed to catalyze the last step in xanthommatin synthesis. An enzyme activity peak was found at the onset of xanthommatin formation, however, a second and much larger peak is found at the time of drosopterin synthesis.

Obviously, several types of interactions between the two pathways must exist.

MATERIALS AND METHODS

Flies were grown at $22 \pm 1°C$ in 0.2 liter milk bottles on standard agar-corn meal-yeast media with tegosept added as fungicide. Phenylalanine crystals (Sigma) were implanted into females 0-3 hours after eclosion. Controls and implant flies were from same culture, and were kept together in one bottle with males for 10 days, several times transferred to fresh food. Heads from 0 day and 10 day old flies were extracted in 30% ethanol, made pH 2 with H Cl[19]. Two dimensional thin-layer chromatography on Merck Cellulose glass plates (Avicel microcrystalline 5757, and DC-Fertig-platten Cellulose 5716). The activity of the reflected fluorescence from each spot was measured from the TLC-plates with the PMQ II Zeiss Spectrophotometer equipped with the chromatogram scanning attachment and a recorder, the monochromator set for the peak of the fluorescence emission curve for each spot; for aurodrosopterins 538 nm, for drosopterin and isodrosopterin 542 nm, for neodrosopterin 555 nm. Fraction (e) was not studied here. Absorption of total drosopterins in the head extracts was determined with a Gilford spectrophotometer at 485 nm.

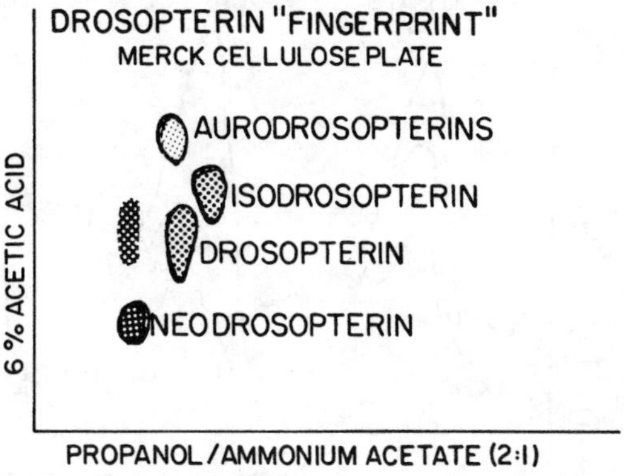

RESULTS

My experimental studies presented here will investigate the effects of the ommochrome pathway metabolites and of the endproduct xanthommatin on the phenylalanine dependent augmentation of drosopterins in several double mutants.

The three ommochrome pathway mutants vermilion (=v), cinnabar (=cn), and scarlet (=st) were combined with mutants controlling the dro-

DROSOPTERIN "FINGERPRINT"
MERCK CELLULOSE PLATE

AURODROSOPTERINS

ISODROSOPTERIN

DROSOPTERIN

NEODROSOPTERIN

6 % ACETIC ACID

PROPANOL / AMMONIUM ACETATE (2:1)

Fig. 1: Fluorescent Fingerprint Pattern of Drosopterins on two-dimensional thin-layer plates.
1st dim. 4 hours in acetic acid, 2nd dim. 18 hours in propanol / 2% ammonium acetate. 18°C.

sopterin biosynthesis. One series studied the mutant ruby (=rb) compared to v rb, to rb cn, and to rb st, each with phenylalanine implant and the related controls. A second series presented here, studied the mutant orange^{66k} (= or^{66k}) compared to v or^{66k}, to cn or^{66k}, to cn or^{66k}, and to or^{66k}st. Additional experiments with the mutant garnet^{70k} (= g^{70k}) and pilot experiments with other drosopterin mutants confirm the results, however, will not be described here. The flies with a single mutant, rb and or^{66k} respectively, have a normal ommochrome pathway and synthesize the brown xanthommatin. The double mutant combinations with v accumulate tryptophan due to the lack of tryptophan oxygenase activity. The mutant cn causes accumulation of kynurenine due to the lack of kynurenine hydroxylase activity. The mutant st has low amounts of hyroxylkynurenine and it was reported that st has a defective transport system for xanthommatin precursors[20,21]. All three mutants, v, cn, and st lack the brown xanthommatin and their eye color is dependent only on the amount of the red drosopterins.

Presence or absence of xanthommatin biosynthesis:

Comparison of flies with a single drosopterin controlling mutant gene to the double mutant flies, which cannot synthesize xanthommatin, demonstrates an augmentation of drosopterin synthesis in response to the phenylalanine implant in the same order of magnitude for all four major red pigments. As in my earlier experiments, the aurodrosopterins show the strongest increase. A tracing from the actual recorded scanning curves of the emitted fluorescence of the aurodrosopterins is given in Fig. 2.: (a) for the 0-3 hour old female flies, at time zero of the implantation experiment, (b) for 10 day old control flies, (c) for 10 day old females with the

144

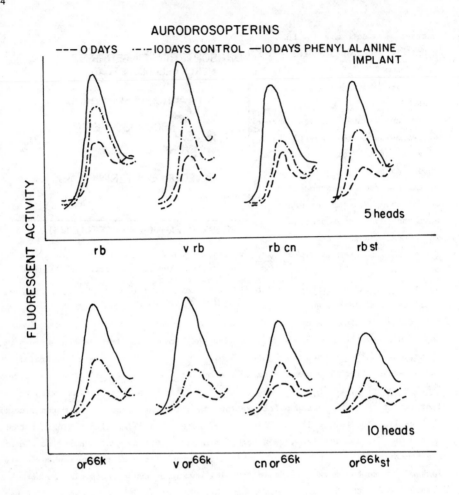

Fig. 2.: Tracing of recorded curves of emitted fluorescence from the aurodrosopterin spots on TLC-plates for 2 single and 6 double mutants from the ruby and orange[66k] series.

phenylalanine implants. Similar, although less extensive increases can be seen in the recorded fluorescence curves for the drosopterin spots and for the isodrosopterin spots; the neodrosopterin spots require further analysis because of the base line fluorescence in this region of the TLC-plates.

Presence or absence of ommochrome pathway metabolites:

The comparison of TLC-plates from v rb flies, cn rb flies, and rb st flies, as well as from v or[66k] flies, cn or[66k] flies, and or[66k]st flies shows some difference in synthesis of total drosopterins, which is also seen in many other double mutant flies with $\underline{v}$, $\underline{cn}$, and $\underline{st}$ ($\underline{st}$ always has the lowest amount of drosopterins). Because these are not isogenic fly stocks* the difference could depend on either the genetic background or on the specific pleiotropic effect of the $\underline{v}$, $\underline{cn}$, or $\underline{st}$ mutant genes -- in modern terms, on pathway interactions of their metabolites. However, the response to the phenylalanine implant in all cases is of the same magnitude for the drosopterin, the isodrosopterin, and the aurodrosopterin (Fig. 2).

The quantitative evaluation of the recorded curves of $\underline{in\ situ}$ fluorescence on the TLC-plates will be discussed in a more detailed publication.

SUMMARY

In this comparative study with the $\underline{ruby}$ and $\underline{orange}^{66k}$ drosopterin controlling mutants, the phenylalanine crystal implants into the abdomen of the newly eclosed flies cause a similar increase of drosopterins in the presence and in the absence of the brown xanthommatin pigment. Furthermore, the presence or absence of the substrates or products of the ommochrome mutant $\underline{vermilion}$ and of $\underline{cinnabar}$, as well as the defective transport caused by the $\underline{scarlet}$ mutant gene, do not effect the epigenetic modulation of the synthesis of drosopterins by phenylalanine. This indicates the independence of the postulated phenylalanine hydroxylase mechanisms from xanthommatin biosynthesis and from ommochrome pathway metabolites.

ACKNOWLEDGEMENTS

This study was supported partially by a grant from the University of Connecticut Research Foundation. Part of this study was done at the Genetics Institute of the University of Giessen, Germany during a leave from the University of Connecticut.

---

*It must be kept in mind that in none of my own comparative studies of the eye color mutants, nor in the publications quoted here, the flies with one or more mutants have been made isogenic in respect to the genetic background. My earlier, mostly unpublished study of several isogenic fly stocks with the $\underline{rosy}$ mutant, demonstrated that the effect of the genetic background was substantial in respect to the red eye pigments quantity[22]. The tremendous work, and the still existing uncertainty about the precisely isogenic part of the genotypes, made the large scale breeding of isogenic multiple mutant stocks inadvisable. However, the modulating effect of the genetic background must be considered in any discussion of quantitative data on the enzyme activity studies as well as in measuring substrate and/or product concentrations.

REFERENCES

1. Schwinck, I. (1971) Genetics 68, s59.

2. Schwinck, I. and Mancini, M. (1973) Archiv für Genetik 46, 41-52.

3. Schwinck, I. (1965) Zeitschr. für Naturforschung 20b, 322-326.

4. Schwinck, I. (1966) Zoolog. Anzeiger Suppl. 30, 382-390.

5. Schwinck. I. (1973) Genetics 74, s254.

6. Schwinck, I. (1976) in Chemistry and Biology of Pteridines, 5th Symposium Konstanz 1975, W. Pfleiderer e., Walter de Gruyter, Berlin-New York, pp. 919-930.

7. Schlobach, H. and Pfleiderer, W. (1971) Angew. Chemie 83, 440-441.

8. Rokos, K. and Pfleiderer, W. (1975) Chem. Ber. 108, 2728-2736.

9. Rokos, K. and Pfleiderer, W. (1976) in Chemistry and Biology of Pteridines, 5th Symposium Konstanz 1975, W. Pfleiderer ed., Walter de Gruyter, Berlin-New York, pp. 934-938.

10. Theobald, H. und Pfleiderer, W. (1977) Tetrahedron Letters 10, 841-844.

11. Viscontini, M., Hadorn, E. und Karrer, P. (1957) Helvet. Chim. Acta 40, 579-585.

12. Lindsley, D. L. and Grell, E. H. (1968) Genetic Variations of Drosophila melanogaster, Carnegie Inst. of Washington Publications No. 627.

13. Hadorn, E. and Schwinck, I. (1956) Nature 177, 940-941.

14. Hadorn, E. and Schwinck, I. (1956) Zeitschr. für induktive Abstammungs- und Vererbungslehre 87, 528-553.

15. Parisi, G., Carfagna, M., and D'Amora, D. (1976) J. Insect Physiol. 22, 415-423.

16. Parisi, G., Carfagna, M., and D'Amora, D. (1976) Insect Biochem. 6, 567-570.

17. Parisi, G., D'Amora, D. and Franco, A.R. (1977) Insect. Biochem. 7, 1-2.

18. Yamamoto, M., Howells, A. J. and Ryall R. L. (1976) Biochem. Genetics 14, 1077-1090.

19. Ephrussi, B. and Herold, J. L. (1944) Genetics 28, 148-175.

20. Sullivan, D. T. and Sullivan, M. C. (1975) Biochem. Genetics 13, 603-613.

21. Howells, A. J., Summers, K. M., and Ryall, R. C. (1977) Biochem. Genetics 15, 1049-1059.

22. Schwinck, I. (1961) Drosophila Information Service 36.

BIOSYNTHESIS OF BIOPTERIN BY CHICKEN ENZYME PREPARATIONS

K. TANAKA, M. AKINO, Y. HAGI AND T. SHIOTA

Department of Microbiology, University of Alabama in Birmingham, Alabama 35294 U.S.A.

ABSTRACT

A chicken kidney preparation which catalyzes the conversion of D-erythrodihydro-neopterin triphosphate (H_2NP-PPP) to dihydrobiopterin in the presence of Mg^{2+} and NADPH was studied. This system was fractionated to obtain fraction A which catalyzes the conversion of H_2NP-PPP to sepiapterin in the presence of Mg^{2+} and NADPH and fraction B which catalyzes the conversion of sepiapterin to dihydrobiopterin in the presence of NADPH. Fraction A was further fractionated into fraction A2 which catalyzes the conversion of H_2NP-PPP to an unknown intermediate, compound X, in the presence of Mg^{2+} and into fraction A1 which catalyzes the conversion of compound X to sepiapterin in the presence of NADPH. Results of experiments performed to characterize compound X indicate that this compound is extremely labile, yielding pterin and pyruvic acid. This information suggests that compound X is 6-(1',2'-dioxopropyl)-7,8-dihydropterin. Other properties of this enzyme system are also described.

INTRODUCTION

Recently enzyme systems which synthesize sepiapterin and biopterin have been demonstrated in liver, kidney and Drosophila preparations[1-6]. Results obtained with these preparations indicate that GTP is utilized for the production of H_2NP-PPP and formic acid as in bacteria[7]. H_2NP-PPP thus formed is subsequently converted to sepiapterin by a Drosophila preparation or to dihydrobiopterin by a golden hamster kidney preparation, each in the presence of Mg^{2+} and NADPH.

In this presentation, we wish to report results obtained with fractions A1 and A2, and describe an intermediate produced from H_2NP-PPP by fraction A2 which is utilized by a fraction A1 for sepiapterin synthesis.

METHODS AND MATERIALS

GTP cyclohydrolase which was partially purified from extracts of Escherichia coli[8] was used to prepare [^{14}C (U)]H_2NP-PPP from [^{14}C (U)]GTP.

Sepiapterin and pterin were identified by thin layer chromatography (TLC) using five different solvent systems[2] and by high performance liquid chromatography (HPLC; Waters) using a μBondapack C18 column (Waters).

Table 1 shows the mobilities and the peak elution volumes of compounds studied. These compounds were detected by their fluorescence, absorbance or radioactivity.

A complete reaction mixture consisted of: [^{14}C (U)H_2-NP-PPP, 61.7 μM (7.4 x 10^4 dpm); Fr. A1, 505 μg of protein; Fr. A2, 390 μg of protein; $MgSO_4$ 0.5 mM; NADPH, 1 mM, 2-mercaptoethanol, 500 mM and Tris buffer (pH 7.4), 25 mM. Total volume was 0.3 ml. Reaction mixtures were incubated at 37° for 60 min. After incubation, four volumes of cold ethanol were added, the mixture centrifuged and the supernatant fluid

TABLE 1   Peak elution volumes and Rf values of compound studied

Compound	HPLC			TLC		
	Methanol 20%		Pic A[1]) in water	Solvent	B Rf	C
		ml		A		
Sepiapterin	6.5			0.34	0.43	0.50
Pterin	3.5		> 16.0	0.52	0.38	0.54
Pyruvic acid			12.0			

[1) Pic A reagent is tetrabutylammonium phosphate, 0.005 M (Waters Associates)

evaporated to dryness. The residue was dissolved in 0.05 - 0.5 ml water. This material was subjected to TLC or HPLC treatment.

RESULTS

Partial fractionation and purification of chicken kidney homogenates--An ammonium sulfate preparation (40% to 65% saturation) from a chicken kidney homogenate was applied to an Ultrogel AcA34 (LKB) column. The fractions collected were assayed for their activity to convert $[^{14}C$ (U)]H_2NP-PPP to $[^{14}C$ (U)]sepiapterin in the presence of NADPH and $MgSO_4$ and also to convert sepiapterin to biopterin in the presence of NADPH. Results show that the gel filtration step separated the biopterin synthesizing enzyme system into two fractions; fraction A which utilized $[^{14}C$ (U)]H_2NP-PPP to produce sepiapterin and fraction B which utilized sepiapterin to produce dihydrobiopterin

The products of the reactions catalyzed by fraction A and fraction B were identified by thin-layer chromatography using five solvent systems. The product formed by fraction A showed the same mobility as sepiapterin and that by fraction B as biopterin. The identity of these products were further substantiated by the similarity of their absorption spectra to authentic sepiapterin and dihydrobiopterin.

Fraction A obtained from an Ultrogel AcA34 column chromatography was subjected to a DEAE Sephadex A50 column chromatography. Each fraction collected was incubated with $[^{14}C$ (U)]H_2NP-PPP, Mg^{2+}, NADPH and a preparation of either fraction A1 or fraction A2 and the mixture was assayed for $[^{14}C$ (U)]sepiapterin production. The use of a previously prepared fraction A1 or fraction A2 was necessary to assay for the presence of the complimentary fraction.   The results presented in Fig. 1 indicate that fraction A was separated into two, Fr. A1 and Fr. A2. When heated at 100^0 for 1 min., the activity of Fr. A1 was completely eliminated whereas the activity of Fr. A2 was unchanged.

In Table 2, the results of an experiment testing the effect of magnesium,NADPH and 2-mercaptoethanol on sepiapterin synthesis in the presence of both Fr. A1 and Fr. A2 are presented. The results show that the combination of Fr. A1 and Fr. A2 requires the presence of Mg^{2+} and NADPH and is stimulated by 2-mercaptoethanol. In the presence of H_2NP-PPP, $MgSO_4$, NADPH, 2-mercaptoethanol, and a constant amount of Fr. A2 or Fr. A1, the amount of sepiapterin synthesized increased with increasing amounts of Fr. A1 or Fr. A2, respectively (Fig. 2).

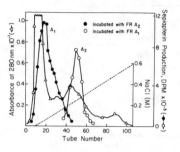
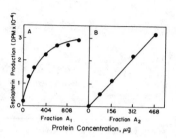

Fig. 1 (left) DEAE-Sephadex A-50 chromatography of Fraction A
Fig. 2 (right) Requirement for Fr. A1 and Fr. A2 for sepiapterin synthesis

TABLE 2 Effect of magnesium, NADPH and 2-mercaptoethanol on the sepiapterin synthesis

Incubation mixture	Sepiapterin production
Complete	DPM 8,974
minus Mg^{2+}	445
minus NADPH	601
minus Mg^{2+} and NADPH	368
plus 2-mercaptoethanol (500 mM)	29,417

Sepiapterin was determined by TLC

Since both Fr. A1 and Fr. A2 were required for sepiapterin synthesis, a two stage experiment was performed in order to determine the sequence of the reactions catalyzed by Fr. A1 and Fr. A2. The results presented in Table 3 indicate that Fr.A2 catalyzes the conversion of $[^{14}C$ (U)]H_2NP-PPP to an unknown intermediate, compound X, which in the presence of Fr. A1 is converted to sepiapterin.

The effect of NADPH and $MgSO_4$ on the synthesis of a radioactive intermediate of sepiapterin from $[^{14}C$ (U)]H_2NP-PPP by Fr. A2 was studied. After incubation, the reaction mixture was applied to a DEAE-Sephadex A-25 column and the column was eluted by a gradient of LiCl. In Fig. 3 the elution profiles of reaction mixtures without cofactors (A), and with NADPH (B) show a major single radioactive peak (peak 3). The reaction mixture containing NADPH and Mg^{2+} (C) or only Mg^{2+} (D) gave a profile with three radioactive peaks, peaks 1, 2 and 3. The analyses of these radioactive peaks in-

TABLE 3 Sequence of reactions catalyzed by Fr. Al and Fr. A2

Reaction Mixture	Additions made in the first incubation	Additions made in the second incubation	Sepiapterin production DPM
1	Fr. A2	None	610
2	None	Fr. Al + Fr. A2	9,725
3	Fr. Al	Fr. A2	885
4	Fr. Al	None	0
5	Fr. A2	Fr. Al	7,020
6	Fr. Al + Fr. A2	None	12,146
7	None	None	0

Each reaction mixture contained the usual reagents during the first incubation period and Fr. Al, (3.25 mg of protein) and/or Fr. A2 (187 µg of protein) as indicated. At the end of 30 min, each tube from the first incubation period was placed in a boiling water bath for 1 min, cooled and additions were made as indicated above for the second incubation period. The tubes were incubated at 37° for an additional 30 min. Sepiapterin was determined by HPLC.

dicated that peak 1 did not contain either dihydroneopterin or sepiapterin, peak 2 did not contain neopterin, and that peak 3 contained unreacted radioactive H_2NP-PPP. These results suggest that the utilization of H_2NP-PPP by Fr. A2 required Mg^{2+}.

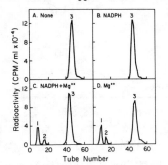
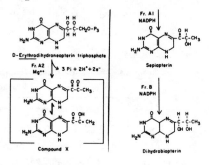

Fig. 3 (left) DEAE-Sephadex A-25 chromatography of A2 reaction mixture
Fig. 4 (right) Proposed pathway of dihydrobiopterin biosynthesis

One of the type of compounds tested as a possible intermediate was a dihydropterin bearing a carbonyl function, other than sepiapterin, which may be reactive with 2,4-dinitrophenylhydrazine (DNP). An A2 reaction mixture similar to that described in Fig. 3D was incubated, treated with DNP and extracted with a 1:1 mixture of 1-butanol-ethyl acetate. Radioactivity was found in both the organic and aqueous layers. A TLC analysis of the organic layer showed three radioactive spots. The spot migrating with a Rf value of 0.62 corresponded to pyruvate hydrazone (Table 4). A TLC analysis of

TABLE 4 TLC analysis of A2 reaction products after a 2,4-dinitrophenylhydrazine treatment

	Organic layer Rf			Aqueous layer Rf
Reaction Mixture	0.62	0.18	0.0	0.54
			cpm	
Complete	840	70	180	2,800
w/o Mg^{2+}	10	0	170	5
w/o Fr A2	5	0	120	10

the aqueous layer gave a blue fluorescent spot migrating as pterin. These results were confirmed by using four additional solvents. The formation of these radioactive materials was dependent upon Mg^{2+} but not upon NADPH.

In order to obtain information on the nature of compound X, the A2 reaction mixture was increased ten-fold and processed as in Fig. 3D. Pooled samples from each peak fraction were tested as soon as possible for sepiapterin synthesis in the presence of Fr. Al and NADPH and subjected to TLC and HPLC. The results of this experiment are presented in Table 5. Only peak 1 contained a compound which was converted to sepiapterin. When a sample of peak 1 was treated with acid and then analyzed by TLC, several fluorescent materials were observed. Of these, a substance with the highest radioactivity (ten-fold greater than a second ranked radioactive compound) moved on TLC as pterin. HPLC analysis showed that a major radioactive peak was eluted like pterin when 20% methanol was employed. Furthermore the UV absorption spectra of the fluorescent material were similar to those obtained with authentic pterin. HPLC analysis also showed that another major radioactive material which was not fluorescent was eluted in a position similar to that of pyruvate with Pic A reagent.

TABLE 5 Analyses of peak 1

Peak	Substrate for sepiapterin	Pterin HPLC		TLC	Pyruvate HPLC
		Solvent[1] 20% MeOH Dpm x 10^{-6}	A	C	Solvent Pic A
1	0.6	3.8	6.1	6.9	1.5
2	0				
3	0				

[1] Reference (2)

In other experiments, when α- or γ-^{32}P-H$_2$NP-PPP was used as the substrate, no radioactivity was detected in peak 1. Furthermore, a phosphorylated intermediate such as neopterin-3'-monophosphate or neopterin-2', 3'-cyclic monophosphate has not been found in reaction mixtures. Additional experiments showed that none of the four isomers of dihydroneopterin, or the four isomers of dihydroneopterin-3' -monophosphate or D-erythroH$_2$neopterin-2', 3' -cyclic-monophosphate were utilized as a precursor of sepiapterin when incubated in a system which consists of Fr. A1, Fr. A2, NADPH and MgSO$_4$.

The results presented in Fig. 3 and in Tables 4 and 5 suggest that H$_2$NP-PPP in the presence of Fr. A2 and Mg^{2+} may undergo several reactions, one of which is an oxidation step. Accordingly, [^{14}C (U)]H$_2$NP-PPP, Mg^{2+} and Fr. A2 were incubated with either flavin adenine dinucleotide, flavin mononucleotide, NAD$^+$, NADP$^+$, NADH, NADPH, dihydrofolate or lipoic acid. These electron carriers at 1×10^{-3} M and 1×10^{-4} M did not stimulate the production of radioactive compound X.

Finally, it is proposed in Fig. 4 that H$_2$NP-PPP in the presence of Fr. A2 and Mg^{2+}, undergoes dephosphorylation and oxidation resulting in compound X. Presently the details of these reactions are not known. The identification of pterin and pyruvate as degradation products of compound X suggests that this compound has a structure of 6-(1',2'-dioxopropyl)7,8-dihydropterin[9]. The facts that this reaction requires Mg^{2+} and that utilization of compound X by Fr. A1 for sepiapterin synthesis requires NADPH support the reactions shown in Fig. 4.

REFERENCES:
1. K. Fukushima, I. Eto, D. Saliba and T. Shiota. Biochem. Biophys. Res. Commun. 65: 644 (1975).
2. I. Eto, K. Fukushima, and T. Shiota. J. Biol. Chem. 251: 6505 (1976).
3. K. Fukushima, W. Richter, Jr., and T. Shiota. J. Biol. Chem. 252: 5750 (1977).
4. C.L. Fan, G.G. Krivi and G.M. Brown. Biochem. Biophys. Res. Commun. 67: 1047 (1975)
5. C.L. Fan, L.M. Hall, A.J. Skrinska and G.M. Brown. Biochem. Genetics 14: 271 (1976).
6. C.L. Fan. and G.M. Brown. Biochem. Genetics 14: 259 (1976).
7. T. Shiota in Comp. Biochem. edited by M. Florikin and E.H. Stotz. Elsevier Publishing Co. New York. vol. 21 p. 111 (1971).
8. J.J. Yim and G.M. Brown. Biochem. Genetics 14; 259 (1976).
9. A. Suzuki, and M. Goto. Biochem. Biophys. Acta 304: 222 (1973).

This work was supported by NSF-PCM Grant 7709884

THE BACTERIAL CATABOLISM OF PTERIDINES

Motoo Tsusue, Shin'ichiro Takikawa and Chizuko Kitayama Yokokawa
Biological Laboratory, Kitasato University, Sagamihara City, 228, Japan

ABSTRACT

A pterin deaminase catalyzing hydroxylative deamination of various pteridines was found in bacteria, and partially purified from bacterial extracts. Specific activity was raised 90-fold over that of the crude extract. The pH optimum is around 7.3 and K_m value for 6-carboxypterin is 1.3 mM. The enzyme deaminates pterin, 6-carboxypterin, biopterin, 6-methylpterin, 7-methylpterin, xanthopterin, 6-hydroxymethylpterin, sepiapterin, isosepiapterin, folic acid, and 6,7-dimethylpterin to their corresponding lumazines, whereas guanine, 7-carboxypterin, leucopterin, isoxanthopterin and 6-methylisoxanthopterin do not serve as substrate. The enzyme is inhibited by PCMB and 8-azaguanine.

INTRODUCTION

Many types of bacteria were found to decompose sepiapterin under aerobic conditions[1]. When added to bacterial media, the yellow color of sepiapterin gradually decreased during the stationary phase as seen in figure 1. During the disappearence of the yellow color a new bright blue fluorescing substance was produced. The blue fluorescent compound was purified and the chemical structure was shown to be 6-[(1S)-1-carboxyethoxy]pterin[2]. This fact may indicate that bacteria have the enzyme system which can catalyze the intramolecular conversion of the lactyl group of sepiapterin.

Another metabolic pathway for sepiapterin in bacterial cells involves a new pterin deaminase. When the pigment was incubated with crude bacterial extracts, sepialumazine was found on paper chromatograms with various solvents systems. This paper reports the characterization of this bacterial pterin deaminase.

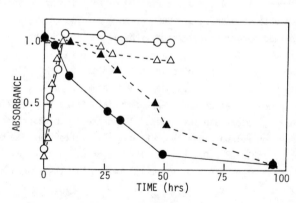

Fig. 1. Decomposition of sepiapterin by <u>Bacillus megaterium</u> and <u>Bacillus subtilis</u>.

o: <u>Bacillus megaterium</u>. Δ: <u>Bacillus subtilis</u>.
Open symbols: growth curve determined by absorbance at 660 nm. Solid symbols: decomposition of the pigment determined by absorbance at 420 nm.

MATERIALS AND METHODS

Bacteria. Bacillus megaterium 63 and Bacillus subtilis 216 were supplied by Dr. Irie of the National Institute of Animal Industry (Japan). Although Bacillus megaterium IFO 12108 showed the same enzyme specific activity as Bacillus megaterium 63, the latter showed a better yield than the former in the same culture system. Therefore the latter was chiefly utilized as the enzyme source.

Culture Conditions. Bacteria were cultured at 36°C with brain-heart infusion (Eiken) under aerobic conditions. After 24 hr growth, cells were harvested by centrifugation. Approximately 15g (wet weight) of cells per liter of medium were obtained. Cells can be stored at -20°C without appreciable loss of enzyme activity.

Chemicals. Sepiapterin and isosepiapterin were prepared by a previously reported method[3]. Sepialumazine and isosepialumazine were prepared enzymatically by a previously described method[4]. Other pterins were the gifts of Prof. Matsuura of Nagoya University.

Ammonia measurement. Ammonia was determined by the alkaline-phenol method[5], using Conway's micro-diffusion technique.

Protein determination. Protein was determined by the method of Lowry et al.[6], using bovine serum albumin as the protein standard.

RESULTS

Enzyme assay. The enzyme has low substrate specificity and deaminates many pterins. 6-Carboxypterin was conveniently utilized to devise a spectrophotometric assay method of enzyme activity, since the acid has high affinity for the enzyme and the substrate was easily obtained by oxidative decomposition of commercially available folic acid. The differential spectrum of 6-carboxypterin and 6-carboxylumazine shows a sharp peak at 360 nm in 0.1 M potassium phosphate buffer, pH 7.0. The enzyme activity was, therefore, determined spectrophotometrically based on the spectral difference at 360 nm at neutral pH.

The standard reaction mixture contained the following components: 6-carboxypterin, 0.25 μmole; potassium phosphate buffer, pH 7.0, 0.1 mmole, and enzyme solution, in a final volume of 1.0 ml. After incubation at 25°C for an appropriate time, the reaction was stopped by heating on a boiling water-bath for 3 min. The decrease in absorbance at 360 nm relative to the 0-time control was measured. From a calibration curve, the amount of reacted substrate was calculated. One unit of the enzyme was defined as the amount which deaminates 1 nmole of 6-carboxypterin per 10 min under the standard assay conditions.

Purification of pterin deaminase.

All subsequent procedures were carried out at 4°C and the buffers used contained 5 mM 2-mercaptoethanol.

Crude extract. Fifty grams of the frozen cells were thawed and suspended in 100 ml of 0.02 M potassium phosphate buffer, pH 7.0, containing 0.1 mM phenylmethylsulfonyl fluoride. The suspension was sonicated for 5 min at 20 KC, 150 W by a Sonore S sonicator. The sonicated suspension was centrifuged and the supernatant fluid was used as crude extract.

Protamine treatment. To the crude extract 0.1 volume of 2 % protamine sulfate was added dropwise with stirring to remove nucleic acid. The precipitate was centrifuged off.

Ammonium sulfate fraction. After addition of ammonium sulfate between 30 to 60 % saturation, the precipitate was dissolved in a small volume of 0.01 M potassium phosphate buffer, pH 7.0. Ammonium sulphate was removed by gel filtration.

Column chromatography on DEAE-cellulose. The eluate was applied to a DEAE-cellulose column equilibrated with 0.01 M potassium phosphate buffer, pH 7.0. After the column was washed with 100 ml of the buffer, a 400 ml linear gradient of NaCl in buffer (0-0.5 M) was applied to the column. The active fractions were combined.

Column chromatography on hydroxylapatite. The combined solution was applied to a hydroxylapatite column equilibrated with 0.01 M potassium phosphate buffer, pH 7.0. After the column was washed with buffer, proteins were eluted by a 200 ml linear gradient of potassium phosphate buffer (pH 7.0, 0.01-0.2 M). The active fractions were combined and concentrated by ultrafiltration.

Table 1
SUMMARY OF PURIFICATION
procedures for bacterial pterin deaminase. Fifty grams of wet cells were used as a starting material.

Purification step	Volume (ml)	Total activity (units)	Total protein (mg)	Specific activity (units/mg)	Yield (%)
Crude extract	120	2,037	1,048	1.9	100
Protamine treatment	127	1,609	1,010	1.6	79
Ammonium sulfate	25	2,241	361	6.2	110
DEAE-cellulose	30	1,263	34	37.2	62
Hydroxylapatite	20	407	2.4	170	20

The purification procedures and results are summarized in Table 1. The specific activity of the final preparation was raised about 90-fold over the crude extract. In all sebsequent work the purified enzyme was immediately used, since the enzyme was rather unstable and activity decreased to about 80 % after standing overnight at 4°C. With freeze storage, activity was maintained for several months, but the effect of freezing and thawing caused severe loss of activity.

Determination of molecular weight. The molecular weight of the enzyme was estimated by gel filtration through a Sephadex G-150 column. Based on a calibration curve with marker proteins, the molecular weight of the enzyme was calculated to be 110,000.

Enzyme kinetics. Under the standard assay conditions, 6-carboxylumazine production in the reaction mixture was linear for at least 30 min, and the initial velocity was proportional to the enzyme concentration. Based on the double reciprocal plot of initial velocity versus substrate concentration, a K_m value of the deaminase for 6-carboxypterin was calculated to be 1.3 mM.

Inhibitors. The inhibitory effect of several compounds on the deaminase activity was studied under the standard assay conditions. As shown in Table 2, the enzyme was inhibited considerably by 1 mM 8-azaguanine and p-chloromercuribenzoate (PCMB). The inhibitory effect of fluoride, cyanide, guanine and amethopterin was very little or nil at the conditions tested.

Table 2

Effect of inhibitors on bacterial deaminase

Compound	Final concentration (M)	Inhibition (%)
8-Azaguanine	10^{-4} 10^{-3}	13 58
PCMB	10^{-4} 10^{-3}	9 69
KCN	10^{-2}	12
KF	10^{-4} 10^{-3}	0 4
Guanine	10^{-3}	0
Amethopterin	10^{-4}	0

pH Optimum. The rate of ammonia production for 60 min in a veriety of buffers over a pH range of 5.5 to 9.0 was determined. The optimum pH of the enzyme for both pterin and 6-carboxypterin is at 7.3.

Substrate specificity. Various pterins were incubated with the enzyme and the reaction products were analyzed by paper chromatography and electrophoresis. Besides sepiapterin and 6-carboxypterin the following pterins were active as substrate: pterin, xanthopterin, biopterin, 6-methylpterin, 6-hydroxymethylpterin, 6,7-dimethyl-pterin, 7-methylpterin, isosepiapterin. However, 7-carboxypterin, isoxanthopterin and 6-methylisoxanthopterin were inactive as substrates. Ammonia was also detected with the pterins which were active as substrate. Pterin and 6-carboxypterin had the highest affinity for the enzyme among the tested pterins. Biopterin, 6-methylpterin, xantho-pterin, 6-hydroxymethylpterin, sepiapterin, isosepiapterin, folic acid and 6,7-di-methylpterin had lower affinity gradually (6,7-dimethylpterin being the lowest).

Balance study. When 6-carboxypterin was used as a substrate, nearly equivalent moles of 6-carboxylumazine and ammonia were detected. The enzyme was active under anaerobic conditions as well. These facts indicate the enzyme catalyzes the hydroxy-lative deamination of pterins without involvement of atmospheric oxygen. No guanase

Table 3

Comparison of properties of pterin deaminases

Material	pH Optimum	Substrate	Not deaminated	Inhibitor	Purity	Literature
Alcaligenes metalcaligenes	6.3-6.7	pterin 6-carboxypterin 6-methylpterin 6-hydroxymethylpterin neopterin folic acid	xanthopterin 7-methylpterin 7-carboxypterin 6,7-dimethylpterin	PCMB KF	20-fold +guanase	Levenberg & Hayaishi, (1959)[7]
Rat liver	6.5	pterin tetrahydropterin isoxanthopterin	xanthopterin biopterin neopterin 6-carboxypterin	KCN 8-azaguanine	23-fold +guanase	Rembold & Simmersbach (1969)[8]
Bombyx mori	6.6	isoxanthopterin	xanthopterin pterin 6-carboxypterin dihydropterin 7-carboxypterin	KCN KF xanthopterin guanine	3-fold -guanase	Gyure, (1974)[9]
Bombyx mori	8.0	sepiapterin isosepiapterin 6-acetyldihydropterin	xanthopterin pterin 6-methylpterin isoxanthopterin	KF PCMB 8-azaguanine xanthopterin	1,500-fold -guanase	Tsusue (1971)[4]
Bacillus megaterium	7.3	pterin 6-carboxypterin biopterin xanthopterin 6-hydroxymethylpterin sepiapterin isosepiapterin folic acid 6,7-dimethylpterin 7-methylpterin	isoxanthopterin leucopterin 6-methyl- isoxanthopterin 7-carboxypterin	PCMB 8-azaguanine	90-fold -guanase	present paper

activity was found in the purified enzyme.

DISCUSSION

Several pterin deaminases, which catalyze the hydrolitic conversion of pterins to corresponding lumazines, have been reported in bacteria[7], mammal[8] and insects[4,9]. The enzymatic properties of these deaminases are summarized in Table 3. One of the characteristic properties of the present enzyme is its rather low specificity for pterin substrates: it can deaminate a wide variety of pterins whether they are aromatic or dihydrotypes. Previously reported characteristics of bacterial[7], insect[9], and mammalian[8] pterin deaminases are a pronounced enzyme instability and pH optima near 6.5. Silkworm sepiapterin deaminase[4] on the other hand is a stable enzyme and its pH optimum is 8.0. The present bacterial deaminase shows intermediate properties in that its pH optimum is 7.3 and it is rather unstable enzyme.

In the case where sepiapterin was added to the culture medium of various bacteria, the yellow fluorescence of the pigment faded away within a few days. This fact indicates that sepiapterin was metabolized by the bacterial cells. Among the megaterium tested, megaterium 63 and IFO 12108 showed the deaminase activity, but IFO 3970, IFO 3003 and IFO 12068 did not. This indicates that deamination is not the sole metabolic pathway for sepiapterin. The formation of 6-[(1S)-1-carboxyethoxy]-pterin[2] is another metabolic product of sepiapterin catabolism. All these pterin pathways occur during the bacterial stationary phase. The significance of these metabolic pathways for bacteria is not yet known and must await further studies.

ACKNOWLEDGEMENT

We thank Dr. Wm Gyure of North Central Bronx Hospital, USA, for his help in preparation of this manuscript.

REFERENCES

1. Kitayama, C., and Tsusue, M., (1975) Agr. Biol. Chem., 39, 905-906.
2. Matsuura, S., Sugimoto, T., Kitayama, C., and Tsusue, M., (1978) J. Biochem. (Tokyo), 83, 19-25.
3. Sugiura, K., Takikawa, S., Tsusue, M., and Goto, M., (1973) Bull. Chem. Soc. Japan, 46, 3312-3313.
4. Tsusue, M., (1971) J. Biochem. (Tokyo), 69, 781-788.
5. Hatano, H., and Kirita, T., (1958) in Special Colorimetry (Nankodo, Tokyo).
6. Lowry, O. H., Rosebrough, N. J., Farr, A. L., and Randall, R. T., (1951) J. Biol. Chem., 193, 265-275.
7. Levenberg, B., and Hayaishi, O., (1959) J. Biol. Chem., 234, 955-961.
8. Rembold, H., and Simmersbach, F., (1969) Biochem. Biophys. Acta, 184, 589-596.
9. Gyure, W. L., (1974) Insect Biochem., 4, 113-121.

DIHYDROXANTHOPTERIN IN URINE FROM NORMALS AND FROM PHENYLKETONURIA
AND ITS VARIANTS

BRUCE M. WATSON, W.L.F. ARMAREGO[*], P. SCHLESINGER, R.G.H. COTTON &
D. M. DANKS
Genetics Research Unit, Royal Children's Hospital Research Foundation,
Parkville, 3052, Australia
[*]John Curtin School of Medical Research, Canberra, Australia

INTRODUCTION

Elevated levels of a pterin, believed to be 7,8-dihydroxanthopterin,
have been demonstrated in urine from patients with phenylketonuria (PKU)
and a patient with dihydropteridine reductase (DHPR) deficiency[1]. This
pterin was readily converted to xanthopterin the yellow fluorescence of
which enabled it to be detected and investigated. In patients with
PKU dietary restriction of phenylalanine, the standard therapy to prevent mental retardation, decreased the level of 7,8-dihydroxanthopterin
in urine.

It has been reported that phenylalanine could affect pterin metabolism[2] and that pterin metabolism was affected in PKU[3,4]. 5,6,7,8-
tetrahydrobiopterin is the essential cofactor for phenylalanine hydroxylase, tyrosine hydroxylase and tryptophan hydroxylase[5,6]. DHPR is
required for the regeneration of 5,6,7,8-tetrahydrobiopterin after
hydroxylation and may be required for the de novo synthesis of 5,6,7,8-
tetrahydrobiopterin.

METHODS

High voltage electrophoresis (HVE) was performed as previously
described[1] and migration of pterins was expressed relative to quinine
(R_Q). Thin layer chromatography (TLC) was performed on cellulose in
3% ammonium chloride and 0.1M K_2HPO_4. Ascending paper chromatography
was performed on Whatman 3MM paper in 3% ammonium chloride, 5% acetic
acid, and 0.1M K_2HPO_4. Xanthopterin (6,7-^{14}C) was synthesised by
W.L.F. Armarego using a modification of the method of Albert and Wood[7]
and reduced with sodium borohydride to produce 7,8-dihydroxanthopterin
(6,7-^{14}C).

RESULTS

Preliminary studies revealed that the pterin in urine migrated
during HVE to R_Q 0.15 and was converted to a yellow fluorescent compound
when the paper was dried. After elution this compound migrated during

160

HVE to R_Q 0.20 and when mixed with urine HVE clearly separated it from the pterin in urine. Yellow fluorescence was not observed at R_Q 0.15 after HVE of solutions containing biopterin, 7,8-dihydrobiopterin or 5,6,7,8-tetrahydrobiopterin. Yellow fluorescence was observed at R_Q 0.15 after HVE of 5,6,7,8-tetrahydropterin which is known to be oxidised to 7,8-dihydroxanthopterin[8].

The pterin in urine from patients with DHPR deficiency and PKU was identical to 7,8-dihydroxanthopterin in the following ways :-
1. Comigration on HVE; R_Q = 0.15
2. Cochromatography in the two TLC systems
3. Neither was fluorescent when viewed immediately after HVE or TLC
4. Both were oxidised to xanthopterin.

After HVE the pterin in urine formed a compound shown to be identical to xanthopterin in the following ways :-
1. Comigration on HVE; R_Q = 0.20.
2. Cochromatography in the two TLC systems and the three paper chromatography systems.
3. Fluorescence spectra in 0.1M NaOH.
4. Oxidation product after treatment with xanthine oxidase[9] migrated with leucopterin on HVE and the three paper chromatography systems.
5. Reduction product after treatment with sodium borohydride migrated with 7,8-dihydroxanthopterin on HVE.

Investigation of urine from normal adults and children revealed a compound which comigrated with 7,8-dihydroxanthopterin during HVE and was converted to a compound with the same fluorescent spectrum as xanthopterin in 0.1M NaOH.

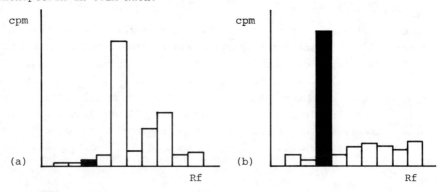

■ Region of putative 7,8-dihydroxanthopterin.

Fig.1. TLC in 0.1M K_2HPO_4 of PKU urine mixed with (a) xanthopterin (6,7-^{14}C) and (b) 7,8-dihydroxanthopterin (6,7-^{14}C).

Administration of a 7 g oral phenylalanine load to three normal adults significantly increased the amount of 7,8-dihydroxanthopterin in their urine.

Experiments with labelled pterins were performed by Dr. W. L. F. Armarego to confirm that the pterin in urine was 7,8-dihydroxanthopterin rather than an adduct or hydrate of xanthopterin. Xanthopterin $(6,7-{}^{14}C)$ was added to PKU urine and stored at $2^{\circ}C$. An aliquot was separated on TLC in 0.1M K_2HPO_4 after 24 hours and 48 hours. After 24 hours the radioactivity was predominantly recovered from the position of xanthopterin (Fig.1a), while the presence of several radioactive bands suggested that much of the xanthopterin added was found to other compounds in the urine. After 48 hours the proportion of the counts in the xanthopterin band dropped by 50%, while that of the 7,8 dihydroxanthopterin band was not significantly altered. An aliquot of 7,8-dihydroxanthopterin $(6,7-{}^{14}C)$ added to PKU urine was separated on TLC in 0.1M K_2HPO_4 after two hours at $2^{\circ}C$. The major radioactive band corresponded to the position of 7,8-dihydroxanthopterin (Fig.1b).

A sample of 5,6,7,8-tetrahydrobiopterin was mixed with distilled water or freshly voided urine and either frozen or incubated in the dark at $37^{\circ}C$ for seven hours. HVE of the solutions revealed that 7,8-dihydroxanthopterin was produced from 5,6,7,8-tetrahydrobiopterin by mixing with either urine and freezing or water and incubating at $37^{\circ}C$. Maximum production of 7,8-dihydroxanthopterin occurred when 5,6,7,8-tetrahydrobiopterin was incubated with urine. When this protocol was repeated with 7,8-dihydrobiopterin, produced by alkaline reduction of biopterin with zinc[10], no 7,8-dihydroxanthopterin was produced.

DISCUSSION

The evidence presented indicates that the pterin elevated in urine from DHPR deficient and PKU patients is 7,8-dihydroxanthopterin. The studies with xanthopterin $(6,7-{}^{14}C)$ clearly show that the pterin in urine is not an adduct or hydrate of xanthopterin and confirm its identification as 7,8-dihydroxanthopterin. Isolation of 7,8-dihydroxanthopterin from urine is difficult due to its instability but this work is in progress and is necessary for confirmation.

The recovery of a compound with a fluorescent spectrum identical to xanthopterin from the position of 7,8-dihydroxanthopterin after HVE constitutes good evidence for the presence of 7,8-dihydroxanthopterin in normal urine. Thus 7,8-dihydroxanthopterin appears to be a normal metabolite in urine, which is abnormally elevated in patients with DHPR deficiency or PKU.

The incubation studies reported indicate that 5,6,7,8-dihydro-biopterin, but not 7,8-dihydrobiopterin, may give rise to 7,8-dihydro-xanthopterin while urine is stored in the bladder. Thus 7,8-dihydro-xanthopterin in urine may reflect the excretion of 5,6,7,8-tetrahydro-biopterin by the kidney. This suggestion is consistent with the studies of Rembold on the catabolism of pterins[8].

In patients with PKU dietary restriction of phenylalanine decreased the amount of 7,8-dihydroxanthopterin in urine[11] (Fig.2). The regress-ion line shown for the patients with PKU was calculated by the method of least squares and the correlation coefficient was 0.94. In contrast the DHPR deficient patient maintained elevated levels of 7,8-dihydro-xanthopterin in urine, although serum and urine phenylalanine were within the range for well controlled PKU patients. The three normal adults investigated had increased 7,8-dihydroxanthopterin in urine after oral phenylalanine loading. Thus both PKU children and normal

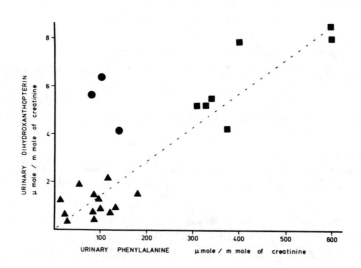

Fig.2. Relationship between 7,8-dihydroxanthopterin and phenylalanine in urine from PKU patients before (■) and during (▲) dietary restriction of phenylalanine and the DHPR deficient patient (●).

adults showed a causal relationship between oral phenylalanine intake and 7,8-dihydroxanthopterin in urine. It seems probable that in normal adults and PKU children elevation of serum phenylalanine either stimulates the de novo synthesis of 5,6,7,8-tetrahydrobiopterin or perturbs the pathway in some unknown way. These results are similar to the response of serum Crithidia factor levels reported by Leeming et al[3]. The observations in normal individuals were not extended to allow formal regression analysis as we do not believe it is possible to mimic in normal individuals the chronic hyperphenylalaninemia present in PKU.

The origin of 7,8-dihydroxanthopterin in the urine of the patient with DHPR deficiency is not as readily explained. The dramatic decrease in this patient's serum phenylalanine after administration of 5,6,7,8-tetrahydrobiopterin[12] supports the suggestion that DHPR deficiency is likely to cause deficiency of 5,6,7,8-tetrahydrobiopterin in plasma rather than excess. In DHPR deficiency its substrate, para quinonoid dihydrobiopterin would be expected to accumulate and may give rise to 7,8-dihydroxanthopterin in urine. Further investigation is required to determine whether DHPR is required for the de novo synthesis of 5,6,7,8-tetrahydrobiopterin or merely for its regeneration after hydroxylation. Elucidation of the pathway for de novo synthesis of 5,6,7,8-tetrahydrobiopterin should reveal the nature of the gross disturbance of pterin metabolism in DHPR deficiency and the origin of 7,8-dihydroxanthopterin in the urine of these patients.

Xanthopterin was first reported in urine by Koschara[13]. It was later revealed that free xanthopterin is not present in urine and the precursor in urine of the xanthopterin observed was termed "pro-xanthopterin"[14]. It is interesting to speculate that the "pro-xanthopterin" reported may have been 7,8-dihydroxanthopterin, particularly as they are both converted to xanthopterin under similar conditions.

Analysis of 7,8-dihydroxanthopterin in urine aids the diagnosis of DHPR deficiency and the management of PKU. Further investigation of pterin metabolism may elucidate the cause of mental retardation in these inborn errors of metabolism. This appears to be the first report of 7,8-dihydroxanthopterin in human urine.

REFERENCES

1. Watson, B.M., Schlesinger, P. and Cotton, R.G.H. (1977) Clin.Chim.Acta. 78, 417-423.
2. Schwink, I. (1965) Zeitschr. für Naturforschung, 20b, 322-326.

3. Leeming, R.J., Blair, J.A., Green, A. and Raine, D.N. (1976) Arch.Dis.Child., 51, 771-777.

4. Kaufman, S. (1958) Science, 128, 1506-1508.

5. Kaufman, S. (1964) in Pteridine Chemistry, Proceedings of the Third International Symposium, Pergamon Press, Oxford. pp. 307-326.

6. Kaufman, S. (1974) Ciba Foundation Symposium 22, 85-115.

7. Albert, A. and Wood, H.C.S. (1952) J.Appl.Chem. 591.

8. Rembold, H. (1970) in Chemistry and Biology of Pteridines, Proceedings of the Fourth International Symposium, International Academic Printing Co., Tokyo. pp. 163-178.

9. Chippel, D. and Scrimgeour, K.G. (1970) Can.J.Biochem., 48, 999-1099.

10. Kaufman, S. (1967) J.Biol.Chem. 242, 3934-3943.

11. Schlesinger, P. Watson, B.M., Cotton, R.G.H. and Danks, D.M. (1978) Submitted to Clin.Chim.Acta.

12. Danks, D.M., Schlesinger, P., Firgaira, F., Cotton, R.G.H., Watson, B.M., Rembold, H. and Hennings, G. (1978). Paediatric Research (In press).

13. Koschara, W. (1936) Z. für Physiol.Chemie. 2403, 127-151.

14. Floystrup, T., Schou, M.A. and Kalckar, H.M. (1949) Acta. Chem.Scand., 3, 985-986.

IN VIVO METABOLISM OF DEUTERO-L-PHENYLALANINE AND DEUTERO-L-TYROSINE AND LEVELS
OF TETRAHYDROBIOPTERIN IN THE BLOOD OF TUMOR BEARING ORGANISMS

IRMGARD ZIEGLER AND NIKOS KOKOLIS

Institut für Toxikologie und Biochemie der Gesellschaft für Strahlen- und
Umweltforschung, Arcisstr.16, 8000 München 2 (FRG)

ABSTRACT

The levels of tetrahydrobiopterin in all tumor patients tested average 200 fold
more than that for the control. However, in experimental tumor rats the turnover
rate of phenylalanine hydroxylase was found to be decreased under in vivo conditions. Kinetic data indicate that about 20% of the tyrosine is constantly withdrawn
from its normal catabolic pathway. These metabolic changes result in elevated blood
levels of phenylalanine and of free and protein bound tyrosine in tumor patients
and in experimental tumor rats. In the case of melanoma, the analytical data agree
with the view that withdrawal of tyrosine from normal catabolism takes place as
long as melanosomes are present for final melanin synthesis.

INTRODUCTION

The Crithidia active substance of human blood ascribed to biopterin, was found
to be as low as 1.9 ng/ml[1]. It is generally accepted that it is not derived from
folic acid degradation[2,3], but is synthesized de novo from the purine precursor[4].
Starting from experiments with neoplastic cell growth during the regeneration process
in Triturus[5], we focused our attention on the levels of tetrahydrobiopterin in the
blood of tumor animals and of tumor patients. Those results in turn precipitated
a study of phenylalanine and tyrosine metabolism in vivo by using both as deuterated
compounds. The levels of both amino acids in the blood also were quantitatively
determined.

MATERIALS AND METHODS

Pterin and amino acid analysis. Blood sampling(rats:Wistar and Holtzman strains;
mice: NMR I) and preparation, the paper chromatographic separation and fluorometric
determination of tetrahydrobiopterin, and the quantitative analysis of free amino
acids by automated amino acid analyzer are described in[6]. The determination of free
and of protein bound tyrosine, using the reaction with 1-nitrosonapthol(2) proved
to be most specific[6]. P values were obtained by Student's t test.
In vivo metabolism of phenylalanine and tyrosine. Both these ring-deuterated amino
acids were injected i.p.,and the deuterium in the water fraction of the blood was
determined by mass spectrometry[7]. The slight modifications of this method and the
basis for calculation of turnover rates are described in[8].

RESULTS

Quantitative determination of tetrahydrobiopterin. Using the fluorometric method, the amount of ⟨2ng/ml in control persons[1] can not be traced. However, in all tumor patients tested considerable amounts had accumulated (table 1). The range may vary widely within different cases of the same carcinoma (e.g.bronchogenic carcinoma), seemingly dependent on the status of illness. In samples of 6 additional tumor patients, calibration curves with pterincarbonic acid (6) indicate that the tetrahydrobiopterin concentration per ml in whole blood averages 400 ng (S.D.= ± 155). This means that it is more than 200 times greater than the control value[1].

TABLE 1

AMOUNT OF TETRAHYDROBIOPTERIN IN CONTROL AND IN TUMOR BEARING PERSONS
Arbitrary fluorometric units

	erythrocytes (0.5 ml)	S.D.	serum (0.2 ml)	S.D.
Controls	7.5	5.0	0	
Tumor patients[a]	644.0	± 210.6	236.4	± 124.9
Bronchogenic carcinoma (4 cases)	1 416.0	± 1 285.6	376.0	± 327.2
Melanoblastoma (eye) (2 cases)	25 000, 4 000		1 200, 1 000	

[a]Epidermal foot carcinoma, epidermal nose carcinoma, breast carcinoma (adeno carcinoma), oesophageal carcinoma, pharynx carcinoma, carcinoma of the larynx, lung carcinoma, Hodgkin's disease.

Quantitative determination of tyrosine and phenylalanine. As seen in table 2,free + protein bound tyrosine definitely show elevated levels in tumor patients.

TABLE 2

AMOUNT OF FREE + PROTEIN-BOUND TYROSINE IN THE BLOOD OF CONTROL AND OF TUMOR BEARING PERSONS
Determination: reaction using 1-nitrosonaphthol (2)

	nmoles/ml blood	S.D.	P value
Controls	299.0	± 27.14	
Tumor patients[a]	647.66	± 152.12	⟨ 0.001

[a]Osteogenic sarcoma, mamma carcinoma (2 cases), teratoma of testicle, Hodgkin's disease, reticulum cell carcinoma.

A similar increase for free tyrosine alone (P= ⟨0.01) was found in all cases investigated (metastatic breast carcinoma, myeloma, Hodgkin's disease, colon carcinoma, lymphosarcoma).

Automated amino acid analysis confirmed the results above and furthermore showed that the levels of phenylalanine are also increased. No change occurs with respect to the amount of total free amino acids (table 3).

TABLE 3

AMOUNT OF FREE TYROSINE AND OF FREE PHENYLALANINE IN THE BLOOD OF CONTROL AND OF TUMOR BEARING PERSONS

Automated amino acid analysis; values are given in nmoles/ml blood

	total amino acids	S.D.	phenyl-alanine	S.D.	tyrosine	S.D.
Controls	2 149.0	± 232.1	26.2	± 15.3	111.9	± 48.6
Tumor patients[a]	2 282.5	± 252.3	57.5	± 16.4[b]	304.8	± 64.4[c]

[a]Tumor patients are the same as listed in table 2; [b] P = < 0.001; [c]P = < 0.01

Clearly elevated levels of free phenylalanine and tyrosine were found also in experimental tumor rats (Ascites AH 130, Guerin T-8).

A most different situation, however, was found in the case of melanomas. On the one hand, patients with melanomas are characterized by exceedingly high levels of tetrahydrobiopterin(table 1); on the other hand, in mice with Harding Passey melanomas, tyrosine + m-tyrosine, which comprise 5.0% of the total free amino acids (S.D.= ± 0.5), drop to 3.7% (S.D.= ± 0.6), whereas phenylalanine stays at the same level: 2% in the controls (S.D.= ± 0.3) and 2.3% in melanoma animals (S.D.= ± 0.15).

In vivo metabolism of deutero-L-phenylalanine and deutero-L-tyrosine.

Rate of phenylalanine hydroxylation and of tyrosine catabolism. From table 4 it is evident that both these rates are reduced in tumor animals. The hydroxylation step is the rate-limiting one not only in the control animals, but also in the tumor animals.

TABLE 4

DEUTERIUM RELEASE INTO THE BODY WATER OF RATS (oo) AFTER INJECTION OF (^{2}H)-PHENYLALANINE AND OF (^{2}H)-TYROSINE RESPECTIVELY

Application: 200 mg/kg; blood drawn 1 h after injection

	ppm phenylalanine degraded/mmol inj.	S.D.	ppm tyrosine degraded/ mmol injected	S.D.
Controls	5.65	± 0.46	26.33	± 1.07
Tumor animals[a]	3.12	± 0.73[b]	23.10	± 1.04[c]

[a]Multiple cases of Jensen sarcoma and Ascites hepatoma; [b]P= < 0.001; [c]P= < 0.01

From 2 - 14 days following the injection of Yoshida ascites hepatoma 130, the hydroxylation rate steadily decreases, finally dropping to 8% of that of the control.

Time course of phenylalanine hydroxylation and tyrosine catabolism. Blood was
drawn after 30, 60, and 120 min after injection of the deuterated compound. Both
rates level off with time since the substrate concentrations decrease; the plateau
is reached after 60 min. Relative to the control in tumor rats the hydroxylation
rate increases with time (fig.1). This indicates that the turnover rate of the enzyme is decreased. Thus D_2O formation catches up with time, whereas in the controls
it had already levelled off. In contrast, the relative percentage to normal D_2O
formation from deuterated tyrosine stays nearly constant during the whole period.
This does not indicate a lowered turnover rate of enzymes involved in the catabolic
pathway, but rather suggests a steady elimination of tyrosine itself or of an
intermediate compound en route to D_2O.

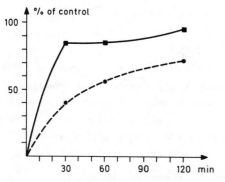

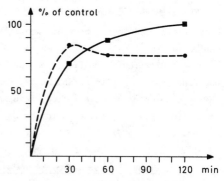

Fig.1 Percentage of phenylalanine hydroxylation ●—● and of tyrosine catabolism ■—■
in relation to control. Wistar ♂♂; Yoshida
ascites hepatoma 180, 8 days after inoculation. 200 md deut.amino acid/kg

Percentage of phenylalanine catabolism
●---● and of tyrosine catabolism
■—■ in relation to control. NMR I ♂♂;
weight 30-35g; Harding Passey melanoma;
200 mg deuterated amino acid/kg

Among tumor animals melanoma-bearing mice display a number of variations. - The
D_2O formation from tyrosine is lowered (though tyrosinase action liberates half the
amount of D_2O compared to total catabolism), but it catches up with time (fig.2).
This can be explained by the prerequisites of melanin synthesis: after injection,
parts of the tyrosine overload are withdrawn from normal catabolism and used for
melanin formation. For its final synthesis melanosomes are needed, whose new synthesis requires hours[9]. Thus their amount present at injection time sets the thresh-
hold level for withdrawal of tyrosine. Thereafter, the tyrosine approaches normal
degradation rate. - The steadily lowered level of D_2O formation after application
of deuterated phenylalanine cannot be used as evidence of whether or not the
hydroxylase is impaired. But it mirrors the fact that parts of the tyrosine delivered by the possibly impaired hydroxylase are immediately used up in melanin
synthesis. This much lower delivery as compared to the overload caused by injected

deuterated tyrosine, seemingly does not result in saturation of the melanosomes
during the time period measured.

ppm aminoacid catabolized

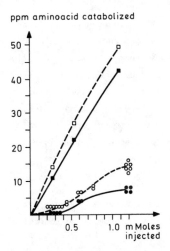

Fig.3 Rate of tyrosine catabolism in controls ▫---▫ , in
tumor rats ▪—▪; of phenylalanine hydroxylation in controls
o--o, in tumor rats ●—● .
Wistar ♂♂, Yoshida ascites
hepatoma 130, 8 days after inoculation. Blood drawn 1 h
after injection.

Substrate kinetics. In the controls the substrate
kinetics of tyrosine catabolism are a linear function of the amount of tyrosine injected (fig.3).
In tumor rats, the percentage to normal D_2O formation increases from 77% to 87% with the amount
of tyrosine injected. Since Lineweaver-Burk plots
do not indicate a competitive inhibition, the
data are consistent with the view that tyrosine
or one of its catabolic intermediates is withdrawn
from the route to D_2O formation. As is expected,
this process has a substrate affinity of its own
and its saturation seems to take place at a relatively low tyrosine concentration. Thus at high
tyrosine concentrations, overspill results in
an approach to normal D_2O formation rates.
In contrast to normal hyperbolic tyrosine catabolism, phenylalanine hydroxylation shows sigmoidal
kinetics (fig.3). Thus a homotropic activation,
previously demonstrated by in vitro experiments[10],
is also shown to occur under in vivo conditions.
Although the turnover rate is clearly decreased
in tumor animals, the kinetic behaviour remains
unchanged.

DISCUSSION

With respect to diagnostic application these results stimulate the need for
further quantitative determinations of tetrahydrobiopterin, tyrosine, and phenylalanine in the blood, or of pterin-6-aldehyde[6] in urine in even more tumor cases,
and for comparison with a manifold of other diseases, e.g. acute infections. Three
to four fold increases in blood biopterin content in uremia or in alcoholic liver
disease[1] or 15 fold increase after methotrexate application[11] do not approach the
levels found in cases of tumor. Separate investigations are especially needed with
respect to PKU, where lowered phenylalanine hydroxylase activity occurs and where
elevated levels of Crithidia active pterin give rise to urinary dihydroxanthopterin[12].

We are aware that the analytical data prompt more questions than they are solving.
Whether the elevated levels of tetrahydrobiopterin, most probably resulting from
tumor specific folic acid degradation[6], and the impairment of phenylalanine

hydroxylase, which seems to be present in tumor tissue with a different isozyme[13], represent primary or subsequent stages during tumor growth needs further investigation. At this point only the following generalization may be put up for discussion: Withdrawal of tyrosine from its normal catabolic pathway seems to be one of the characteristics of tumor-bearing organisms. - Catechol amine accumulation in cases of neuroblastoma, ganglioneuroma or pheochromocytoma[14], melanin formation in melanoma, and accumulation of hydroxyphenylacetic acid derivatives in islet cell tumor[15] are cases of "specialized" tyrosine usage. A detailed characterization of their respective tyrosine hydroxylase and tyrosinase is needed. In tumor cases, where this does not occur, tyrosine in its free or protein-bound form is simply stored. In both cases, however, the rate of complete tyrosine catabolism is decreased in tumor organisms.

ACKNOWLEDGEMENTS

We are indebted to Dr.W.Stichler,GSF, for mass spectrometric deuterium determination, and to Dr.H.Kummermehr, GSF, for providing Harding Passey melanoma. The sources of all other animals and of patients are listed in[5,8].

REFERENCES

1. Baker,H.,Frank,O.,Bacchi,C.J.and Hutner,S.H.(1974) Amer.J.Clin.Nutr.,27,1247-53.
2. Fukushima,K.,Eto,I.Richter,W.,Goodson,S. and Shiota,T.(1975) in Chemistry and Biology of Pteridines,Pfleiderer,W. ed., de Gruyter, Berlin, pp.247-263.
3. Halpern,R.,Halpern,B.C.,Stea,B.,Dunlap,A.,Conklin,K.,Clark,B.Ashe,H.Sperling,L., Halpern,J.,Hardy,D. and Smith,R.(1977) Proc.Natl.Acad.Sci.(USA),74, 587-591.
4. Buff,K. and Dairman,W.(1975) in Chemistry and Biology of Pterdines, Pfleiderer, W. ed., de Gruyter, Berlin, pp. 273-283.
5. Kokolis,N.,Mylonas,N.and Ziegler,I.(1972) Zeitschr.f.Naturforschg.,27b,285-291.
6. Kokolis,N. and Ziegler,I. (1977) Cancer Biochem.Biophys., 2, 79 - 85.
7. Milstien,S. and Kaufman,S. (1975) J.Biol.Chem., 250, 4782 - 4785.
8. Ziegler,I.,Kokolis,N. and Stichler,W. (1977) Cancer Biochem.Biophys.,2,71-77.
9. Brumbaugh,J.A. and Schall,D.G. (1977) J.Exp.Zool., 202, 163 - 170.
10. Ayling,J.E. and Helfand,D.G. (1975) in Chemistry and Biology of Pteridines, Pfleiderer, W. ed., de Gruyter, Berlin, pp. 305 - 320.
11. Leeming,R.J.,Blair,J.A.,Melikian,V.and O'Gorman,D.(1976) J.Clin.Path.,29,444-451.
12. Watson,B.M.,Schlesinger,P. and Cotton,R.G.H.(1977) Clin.chim.Acta, 78, 417-423.
13. Tourian, A. (1976) Biochem.Biophys.Res.Comm., 68, 51 - 55.
14. Hinterberger,H. and Bartholomew,R,J. (1969) Clin.chim.Acta, 23, 169 - 175.
15. Axelsson,S., Cegrell,L. and Rosengren,A.M. (1970) Experientia, 26, 998 - 999.

NON-PTERIDINE COFACTORS FOR PHENYLALANINE HYDROXYLASE

S. W. BAILEY and J. E. AYLING
University of Texas at San Antonio, San Antonio, Texas 78285

The most striking feature of tetrahydrobiopterin, cofactor of aromatic amino acid hydroxylases[1] (Fig. 1), is its highly activated pyrimidine nucleus. That the general lability to oxidation of tetrahydropterins is contained in this part of the molecule is demonstrated by early work on substituted pyrimidines[2]. With this in mind, an extrapolation of previous studies[3] of the effectiveness of tetrahydrobiopterin analogs in the reaction of phenylalanine hydroxylase has provided a useful new probe of enzymatic hydroxylation mechanisms.

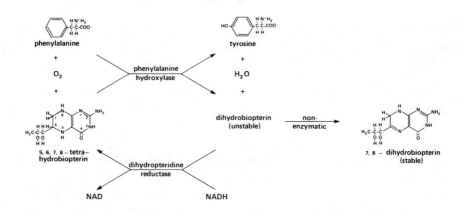

Fig. 1. Function of tetrahydrobiopterin as cofactor in enzymatic hydroxylation of aromatic amino acids.

That the dihydroxypropyl group of tetrahydrobiopterin (I, Fig. 2) is not necessary for catalytic activity has already been demonstrated by its replacement with a methyl group[4] (II, Fig. 2) which, although eliminating several regulatory properties[5], does not significantly alter the maximum rate of enzymatic hydroxylation. With tetrahydropterin (III, Fig. 2) as cofactor phenylalanine hydroxylase no longer couples oxidation of cofactor to hydroxylation of phenylalanine[3]. However, tyrosine is still produced at 20% of the rate as with tetrahydrobiopterin (Fig. 2).

	R	K_m	Rel. V_{max}
A.	I. $CH_3CHOHCHOH-$	20 μM	1
	II. CH_3	80 μM	1
	III. H	130 μM	0.2
	V. C_6H_5	3 μM	0.2
B.	IV. H	50 μM	0.008
	VI. $C_6H_5CH_2$	3 μM	0.002

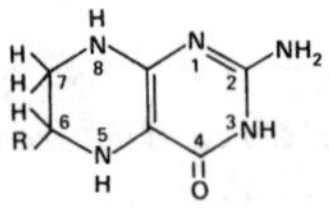

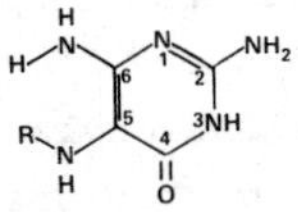

Fig. 2. A. 6-Substituted pterins, and, B. 5-substituted 2,6-diamino-4-pyrimidinones, active as cofactors for phenylalanine hydroxylase. The K_m values are apparent K_m's measured at 1 mM phenylalanine and atmospheric O_2, at 27° and pH 7.4.

We wished to determine, by further structural modifications, to what extent the sigma bonded 6 and 7 carbon atoms of the tetrahydropterin ring contribute to the cofactor properties. As an alkyl group these atoms add slightly to the general activation of the pyrimidine ring (pK of 2,5,6-triamino-4-pyrimidinone N-5 = 5.1[6]; pK of tetrahydropterin N-5 = 5.6[7]), and restrict the degrees of freedom of the 5 and 8 nitrogens. Our recent studies on the retention of configuration at the 6-carbon atom of tetrahydrobiopterin[8] have conclusively confirmed[9,10] that the hydrogens on the 6-carbon, as well as those on the 7-carbon[9], are not utilized in the enzymatic reaction.

Cofactor activity of substituted pyrimidines
    To test the possibility that the complete pyrazine ring of tetrahydropterin may not be an absolute requirement for cofactor function, 2,5,6-triamino-4-pyrimidinone (IV, Fig. 2) was added to a mixture containing phenylalanine and phenylalanine hydroxylase. Indeed, this pyrimidine is capable of supporting enzyme catalyzed p-tyrosine formation, at a rate which is about 1% that of tetrahydrobiopterin, or 4% that of tetrahydropterin (III)(Fig. II). The reaction with 2,5,6-triamino-4-pyrimidinone is uncoupled(i.e. more cofactor oxidized than tyrosine formed), as also is the reaction with tetrahydropterin[3], and

this contributes partly to the decreased tyrosine formation. A new assay which can detect picomole quantities of tyrosine has been developed to facilitate the measurement of these low rates[11].

The affinity (K_m) of 2,5,6-triamino-4-pyrimidinone (IV) for phenylalanine hydroxylase is between that of tetrahydrobiopterin (I) and tetrahydropterin (III) (Fig. 2). However, concentrations of the pyrimidine cofactor above 0.2 mM begin to inhibit, prohibiting accurate measurements of apparent K_m, as well as of V_{max}. Thus the values given are at best an approximation, but they are sufficient to indicate that the 6 and 7 carbon atoms contribute very little to the overall binding of the cofactor.

That appropriately substituted pyrimidines can participate as co-factors in enzymatic hydroxylation opens new paths of investigation of the forces involved in cofactor binding, the nature of the transition states, and the mechanism of enzymatic oxygen activation. Toward these ends we have synthesized series of new pyrimidines and are study-ing their chemical properties and interactions with phenylalanine hydr-oxylase. Since there are orders of magnitude differences in reactivit-ies of some of these compounds a high degree of purity has been ascert-ained by high pressure liquid chromatographic analysis. An example of the power of this approach with pyrimidines is illustrated by the following study.

Mechanism of enzymatic oxygen activation

There are currently several hypotheses for the mechanism of activat-ion of molecular oxygen by flavin mediated oxygenases[12-16]. These theories differ with respect to the initial point of attack of the oxygen, usually one of the bridgehead carbons, and the nature of the functionality containing the oxygen, e.g. hydroperoxide, oxaziridine, vinylogous ozone. The common features of dihydroflavin and tetrahydro-biopterin have lead to the suggestion that tetrahydrobiopterin may function in the hydroxylation of aromatic amino acids analogously to flavins. In the hypothesis of Hamilton[17] (Fig. 3) an oxenoid reagent is created from dihydroflavin or tetrahydrobiopterin by attack of oxygen at position 4a (8a also suggested), followed by cleavage of the 4a - 5 bond, possibly facilitated by enzymatic protonation. The res-ulting vinylogous ozone, or perhaps cyclic trioxide[18], with sufficient resonance delocalization, might create electrophilic oxygen and/or lower the transition energy of oxenoid attack on an aromatic system. Following oxygen transfer the pyrazine ring would recyclize by Schiff's base condensation forming a 4a - OH intermediate. This 4a - OH inter-

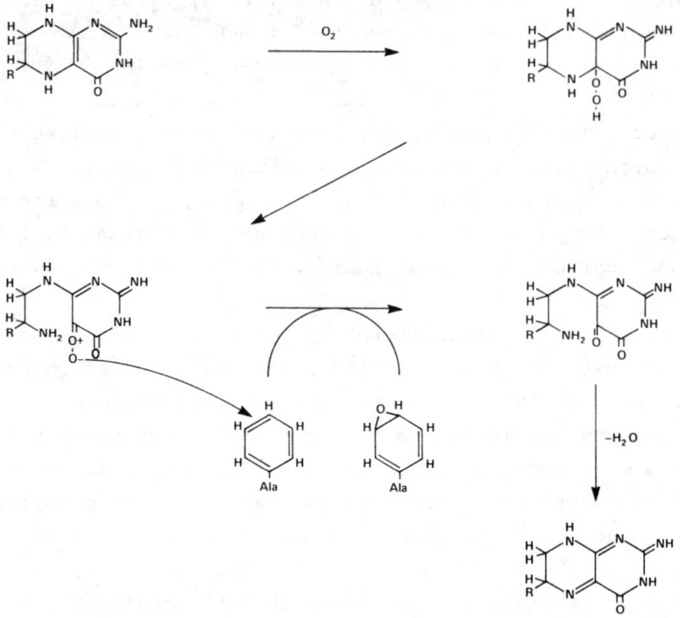

Fig. 3. Mechanism of oxygen activation by tetrahydropterins proposed by Hamilton[17].

mediate, a common end product of several of the proposed activation schemes[12,14,16], then dehydrates to a form which can be reduced by NADH (Fig. 3, Fig. 1).

We have used a pyrimidine cofactor to directly test this hypothesis. If during phenylalanine hydroxylation the mechanism proposed by Hamilton is operating, and an appropriately substituted pyrimidine (equivalent to a tetrahydropterin, minus carbon 7) is supplied as cofactor, it should be cleaved, at least temporarily, to two separate molecules, - an oxidized pyrimidine and an amine (Fig. 4). The detection of this amine, if produced specifically by phenylalanine dependent utilization of cofactor, and not by any auto-oxidation process, would provide convincing evidence for a theory which involves cleavage of the 4a - 5 bond.

A specific pyrimidine probe for this experiment was chosen after considering that the structure must be compatible with our knowledge of cofactor binding requirements and that the resulting amine must be detectable in picomole quantities in the presence of all other amines, such as phenylalanine and tyrosine, present in the reaction. This

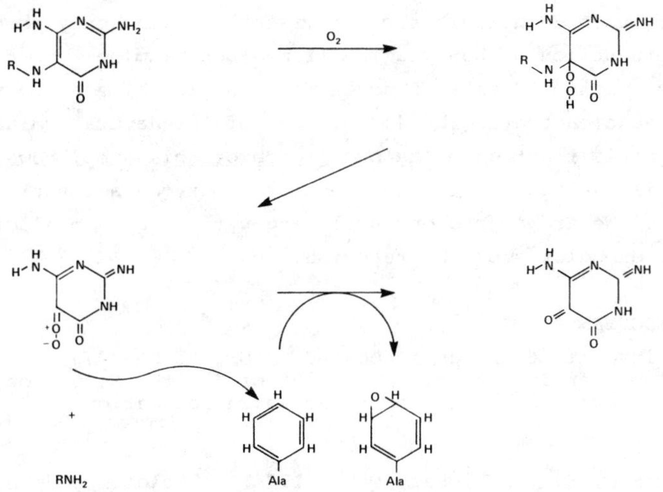

Fig. 4. Mechanism of oxygen activation proposed by Hamilton as applied to pyrimidines.

level of sensitivity in detecting the amine was required because (a) pyrimidines function more slowly in the hydroxylation reaction than do tetrahydropterins, and (b) a large percentage of the initially cleaved products might recombine and thus escape detection.

6-Phenyltetrahydropterin (V, Fig. 2) possesses a very high affinity for the catalytic site and a maximum velocity similar to that of tetrahydropterin (III, Fig. 2). The analogous pyrimidine (i.e. lacking the 7 - carbon), 5-benzylamino-2, 6-diamino-4-pyrimidinone (VI, Fig. 2), was therefore tested for cofactor activity. This pyrimidine also proved to be active with phenylalanine hydroxylase but, as with other pyrimidines with cofactor activity, catalyzes an uncoupled reaction. Although the pyrimidine reacts a hundred times slower than 6-phenyltetrahydropterin, both compounds have the same high affinity (K_m = 3 µM) (Fig. 2). With this pyrimidine the resulting product of a ring opening mechanism would be benzylamine. A high pressure liquid chromatographic system was used to separate the reactants, followed by general amine detection by o-phthalaldehyde.

When oxidized with iodine, 5-benzylamino-2,6-diamino-4-pyrimidinone readily hydrolyzes to benzaldehyde and 2,5,6-triamino-4-pyrimidinone. When allowed to auto-oxidize in air at neutral pH the same products are formed. In the phenylalanine hydroxylase reaction, however, about one

third of the pyrimidine cofactor consumed by the enzyme yielded benzylamine, with tyrosine being formed at a similar rate. No benzylamine was
detected in an identical reaction mixture lacking only phenylalanine.

The production of benzylamine from 5-benzylamino-2, 6-diamino-4-pyr-
imidinone when used as a cofactor for phenylalanine hydroxylase highly
implicates cleavage of the 4a - 5 bond of the natural cofactor during
the enzymatic reaction. The occurrence of this step, however, does not
necessarily validate the other details of oxygen activation proposed by
Hamilton. We are at present utilizing pyrimidines to elucidate the
other intermediates of the reaction.

ACKNOWLEDGEMENTS

This investigation was supported by Grants CA-20708, awarded by the
National Cancer Institute, Department of Health, Education, and Welfare,
and AX-706 awarded by the Robert A. Welch Foundation.

REFERENCES

1. Kaufman, S. and Fisher, D.B. (1974) in Molecular Mechanisms of Oxy-
    gen Activation, Hayaishi, O. ed. Academic Press, NY pp. 285-369.

2. Brown, D.J. (1962) The Pyrimidines, Wiley Interscience, NY p. 335.

3. Ayling, J.E., Boehm, G.R., Textor, S.C. and Pirson, R.A. (1973)
    Biochemistry, 12, 2045-2051.

4. Kaufman, S. and Levenberg, B. (1959) J. Biol. Chem.,234, 2683-2688.

5. Ayling, J.E. and Helfand, G.H. (1975) in Chemistry and Biology of
    Pteridines, Pfleiderer, W. ed., W. de Gruyter, Berlin, pp. 305-319.

6. Pohland, A., Flynn, E.H., Jones, R.G. and Shive, W. (1951) J. Am.
    Chem. Soc., 73, 3247-3252.

7. Bobst, A. and Viscontini, M. (1966) Helv. Chim. Acta, 49, 875-883.

8. Ayling, J.E. and Bailey, S.W. (1978) Fed. Proc., 37, 1345.

9. Kaufman, S. (1964) J. Biol. Chem., 239, 332-338.

10. Scrimgeour, K.G. (1975) in Chemistry and Biology of Pteridines,
    Pfleiderer, W. ed., W. de Gruyter, Berlin, pp 731-751.

11. Bailey, S.W. and Ayling, J.E., manuscript in preparation.

12. Berends, W., Posthuma, J., Sassenkach, J. and Mager, H. (1966) in
    Flavins and Flavoproteins, Slater, E.C. ed., Elsevier, NY, p. 22.

13. Orf, H. and Dolphin, D. (1974) Proc. Nat. Acad. Sci.,71, 2646-2650.

14. Dmitrienko, G.I., Snieckus, V. and Viswanatha, T. (1977) Biorganic
    Chemistry, 6, 421-429.

15. Hemmerich, P. and Wessiak, A. (1976) in Flavins and Flavoproteins,
    Singer, T.P. ed., Elsevier, NY, pp 9-22.

16. Hamilton, G.A. (1971) in Progress in Biorganic Chemistry, Kaiser,
    E.T. and Kezdy, T.J., eds. Wiley Interscience, NY, Vol. I, p 83.

17. Hamilton, G.A. (1974) in Molecular Mechanisms of Oxygen Activation,
    Hayaishi, O. ed., Academic Press, NY, pp. 405-451.

18. Keay, R.E. and Hamilton, G.A. (1976) J. Am. Chem. Soc., 98, 6578-
    6582.

AFFINITY CHROMATOGRAPHY OF PHENYLALANINE HYDROXYLASE AND
DIHYDROPTERIDINE REDUCTASE ON PTERIN AND NAPHTHOQUINONE ADSORBENTS

RICHARD G. H. COTTON & IAN G. JENNINGS
Genetics Research Unit, Royal Children's Hospital Research Foundation,
Parkville, 3052, Australia

Affinity Chromatography of enzymes allows considerable savings in
time of purification. It is hoped the adsorbents described here will
help in the efficient elucidation of the molecular defects in phenylketonuria and in dihydropteridine reductase deficiency.

1. Phenylalanine hydroxylase.

Earlier papers described the synthesis[1] and use[2,3] of a 6,7-dimethyl
5,6,7,8-tetrahydropterin CH-Sepharose 4B adsorbent for the purification
of phenylalanine hydroxylase. Recently a 5-methyl tetrahydrofolate AH-
Sepharose 4B adsorbent has been used for the purification of rat hepatoma phenylalanine hydroxylase[4]. Otherwise there has only been one
report of an affinity adsorbent being applied to any of the pterin dependent aromatic amino acid hydroxylases, 3 iodotyrosine-Sepharose 4B
for tyrosine hydroxylase[5].

The Me_2PH_4* adsorbent[1] was until recently used[2,3] with little idea
of structure. However recent experiments[6] have indicated a possible
structure.

The initial intention was to couple, using a carbodiimide, the 2-
amino group to the carboxyl of CH-Sepharose 4B. However as no coupling
occurs[6] when the N(5) atom is blocked by a formyl group (see below) it
appears the 2-amino group is not reactive under these conditions. However coupling does occur when Me_2PH_4 is reacted as revealed by the
production of fluorescent compounds after hydrolysis of the gel[1] and by
its biological activity[1].

That the structure is that in Fig.1 and analogous to that of leucovorin (Fig.1) is supported by four independent lines of evidence[6].

(a) Synthesis of a model for the adsorbent by replacing CH-Sepharose
4B by formic acid for the coupling. The major product of this coupling
was shown to be 5-formyl Me_2PH_4 by comparison with authentic material
(kindly provided by Dr. J.Bieri) on 6 separation systems and by mass
spectral analysis.

---

*Abbreviations. PH_4: 5,6,7,8-tetrahydropterin, Me_2PH_4: 6,7-dimethyl
PH_4, BH_4: 5,6,7,8-tetrahydrobiopterin, FH_4 : 5,6,7,8-tetrahydrofolate,
$5MeFH_4$: 5-methyl FH_4, $BH_2$7,8: 7,8-dihydrobiopterin, $Me_2PH_2(7,8)$:7,8-
dihydro 6,7-dimethyl pterin. DTT: dithiothreitol, $MePH_4$: 6-methyl PH_4.

(b) Identity of hydrolysis products from 5-formyl Me_2PH_4 and the adsorbent on 3 separation systems. A considerable proportion of the hydrolysis products are in the tetrahydro form.

(c) 5-formyl Me_2PH_4 does not couple under the standard coupling conditions, indicating that the N(5) is the likely atom of attachment in the adsorbent.

(d) The active pterin moiety in the adsorbent was suspected to be the same as that in leucovorin. Thus an adsorbent was constructed from leucovorin and AH-Sepharose 4B by carbodiimide coupling. As the elution profile[6] of this adsorbent and that of Me_2PH_4 adsorbent under the same conditions were almost identical it was presumed the active pterin moieties were nearly identical. A different performance[4,6] of a 5-methyl tetrahydrofolate - AH-Sepharose 4B adsorbent[6] suggests the pterin moiety in this case is different (possibly 5,6-dihydro). Folate and methotrexate (i.e. oxidized pterins) adsorbents constructed and used similarly were not active. Carbodiimide treated CH-Sepharose was not active.

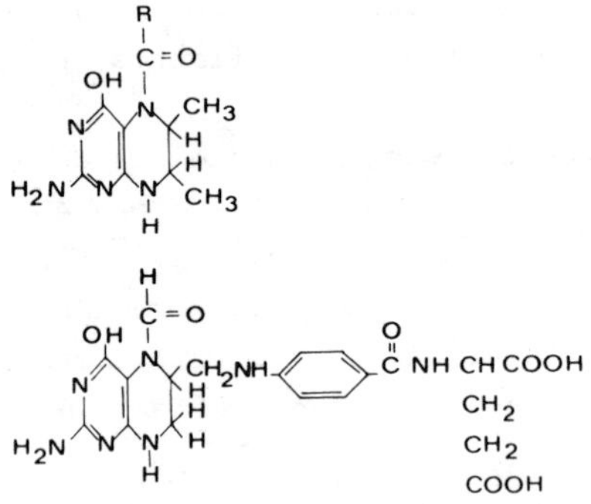

Fig.1. The postulated structure of a Me_2PH_4–CH-Sepharose 4B adsorbent (upper) compared with the structure of 5-formyl FH_4 (leucovorin) (lower). R = pentanyl Sepharose 4B.

Thus we presume the coupling at N(5) serves to fortuitously stabilize the Me_2PH_4 in the tetrahydro state necessary for binding of phenylalanine hydroxylase.

The binding of phenylalanine hydroxylase to leucovorin and 5-methyl tetrahydrofolate adsorbents is interesting as these pterins are neither inhibitors nor cofactors for phenylalanine hydroxylase (evidence reviewed in Ref.6). It is possible that the binding is due to the high salt (0.8N NaCl) present during the operation of the column.

In the earlier publication[2] it was noted that considerable phenylalanine hydroxylase (Peak 1), while initially retarded by the Me_2PH_4 adsorbent column was not retained during the high salt wash. Many manipulations were tried to achieve strong binding. It was disappointing, though interesting, that leucovorin adsorbent behaved in the same way, as this indicated that construction of the adsorbent by a "different route" still gave rise to the same problem. Thus it is unlikely that multiple species of pterin in the Me_2PH_4 adsorbent are responsible for "loose" attachment of peak 1.

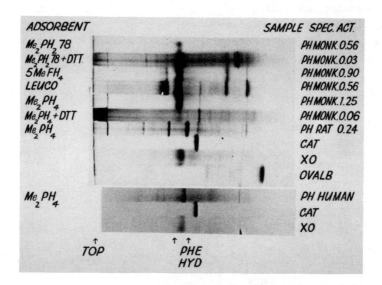

Fig.2. Analysis of phenylalanine hydroxylase (PH)(purified from various species on various affinity adsorbents) and molecular weight markers by native gradipore electrophoresis[6]. Arrows indicate the phenylalanine hydroxylase area (PHE HYD) and the top of the gel. Molecular weight markers are catalase (CAT) 232,000, ovalbumen (OVA) 45,000 and xanthine oxidase (XO) 275,000. MONK = Monkey. K. H. Choo is thanked for the photo of the human protein.

Many different adsorbents were made from different reduced pterins and CH-Sepharose 4B (or AH-Sepharose 4B for tetrahydrofolate species) to see if (a) their removal of phenylalanine hydroxylase was more efficient than that of Me_2PH_4 adsorbent (b) peak 1 could be retained for specific removal by phenylalanine. The following pterins when coupled[1,6] were able to remove a similar amount of enzyme to the Me_2PH_4 adsorbent under the standard conditions:- Me_2PH_2 (7,8), BH_2 (7,8), BH_4, PH_4, $MePH_4$, 5-formyl FH_4 and $5MeFH_4$. The naphthoquinone adsorbent (see below) was slightly less active in removal than these pterins under the same conditions. Only $5MeFH_4$ AH-Sepharose 4B showed any reduction in the amount of Peak 1[4,6]. The two hitherto undescribed tetrahydrofolate adsorbents are likely to be useful in the study of folate metabolizing enzymes.

It is interesting that the strong contaminants purified by the Me_2PH_2 (7,8) +DTT protocol (Fig.2) are not present in material purified by the Me_2PH_4 +DTT protocol (Fig.2). This may indicate a lack of significant Me_2PH_2 (7,8) moiety in the Me_2PH_4 adsorbent.

The degree of purification of phenylalanine hydroxylase obtainable in a single step from rat, monkey and human liver on several different pterin adsorbents can be seen in Fig.2.

2. Dihydropteridine reductase.

Early work[7,8] had indicated the strong inhibition of phenylalanine hydroxylase by 1,2-naphthoquinone. Consequently an adsorbent was constructed[9] by reacting 1,2-naphthoquinone 4-sulphonic acid with AH-

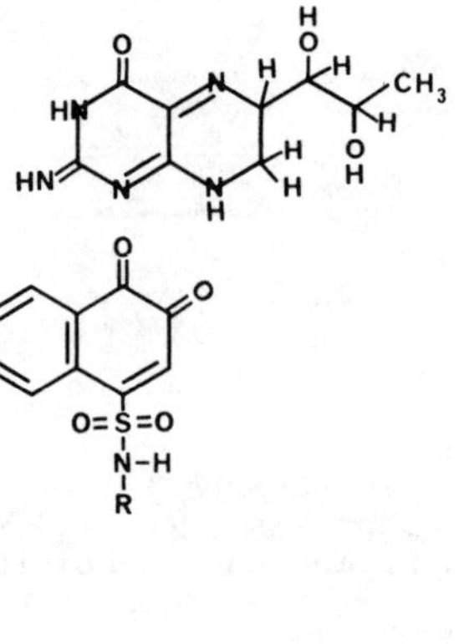

Fig.3. The suggested structure for 1,2-naphthoquinone 4-sulphonic acid AH-Sepharose adsorbent (lower) compared with the structure of p-quinonoid dihydrobiopterin (upper), the substrate for dihydropteridine reductase. R = hexanyl Sepharose 4B.

Sepharose 4B using a water soluble carbodiimide. There was some removal of phenylalanine hydroxylase from a crude monkey liver extract under the standard conditions but the removal of dihydropteridine reductase (DHPR) was substantial[9]. This ability was developed to obtain a substantial purification in a single step[9]. A control adsorbent prepared in the same way with the 1,2-naphthoquinone sulphonic acid omitted did not remove activity from a crude extract.

The property of the adsorbent which allows it to remove DHPR activity from a crude liver extract seems stable for at least 10 months. However the property allowing elution appears to vary with time and gel batch. Thus the original elution protocol[9] changed so activity (similarly highly purified) was eluted with the first pH10.9 buffer wash. Any enzyme retained after this wash could be removed with 2mM DTT in column buffer 1[9] which presumably reduces the adsorbent. Hydrogen peroxide (1mM) in column buffer 1[9] was also effective in eluting activity presumably by oxidizing NADH assumed to be bound to DHPR. The variability in the elution may be due to the reactivity of 1,2-naphthoquinone[10].

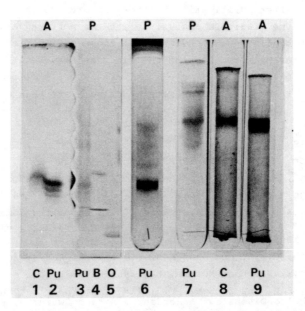

Fig.4. Analysis of human dihydropteridine reductase purified using a 1,2-naphthoquinone 4-sulphonic acid AH-Sepharose 4B adsorbent. A = activity stain and P = protein stain. Samples are either of purified protein (Pu) or crude extract (C). Analysis was by gradipore electrophoresis pH8.7 (samples 1-5) dodecyl sulphate disc electrophoresis (sample 6) or disc electrophoresis at pH9.4 (samples 7-9). The molecular weight markers are ovalbumen (45,000)(O) and bovine serum albumen (67,000)(B).

Unanswered questions are 1. the structure of the adsorbent and 2. the reason for the binding of DHPR so specifically[9] and strongly[9] to the adsorbent.

The structure of the adsorbent may be that shown in Fig.3. However it is possible the amino group of AH-Sepharose 4B has displaced the 4-sulphonic group[10] or that a Schiffs base may have been formed at $C(2)$[10]. Model studies are necessary to resolve this problem.

The structure of p-quinonoid dihydrobiopterin (Fig.3) when compared with that of 1,2-naphthoquinone reveals some similarities. The configuration of the two compounds around atoms 1,2,3,4 of 1,2-naphthoquinone and 4,4a,8a and 1 respectively of p-quinonoid dihydrobiopterin are remarkably similar and may form the basis for the biological activity of the naphthoquinone adsorbent.

The degree of purification that can be obtained in a single step is illustrated in Fig.4. for the human dihydropteridine reductase. Pure enzyme can be obtained with a single further step (F. Firgaira personal communication).

It is interesting that both phenylalanine hydroxylase and DHPR recovered after purification by these adsorbents show tetramer structure[6,9] in the gradipore analysis. Other reports have only demonstrated a dimeric species. The kinetics of these tetramer species is likely to be different from those of the dimer and may reflect the in vivo state.

Dr. R. Truscott and Professor B. Halpern are thanked for solid probe mass spectral studies.

REFERENCES

1. Cotton, R.G.H. (1974) FEBS Letters, 44, 290-292.
2. Cotton, R.G.H. and Grattan, P.J. (1975) Eur.J.Biochem., 60, 427-430.
3. Cotton, R.G.H. and Danks, D.M. (1976) Nature, 260, 63-64.
4. Choo, K.H. and Cotton, R.G.H. (1978) Submitted Somatic Cell Genetics.
5. Lloyd, T. and Kaufman, S. (1974) Biochem.Biophys.Res.Comm. 59, 1262-1269.
6. Cotton, R.G.H. and Jennings, I. (1978) Eur.J.Biochem. 85, 357-363.
7. Zannoni, V.G. and Moraru, E. (1969) FEBS Proc.Meet. 19, 347-354.
8. Ladu, B.N. and Zannoni, V.G. (1967) in Phenylketonuria and Allied Metabolic Diseases. Anderson, J.A. and Swainman, K.F. eds., U.S. Govt. Printing Office, pp.193-204.
9. Cotton, R.G.H. and Jennings, I. (1978) Eur.J.Biochem. 83, 319-324.
10. Mason, H.S. (1955) Advances in Enzymology 16, 105-184.

COFACTOR ACTIVITY OF DIASTEREOISOMERS OF TETRAHYDROBIOPTERIN

HIROYUKI HASEGAWA, SHUNSUKE IMAIZUMI, AND ARATA ICHIYAMA

Department of Biochemistry, Hamamatsu University· School of Medicine
Handa-cho, Hamamatsu 431-31, Japan

TAKASHI SUGIMOTO AND SADAO MATSUURA

Department of Chemistry, College of General Education, Nagoya
University, Furo-cho, Chikusa-ku, Nagoya 464, Japan

KAZUHIRO OKA, TAKESHI KATO, AND TOSHIHARU NAGATSU

Department of Life Chemistry, Graduate School at Nagatsuta, Tokyo
Institute of Technology, Nagatsuta-cho, Midori-ku, Yokohama 227, Japan

MIKI AKINO

Department of Biology, Tokyo Metropolitan University
Fukasawa, Setagaya-ku, Tokyo 158, Japan

INTRODUCTION

Pterin-dependent aromatic amino acid hydroxylases have been studied
using chemically reduced 5,6,7,8-tetrahydropterins (PH_4) such as 6,7-
dimethyltetrahydropterin ($DMPH_4$), 6-methyltetrahydropterin ($6MPH_4$) and
tetrahydrobiopterin (BPH_4) as cofactor. ℓ-erythro-BPH_4 (6-[ℓ-erythro-
1',2'-hydroxypropyl]-tetrahydropterin) is the natural cofactor of the
amino acid hydroxylases. The full expression of regulatory properties
of these enzymes has been shown to be dependent on the structure of the
side chain at the 6 position[1,2,3].

In the chemical reduction of 6-substituted pterins, however, an asymmetric center is introduced at this carbon resulting in the formation
of two diastereoisomers and the effects of the stereochemical structure
on properties of the enzymes have been until recently elusive. Since
BPH_4 cofactor is produced from 7,8-dihydrobiopterin (7,8-BPH_2) in the
living cells by the action of dihydrofolate reductase (DFR), this study
was undertaken to determine the stereochemical structure at the 6 position of enzymically reduced $6MPH_4$ and ℓ-erythro-BPH_4 and to examine the
properties of bovine adrenal tyrosine and bovine pineal tryptophan
hydroxylases with the natural ℓ-erythro-BPH_4 as cofactor. While this
study was in progress, Bailey and Ayling reported a separation of the
6-diastereoisomers of ℓ-erythro-BPH_4 by a high pressure liquid chromatography and a comparison of the "natural" and "unnatural" ℓ-erythro-
BPH_4 as cofactor of phenylalanine hydroxylase[4].

MATERIALS AND METHODS

Materials and Enzymes. Enzymically reduced $6MPH_4$ and ℓ-erythro-BPH_4
were obtained by reduction of corresponding 7,8-dihydropterin (7,8-PH_2)

with NADPH and bovine liver DFR followed by isolation by CM-Sephadex
C-25 (H$^+$) column chromatography. NADH-dependent dihydropteridine reductase (DPR) was purified from bovine liver by the method of Hasegawa[5].
In the course of the purification of NADH-dependent DPR, NADPH-dependent DPR, DFR and NADH-dependent DPR were eluted from DEAE-Sephadex A-50
column in that order and separated from each other. DFR thus obtained
was further purified by hydroxylapatite column chromatography to be free
of any DPR activity. Tyrosine hydroxylase was partially purified from
bovine adrenal medulla as described previously[3]. Tryptophan hydroxylase
was partially purified from bovine pineal gland as described previously[6]
except that P- and DEAE-Cellulose steps were omitted and Sephadex G-200
was replaced by Sephadex G-100.

Methods. Tyrosine hydroxylase reaction was carried out at 30° for 15
min in air under conditions described previously[3] except that non-radioactive L-tyrosine was used as substrate and L-Dopa formed was estimated
fluorometrically. Tryptophan hydroxylase activity was determined with
L-phenylalanine-4-T as substrate (bovine pineal tryptophan hydroxylase
catalyzes reactions of both L-tryptophan and L-phenylalanine at a comparable rate[6]). Before each assay, the enzyme was activated[7] by preincubation at pH 8.1 and 30° for 120 min under N_2 in the presence of
5 mM dithiothreitol, 50 µM $Fe(NH_4)_2(SO_4)_2$ and a glucose dehydrogenase
preparation (about 1 mg/ml) purified from beef liver according to the
method of Strecker[8]. Under these conditions, the activated enzyme was
stable for more than 1 h. Reactions with the activated enzyme were cal-
ried out at 30° and pH 7.0 for 1 min in air and THO formed was determined by the method of Guroff and Abramowitz[9] except that THO was
evapolated from the reaction mixture under a reduced pressure and
collected at - 70°. Separation of 6-diastereoisomers of ℓ-erythro-BPH$_4$
by a high pressure liquid chromatography on Partisil-SCX was carried out
according to the method of Bailey and Ayling[4].

RESULTS

The Stereochemical Structure at 6 Position of Tetrahydropterin Cofactors. (2S)- and (2R)-1,2,3,4-Tetrahydro-2-methylquinoxaline ([2S]-2MQH$_4$
and [2R]-2MQH$_4$) were synthesized starting from o-nitrofluorobenzene and
L- or D-alanine as outlined in Fig. 1 and served as model compound for
(6S)- and (6R)-6MPH$_4$, respectively. The structure of the final products, (2S)- and (2R)-2MQH$_4$, was identified by elementary analysis and
the comparison of UV and IR spectra with those of authentic, optically
inactive 2MQH$_4$. When CD spectra of various tetrahydropterin cofactors
were compared with those of the model compounds, enzymically reduced
6MPH$_4$ and ℓ-erythro-BPH$_4$ and ℓ-erythro-BPH$_4$ isolated from chemically

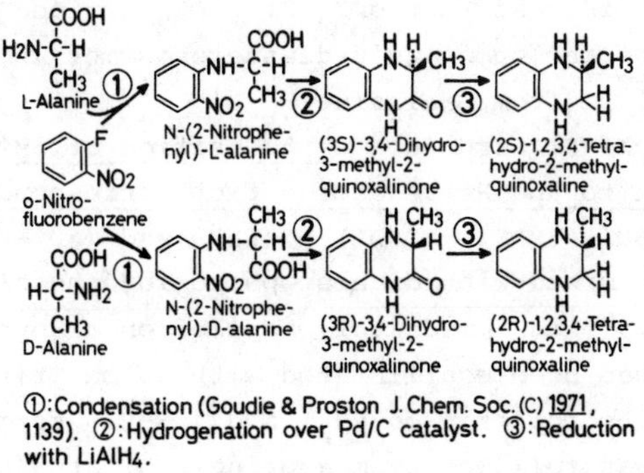

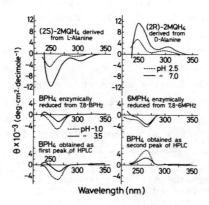

Fig. 1.   Synthesis of (2S)- and (2R)-1,2,3,4-tetrahydro-2-methylquinoxaline as model compound of (6S)- and (6R)-6MPH₄.

reduced ℓ-erythro-BPH₄ as the first peak of high pressure liquid chromatography ("natural isomer" according to Bailey and Ayling[4]) displayed a similar pattern with those of (2S)-2MQH₄ derived from L-alanine. CD spectra of ℓ-erythro-BPH₄ obtained as the second peak (unnatural isomer [4]) showed an opposing pattern and were similar to those of (2R)-2MQH₄ derived from D-alanine (Fig. 2). Chemically reduced 6MPH₄ gave no signal and much smaller signals were observed with freshly prepared chemically reduced ℓ-erythro-BPH₄ indicating the main contribution of the asymmetric 6 carbon to the CD spectra. Above results thus indicated that the stereochemical structure of enzymically reduced 6MPH₄ and ℓ-

Fig. 2.   CD spectra of tetrahydropterins in comparison with those of (2S)- and (2R)-tetrahydro-2-methylquinoxaline. HPLC : High Pressure Liquid Chromatography.

erythro-BPH$_4$ is same as that of (2S)-2MQH$_4$ derived from L-alanine and the structure of the opposite 6-diastereoisomer is same with that of (2R)-2MQH$_4$ derived from D-alanine.

The Stereochemical Structure at 6 Position of 6MPH$_4$ and ℓ-erythro-BPH$_4$ after Oxidation to and Re-reduction from Corresponding quinonoid Dihydropterin. (6DL)-6MPH$_4$*, (6DL)-, (6L)- and (6D)-BPH$_4$ (2.7 - 7.0 μmol) were separately mixed with dichlorophenolindophenol (DCPIP, final 1.75 mg/ml) at pH 7.5, and immediately applied on a Sephadex G-25 column (0.9 x 5 cm) which had been equilibrated with 50 mM Tris-Cl, pH 7.0. Elution of quinonoid dihydropterin (q-PH$_2$) and 7,8-PH$_2$ formed from q-PH$_2$ during the procedure was followed by measuring O.D. at 340 nm (isosbestic point of q-PH$_2$ and 7,8-PH$_2$) and in some experiments q-PH$_2$ content by the NADH-DPR system. Peak fraction of q-PH$_2$-eluate was immediately mixed with DPR and slight excess of NADH, and incubated for 1 min**. PH$_4$ formed was then isolated by CM-Sephadex C-25 (H$^+$) column chromatography. Examination of the 6-stereostructure of the isolated tetrahydropterins by CD spectrophotometry and high pressure liquid chromatography revealed that the stereostructure of 6MPH$_4$ and BPH$_4$ at the 6 position is retained during oxidation and reduction cycle through q-PH$_2$

Reactivities of (6L)- and (6D)-BPH$_4$ with Bovine Adrenal Tyrosine Hydroxylase. Kinetic experiments on tyrosine hydroxylase purified from the soluble fraction of bovine adrenal medulla were carried out in air with 50 μM L-tyrosine as substrate and varied concentrations of (6L)- or (6D)-BPH$_4$ or with 130 μM (6L)- or (6D)-BPH$_4$ as cofactor and varied concentrations of L-tyrosine. The results were summerized in Table I. The Lineweaver-Burk plot against the reciprocal concentration of (6L)-BPH$_4$ deviated downward in the vicinity of ordinate and two different Km values were obtained for (6L)-BPH$_4$ depending on whether the concentration of BPH$_4$ is lower or higher than about 0.25 mM. The plot against the reciplocal concentration of (6D)-BPH$_4$ appeared to be linear under conditions employed. The second (higher) Km value for (6L)-BPH$_4$ was close to Km obtained for (6D)-BPH$_4$. The substrate inhibition by relatively high concentrations (over approximately 50 μM) of L-tyrosine[3] was observed in the present study only with (6L)-BPH$_4$ as cofactor. Km for L-tyrosine with (6L)- and (6D)-BPH$_4$ as cofactor did not differ significantly and

---

* In the following section of this manuscript, 6MPH$_4$ and ℓ-erythro-BPH$_4$ having the same 6-stereostructure with that of (2S)-2MQH$_4$ are abbreviated as (6L)-6MPH$_4$ and (6L)-BPH$_4$, and the tetrahydropterins having opposite stereostructure as (6D)-6MPH$_4$ and (6D)-BPH$_4$.

** Under the conditions employed, the reduction of q-PH$_2$ to PH$_4$ was sufficiently rapid that the addition of DPR accelerated the velocity only slightly. The 6-stereospecificity of DPR is therefore remained to be studied kinetically.

Table I. Kinetic constants of bovine adrenal tyrosine hydroxylase.

BPH$_4$ used as cofactor	Km for BPH$_4$ at 50 µM L-Tyr	Km for L-Tyr at 130 µM BPH$_4$	Vmax $\left(\begin{array}{c}\text{L-Tyr} = \\ 50\ \mu M \\ \text{BPH}_4 \to \infty\end{array}\right)$ $\left(\begin{array}{c}\text{BPH}_4 = \\ 130\ \mu M \\ \text{L-Tyr} \to \infty\end{array}\right)$		Inhibition by L-Tyr over 50 µM
	(µM)	(µM)	(nmol/min/mg protein)		
(6L)-ℓ-erythro-BPH$_4$	72 ± 3* 28 ± 5**	12.0 ± 4	10.0 ± 0.1* 8.9 ± 0.5**	8.7 ± 1.2	(++)
(6D)-ℓ-erythro-BPH$_4$	77 ± 9	9.0 ± 0.4	7.0 ± 0.3	3.0 ± 0.03	N.D.

* When [(6L)-BPH$_4$] is over 248 µM, ** When [(6D)-BPH$_4$] is below 248 µM, N.D. : Not detectable under conditions employed.

Vmax with (6L)-BPH$_4$ as cofactor was slightly higher than that with (6D)-BPH$_4$.

Reactivities of (6L)- and (6D)-BPH$_4$ with Bovine Pineal Tryptophan Hydroxylase. Initial velocity studies on tryptophan hydroxylase were carried out in air in a combination of 10 different (6L)-BPH$_4$, (6D)-BPH$_4$, (6DL)-6MPH$_4$ or (6L)-6MPH$_4$ and 5 different L-phenylalanine concentrations. The kinetic constants (Vmax and Km) were tentatively calculated on the assumption that the enzyme is saturated by 20.9% O$_2$ under every condition used***. As in the case of tyrosine hydroxylase, inhibition by high concentrations (over approximately 50 µM) of L-phenylalanine was most conspicuous when (6L)-BPH$_4$ was used as cofactor. Two different Km values were observed for (6L)-BPH$_4$ depending on whether the concentration of (6L)-BPH$_4$ is lower or higher than about 25 µM and this phenomenon was independent of phenylalanine concentration. The Lineweaver-Burk plot against the reciprocal concentration of (6D)-BPH$_4$ was linear under conditions employed. In contrast to phenylalanine[4] and tyrosine hydroxylases, however, much higher Km value was calculated for (6D)-BPH$_4$ than that for (6L)-BPH$_4$ and Vmax with (6L)- and (6D)-BPH$_4$ as cofactor did not differ significantly. Km for L-phenylalanine with (6D)-BPH$_4$ as cofactor was slightly higher than that with (6L)-BPH$_4$. No significant difference was detected between (6L)- and (6DL)-6MPH$_4$. These results are summarized in Table II.

SUMMARY

6MPH$_4$ and ℓ-erythro-BPH$_4$ enzymically reduced from corresponding 7,8-

*** Kinetic experiments with varied concentrations of O$_2$ will be performed in the near future.

Table II. Kinetic constants of bovine pineal tryptophan hydroxylase.

BPH$_4$ used as cofactor	Km for BPH$_4$ at 20.9% O_2	Km for L-Phe at 20.9% O_2	Vmax at 20.9% O_2	Inhibition by L-Phe (over 50 µM)
	(µM)	(µM)	(nmol/min/ 5 µl enzyme)	
(6L)-ℓ-erythro-BPH$_4$ over 25 µM	46	41	3.0 - 3.4	(++)
(6L)-ℓerythro-BPH$_4$ below 25 µM	24	25	1.6 - 2.2	(++)
(6D)-ℓ-erythro-BPH$_4$	430*	120	2.8 - 3.1*	N.D.

* Approximate value,   N.D. : Not detectable under conditions used.

PH$_2$ by the action of DFR showed a same pattern of CD spectra with those of (2S)-tetrahydro-2-methylquinoxaline, a model compound synthesized from o-nitrofluorobenzene and L-alanine. The results together with the finding by Mathews and Huennekens[10] that ℓ,L-tetrahydrofolate is formed by the enzymic reduction of 7,8-dihydrofolate indicated that the natural cofactor of aromatic amino acid hydroxylases is the (6L)-isomer of ℓ-erythro-BPH$_4$. (6L)-ℓ-erythro-BPH$_4$ was a better cofactor for both tyrosine and tryptophan hydroxylases than the (6D)-isomer and only with this natural cofactor possible regulatory mechanisms of these enzymes (substrate inhibition and two different Km for the cofactor) were evident.

REFERENCES

1. Kaufman, S. and Fisher, D.B. (1974) in Molecular Mechanisms of Oxygen Activation (O. Hayaishi, ed) pp. 285-369, Academic Press.

2. Ayling, J.E. and Hefland, G.D. (1975) in Chemistry and Biology of Pteridines (W. Pfleiderer, ed) pp. 305-319, Walter de Gruyter.

3. Numata (Sudo), Y., Kato, T., Nagatsu, T., Sugimoto, T. and Matsuura, S. (1977) Biochim. Biophys. Acta 480, 104-112.

4. Bailey, S.W. and Ayling, J.E. (1978) J. Biol. Chem. 253, 1598-1605.

5. Hasegawa, H. (1977) J. Biochem. 81, 169-177.

6. Nukiwa, T., Tohyama, C., Okita, C., Kataoka, T. and Ichiyama, A. (1974) Biochem. Biophys. Res. Communs. 60, 1029-1035.

7. Ichiyama, A., Hori, S., Mashimo, Y., Nukiwa, T. and Makuuchi, H. (1974) FEBS Letters 40, 88-91.

8. Strecker, H.J. (1955) in Method in Enzymology Vol I (S.P. Colowick and N.O. Kaplan, ed) pp. 335-339, Academic Press.

9. Guroff, G. and Abramowitz, A. (1967) Anal. Biochem. 19, 548-555.

10. Mathews, C.K. and Huennekens, F.M. (1960) J. Biol. Chem. 235, 3304-3308.

STUDIES ON THE COFACTOR OF PHENYLALANINE HYDROXYLASE
IN SOME TRANSPLANTABLE RAT ASCITES HEPATOMAS

SETSUKO KATOH, TERUMI SUEOKA AND SHOZO YAMADA
Department of Biochemistry, Josai Dental University, Sakado-shi,
Saitama-ken, 350-02 (JAPAN)

SUMMARY

We have investigated the phenylalanine hydroxylase activity and
pteridine cofactor metabolism in ascites tumor cells of several transplantable rat ascites hepatomas (AH 13, 41C, 60C, 66 and 109A). In
these lines, the ascites cells did not show phenylalanine hydroxylase
activity but maintained pteridine-metabolizing system even though the
system showed lower ability than that in normal liver. Dihydropteridine
reductase, dihydrofolate reductase and sepiapterin reductase were 6-10%,
12-44 % and 16-86 % in activity/g cell, respectively, of the activities
in normal liver. Pteridine cofactor was found in about 15 % activity
of normal liver. The lowering was mostly observed in the activities of
dihydropteridine reductase and cofactor.

INTRODUCTION

The activity of phenylalanine hydroxylase is one of the differentiated functions of mammalian hepatic tissue. This enzyme activity is
not expressed in tissue culture either normal or cancerous hepatic
origin except two lines of minimal deviation hepatomas[1]. This defect
of phenylalanine hydroxylase activity is, in appearance, also observed
in the liver of classical phenylketonuria[2] and of the fetal rat of
early stage[3]. It was reported in classical phenylketonuria that
pteridine cofactor and dihydropteridine reductase which are required
in the phenylalanine hydroxylation[4] are present in normal amount[5].
However, it is unknown about the pteridine metabolism in the cultured
hepatic cell lines.

We have found in this study that phenylalanine hydroxylase activity
is also defective in the ascites tumor cells of several lines of transplantable rat ascites hepatomas (AH 13, 41C, 60C, 66 and 109A). To get
some insight for cancerous sisuation and expression mechanism of
phenylalanine hydroxylation in hepatocyte, we have studied on the
pteridine cofactor and its metabolizing enzymes in these ascites tumor
cells of AH-hepatomas in the following items : (1) phenylalanine
hydroxylase activity (2) dihydropteridine reductase activity

(3) activities of another two NADPH-mediated pteridine metabolizing enzymes concerning with the supply or regulation of the cofactor, such as dihydrofolate reductase[a] and sepiapterin reductase[b]: (tetrahydrobiopterin $\overset{a}{\rightleftharpoons}$ dihydrobiopterin $\overset{b}{\rightleftharpoons}$ sepiapterin)[6,7] (4) presence of cofactor.

MATERIALS AND METHODS

Servival times of five malignant lines of AH-hepatomas are one week in AH 13 and AH 66, and two weeks in AH 41C, 60C and 109A, respectively.

Ascites cells of each line were collected from male Donryu rat at 4th day after intraperitoneal inoculation of about 10^7 cells per animal. An equivalent weight of ascites tumor cells or liver was collected from each animal and was pooled from 8-9 animals to prepare the extract for enzyme assay in each line. Enzyme was extracted with 3 vol of 0.03M phosphate buffer pH7.3 and centrifuged at 17,000×g for 40 min for photometric assay and at 100,000×g for 60 min for radioisotopic assay. Cofactor was extracted with 2 vol of water[8].

RESULTS AND DISCUSSION

Phenylalanine hydroxylase activity. Activity of this enzyme was not found in ascites tumor cells in all lines of ascites hepatomas examined (Table 1). The activity was not measurable in these cells even by the incubation at 37°C for 40 min or by radioisotopic procedures described in Fig.2 and Table 4 with the use of 0.2 μmole of 6-methyltetrahydropte-rin (6MPH$_4$) as cofactor. The activity could not be detected in ascites cells up to the last stage of animal (Fig.1). And it is considered that phenylalanine hydroxylase is also deficient in the ascites tumor cells of these AH hepatomas as observed in cultured hepatic cells. But in the host liver in all lines tested, this enzyme was observed in

TABLE 1   ASSAY OF PHENYLALANINE HYDROXYLASE IN ASCITES TUMOR CELLS

Lines of Hepatoma	Activity tyrosine formation (μ moles/hr/mg protein)	
	hepatoma cell	host liver
AH 13	0	1.077
41 C	0	0.865
60 C	0	0.875
66	0	0.618
109 A	0	0.871
Normal liver	1.025	

The assay was based on the nonenzymatic regeneration of 6MPH$_4$ from quinonoid di-hydroform by dithiotheritol (DTT) (9). Tyrosine formed (at 25°C, 60min) was measured by nitrosonaphtol method (10).

TABLE 2   ACTIVITY OF DIHYDROPTERIDINE REDUCTASE IN ASCITES TUMOR CELLS

Lines of Hepatoma	Activity (ΔA_{550}/hr)			
	per mg protein	per g cell (tissue)	per cell $\times 10^{-8}$	No. of cells (per g cell) $\times 10^8$
AH 13	3.20 [16]	121.0 [7]	27.8 [1.7]	(4.36)
AH 41 C	4.07 [20]	153.3 [9]	33.0 [2.0]	(4.64)
AH 60 C	3.78 [18]	102.9 [6]	26.1 [1.6]	(3.95)
AH 66	6.15 [30]	168.0 [10]	39.2 [2.4]	(4.35)
AH 109 A	3.30 [16]	125.6 [8]	28.4 [1.7]	(4.43)
Normal liver	20.57 [100%]	1637.4 [100%]	1637.4 [100%]	(1.0[a])

The activity was measured at A_{550} on the 6MPH$_4$-dependent
reduction of cyt c(ox) in the presence of NADH at 25°C (11).
[a]The number of parencymal cells in adult rat liver per g
tissue reported by Greengard et al (12).

almost normal level (Table 1).

Dihydropteridine reductase activity. Table 2 showes the presence of
the activity of this enzyme in the ascites cells of all 5 lines of AH
hepatoma. Specific activity is 16-30 % of normal liver activity. But
total activity of this enzyme is ultimately quite low; it is 6-10 % per
g cell and 1.6-2.4 % per cell of liver activity.

The progressive increase in dihydropteridine reductase activity was
found up to the 4th day of the proliferation phase of ascites cells in
AH 13, and then the activity gradually decreased (Fig.1). Similar
patterns of activity curve were observed in dihydrofolate reductase and
sepiapterin reductase but more high and sharp in the peak. It is interesting that not only dihydrofolate reductase but also sepiapterin
reductase exhibits tipical form of log-phase-enzymes (Fig.1). As the
three enzymes reached at maximum level in the activity at 3rd-4th day
after inoculation, the measurements of enzyme activity and amount of
cofactor were made at this stage.

Activities of dihydrofolate reductase and sepiapterin reductase.
Some of the lines of AH hepatomas showed same or higher level of the
enzymes in specific activity comparring with those of liver. But total
activities of them were 12-44 % per g cell (3-10 % per cell) in
dihydrofolate reductase and 16-86 % per g cell (7-20 % per cell) in
sepiapterin reductase, respectively, of those in the liver enzymes
(Table 2). The rate of decrease in the activities of the two enzymes
was not remarkable than that of dihydropteridine reductase.

192

Fig. 1. Activities of phenylalanine hydroxylase, dihydropteridine reductase, dihydrofolate reductase and sepiapterin reductase in the ascites tumor cells of AH 13
during the days after inoculation.

One assay represents the
level in the mixture of
cells from 3-4 animals
of the same stage.

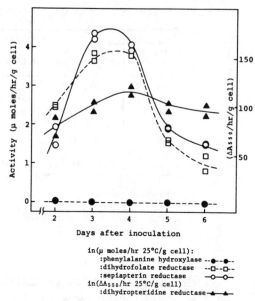

Days after inoculation

in(μ moles/hr 25°C/g cell):
    :phenylalanine hydroxylase --●--●--
    :dihydrofolate reductase --□--□--
    :sepiapterin reductase   --○--○--
in(ΔA_{550}/hr 25°C/g cell)
    :dihydropteridine reductase--▲--▲--

TABLE 3   ACTIVITIES OF DIHYDROFOLATE REDUCTASE AND SEPIAPTERIN
REDUCTASE IN ASCITES TUMOR CELLS

Lines of Hepatoma	dihydrofolate reductase (μ moles/hr)		sepiapterin reductase (μ moles/hr)	
	per mg	per g cell (tissue)	per mg	per g cell (tissue)
AH 13	0.100[109]	3.78[44]	0.149[204]	5.63[86]
AH 41 C	0.048[52]	1.81[21]	0.112[153]	4.22[65]
AH 60 C	0.024[26]	1.04[12]	0.039[53]	1.06[16]
AH 66	0.092[100]	2.51[29]	0.095[130]	2.59[40]
AH 109 A	0.054[59]	2.05[24]	0.050[68]	1.90[29]
Normal liver	0.092[100%]	8.52[100%]	0.073[100%]	6.53[100%]

Two enzyme activities were determined by photometrically
at A_{340} (13) and A_{420} (14), respectively at 25°C.

Presence and amount of cofactor activity. Presence of cofactor was
exactly confirmed in the ascites tumor cells of AH 13 and AH 66. Clear
formation of ^{14}C-tyrosine was observed by paper chromatography in the
hydroxylation system containing ^{14}C-phenylalanine as substrate (Fig.2).

The amount of cofactor in the ascites cells of these lines was determined in the activity of ^{3}H-phenylalanine hydroxylation[17] at 4th day
after inoculation (Table 4). The levels of cofactor activities were
both about 15 % of liver activity. These levels seemed to decrease
rapidly after 4th day of inoculation.

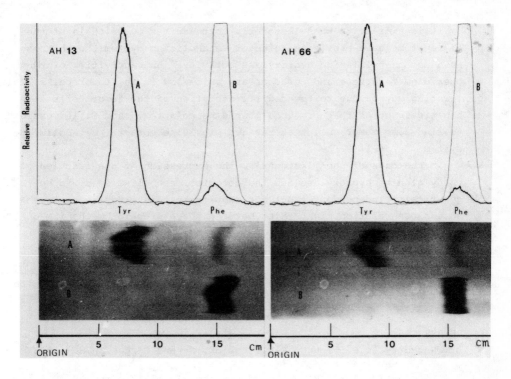

Fig. 2. Presence of cofactor in ascites tumor cells of AH 13 and AH 66 showed by ^{14}C-tyrosine formation by paper chromatography.

(A) complete system (B) the system with boiled enzyme. Complete system (250μl, pH6.8):0.25μCi L-^{14}C(U)-phe(0.5Ci/mmol), L-phe 0.05μmol, DTT 2μmol, rat liver phenylalanine hydroxylase (2nd (NH$_4$)$_2$SO$_4$ fractionation (8)) and cofactor extract of cells. Incubation:25°C for 60min. Paper chromatography:2-propanol/water/NH$_4$OH(8:1:1), 18hrs. Radioisotope on the paper was exposed with X-ray film.

TABLE 4   ASSAY OF PHENYLALANINE HYDROXYLASE COFACTOR IN ASCITES TUMOR CELLS OF AH 13 AND AH 66

Lines of Hepatoma	Amount	Counts per minute in expt. No.		Tyrosine formation n moles/hr/g cell (tissue) in expt. No.	
		1	2	1	2
None	—	334	369	—	—
AH 13 cell	150 μl	1513	1835	18.2	23.3
AH 66 cell	150 μl	1796	1949	22.7	25.1
Normal liver	30 μl	2315	2721	137.5	165.9

The reaction mixture and the incubation were same as described in Fig.2 except with 0,1μCi L-4-^{3}H-phe(27Ci/mmol) as isotopic substrate(15) and with one-half vol of rat liver enzyme. Each value represents the mean of duplicate determinations in ascites tumor cells from 3 animals.

It is similar to phenylketonuria that ascites tumor cells of the AH hepatoma have pteridine cofactor metabolizing system though these have not phenylalanine hydroxylase activity. But activities of dihydropteridine reductase and cofactor are quite low in the tumor cells. This lowering may be due to the dedifferentiation of the tumor cells in hepatic function that produces pteridine cofactor. And it is possible to find some tumor cell that has not pteridine cofactor metabolizing system.

In the case of phenylketonuria, the expression of the function of phenylalanine hydroxylase and the cofactor metabolism seems to be genetically independent. But our results in this study suggests that some close relation might exist between the expression mechanism of this enzyme and of pteridine cofactor metabolism.

ACKNOWLEDGEMENT

The authors wish to thank Sasaki Institute (Tokyo) for kindly suppling five lines of AH hepatomas.

REFERENCES

1. Haggerty, D.F., Young, P.L., Popjak, G. and Carnes, W.H. (1973) J. Biol. Chem, 248, 223-232.

2. Mitoma, C., Auld, R.M. and Udenfriend, S. (1957) Proc. Soc. Exp. Biol. Med, 94, 634-635.

3. Tourian, A., Treiman, D.M. and Carr, J.S. (1972) Biochim. Biophys. Acta, 279, 484-490.

4. Kaufman, S. (1971) in Advan. in Enzymol, Meister, A. ed, Interscience Publishers, New York, 35, 245-319.

5. Kaufman, S. (1958) Science, 128, 1506-1508.

6. Matsubara, M., Katoh, S., Akino, M. and Kaufman, S. (1966) Biochim. Biophys. Acta, 122, 202-212.

7. Kaufman, S. (1967) J. Biol. Chem, 242, 3934-3943.

8. Kaufman, S. and Fisher, D.B. (1970) J. Biol. Chem, 245, 4745-4750.

9. Bublitz, C. (1969) Biochim. Biophys. Acta, 191, 249-256.

10. Udenfriend, S. and Cooper, J.R. (1952) J. Biol. Chem, 196, 227-233.

11. Hasegawa, H. (1977) J. Biochem, 81, 167-177.

12. Greengard, O., Federman, M. and Knox, W.E. (1972) J. Cell Biol. 52, 261-272.

13. Mathews, C.K., Scrimgeour, K.G. and Huennekens, F.M. (1963) in Methods in Enzymol, Colowick, C.K. and Kaplan, N.O. eds, Academic Press, London, 6, pp.364-368.

14. Katoh, S. (1971) Arch. Biochem. Biophys, 146, 202-214.

15. Guroff, G. (1971) in Methods in Enzymol. McCormick, D.B. and Wright, L.D. eds, Academic Press, New York, 18B, pp.600-605.

RECENT STUDIES ON NADPH-DIHYDROPTERIDINE REDUCTASE FROM BOVINE LIVER

NOBUO NAKANISHI[*], HIROYUKI HASEGAWA[**], and MIKI AKINO[***]

*Department of Biochemistry, Josai Dental University, Sakado, Saitama
350-02 ; **Department of Biochemistry, Hamamatsu University School of
Medicine, Hamamatsu 431-31 ; ***Department of Biology, Tokyo Metropolitan University, Setagaya, Tokyo 158, Japan

ABSTRACT

NADPH-dihydropteridine reductase, which is rather specific for NADPH
than NADH in catalyzing the reduction of quinonoid-dihydropterin, was
purified to homogenity from bovine liver, and properties of the enzyme
were studied comparing with those of NADH-dihydropteridine reductase
[EC 1.6.99.7]. The molecular weight of NADPH-dihydropteridine reductase was determined to be 70,000. These two enzymes were distinguish-
able from each other with respect to their physical and catalytic
properties. NADPH was more effective than NADH for tyrosine formation
when NADPH-dihydropteridine reductase was used in the phenylalanine
hydroxylation system, whereas NADH was more effective than NADH when
NADH-dihydropteridine reductase was used.

INTRODUCTION

Tetrahydropterin is known to participate as an essential cofactor
in the enzymic hydroxylation of aromatic amino acids such as phenylalanine, tyrosine and tryptophan[1]. The phenylalanine hydroxylation
system consists of two essential enzymes, phenylalanine hydroxylase
[EC 1.14.16.1] and dihydropteridine reductase [EC 1.6.99.7]. Tetrahydropterin is oxidized to quinonoid-dihydropterin during the hydroxylation reaction, and the quinonoid-dihydropterin is reduced back to
the tetrahydro form by dihydropteridine reductase in the presence of
reduced pyridine nucleotide[1]. Concerning the pyridine nucleotide
specificity of the phenylalanine hydroxylation system, contradictory
observations were reported by Mitoma[2] and by Kaufman[3], respectively.
Thereafter, the specificity of the system has not unequivocally been
determined. In 1969, Nielsen et al[4]. determined the pyridine nucleotide
specificity of dihydropteridine reductase for the first time that
NADH was more effective than NADPH. The result was confirmed by other
investigators[5,6,7]. Furthermore, dihydropteridine reductase was suggested to utilize NADH in vivo by the observation that the enzyme
mostly exists as a binary complex with NADH in the crude extract of

6-methyl-5,6,7,8-tetrahydropterin ($6MPH_4$) by the method of Hasegawa[7].
The concentration of q-$6MPH_2$ was estimated using NADH-dihydropteridine
reductase; cytochrome c reduction was followed in the presence of
fixed amount of the enzyme and limiting amount of q-$6MPH_2$. The concentration of q-$6MPH_2$ was assumed to be equivalent to that of $6MPH_4$
which gives the same reduction velocity of cytochrome c under the
assay conditions. A half life of q-$6MPH_2$ in 40 mM Tris-HCl, pH 7.0
at 20°C was calculated to be 33 min by this method.

RESULTS AND DISCUSSION
Purification and Properties
The flow-though fraction from a DEAE-Sephadex A-50 column (40 mM
K-phosphate, pH 7.4) in the purification procedure of bovine liver
NADH-dihydropteridine reductase[7] was used as starting material for the
purification of NADPH-dihydropteridine reductase. The fraction was
concentrated and chromatographed on a Sephadex G-100 column. The
column eluate containing bulk of the enzyme activity was further purified by successive column chromatography on CM-Sephadex C-50, and DEAE-
Sephadex A-50 (40 mM Tris-HCl, pH 8.0). The final enzyme preparation
gave a single protein band when subjected to polyacrylamide gel
electrophoresis in the presence or absence of sodium dodectl sulfate.

The molecular weight of NADPH-dihydropteridine reductase was determined to be 70,000 by the method of Hedrick and Smith[10], and by gel
filtration through a Sephadex G-100 column.

In the purification of NADPH-dihydropteridine reductase, when the
step of Sephadex G-100 column was omitted and the flow-through fraction from a DEAE-Sephadex column (40 mM K-phosphate, pH 7.4) was
directly applied to a DEAE-Sephadex A-50 column (40 mM Tris-HCl, pH
8.0), two or more peaks of the enzyme activity appeared (Fig.2).
Occasionally, two activity bands were also recognized when analyzed by
gel electrophoresis (Fig.3-A). However, the active fractions from the
column were subjected to Sephadex G-100 column chromatography, the
enzyme activity was eluted as a single peak, and the active fraction
migrated as a single activity band on the gel (Fig.3-B). In the case
of NADH-dihydropteridine reductase, Hasegawa[7] reported that four
activity peaks of the enzyme were noticed when the crude preparation
was applied to a CM-Sephadex C-50 column. Similarly, multi-distribution of the NADPH-dihydropteridine reductase activity on the DEAE-
Sephadex A-50 column chromatography suggests existence of multiple
enzyme forms. For example, the existence of the enzyme-NADPH complex
was suggested by the observation that one of the peaks from the column

bovine liver, and that the enzyme-NADPH complex is not detectable in the extract[7].

Recently, we found another type of dihydropteridine reductase which is rather specific for NADPH[8]. Hence, we called the new enzyme and dihydropteridine reductase so far been studied [EC 1.6.99.7] as NADPH-dihydropteridine reductase and NADH-dihydropteridine reductase, respectively. The pyridine nucleotide specificity of regenerating system of tetrahydropterin from quinonoid-dihydropterin depended on the type of dihydropteridine reductase employed in the system. It is likely that tetrahydropterin is regenerated from quinonoid-dihydropterin in two different ways in vivo, i.e., by NADPH-dihydropteridine reductase and NADPH (Fig.1, reaction **b**), or by NADH-dihydropteridine reductase and NADH (Fig.1, reaction **c**).

In the present report, we describe results of recent studies on NADPH-dihydropteridine reductase. Efficiency of tyrosine formation in the phenylalanine hydroxylation system is also examined using NADPH-dihydropteridine reductase or NADH-dihydropteridine reductase.

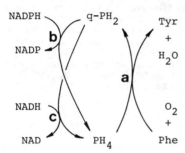

Fig. 1. Schematic representation showing oxidoreduction of pteridine cofactor in the phenylalanine hydroxylation system. The reaction **a**, **b**, and **c** are those catalyzed by phenylalanine hydroxylase, NADPH-dihydropteridine reductase, and NADH-dihydropteridine reductase, respectively. PH_4 and q-PH_2 represent tetrahydropterin and quinonoid-dihydropterin respectively.

MATERIALS AND METHODS

NADPH-dihydropteridine reductase and NADH-dihydropteridine reductase were assayed as described previously[7,8]. The pterin-substrate was usually added to the reaction mixture as a tetrahydro form[5-8]. Quinonoid-dihydropterin was also used for enzyme assay. NADPH-dihydropteridine reductase on polyacryla,ide gel after electrophoresis was stained for the activity by the previous method[8]. Phenylalanine hydroxylase was prepared from rat liver according to Kaufman et al[9]. Purification was performed up to the 2nd ammonium sulfate fractionation. 6-Methyl-quinonoid-dihydropterin (q-6MPH$_2$) was prepared from

showed fluorescence presumably due to NADPH. This possibility was supported by the fact that purified NADPH-dihydropteridine reductase formed an enzyme-NADPH complex which was not separated by passage through a Sephadex G-25 column.

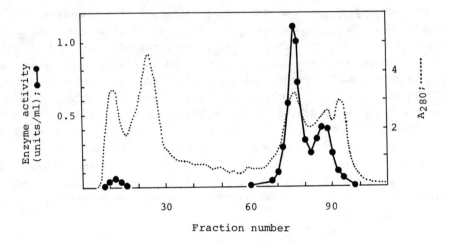

Fig. 2. Multi-distribution of NADPH-dihydropteridine reductase activity on a DEAE-Sephadex A-50 column chromatography. The flow-through fraction (=starting materil) prepared from 1 kg of bovine liver (about 30 ml) was directly applied to a DEAE-Sephadex A-50 column (3 x 27 cm) equilibrated with 40 mM Tris-HCl, pH 8.0. After washing the column with 300 ml of the buffer, protein was eluted with linear KCl gradient in the buffer (0-0.2 M, 700 ml). The flow rate was 25 ml/hr and 10-ml fractions were collected.

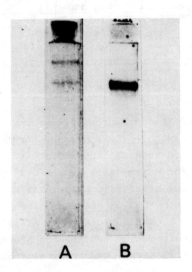

Fig. 3. NADPH-dihydropteridine reductase activity on polyacrylamide gel.
A: The eluate from a DEAE-Sephadex A-50 column (40 mM Tris-HCl, pH 8.0). B: The eluate from a Sephadex G-100 column.
After electrophoresis, each gel was incubated at 30°C for 15 min in a solution containing 40 mM Tris-HCl, pH 7.6, 1 mg of MTT-tetrazolium, freshly prepared quinonoid-dihydropterin (about 10 μM) and 125 μM NADPH.

With use of $6MPH_4$, K_m value of NADPH-dihydropteridine reductase for NADPH was determined to be 1.4 μM. K_m for NADH was greater than 500 μM. With use of NADPH and $6MPH_4$, K_m value of the enzyme for $q-6MPH_2$ was determined to be 1.4 μM. The value well agreed with that (1.5 μM) determined by adding $q-6MPH_4$ to the reaction mixture confirming that quinonoid-dihydro form of pterin is the substrate of NADPH-dihydropteridine reductase.

Each antibody to NADPH-dihydropteridine reductase and NADH-dihydropteridine reductase was prepared by intradermal injection of each enzyme in to rabbit. NADPH-dihydropteridine reductase did not cross react with anti-NADH-dihydropteridine reductase antibody, and vice versa, indicating structural difference of these reductases.

Efficiency of Tyrosine Formation

The efficiency of tyrosine formation in the phenylalanine hydroxylation system was compared using two types of dihydropteridine reductase (TABLE 1). The reaction mixture contained excess phenylalanine hydroxylase from rat liver, and limitting amount of NADPH-dihydropteridine reductase or NADH-dihydropteridine reductase, NADPH or NADH, and $6MPH_4$. Since the hydroxylase preparation was contaminated with NADH-dihydropteridine reductase activity, tyrosine formation in the presence of NADH and NADPH-dihydropteridine reductase was higher than that expected. However, the efficiency of tyrosine formation

TABLE 1   EFFECT OF COMBINATION OF DIHYDROPTERIDINE REDUCTASES WITH NADPH OR NADH ON TYROSINE FORMATION

Tetrahydropterin regenerating enzyme	Tyrosine formed (nmol)	
	NADPH	NADH
NADPH-dihydropteridine reductase	0.729	0.552
NADH-dihydropteridine reductase	0.280	0.802

Tyrosine formation was measured according to Guroff et al.[11] The reaction mixture contained 25 μmol of K-phosphate, pH 6.8, 50 nmol of L-phenylalanine, 0.1 μCi of [4-^{3}H]phenylalanine (27 Ci/mmol), 0.25 nmol of $6MPH_4$, 5 nmol of NADPH or NADH, 0.01 unit of NADPH-dihydropteridine reductase or NADH-dihydropteridine reductase, and phenylalanine hydroxylase in excess in a final volume of 250 μl. Incubation was performed at 25°C for 15 min.

depended on the combination of respective dihydropteridine reductase with reduced pyridine nucleotide. When NADPH-dihydropteridine reductase was used, NADPH was more effective than NADH for tyrosine formation. On the contrary, when NADH-dihydropteridine reductase was used, NADH was more effective than NADPH.

The pyridine nucleotide specificity of the phenylalanine hydroxylation system, and other tetrahydropterin-dependent hydroxylation systems in vivo should be examined including NADPH-dihydropteridine reductase as an another essential component of the systems.

ACKNOWLEDGEMENT

We wish to thank Dr. Setsuko Katoh of Josai Dental University for her interest in this work and for helpful discussion.

REFERENCES

1. Kaufman,S. and Fisher,D.B. (1974) in Molecular Mechanisms of Oxygen Activation, Hayaishi,O., ed., Academic Press, New York, pp. 285-369

2. Mitoma,C. (1956) Arch. Biochem. Biophys. 60, 476-484

3. Kaufman,S. (1957) J. Biol. Chem. 226, 511-524

4. Nielsen,K.H., Simonsen,V., and Lind,K.E. (1969) Eur. J. Biochem. 9, 497-502

5. Craine,J.E., Hall,E.S., and Kaufman,S. (1972) J. Biol. Chem. 247, 6082-6091

6. Cheema,S., Soldin,S.J., Knapp,A., Hofmann,T., and Scrimgeour,K.G. (1973) Can. J. Biochem. 51, 1229-1239

7. Hasegawa,H. (1977) J. Biochem. 81, 169-177

8. Nakanishi,N., Hasegawa,H., and Watabe,S. (1977) J. Biochem. 81, 681-685

9. Kaufman,S. and Fisher,D.B. (1970) J. Biol. Chem. 245, 4745-4750

10. Hedrick,J.L. and Smith,A.J. (1968) Arch. Biochem. Biophys. 126, 155-164

11. Guroff,G. and Abramowitz,A. (1967) Anal. Biochem. 19, 548-555

TYROSINE HYDROXYLASE AND A PTERIDINE COFACTOR INVOLVED IN THE CONVERSION OF THYROXINE TO TRIIODOTHYRONINE?

HARTMUT ROKOS and EKKEHARD SCHEIFFELE

Research Laboratory, Henning Berlin GmbH, Komturstr. 19/20, D-1000 Berlin 42 (Germany)

ABSTRACT

Tyrosine hydroxylase from adrenal medulla failed to produce 3.3'.5-triiodo-L-thyronine from L-thyroxine. In rat liver tyrosine hydroxylase and 5'-deiodinase were present, however both enzyme activities were selectively inhibited by α-Me-Tyr and PTU, respectively. In a bovine liver preparation only high 5'-deiodinase activity was found. No tetrahydropteridine was required as cofactor. Therefore, 5'-deiodination of T_4 is not mediated by tyrosine hydroxylase but by a thyroxine 5'-deiodinase, which is dependent upon thiol compounds.

INTRODUCTION

T_4 (<u>1</u>) and T_3 (<u>2</u>) are secreted by the thyroid gland[1]. However most of T_3, which is the hormone with the higher thyromimetic activity, is formed by 5'-deiodination of T_4 in peripheral tissues. A possible role of T_4 soleley as prohormone for T_3 is discussed[2]. 5-Deiodination of T_4 leads to reverse T_3 (<u>3</u>), which is practically devoid of thyroid hormone activity[1,2].

$$\underline{1} \quad R^{5'} = I, \quad R^5 = I$$

$$\underline{2} \quad R^{5'} = H, \quad R^5 = I$$

$$\underline{3} \quad R^{5'} = I, \quad R^5 = H$$

Tyrosine hydroxylase (EC 1.14.16.2) has been reported[3-6] to be the enzyme responsible for deiodination of T_4 at 5'-position. α-Me-Tyr reduced in newborn sheep the T_3 surge after cord cutting, thus, according to the authors[7], proving tyrosine hydroxylase involvement in $T_4 \rightarrow T_3$ conversion.

However, this seems unlikely because (i) tyrosines with halogen in ortho-position to the hydroxy group are among the most potent inhibi-

Abbreviations: T_4 = L-thyroxine, T_3 = 3.3'.5-triiodo-L-thyronine, rT_3 = 3.3'.5'-tri-iodo-L-thyronine, α-Me-Tyr = α-methyl-L-tyrosine, PTU = 6-propylthiouracil, $DMPH_4$ = 6.7-dimethyltetrahydropterin, ANS = 8-anilino-1-naphthalene sulphonic acid, DTE = 1.4-dithioerythritol

tors of tyrosine hydroxylase[8-10]; (ii) not T_3 but a hydroxylated T_3 should be the reaction product of tyrosine hydroxylase with T_4 ; (iii) Udenfriend et al .[11] observed specific hydroxylation of L-tyrosine by tyrosine hydroxylase. In contrast to this finding, formation of D-T_3 from D-T_4 has been reported[12,13]; (iv) tyrosine hydroxylase has an absolute requirement of a tetrahydropteridine cofactor[11, 14].

Already in 1954 formation of T_3 from T_4 was demonstrated by Albright et al .[15]in kidney slices. Renewed interest in conversion led to the use of rat liver homogenate as in vitro system with high T_3-forming activity by many authors[12,16-23], the nature and sub-cellular localisation of the enzyme being much disputed.

Therefore in vitro experiments with tyrosine hydroxylase were undertaken to allow a clear decision about its involvement in $T_4 \rightarrow T_3$ conversion[24].

MATERIALS AND METHODS

Usual chemicals were analytical grade, others were purchased as given: L-$[3,5-^3H]$tyrosine, 1776 GBq/mmol (New England Nuclear), DTE (Merck), ANS (Serva), catalase (Boehringer), PTU (Degussa), α-Me-Tyr (Hässle, Sweden); T_3 and T_4, puriss. quality (Henning Berlin).

TLC. Precoated silica plates (Merck); ethyl acetate / methanol/ 2 M NH_3 (50/20/10 by vol).

$DMPH_4$ was synthesized by the method of Viscontini[25]: 6.7-dimethylpterin (117 mg) was added to Pt (prepared from 50 mg of PtO_2) in CF_3COOH (15 mL) and reduced with H_2 for 30 min. After filtration, conc. H_2SO_4 (40 μL) in ethanol (1 mL) was added. Precipitation was completed by addition of 30 mL of ether to give 164 mg product. H_4Folic acid and H_4biopterin were prepared by the same method.

Tyrosine hydroxylase. The procedure of Kaufmann et al.[14] was followed with minor modifications. Minced adrenal medulla (or liver) was homogenized (glass-teflon Potter 100 μm) in 3 vol buffer A (o.3 M sucrose, 4 mM phosphate pH 7.5, 5 mM mercaptoethanol). The supernatant ("Homogenate") after centrifugation (30 min) at 1500 g was then centrifuged at 30000 g to give the "Supernatant Fraction" (which was used for soluble tyrosine hydroxylase preparation[11]) and the pellet. The latter was resuspended in 3 vol buffer (15 mM KCl, 5 mM mercaptoethanol) and centrifuged at 30000 g - using the pellet, this was repeated twice. Then resuspension was in 3 vol buffer (0.1 Mphosphate pH 6.2, 5 mM mercaptoethanol), after centrifugation at 30000 g - this was again repeated twice. Finally, the pellet was resuspended in 3 vol buffer A to give a purified "Particulate fraction".

<u>Tyrosine hydroxylase assay</u>. The incubation mixture contained 53 mM K-phosphate (pH 6.2), 16 mM DTE, catalase 2600 units, 0.66 mM $DMPH_4$, 28 nM L-$[3,5-^3H]$tyrosine; total volume 300 μL. Incubation was at 25°C for various times, then 5 μL of the mixture were spotted on chromatography paper (Schleicher-Schüll 2243 b) within segments (1.5 x 2.0 cm). After drying and equilibration (in a desiccator over NaOH) the rectangles were cut out, placed in scintillation vials and eluted with 1 mL of 2 M NH_3. 10 min thereafter, 10 mL of Brays solution were added.

<u>$T_4 \rightarrow T_3$ conversion assay</u>. 2 μM T_4, 3.2 mM DTE, 3.2 mM EDTA, 65 mM K-phosphate (pH 7.5), total volume 625 μL; 37° C. Reaction was initiated by adding T_4 solution after preincubation of enzyme (10 min, room temp.) with an inhibitor or its solute; it was stopped by adding 100 μL to 200 μL of cold ethanol (for blanks immediately after T_4 addition). This mixture was kept overnight at -20°C, then centrifuged; 5-20 μL of the supernatant were used for T_3-RIA.

<u>T_3-RIA</u>. The assay was run in 80 mM barbital buffer (pH 8.4), containing 1 g/L bovine serum albumin. Each tube (Eppendorf) contained 20 μL T_3 standard solution (T_3 5-160 pg) or 5-20 μL ethanol extract, ca. 6 pg $[^{125}I]T_3$ (spec. activity ca. 100 GBq/mg), 84 μg ANS, 60 μL anti-rabbit gammaglobulin serum (donkey). Incubation was started by adding 100 μL T_3-antiserum (rabbit, final dil. 1:210000); total assay volume 420 μL. After 2 h at room temperature, protected from light, 0.6 mL of H_2O was added. After centrifugation at 4500 g for 10 min, the precipitate was washed with 1.1 mL of H_2O, recentrifuged and counted in a γ-counter (BF 6000; Berthold-Frieseke).

Protein was determined by the Lowry procedure[26].

RESULTS

Tyrosine hydroxylase activity in the bovine adrenal medulla preparation was first determined by standard methods (by using L-$[3.5-^3H]$tyrosine as substrate and measuring the tritiated water formed[14] or by following the oxidation of $DMPH_4$ photometrically[14,27] at 335 nm). A more simple method in which aliquots of the incubation mixture were spotted on paper and the remaining radioactivity was counted after drying gave identical results, therefore we used this routinely.

We replaced mercaptoethanol[11] as reducing agent for the quionoid dihydropterin to regenerate $DMPH_4$ by dithioerythritol. This made the system less sensitive to peroxide, omission of catalase (or Fe^{2+}) led to a 45% decrease in enzyme activity, whereas it was rendered totally inactive with mercaptoethanol. For phenylalanine hydroxylase DTE offers full protection against peroxides[28].

Table 1
Tyrosine hydroxylase activity
(bovine adrenal medulla, 0.96 mg; Δ cpm ^{3}H
after 10 min, 25°C)

complete assay	1430
no enzyme	80
no $DMPH_4$	90
no catalase	800
80 µM α-Me-Tyr	300
80 µM PTU	1320

Table 2
T_4 5'-deiodinase activity
(bovine liver, 0.8 mg; Δ ng T_3 after
30 min, 37°C)

complete assay	31.4
no enzyme	0
no EDTA	17.7
no DTE	0
40 µM α-Me-Tyr	30.6
40 µM PTU	7.5

No T_3 formation from T_4 could be detected with this particulate tyrosine hydroxylase preparation under standard assay conditions. T_3 was
determined by a double-antibody radioimmunoassay using specific T_3-an-
tibodies raised in rabbits and precipitating donkey anti-rabbit antiserum. Also incubation of $[^{125}I]T_4$ with particulate tyrosine hydroxylase revealed no T_3 after chromatography and autoradiography.

A preparation of soluble tyrosine hydroxylase, after ammonium sulphate precipitation[11], also failed to catalyse formation of T_3.

α-Me-Tyr[8,9] at 80 µM almost completely inhibited our praticulate enzyme preparation. However, PTU, known as inhibitor of T_3-formation *in
vivo*[1,2] and *in vitro*[12,16-22], had practically no effect on tyrosine
hydroxylase activity; it was also not influenced by T_4 at 80 µM.

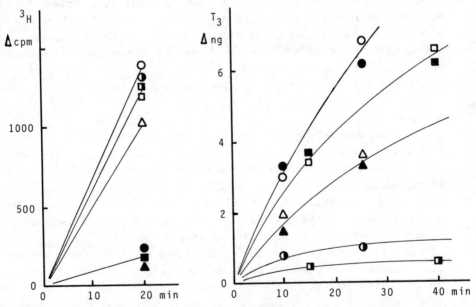

Fig. 1. Tyrosine hydroxylase activity (left) and T_4 5'-deiodinase activity (right) in
rat liver, standard assay conditions (pH 6.2). ☐ Homogenate, ○ Pellet, △ Supernatant;
Filled symbols with 80 µM α-Me-Tyr; half-filled symbols with 80 µM PTU.

We were able to demonstrate in rat liver fractions, prepared by the same procedure, both enzyme activities (fig. 1). However, tyrosine hydroxylase and 5'-deiodinase activity were selectively inhibited by α-Me-Tyr and PTU, respectively. This is in accordance with recent reports[20,21] that in rat liver homogenate 5'-deiodinase was not influenced by α-Me-Tyr.

A particulate fraction of bovine liver was free of tyrosine hydroxylase activity. However, the $T_4 \rightarrow T_3$ converting activity was the highest so far reported (7 ng T_3/mg protein/min from 2 μM T_4, which would amount to a conversion of 25% of added T_4 in 30 min). This enzyme preparation was also very stable.

In contrast to tyrosine hydroxylase activity, the T_4 5'-deiodinase activity was unaffected by α-Me-Tyr (40 μM), the absence of oxygen or tetrahydropteridines (DMPH$_4$, H$_4$folate, H$_4$biopterin). Conversely, EDTA improved T_3 formation whereas tyrosine hydroxylase was not affected. The 5'-deiodinase activity in this preparation was totally dependent upon added thiol compounds. While in the absence of DTE no T_3 was formed, we observed a concentration dependent relationship of T_3 formation with DTE.

SUMMARY

In contrast to the mentioning of Dratman *et al.*[3] we could not observe any significant conversion of $T_4 \rightarrow T_3$ by tyrosine hydroxylase *in vitro*. Our notion that tyrosine hydroxylase is not involved in 5'-deiodination of T_4 is supported by the findings that these enzymes can preferentially be blocked by α-Me-Tyr and PTU, respectively.

Since the T_4 5'deiodinating enzymatic activity from bovine liver is strongly dependent upon addition of thiol compounds, these findings suggest that this enzyme represents a transhydrogenase.

ACKNOWLEDGEMENTS

We wish to thank Dr. K. Bauer, TU Berlin, for his help and discussions throughout this work. 6.7-Dimethylpterin and biopterin were the gift of Prof. W. Pfleiderer, University Konstanz.

REFERENCES
1. for reviews see: (1974) Handb. Physiol., 3, Greer, M.A. and Solomon, D.H. eds.
2. Ingbar, S.H. and Braverman, L.E. (1975) Ann. Rev. Med., 26, 443-449.
3. Dratman, M.B., Axelrod, J., Crutchfield, F.L., Coyle, J.T., and Utiger, R. (1973) Proc. Endocrine Soc., p. A-156 (Abstr.).
4. Dratman, M.B. (1974) J. Theor. Biol., 46, 255-270.

5. Dratman, M.B., Crutchfield, F.L., Axelrod, J., Bond, C. and Marsh, E. (1974) Proc. American Thyroid Ass. Meeting, p. T-9 (Abstr.).

6. Sterling, F.H. (1975) N. Engl. J. Med., 293, 309.

7. Sack, J. and Fisher, D.A. (1975) in Perinatal Thyroid Physiology and Disease, Fisher, D.A. and Burrow, G.N. eds., Raven Press, New York, pp. 197-209.

8. McGeer, E.G. and McGeer, P.L. (1967) Can. J. Biochem., 45, 115-131.

9. Lutsky, B.N. and Zenker, N. (1968) J. Med. Chem., 11, 1241-1242.

10. Weinhold, P.A. and Rethy, V.B. (1969) Biochem. Pharmac., 18, 677-680.

11. Nagatsu, T., Levitt, M. and Udenfriend, S. (1964) J. Biol. Chem., 239, 2910-17.

12. Hüfner, M. and Knöpfle, M. (1975) in Biochemical Basis of Thyroid Stimulation and Thyroid Hormone Action, von zur Mühlen, A. and Schleusener, H. eds., Thieme, Stuttgart, pp. 215-220.

13. Flock, E.V., David, D., Hallenbeck, G.A. and Owen, C.A. (1963) Endocrinology, 73, 764-74.

14. Shiman, R., Akino, M. and Kaufman, S. (1971) J. Biol. Chem., 246, 1330-1340.

15. Albright, E.C., Larson, F.C. and Tust, R.H. (1954) Proc. Soc. Exp. Biol. Med., 86, 137-140.

16. Hesch, R.D., Brunner, G. and Söling, H.D. (1975) Clinica Chimica Acta, 59, 209-213.

17. Höffken, B., Ködding, R., Hehrmann, R., von zur Mühlen, A., Jüppner, H. and Hesch, R.D. (1975) in Biochemical Basis of Thyroid Stimulation and Thyroid Hormone Action, von zur Mühlen, A. and Schleusener, H. eds., Thieme, Stuttgart, pp. 204-214.

18. Visser, T.J., van der Does-Tobe, I., Docter, R. and Hennemann, G. (1975) Biochem. J., 150, 489-493.

19. Visser, T.J., van der Does-Tobe, I., Docter, R. and Hennemann, G. (1976) Biochem. J., 157, 479-482.

20. Hüfner, M., Grussendorf, M. and Ntokalou, M. (1977) Clin. Chim. Acta, 78, 251-259.

21. Chopra, I.J. (1977) Endocrinology, 101, 453-463.

22. Cavalieri, R.R., Gavin, L.A., Bui, F., McMahon, F., Hammond, M. (1977) Biochem. Biophys. Res. Commun., 79, 897-902.

23. Chopra, I.J. (1978) Science, 199, 904-906.

24. Rokos, H. and Scheiffele, E. (1977) Ann. Endocrinol. (Paris), 38, 31 A (Abstr.).

25. Bobst, A. and Viscontini, M. (1966) Helv. Chim. Acta, 49, 875-884.

26. Lowry, D.H., Rosebrough, N.T., Faler, A.L. and Randall, R.J. (1951) J. Biol. Chem., 193, 265-275.

27. Mineeva-Vyalykh, M.F. (1976) Vopr. Med. Khim., 22, 274-279.

28. Bublitz, C. (1977) Biochem. Med., 17, 13-19.

INTERACTION OF DIHYDROPTERIN REDUCTASE WITH BLUE DEXTRAN

K.G. SCRIMGEOUR, ANNE TIRPAK AND MICHAEL M. CHAUVIN
Department of Biochemistry, University of Toronto, Toronto, Canada

ABSTRACT

Blue Dextran-agarose is the most suitable "general ligand" matrix
for purification of dihydropterin reductase. Pure reductase with high
activity has been obtained from beef kidney using experimental conditions that separate dihydropterin reductase from other proteins that
bind to the Blue Dextran. In addition, we have found that folate or
amethopterin can elute the reductase from columns of Blue Dextran-agarose. The p-aminobenzoylglutamate portion of the folates is responsible
for this elution. We suggest that folate binds to the NAD^+ site of dehydrogenases, and are measuring the binding of folate to these enzymes.

INTRODUCTION

Quinonoid dihydropterin reductase catalyzes the reduction of quinonoid dihydropterin by the pyridine nucleotide NADH[1,2]. Affinity chromatography of dihydropterin reductase cannot be performed by binding its
specific substrate, a quinonoid dihydropterin, to an insoluble matrix
because this substrate is extremely unstable. Therefore, we have used
the "general ligand" or "group specific" method, with analogues of
either the pterin or the NADH as the affinity ligands. Initial experiments[3] provided purification methods, and also suggested a kinetic
mechanism for the reductase. The requirement for the presence of a
pyridine nucleotide for the binding of the enzyme to amethopterin agarose, but no pterin requirement for its binding to AMP-agarose, indicate that the mechanism is an ordered process in which quinonoid dihydropterin can only bind to the reductase after NADH has been bound, and
that tetrahydrobiopterin is the first product to be released. This
kinetic mechanism has since been verified by inhibition studies[4].

The most useful affinity ligand that we have encountered is Blue
Dextran. Enzymes that contain the dinucleotide (NAD^+) binding domain
interact specifically with the dye moiety of Blue Dextran, Cibacron
Blue F3GA[5]. They are eluted from columns of Blue Dextran-agarose
either by high concentrations of salt or by low concentrations of specific eluants such as NADH, NAD^+ or AMP. The results of our experiments
on the interaction of dihydropterin reductase with Blue Dextran have
provided both a rapid isolation method and evidence that folate and
amethopterin can bind to the NAD^+ domains of dehydrogenases.

MATERIALS AND METHODS

The spectrophotometric assay and the sources of the reagents have been published previously[1,3]. Blue Dextran-agarose was prepared and washed by the method of Ryan and Vestling[6]. The binding and elution of enzymes to Blue Dextran-agarose was determined with small (0.55 x 5.0 cm) columns of the affinity matrix. The buffer used for all experiments was Tris-HCl, pH 7.5 containing 1 mM 2-mercaptoethanol. Eluting ligands were added, as required, to this buffer.

RESULTS AND DISCUSSION

Elution from Blue Dextran-agarose

By column chromatography on Blue Dextran-agarose, we were able to achieve extensive purification (up to 60-fold) of dihydropterin reductase. However, even the most highly purified preparations contained small amounts of contaminating proteins. Whereas 1 M NaCl is required for elution of the reductase, low concentrations of nucleotides provide specific elution (NADH at 0.01 mM, NAD^+ at 1 mM, and AMP at 10 mM). These results predict that dihydropterin reductase contains the large polypeptide unit called the NAD^+ binding domain[5]. The reductase is the smallest protein to have this protein structural element (the NAD^+ domain would be over one-half of each reductase subunit). Additional evidence that Blue Dextran and Cibacron Blue bind to the NADH site of the reductase is their competitive inhibition with respect to NADH ($K_i = 3 \times 10^{-7}$ M)[4].

Preparation of pure reductase

When an enzyme is to be purified by the "general ligand" affinity method, binding and elution conditions must be found to separate the desired enzyme from the other proteins that bind to the matrix. By applying a modification to the affinity procedure, we have succeeded in eluting dihydropterin reductase from Blue Dextran-agarose in pure form. We had previously shown[3] that the presence of 6,7-dimethyltetrahydropterin delays or prevents the elution of reductase from AMP-agarose by NADH. Tetrahydropterin has a similar effect with reductase and columns of Blue Dextran-agarose. We have used this retarding effect with partially purified reductase from beef kidney to separate it from other dehydrogenases. Beef kidney extracts were fractionated by ammonium sulphate precipitation and by chromatography on a column of DEAE-cellulose, and the reductase (approx. 70 mg of protein, with a specific activity of 15 U/mg) was applied to a 4.2 x 4.0 cm column of Blue Dextran-agarose. This column was washed with 60 ml of 1 mM dimethyltetra-hydropterin-0.05 mM NADH in Tris buffer, and then with 120 ml of Tris. These washings removed proteins other than the reductase that were bound to the Blue Dextran. The reductase activity was eluted with a gradient of NAD^+. Most active tubes were electrophoretically pure, and a further 15-fold purification was achieved. This isolation method provides a rapid means for obtaining dihydropterin reductase that possesses high specific activity.

Elution by folate or by amethopterin

During our purification studies using NAD^+ analogues bound to agarose, we observed that folate or amethopterin can specifically elute dihydropterin reductase from these matrices[3]. Neither 6,7-dimethyl-tetrahydropterin nor 6,7-dimethyl-7,8-dihydropterin can effect elution, so that the pterin portion of folate cannot alone be responsible for elution of reductase. Results, summarized in Table 1, indicate that it

TABLE 1

ELUTION OF DIHYDROPTERIN REDUCTASE FROM BLUE DEXTRAN-AGAROSE

Eluting agent	Concentration required for elution
NaCl	1 M
NADH	0.01 mM
Folate or amethopterin	1 mM
p-Aminobenzoylglutamate	10 mM
L-Glutamate	25 mM
p-Aminobenzoate	Ineffective

is primarily the p-aminobenzoylglutamate portion of folate or amethopterin that causes elution of dihydropterin reductase from Blue Dextran-agarose. The data also indicate that the glutamate, the p-aminobenzoate, and the pterin groups of folate all contribute to its elution properties. Since, in order to be a specific eluant, folate must compete for the same binding site of the reductase as does Blue Dextran, we have concluded that folate interacts with the NAD^+ binding domain. This conclusion is supported by the observation that p-aminobenzoyl-glutamate is a weak competitive inhibitor with respect to NADH[4].

Over the past 15 years, there have been many reports that folate and amethopterin inhibit dehydrogenases. Our observations that folate interacts with the NAD^+ binding domain of dihydropterin reductase have suggested that inhibition of dehydrogenases by folate could be a competition between folate and NAD$^+$ or NADH. We have used elution of dehydrogenases by folate from columns of Blue Dextran-agarose as a probe for this type of competition. Both folate and p-aminobenzoyl-glutamate (10 mM-50 mM) can elute either liver alcohol dehydrogenase or heart lactate dehydrogenase from columns of Blue Dextran-agarose. We are currently attempting to determine the extent of interaction of folate with several dehydrogenases. If the inhibition of dehydrogenases by folate can be verified, then binding of folic acid to their NAD$^+$ binding domains can explain the unelucidated non-specific inhibitions by folate. Initial experiments suggest that the binding of folate is weaker than indicated by published inhibition studies. The observed apparent inhibitions by folate may have been caused by stray light artifacts, such as that shown[7] to have been the cause of the incorrect description of NADH as an allosteric regulator of glucose-6-phosphate dehydrogenase.

In conclusion, our studies on affinity chromatography of dihydropterin reductase have provided not only a good isolation method but also support for a kinetic mechanism, evidence for the presence of the NAD$^+$ domain, indication that folate binds to the NAD$^+$ site, and a possible explanation for inhibition of many dehydrogenases by folate.

ACKNOWLEDGEMENTS

This work was supported by the Medical Research Council of Canada. We would like to thank Michele Korri for her assistance.

REFERENCES

1. Cheema, S., Soldin, S.J., Knapp, A., Hofmann, T. and Scrimgeour, K.G. (1973) Can. J. Biochem., 51, 1229-1239.

2. Craine, J.E., Hall, E.S. and Kaufman, S. (1972) J. Biol. Chem. 247, 6082-6091.

3. Korri, K.K., Chippel, D., Chauvin, M.M., Tirpak, A. and Scrimgeour, K.G. (1977) Can. J. Biochem., 55, 1145-1152.

4. Simpson, R.C. and Scrimgeour, K.G. (1978) submitted to Can. J. Biochem.

5. Stellwagen, E. (1977) Accounts of Chem. Research, 10, 92-98.

6. Ryan, L.D. and Vestling, C.S. (1974) Arch. Biochem. Biophys., 160, 279-284.

7. Cavalieri, R.L. and Sable, H.Z. (1973) J. Biol. Chem., 248, 2815-2817.

RAT LIVER DIHYDROPTERIDINE REDUCTASE

STEPHANIE WEBBER and JOHN M. WHITELEY

Scripps Clinic and Research Foundation, La Jolla, CA 92037

Dihydropteridine reductase, which catalyzes the reduction of "quinonoid" dihydro-
pteridines to tetrahydropteridines by means of a reduced pyridine nucleotide,[1] has
been purified to homogeneity from rat liver in 20-30% yield using the procedure
shown in Table 1. The details of this procedure have been described previously,[2]
however, a new step employing a column of Cibacron Blue F3GA-agarose (Biorad Laboratories) has been included, which has given improved reproducibility and a product of
higher specific activity ($\sim$ 100 µg NADH oxidized/min/mg) when assayed by the modified
procedure of Cheema et al.[2,3] The purified enzyme has a MW of 51,000 and is composed
of two identical subunits.

The interaction of this purified dihydropteridine reductase with NADH, NADPH, NAD^+,
$NADP^+$ and the fluorescent $1,N^6$-ethenoadenine derivative of NAD^+ (ε-NAD^+) has been
examined by fluorescence titration. The dissociation constants of the nucleotides
were obtained by measuring the reduction in fluorescence of the reductase (excitation 285 nm, emission 335 nm). Quenching was greatest for the reduced nucleotides
(approximately 70%); in no case was a shift in either excitation or emission wavelength observed. Dissociation constants, shown in Table 2 together with K_m values
for the reduced compounds, were calculated from double reciprocal plots of change
in fluorescence vs. concentration of nucleotide. The low K_m and K_D values for
NADH suggest this is the preferred nucleotide cofactor for this enzymatic reaction.

TABLE 1

PURIFICATION OF RAT LIVER DIHYDROPTERIDINE REDUCTASE

Purification step	Protein (mg)	Enzyme (units)	Specific Activity (units/mg)	Recovery (%)
Acetic acid extract*	4090	1730	0.42	100
DEAE cellulose	806	1159	1.44	67
MTX-Sepharose	32.0	869	27.2	50
Cibacron Blue F3GA-agarose	6.6	536	81.2	31
Sephadex G-100	4.8	450	93.7	26

* From 100g of rat liver.

TABLE 2

DISSOCIATION AND MICHAELIS CONSTANTS FOR

RAT LIVER DIHYDROPTERIDINE REDUCTASE

PYRIDINE NUCLEOTIDE	K_D	K_m
	(M)	(M)
NADH	5.71×10^{-6}	2.9×10^{-5}
NADPH	3.12×10^{-5}	5.0×10^{-4}
NAD^+	2.00×10^{-5}	---
$NADP^+$	1.45×10^{-5}	---
$\varepsilon\text{-}NAD^+$	2.50×10^{-5}	---

If, during the titration of the enzyme and NADH, the nucleotide fluorescence was observed directly (excitation 348 nm, emission 456 nm) a maximum 3-fold enhancement was observed at a 1:1 molar ratio (Fig. 1). In contrast NADPH required 7-8 moles of nucleotide per mole of enzyme to achieve saturation, which suggested non-specific binding. Titration of the reductase with $\varepsilon\text{-}NAD^+$ also showed an equivalence point at a 1:1 molar ratio, although the enhancement of fluorescence in the presence of enzyme was extremely small.

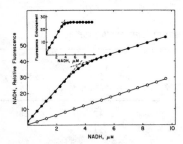

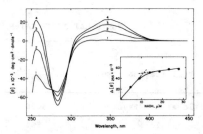

Fig. 1. The fluorescence changes observed when the NADH concentration is increased from 0 to 9.5 µm in the presence (•——•) and absence (o——o) of rat liver dihydropteridine reductase (3.28 µM) (excitation 348 nm; emission, 454 nm). *Inset*, fluorescence enhancement of NADH as a function of nucleotide concentration. Solutions were buffered at pH 7.0 with 0.05 M Tris-hydrochloride, 0.001 M β-mercaptoethanol.

Fig. 2. The CD spectrum at 25°C of rat liver dihydropteridine reductase (10.1 µM) in 0.05 M Tris-hydrochloride buffer, pH 7.0, containing 0.001 M β-mercapto-ethanol; alone (1), and after titration with 4.7 (2), 9.3 (3) and 14.0 (4) µM NADH. *Inset*, the change in molar ellipticity observed at 255 nm as a function of nucleotide concentration.

The binding of NADH and NAD$^+$ was also examined by circular dichroism measurements. The reductase alone showed an overall negative ellipticity (Fig. 2, curve 1), and the major band was centered at 285 nm ([θ] = 54,700 deg. cm^2, dmole^{-1}). Titration of the enzyme with NADH generated a band of positive ellipticity at 255 nm, a sharpening of the negative band at 285 nm, disappearance of the shoulder at 265 nm and a positive extrinsic Cotton effect between 340 and 350 nm. All of the transitions reached a maximum at a 1:1 molar ratio of enzyme to nucleotide as is shown for the 255 nm band in the inset to Fig. 2. No CD changes were observed when the enzyme was titrated with the oxidized nucleotide, NAD$^+$.

Stable complexes formed between dihydrofolate reductase, thymidylate synthetase and their respective substrates and cofactors have been demonstrated previously by altered mobilities during polyacrylamide gel electrophoresis.[4,5] When similar experiments were performed with dihydropteridine reductase preincubated with excess NADH, the formation of an enzyme-cofactor complex was also visible by the appearance of a second band of increased mobility 0.26 compared to the native enzyme 0.21. However, variation in incubation time from 1-120 min at temperatures between 4 and 37°, with up to a 50-fold excess of pyridine nucleotide, failed to demonstrate quantitative conversion to a nucleotide-enzyme complex. In addition, no bands which suggested the formation of a ternary complex were observed when the enzyme and nucleotide were incubated with a 5-fold excess of either the reaction product, 2-amino-4-hydroxy-6,7-dimethyl-5,6,7,8-tetrahydropteridine or the inhibitor, methotrexate.

The possible existence of an unstable 2:1 nucleotide-enzyme complex which is not visible by fluorescence or CD was investigated by equilibrium dialysis experiments. The rate of efflux of ^{3}[H]NADH from a dialyzing mixture of nucleotide and enzyme was compared to the efflux rate of the labeled nucleotide when dialyzed alone. The results analyzed mathematically again, however, supported a 1:1 relationship for the reductase and NADH.[6]

The participation of sulfhydryl groups in the catalytic activity of the reductase has also been examined, with particular reference to their influence on pyridine nucleotide binding. The enzyme is strongly inhibited by both mercuric chloride and p-chloromercuribenzoate (PCMB); complete inactivation is associated with the binding of 6 moles of the latter reagent. This observation is in agreement with amino acid analyses which have shown 3 sulfhydryl groups per subunit or a total of 6 per dimeric enzyme molecule. The loss of activity produced by PCMB can be halted, although not restored by the addition of NADH at any point in the titration. If a 1:1 enzyme-NADH mixture is titrated, the nucleotide affords significant protection from inactivation (80% activity retention) with the binding of only 4 moles of mercurial. Prolonged incubation, however, results in slow denaturation which reaches 50% after 2 h and almost 90% after 24 h.

The combined results of these experiments confirm that a complex is formed between homogeneous rat liver dihydropteridine reductase and only one mole of its preferred cofactor NADH. This result was unexpected as the reductase from this and other sources[2,3,7] consists of two apparently identical subunits and therefore an affinity for two moles of cofactor might be anticipated. It is possible that the rat liver enzyme may indeed possess a second site which is activated only in the presence of the quinonoid dihydropterin substrate; the demonstration of such a property must await the isolation of a stable form of the quinonoid substrate or a high affinity analog. The preliminary thiol-titration experiments suggest that sulfhydryl groups are involved in the maintenance of the catalytic activity of the reductase; there is as yet, however, no evidence for a direct involvement of a thiol group at the active site.

ACKNOWLEDGEMENTS

This investigation was supported by USPHS Grants Nos. CA-11778 and GM-22125. John M. Whiteley is the recipient of a USPHS Research Career Development Award (CA-00106 from the National Cancer Institute.

REFERENCES

1. Kaufman, S. (1971) Adv. Enzymol. 35, 245-319.

2. Webber, S., Diets, T.L., Snyder, W.R. and Whiteley, J.M. (1978) Anal. Biochem. 84, 491-503.

3. Cheema, S., Soldin, S.J., Knapp, A., Hofmann, T. and Scrimgeour, K.G. (1973) Can. J. Biochem. 51, 1229-1239.

4. Neef, V.G., and Huennekens, F.M. (1975) Arch. Biochem. Biophys. 171, 435-443.

5. Aull, J.L., Lyon, J.A. and Dunlap, R.B. (1974) Microchem. J. 19, 210-218.

6. Webber, S. and Whiteley, J.M. (1978) J. Biol. Chem., *in press*.

7. Craine, J.E., Hall, E.S. and Kaufman, S. (1972) J. Biol. Chem. 247, 6082-6091.

INHIBITION OF MYCOBACTERIAL DIHYDROFOLIC REDUCTASE BY 2,4-DIAMINO-6-ALKYLPTERIDINES
AND DEAZAPTERIDINES

W. T. COLWELL, V. H. BROWN, J. I. DEGRAW, AND N. E. MORRISON
Department of Bio-Organic Chemistry, SRI International, Menlo Park, CA 94025; Johns
Hopkins University, Baltimore, MD 21205

ABSTRACT

Four series of antifolate agents have been investigated for their activity against
Mycobacterium species 607--a culturable mycobacterium that shows a drug-response
profile similar to that of *M. leprae*. The series investigated were 2,4-diamino-6-
substituted pteridines, quinazolines, and 1,3,5- and 1,3,8-triazanaphthalenes. The
pteridine compounds were effective inhibitors of isolated DHFR from *M. sp. 607* but
cellular growth inhibition was disappointing. The 1,3,8-triazanapthalenes were
similarly effective against DHFR and were also effective cell growth inhibitors. A
few examples of the relatively unknown 1,3,5-triazanapthalene series were investigated
however the compounds were ineffective in either assay. The quinazoline series,
particularly the 5-methyl-6-alkyl compounds, were exceptionally potent DHFR inhibitors
and were highly effective in the whole cell assay. The latter compounds showed
potentiative synergy when tested in combination with the antileprotic drug diamino-
diphenyl sulfone. Several of the quinazolines were selected for assay against *M.*
leprae in the mouse foot pad.

The synthesis of several series of antifolate compounds was undertaken in attempt
to prepare a compound that could be used in combination with the known antileprotic
diaminodiphenyl sulfone--a PABA competitor--in the treatment of leprosy. The only
direct assay against *M. leprae* is an expensive, lengthy (6-9 months) *in vivo* screen
against the organism harbored in the mouse foot pad.[1] However, a correlation has been
observed between minimum inhibitory concentrations (MIC) for *Mycobacterium species*
607, determined *in vitro*, and dietary MIC's for *M. leprae* growing in the mouse foot
pad.[2] Therefore initial screens chosen for this work were the *in vitro* whole cell
growth inhibition of *M. species 607* and inhibition of the dihydrofolic reductase
(DHFR) from this organism.

The first set of compounds screened were 2,4-diamino-6-substituted pteridines. The
structures and inhibition data for these compounds are shown in Table 1. Since
the mycobacteria do not require exogenous folate, it is likely that they do
not have active transport provision for passing the more polar compounds such as
Aminopterin or Methotrexate through the cell wall. This is apparently demonstrated by
the lack of whole cell inhibition shown by the latter two compounds, although they

TABLE 1

BIOLOGICAL DATA IN *M. sp. 607* FOR 2,4-DIAMINO-6-SUBSTITUTED PTERIDINES AND SEVERAL
OTHER 2,4-DIAMINO DHFR INHIBITORS

Compound	R	Inhibn of Mycobacterial Dihydrofolic Reductase Ki	Km/Ki	Mycobacterial Growth Inhibn MIC, nmol/ml
1	CH_3	5.1×10^{-6}	0.8	>568
2	$n-C_4H_9$	1.0×10^{-9}	4,100	917
3	$(CH_3)_2CHCH_2$	9×10^{-10}	4,560	688
4	$n-C_5H_{11}$	1.2×10^{-9}	3,415	862
5	$(CH_3)_2CH(CH_2)_2$	1.0×10^{-9}	4,100	775
6	$C_6H_5CH_2$	9×10^{-10}	4,560	>794
7	$3,4,5-(OCH_3)_3C_6H_2CH_2$	5×10^{-9}	820	347
8	$3,4,5-(OCH_3)_3C_6H_2(CH_2)_2$	1.8×10^{-8}	230	>281
9	$3,4-(Cl_2)C_6H_3CH_2$	2×10^{-9}	2,050	>311
Trimethoprim		7.0×10^{-8}	58.5	34
Pyrimethamine		7.5×10^{-8}	54.6	101
Aminopterin		1.8×10^{-10}	23,111	742
Amethopterin (Methotrexate)		3.5×10^{-10}	11,714	2200

Km = Michaelis constant for dihydrofolic acid at pH 6.0 and 25° = 4.1×10^{-6}.

possessed the highest Km/Ki ratio among the compounds in Table 1. Potent cell entry
is indicated for the relatively non-polar Trimethoprim and Pyrimethamine as they have
fairly impressive MIC values while having little effect on mycobacterial DHFR. The
structurally related compounds 7, 8, and 9 behave in a similar manner. Compounds 2-6
showed good DHFR activity but poor cell growth inhibition. Comparison of the DHFR
activity for compound 1 with that for 2-6 suggests the presence of a lipophilic region
on the enzyme with a requirement for the 6-substituent to be greater than methyl to
obtain substantial binding. As it had been observed by Shepard that Trimethoprim
alone was without effect against *M. leprae*[3] it was decided to investigate other series
of DHFR inhibitors in an attempt to find compounds with *M. species 607* activity
superior to that shown by this compound.

The bioassay data for some 2,4-diamino-1,3,5- and 1,3,8-triazanaphthalenes are
presented in Table 2. The three 1,3,5-triaza compounds showed promise only for the
compound (10) containing the more complex pteroate sidechain. The 1,3,8-triaza series
displayed impressive DHFR and whole cell inhibition properties. There was little to
differentiate the compounds in this series, but the desirability of a 5-substituent—
such as methyl—and a fairly large, lipophilic-6-substituent was indicated.

TABLE 2

BIOLOGICAL DATA IN *M. sp. 607* FOR 2,4-DIAMINO-1,3,5- AND 1,3,8-TRIAZANAPTHALENES

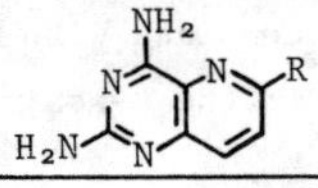

No.	R	Inhibn of Mycobacterial Dihydrofolic Reductase Ki	Km/Ki	MIC µg/ml
10	$-CH_2NH-\bigcirc-COOEt$ 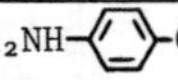	7.8×10^{-10}	5256	30
11	$-CH_3$	1.4×10^{-6}	3.2	>100
12	$n-C_4H_9$	7.6×10^{-8}	54	>100

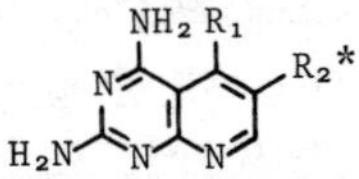

	R_1	R_2			
13	$-CH_3$	$i-C_4H_9$	1.5×10^{-10}	3727	3.6
14	$-CH_3$	$n-C_5H_{11}$	2.1×10^{-10}	5256	3.7
15	$-CH_3$	$n-C_6H_{13}$	3.0×10^{-10}	7345	7.2
16	$n-C_3H_7$	$-C_2H_5$	5.4×10^{-9}	1336	411
17	$-CH_3$	$-CH_2-\bigcirc-Cl$ 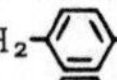	2.1×10^{-10}	5256	3.3
18	$-CH_3$	$-CH_2-\bigcirc-Cl$ 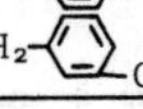	2.3×10^{-10}	5616	2.3

*Compounds provided by the Burroughs-Wellcome Co. See B. S. Hurlbert et al., J. Med. Chem. 11, 703, 708, 711 (1968).

TABLE 3

BIOLOGICAL DATA IN *M. sp. 607* FOR 2,4-DIAMINO-5-METHYL-6-SUBSTITUTED QUINAZOLINES

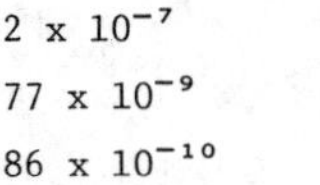

No.	R	Inhibn of Mycobacterial Dihydrofolic Reductase Ki	Km/Ki	MIC, nmol/ml (µg/ml)
19	H	1.5×10^{-6}	2.7	115 (20.0)
20	CH_3	5.2×10^{-7}	7.9	16 (3.0)
21	$n-C_3H_7$	1.77×10^{-9}	2,300	1.8 (0.4)
22	$n-C_4H_9$	2.86×10^{-10}	14,300	3.0 (0.7)
23	$n-C_5H_{11}$	1.79×10^{-14}	2.29×10^8	7.1 (1.75)
24	$i-C_5H_{11}$	(5.62×10^{-16})	(7.29×10^9)	8.2 (2.0)
25	$n-C_6N_{13}$	1.79×10^{-13}	2.29×10^7	15.5 (4.0)

Several 2,4-diamino-5-methyl quinazolines had also been prepared and assayed for mycobacterial activity. The MIC data for the first three members of the series (compounds 19, 20 and 21, Table 3) combined with the previously observed desirability for larger lipophilic substituents in the 6-position encouraged us to put our major effort into this series.

Seven 6-alkyl compounds were assayed in this program (Table 3). Both DHFR potency and MIC values peaked for the intermediate members of the series. Again, the compound (21) possessing the best MIC value was not the most potent DHFR inhibitor. Compounds 23, 24 and 25 however had Km/Ki values ranking with the most potent ever measured against an isolated DHFR.

Further screening was conducted with the 6-n-propyl compound 21 owing to its favorable MIC value and also compound availability. When the 6-n-propyl analog was used in combination with the antileprotic drug diaminodiphenyl sulfone against *M. sp. 607* a pronounced synergistic effect was observed. The optimal MIC requirement of the quinazoline was reduced by eightfold and DDS by 20-fold for mycobacterial growth inhibition. The plot of changing values of MIC's for both drug components according to the method of Rosenoer[4] established that true potentiative synergism was in effect.

Low oral and moderate i.p. toxicity in mice has been demonstrated for these quinazolines. Subsequent screening of n-propyl compound 21 against *M. leprae* in the mouse foot pad has given equivocal results when tested in both alone and in combination with diaminodiphenyl sulfone.

Only weak antibacterial action was shown by the quinazolines when screened against seven other organisms *in vitro*.

REFERENCES

1. Shepard, C. C. (1960) J. Exp. Med., 122, 445.
2. Morrison, N. E. (1971) Int. J. Lepr., 39, 34.
3. Data of C. C. Shepard cited in Ref. 2.
4. Rosenoer, V. (1966) Exp. Chemother., 4, 9.

DETERMINATION OF THE GAMMAGLUTAMYL CHAIN LENGTHS IN THE FOLATES BY A COMBINED ZINC/ACID-PERACID PROCEDURE

CHARLES M. BAUGH, LLOYD MAY, ELEANOR BRAVERMAN and M.G. NAIR

Department of Biochemistry, College of Medicine, University of South Alabama, Mobile, Alabama   36688

ABSTRACT

In the ten years since synthetic pteroylpoly-γ-glutamates have been available,[1-3] evidence suggests that these peptides are the functioning forms of this group of coenzymes.[4,5] Methods developed to determine the length of the glutamyl chains[6,7] have recently proven inadequate.[8,9] A new method incorporating the zinc/acid[7] method followed by a peracid[9] treatment is reported here.

INTRODUCTION

The number of potential structures, minor structural variations, chemical instability and low concentrations of the folates in biological materials preclude the quantitative isolation and identification of each member of the group directly. Without methodology to approach these problems head on, a number of methods have been proposed to allow the gross assessment of the distribution of pteroyl-γ-glutamyl chain lengths irrespective of other structural features. These methods all involve the cleavage of the C^9-N^{10} bond, producing the corresponding p-amino-benzoylglutamates (pABGs) which are then identified by co-chromatography with authentic samples.

The first method to be developed[6] and employed[10,11] used alkaline permanganate. A recent critical evaluation of this method provided evidence that virtually all the folate coenzyme forms were resistant at C^9-N^{10} to alkaline permanganate at room temperature for 20 minutes. Only folic acid (PGA), dihydrofolic acid (DHF), tetrahydrofolic acid

(THF), and 5-formyltetrahydrofolic acid (5-CHO-THF) were cleaved to pABG in reasonable yields.[8]

Similar problems have arisen with a zinc/acid reductive cleavage method[7] which has been used in a number of instances.[12,13] Although a complete evaluation of this method has not been reported, it recently was noted that 5-methyltetrahydrofolate (5-CH_3-THF) was resistant to the zinc/acid method, yielding 5-CH_3-DHF instead of the expected pABG.[9]

Therefore, a new approach to cleavage of folates at C^9-N^{10} was begun. A model compound, 5-CH_3-THF, which was resistant to cleavage in both the existing methods, was used. A method was ultimately perfected using peracetic acid in trifluoroacetic acid (TFA) which cleaved at C^9-N^{10} to pABG quantitatively.[9] We report here the extension of this method to provide a procedure for the quantitative cleavage of all known folate coenzymes without destruction of the pABG products.

MATERIALS AND METHODS

The compound, mixture of compounds, or folate extract to be cleaved is made 50% (v/v) with TFA. Final volumes have varied from 3.0 to 140 ml. The reaction is placed in a 50° water bath for five minutes to promote conversion of 5-CHO-THF to 5,10=CH-THF. Zinc powder, 200 mg, is added and the mixture stirred for 45 minutes at room temperature. Excess zinc, which should persist throughout the reaction time, is removed by filtration into a round bottomed flask. The reaction vessel and filter are washed with small amounts of 50% TFA.

Peracetic acid (40%, FMC Corp.) is diluted into 100% TFA to a final concentration of 100 μmoles/ml and stored in the cold for 24 hours during which time we assume that pertrifluoroacetic acid is formed.[9] The peracid reagent is stable for 2-3 months in the refrigerator.

A 10- to 50-fold excess of the peracid reagent is added to the zinc filtrate and the reaction stirred for 45 minutes at room temperature. The solution is evaporated to dryness under vacuum. The residue is

dissolved in 10 ml water and adjusted to pH 7, then made 0.1 N with
respect to NaOH and placed in a boiling water bath for 15 minutes to
hydrolyze any N-trifluoroacetyl derivatives of pABG which have formed.
The ZnOH present is removed by centrifugation. Authentic marker
compounds are added in the case of bacterial extracts. The alkaline
solution is neutralized, diluted with water and chromatographed on DEAE
cellulose in the chloride form as previously described.[7] The pABG
products are quantitated at 274 nm.[14]

RESULTS AND DISCUSSION

Early in this work it became clear that the zinc/acid procedure was
effective in cleaving fully oxidized forms of folic acid only, with the
exception of THF, which is known to be unstable in acid.[15]

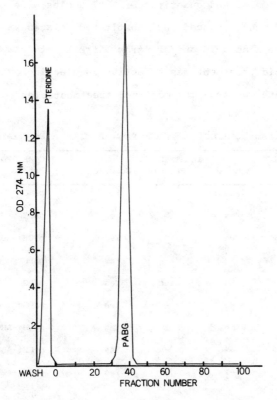

FIGURE 1. Purification of peracid cleavage products of 5-CH3-THF

The treatment of 10 μmoles of 5-CH$_3$-THF (in 5.0 ml 0.1% 2-mercapto-ethanol/0.05 N HCl) with 5.0 ml 100% TFA and 100 μmoles (1.0 ml) peracid reagent for 30 minutes at room temperature produced a clear gold solution. After evaporation to dryness and treatment with 0.1 N NaOH for 15 minutes at 100°, the pH was adjusted to 7.0. This solution was then diluted, applied to a 1.2 x 20 cm DEAE cellulose column and washed with water until the UV monitor returned to baseline. The column was eluted by a linear gradient of one liter each water to 0.5 M NaCl in 12.5 ml fractions. Two UV peaks were obtained; the yellow first peak (see Figure 1), which did not bind to the column, was an unstable pteridine which remains to be identified. The second peak eluted in the expected position for pABG and was so identified spectrally.[14] The pABG peak was pooled and quantitated; 9.97 μmoles were recovered.

A variety of other reduced and substituted folates was prepared and put through the zinc/acid and/or peracid treatment. As shown in Table 1, the zinc/acid treatment was effective in cleaving oxidized folates and methotrexate, whereas the combined treatment cleaved all forms.

TABLE 1

PRODUCTS AND YIELDS OF COMBINED ZINC/ACID-PERACID CLEAVAGE OF FOLATES

FOLATE DERIVATIVE	TREATMENT			COMBINED METHOD RESULTS	
	Zinc/Acid	Peracid	Combined	Product	% Yield
PGA	Yes	No	Yes	pABG	100
PteG$_n$	Yes	No	Yes	pABG$_n$	100
Methotrexate	Yes	No	Yes	p-CH$_3$-ABG	100
THF	–	–	Yes	pABG	100
5-CH$_3$-THF	No	Yes	Yes	pABG	100
5-CH$_3$-THF(G$_7$)	No	–	Yes	pABG$_7$	100
5-CHO-THF	No	?	Yes	p-CH$_3$-ABG	98
5,10-CH$_2$-THF	–	–	Yes	p-CH$_3$-ABG	98
5,10=CH-THF	–	–	Yes	p-CH$_3$-ABG	96
10-CHO-THF	–	–	Yes	pABG	97

There is an indication that 5-CHO-THF is not cleaved directly but only after cyclization to the 5,10=CH-THF and subsequent reduction in the zinc/acid to 10-CH_3-THF, which is then cleaved by the peracid reagent. This conclusion was based on the following: (1) p-CH_3-ABG was the product;[16] (2) less than quantitative yields were obtained when the peracid treatment alone was used; (3) the presence of p-CH_3-ABG was confirmed by Nmr spectroscopy. Presumably due to concentrated buffer present from the preparation of 10-CHO-THF, that compound did not cyclize in these studies[17] and at some stage of the treatment, either the starting compound or the pABG derivative was deformylated to yield pABG as the product.

At this point it seemed that a combination of the two methods could cleave all forms of the folate coenzymes. The problems of sequence for the procedure was considered. Concern that pyrazine ring oxidation in the peracid environment could create subsequent problems, and the fact that adequate yields were obtained when the zinc/acid treatment preceded the peracid established this sequence for routine use. However, arguments for the reverse sequence of reagents can be made.

The cleavage of 5-methyltetrahydropteroylheptaglutamate [5-CH_3-THF(G_7)] and quantitative recovery of $pABG_7$ clearly demonstrated the nondestructive nature of these procedures toward gammaglutamyl bonds.

If these methods are to find use in the study of natural folate distribution with regard to gammaglutamyl peptide lengths, several important considerations must be made. The pABGs and p-CH_3-ABGs of the same chain lengths are poorly resolved from each other as anions. No such pair of compounds can be separated adequately by DEAE cellulose chromatography to permit quantitation of both members. When a suitably labeled folate mixture is cleaved and chromatographed, without carrier, the plot of radioactivity versus fraction number can be used directly to assign chain length. These peaks of radioactivity are very sharp because of the low molar concentration of the labeled material. When these peaks are pooled and divided into two equal portions, one chromatographed with pABG markers and the other with p-CH3-ABG markers, precise alignment of radioactivity and UV provides assignment of the correct structure. Because of the possibility of mixtures of pABG and p-CH3-ABG at any given chain length, studies on separation are also in progress.

REFERENCES

1. Krumdieck, C.L. and Baugh, C.M. (1969) Biochem. 8, 1568-1572

2. Baugh, C.M., Stevens, J.C., and Krumdieck, C.L. (1970) Biochim. Biophys. Acta 212, 116-125

3. Meienhofer, J., Jacobs, P.M., Godwin, H.A. and Rosenberg, I.H. (1970) J. Org. Chem. 35, 4237-4140

4. Baugh, C.M. and Krumdieck, C.L. (1971) Ann. N.Y. Acad. Sci. 186, 7-28

5. Burton, E., Selhub, J. and Sakami, W. (1969) Biochem. J. 111, 793-795

6. Houlihan, C.M. and Scott, J.M. (1972) Biochem. Biophys. Res. Comm. 48, 1675-1681

7. Baugh, C.M., Braverman, E.B. and Nair, M.G. (1974) Biochem. 13, 4952-4957

8. Maruyama, T., Shiota, T. and Krumdieck, C.L. (1978) Anal. Biochem. 84, 227-295

9. Baugh, C.M., Braverman, E.B. Nair, M.G. Horne, D.W., Briggs, W.T. and Wagner, C. (1978) Anal. Biochem. (in press)

10. Buehring, K.U., Tamura, T. and Stokstad, E.L.R. (1974) J. Biol. Chem. 249, 1081-1089

11. Brown, J.P., Davidson, G.E. and Scott, J.M. (1974) Biochim. Biophys. Acta 343, 78-88

12. Hintze, D.N. and Farmer, J.L. (1975) J. Bacteriol. 124, 1236-1239

13. Leslie, G.I. and Baugh, C.M. (1974) Biochem. 13, 4957-4961

14. Kallen, R.G. and Jencks, W.P. (1966) J. Biol. Chem. 241, 5845-5850

15. Zakrezewski, S.F. (1966) J. Biol. Chem. 241, 2957

16. Fu, S.J., Reiner, M. and Loo, T.L. (1965) J. Org. Chem. 30, 1277-1278

17. May, M., Bardos, T.J., Barger, F.L., Lansford, M., Ravel, J.M., Sutherland, J.L. and Shive, W. (1951) J. Am. Chem. Soc. 73, 3067-3075

SYNTHESIS AND ANTIFOLATE ACTIVITY OF 10-DEAZAMINOPTERIN

J. I. DEGRAW, V. H. BROWN, R. L. KISLIUK, AND F. M. SIROTNAK

SRI International, Menlo Park, CA 94025; Tufts University Medical School, Boston, MA 02111; and Memorial Sloan-Kettering Cancer Center, New York, NY 10021

ABSTRACT

10-Deazaminopterin (10-DA) was synthesized and shown to possess very potent antifolate properties. The inhibitory potency of 10-DA and reduced forms against folate dependent bacteria, the transport-pharmacokinetic advantages of this compound and its potent activity against L1210 leukemia and other tumor systems are being reviewed.

The synthetic methodology developed for preparation of 10-DA and related compounds in this area was derived from the classical Boone-Leigh route. Thus 10-DA was synthesized in a 15-step procedure originating from p-carboxybenzaldehyde and proceeding through 10-deaza-4-amino-4-deoxypteroic acid as a key intermediate. A practical synthetic approach originating from 2,4,5,6-tetraminopyrimidine is also presented.

INTRODUCTION

The antimicrobial and antileukemic activities of the potent dihydrofolate reductase inhibitors aminopterin and its N^{10}-methyl derivative, methotrexate (MTX) are well known. MTX has been a major clinical drug for the treatment of leukemias for over twenty years. However, other human cancers are only marginally responsive or unsusceptible to MTX. Various analogs have been made in attempts to improve the potency or therapeutic index of MTX. Recently, we have reported[1] the synthesis and antimicrobial activity of 10-deazaminopterin (10-DA, 1). This compound in which the N^{10}-nitrogen of aminopterin has been replaced by a methylene unit was found to be about as potent an inhibitor as MTX of two folate dependent bacteria, Streptococcus faecium and Lactobacillus casei. Moreover the dihydro and tetrahydro derivatives of 3 were more inhibitory than MTX or its reduced forms, thus making these new analogs among the most potent antifolates known (Table 1). 10-DA and its dihydro derivative were also potent inhibitors of dihydrofolate reductase derived from L. casei. The tetrahydro derivative was a poor inhibitor of the reductase, but a good inhibitor of the bacterial thymidylate synthetase.

10-DA was further tested[2,3] for bioavailability and antitumor activity. In Table 2 the relative s.c. activity of 10-DA and MTX against a variety of murine ascites tumors is shown. Maximum increases in life span for 10-DA vs. MTX at the approximately optimum dose of 12 mg/kg were significantly higher on all five cases and outstanding in the Ehrlich carcinoma, Taper liver tumor and Sarcoma-180. When

TABLE 1

BACTERIAL GROWTH AND ENZYME INHIBITION BY 10-DA AND REDUCED FORMS

| Compound | MIC (ng/ml) for 50% Inhibition | | Molarity for 50% Inhibition | |
	S. faecium	L. casei	Dihydrofolic Reductase[a]	Thymidylate Synthetase[a]
10-DA	0.20	0.02	4.5×10^{-9}	$> 1 \times 10^{-4}$
Dihydro-10-DA	0.01	0.002	4.5×10^{-9}	1×10^{-5}
Tetrahydro-10-DA	0.03	0.007	1.0×10^{-7}	5.7×10^{-6}
MTX	0.15	0.01	3.3×10^{-9}	$> 1 \times 10^{-4}$
Dihydro MTX	0.01	0.009		
Tetrahydro MTX	0.05	0.06		

[a]Derived from L. casei.

TABLE 2

RELATIVE ACTIVITY OF 10-DA AND MTX AGAINST MURINE ASCITES TUMORS

| Compound | Route[a] | Increased Life Span (%) | | | | |
		L1210	P815	Ehrlich	Taper	S-180
MTX	s.c.	149.8	109.1	17.0	41.6	64.0
10-DA	s.c.	171.6	118.4	64.0	84.2	159.6[b]
MTX	p.o.	57.8				
10-DA	p.o.	122.8				

[a]Optimum dose was 12 mg/kg subcutaneous; 6 mg/kg oral.
[b]Two 60-day survivors.

given orally, 10-DA was about 2.1 times more effective than MTX against L1210 at 6 mg/kg. At a dosage of 6 mg/kg against solid tumors the relative tumor volume (10-DA vs. MTX) was 12%/41% for Sarcoma-180, 16%/31% for Taper liver tumor and 20%/30% for Ehrlich carcinoma. The plasma and tissue (tumor, small intestine, marrow) pharmacokinetics were similar for the two drugs. However, the increased efficacy of 10-DA over MTX was attributed to relatively greater accumulation in tumor, but similar persistence of each compound in drug-limiting normal intestinal epithelium. Both compounds compete for the same membrane carrier mechanisms, but with a greater affinity being shown for 10-DA by the tumor carrier. Overall the data suggest an improved delivery for 10-DA and a broader spectrum of antitumor action in mice with a potential for wide clinical application for this new agent.

The initial synthetic route[1,4] for 10-DA was a 15 step process based on the classical Boone-Leigh method for 6-substituted pteridines. Starting from p-carboxy benzaldehyde (2, Scheme 1) a 5% overall yield of the key intermediate 4-amino-4-deoxy-10-deazapteroic acid (3) was obtained. Coupling of 3 with

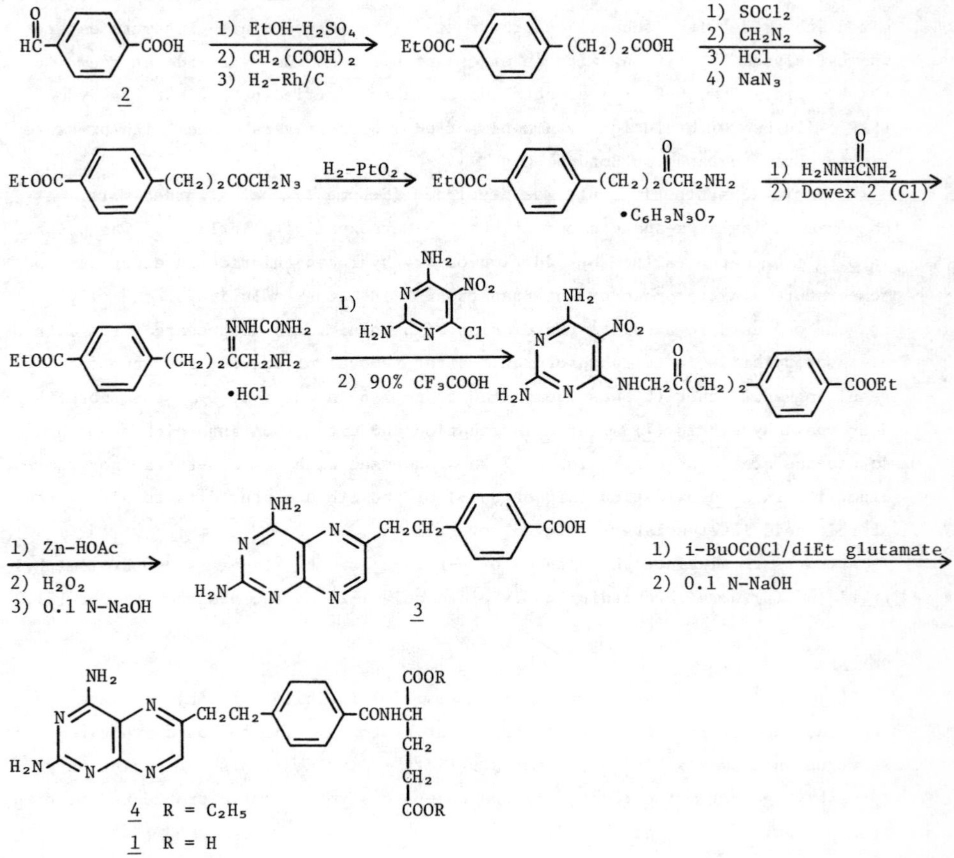

SCHEME 1

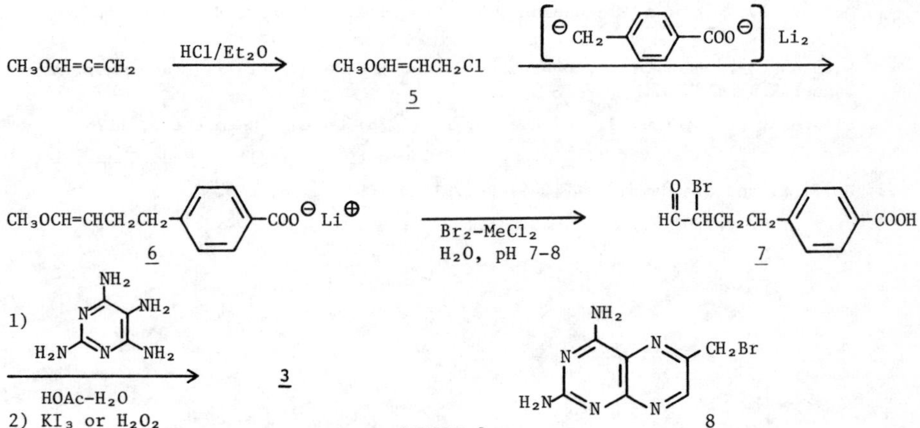

SCHEME 2

diethylglutamate was carried out with activation of the carboxyl group as the mixed anhydride with isobutyl chloroformate. The intermediate glutamate ester (4) was hydrolyzed by stirring with an excess of 0.1 N sodium hydroxide at room temperature. The 10-DA (1) so obtained could be purified by chromatography on DEAE-cellulose with elution by ammonia at pH 9 or by reverse phase high pressure liquid chromatography on Bondpak-C_{18}.

An improved synthetic route was developed (Scheme 2) that afforded more convenience in large-scale preparations. 3-Methoxyallyl chloride (5) was prepared in situ from methoxyallene by addition of dry hydrogen chloride in ether at low temperature via the procedure of Brandtsma.[5] The ether solution of the allyl reagent was used to alkylate the dianion of p-toluic acid as prepared from lithium di-isopropylamide in tetrahydrofuran.[6] After removal of solvent in vacuo the resulting enol ether (6) was brominated at pH 7-8 in water at 0-5° to afford the α-bromoaldehyde acid (7) after acidification and extraction into dichloromethane. An aqueous acetic acid solution of 7 was condensed with 2,4,5,6-tetraminopyrimidine with in situ oxidation (KI_3 or H_2O_2) of the dihydro pteridine to afford the pteroic acid intermediate (3) in 25% overall yield.

Attempts to alkylate the dianion of p-toluic acid by 2,4-diamino-6-bromomethyl-pteridine (8) were unrewarding and yielded only 1-2% of the desired product (3).

SUMMARY

10-Deazaminopterin was found to be a powerful inhibitor of dihydrofolate reductase and of growth in folate dependent bacteria. The compound exhibited broad spectrum antitumor activity against a variety of murine tumors, comparing very favorably against methotrexate. A convenient 4-step synthetic procedure starting from p-toluic acid is described.

REFERENCES

1. DeGraw, J., Kisliuk, R., Gaumont, Y., Baugh, C. and Nair, M. (1974) J. Med. Chem., 17, 552.

2. Sirotnak, F., DeGraw, J., Donsbach, R. and Moccio, D. (1977) Proc. Amer. Assoc. Cancer Res., 18, 37.

3. Sirotnak, F., DeGraw, J. and Chello, P. (1978) Current Chemother., 1128.

4. DeGraw, J., Brown, V., Kisliuk, R. and Gaumont, Y. (1971) J. Med. Chem., 14, 866.

5. Hoff, S. and Brandsma, L. (1969) Rec. Trav. Chim., 88, 845.

6. Creger, P. (1970) J. Am. Chem. Soc., 92, 1396.

8-DEAZA ANALOGS OF FOLIC ACID

J. I. DEGRAW, V. H. BROWN, R. L. KISLIUK, Y. GAUMONT, AND F. M. SIROTNAK
SRI International, Menlo Park, CA 94025; Tufts University Medical School, Boston,
MA 02111; and Memorial Sloan-Kettering Cancer Center, New York, NY 10021

ABSTRACT

Until 1964 it was generally accepted that antifolate activity required a
2,4-diaminopyrimidine structural moiety as in methotrexate or pyrimethamine. It was
then shown that derivatives of homofolate were potent antagonists in folate dependent
bacterial systems. Since that time it has also been shown that isofolate and
8-deazafolate possessed strong antifolate activity. We report here a discussion of
synthetic approaches for development of additional analogs in the 8-deazafolate
series.

A synthetic route was developed which depended on condensation of 2-acetamido-4-
hydroxypyrimidine-6-carboxyaldehyde with suitably substituted dimethyl 2-oxophos-
phonates to form 2-acetamido-4-hydroxy-6-pyrimidinyl enones. Subsequent saturation
of the olefinic ketone, introduction of nitrogen at C-5 via phenylazo coupling and
reductive cyclization afforded the required 1,3,5-triazanaphthalene intermediates.
Removal of blocking groups and attachment of glutamate functionality on pteroic acid
intermediates was accomplished in the usual manner. Special problems encountered in
the synthesis of 8-deazahomofolic acid are discussed.

INTRODUCTION

The synthesis and antimicrobial and enzyme inhibitory activity of homofolic acid
and its tetrahydro derivative were reported several years ago.[1,2] The tetrahydro
compound was found to be a potent growth inhibitor of the folate dependent organism
Streptococcus faecium and a strong inhibitor of bacterial thymidylate synthetase,
but was a poor inhibitor of dihydrofolate reductase. Tetrahydrohomofolic acid and
its 5-methyl derivative showed promising activity as anticancer agents,[3-5] being
active against methotrexate resistant strains in test systems. Isofolate has also
been shown to possess some antifolate activity.[6] The mechanism of action of these
relatively non-toxic 2-amino-4-hydroxypteridine compounds is distinctly different
from 2,4-diaminopteridine inhibitors of the reductase enzyme, such as methotrexate.
Tetrahydrohomofolate was shown to act by interference with folate uptake by cells,[7]
the inhibition of thymidylate synthetase notwithstanding. It is possible that an
active transport system for folic acid, located at the cell wall, is sensitive to
structural variation about N-5 through the connecting bridge to the side chain
phenyl ring in these molecules. In a previous communication[8] we reported on the
synthesis and antibacterial activity of 8-deazafolic acid and its reduced forms.

The interesting spectrum of activity encouraged further exploration in this new series of antifolate compounds.

At the outset, methods suitable for the preparation of 8-deazapterins containing a variety of substituents at position 6 were not available. A new synthetic route was developed[9] (Scheme 1) that used 2-acetamido-4-hydroxy-6-formylpyrimidine (1) as a key intermediate. When 1 was condensed with the sodium salt of dimethyl 2-oxo-heptylphosphonate under conditions of the Emmons-Horner reaction, the pyrimidinyl enone (2) was obtained in 87% yield. Attempts to directly couple 2 or the deacety-lated enone with benzenediazonium chloride failed to give the 5-phenylazo compound. However, reduction of the olefin, hydrolysis and diazonium coupling gave the phenyl-azo, ketone (3). Reductive ring closure with hydrogen-Pd/C gave 6-amyl-8-deazapterin (4), as shown by ultraviolet and ^{13}C-nmr spectra. It is unknown why a fully aromatic product was obtained, although air oxidation on workup or disproportionation of the 7,8-dihydro transitory intermediate may have been responsible. In one run, the tetrahydro compound (5) was obtained. It was unaffected by prolonged exposure to air or aqueous hydrogen peroxide, thus indicating the desired oxidative stability of the tetrahydro derivatives in the 8-deazapterin series.

The model sequence described above was then applied to the synthesis of 8,10-dideazafolic acid (6) (Scheme 2). p-Carbethoxyphenylpropionic acid chloride was used to selectively acylate lithio dimethyl methylphosphonate. The inverse addition of the lithio reagent to the ester acid chloride at -75° took advantage of the greater reactivity of the acid chloride function without exposure of the ester to an excess of lithio reagent. The oxophosphonate (7) so obtained was condensed with the pyrimidine aldehyde (1) to afford the key enone intermediate (8), m.p. 180-182°; NMR, δ, 7.95 (2 H, d, phenyl), 7.40 (4 H, m, olefin + phenyl), 6.45 (1 H, s, pyrim-5-H), 2.25 (3 H, s, Ac). The enone was hydrogenated over a rhodium catalyst and the product subjected to alkaline hydrolysis to give the 2-amino-4-hydroxy-6-pyrimidinyl keto acid (9), $\lambda^{pH\ 13}$ 236, 276 nm. Coupling of 9 with benzene diazonium chloride afforded the 5-phenylazo compound, which underwent reductive cyclization when hydrogenated over a palladium catalyst. As in the model series, the product obtained upon ring closure was the fully aromatic 8,10-dideazapteroic acid (10), $\lambda^{pH\ 13}$ 240, 271, 338 nm.

The deazapteroic acid was directly coupled with diethyl L-glutamate via activation of the carbonyl group as a mixed anhydride via treatment with isobutyl chloroformate. Subsequent hydrolysis of the ester groups by exposure to warm 0.1 N sodium hydroxide gave the target 8,10-dideazafolic acid (6) after chromatography on DEAE-cellulose, $\lambda^{pH\ 13}$ 242, 338 nm.

Table 1 shows the antimicrobial activities of 8,10-dideazafolic acid (6), the deazapteroic acid (10), and the uncyclized keto acid (9). Compounds 6 and 11 were moderately active against S. faecium, but only 6 had much effect against L. casei. None of the compounds showed significant inhibition of methotrexate-resistant strains of the organisms.

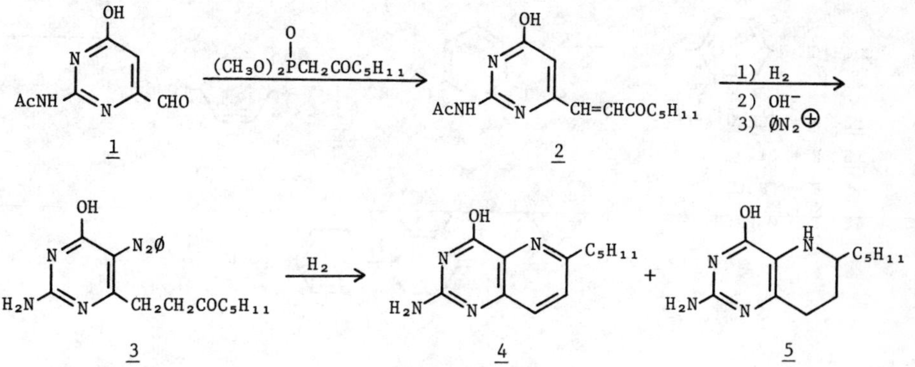

SCHEME 1

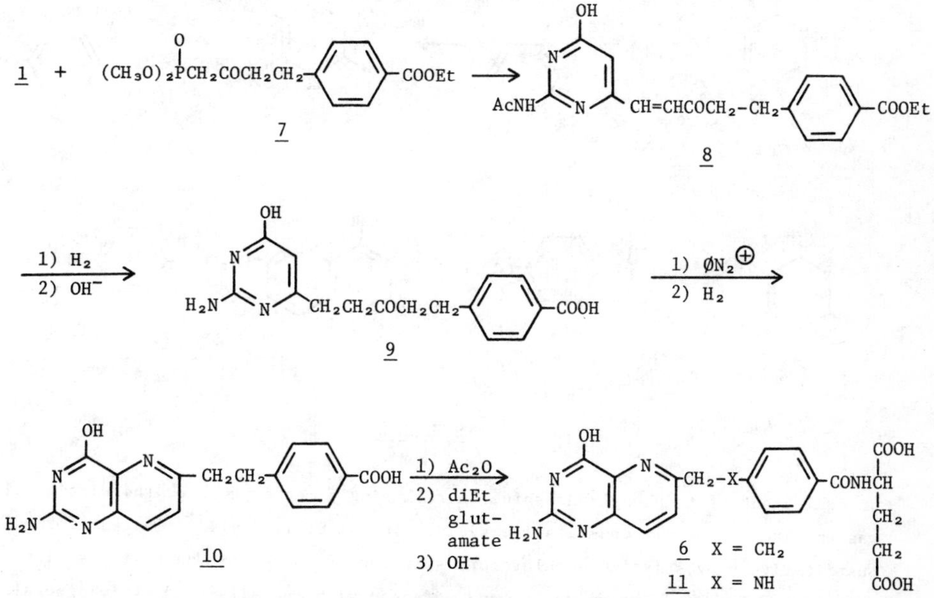

SCHEME 2

Extension of the synthetic route to the synthesis of 8-deazahomofolic acid was then investigated (Scheme 3). Attempted acylation of lithio dimethyl methylphosphonate by the acid chloride (13) in the previous manner failed to yield the required oxophosphonate (12). The nmr spectrum suggested that the product was the cyclized phosphonate 14. The N-formyl blocking group was tried in lieu of the N-acetyl but with similar results. We were unable to obtain the N-COOEt or N-tosyl derivatives.

The acid chloride (13) was then converted to the chloromethyl ketone (15) by treatment with diazomethane and hydrogen chloride. When 15 was allowed to react with

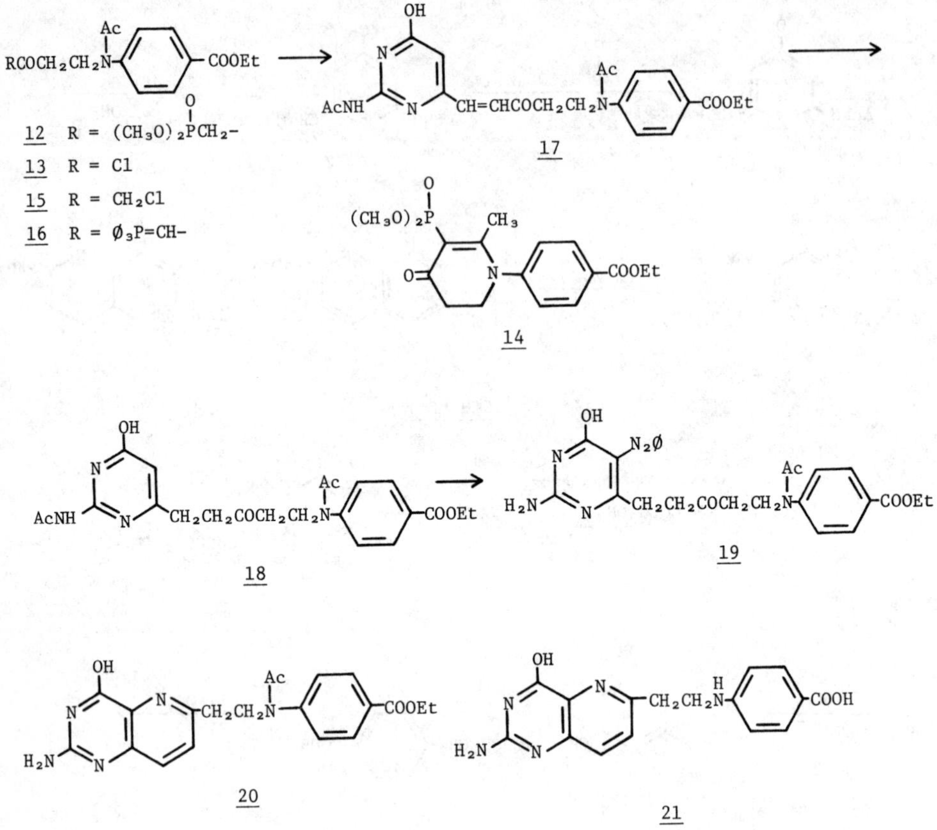

SCHEME 3

an equivalent of triphenyl phosphine in refluxing dimethoxyethane, the Wittig salt
was obtained in nearly quantitative yield. The stabilized ylide (16) was formed
quantitatively by stirring a chloroform solution of the Wittig salt with sodium
carbonate solution. The ylide 16 was condensed with the silylated pyrimidine aldehyde (1) in dimethylformamide at 100° for 16 hours to afford the crystalline enone
(17), m.p. 158-159; NMR, δ, 8.17 (2 H, d, phenyl-2',6'), 7.35 (2 H, d, phenyl-3',5'),
7.05 (2 H, d, olefin), 6.30 (1 H, s, pyrim-5), 2.40 (3 H, s, 2-Ac), 1.95 (3 H, s,
11-Ac). The olefin was saturated by treatment with hydrogen in the presence of
rhodium/carbon to give the dihydro ketone (18) as a syrup identified by its NMR
spectrum.

When 18 was exposed briefly to a warm excess of 0.1 N sodium hydroxide, no
precipitate was obtained upon acidification to pH 4-5. It was apparent that fragmentation of the beta-acetamido ketone had occurred. Similar treatment with three

TABLE 1

BACTERIAL GROWTH INHIBITION BY 8,10-DIDEAZAFOLATES MIC (NG/ML) FOR 50% INHIBITION[a]

Compound	S. faecium (ATCC 8043)	S. faecium MTX-resistant	L. casei (ATCC 7649)	L. casei MTX-resistant
(9)	55.0	> 2,000	880	> 2,000
(10) 8,10-Dideazapteroate	3.4	> 2,000	2,550	> 2,000
(6) 8,10-Dideazafolate	1.4	620	10	> 2,000
(11) 8-Deazafolate	0.15	130	0.6	900
Methotrexate	0.15	10,000	0.01	60,000

[a]Folate 1 ng/ml, MIC denotes Minimum Inhibitory Concentration.

TABLE 2

ACTIVITY OF 8-DEAZAFOLATE IN L1210 LEUKEMIA CELLS

Compound	Growth Inhibition[a] IC_{50} (M x 10^{-6})	FAH_2 Reductase[b] Inhibition Ki (M x 10^{-9})	Transport Influx[b] Ki (M x 10^{-6})
Methotrexate	0.013 ± 0.0003	0.62 ± 0.05	3.5 ± 0.6
(11) 8-Deazafolate	1.33 ± 0.07	1207.3 ± 80	51.9 ± 1.8
Folate	--	2123.3 ± 200	202.0 ± 35

[a]72 hr. cultures in Fisher medium + calf serum (10%) + folate (1 µg/ml).
[b]Competition assay for ^{3}H-methotrexate uptake.

TABLE 3

ANTILEUKEMIC ACTIVITY (L1210) OF 8-DEAZAFOLATE at LD_{10} DOSAGE IN MICE

Compound	Dose (q2d x 5)	Average Survival Time (days)	Increase Life Span (%)
Control	--	6.7 ± 0.7	--
Methotrexate	48	20.7 ± 2.3	+209
(11) 8-Deazafolate	120	10.1 ± 1.4	+51

equivalents of 0.1 N sodium hydroxide, but at 0°, gave the same result. Treatment of 18 with three equivalents of 0.1 N ammonia at 0° caused saponification of the ester but did not affect the 2-acetamido group. When conducted at room temperature, this hydrolytic medium again failed to cleave the 2-acetamido and caused the appearance of a third methyl signal in the nmr spectrum besides the N_2-N_{11}-acetamidos.

Acid hydrolysis of the 2-N-acetyl could be effected with ethanolic hydrogen chloride and subsequent coupling with benzene diazonium chloride gave the 5-phenylazo keto ester (19). Hydrogenation over a palladium catalyst afforded a product regarded as the 11-N-acetyl-8-deazahomopteroate (20). This compound was hydrolyzed in hot 10% NaOH to 8-deazahomopteroic acid (21); $\lambda^{pH\ 13}$ 278, 340 (sh); pH 1 245, 305 nm in agreement with 11. Incorporation of the glutamate moeity is currently under study.

8-Deazafolic acid (11) was found (as expected) to be inactive as an inhibitor of L1210 dihydrofolate reductase, but was transported four times as well as folic acid into L1210 cells in tissue culture (Table 2). However, methotrexate was 15 times more competitive than 11 for this active transport. Compound 11 was about 1/100 as potent as MTX for growth inhibition of the L1210 cells in culture. Yet when tested in mice (Table 3) infected with L1210, 11 showed a T/C of 151 which is well into the active compound range and is about equal to tetrahydrohomofolate. The acute toxicity is only about 1/3 that of MTX.

SUMMARY

Synthetic methods for analogs of 8-deazafolic acid are presented. While 8-deazafolic acid was found to be a potent inhibitor of *S. faecium*, the 8,10-dideaza analog was only about 1/10 active. 8-Deazafolic acid was only 1/100 potent as metho- trexate as an inhibitor of cell growth in L1210 culture. However, the compound showed significant activity against L1210 leukemia in mice.

ACKNOWLEDGEMENTS

This work was supported by Grant No. CA 16533, National Cancer Institute, DHEW.

REFERENCES

1. Goodman, L., DeGraw, J., Kisliuk, R., Friedkin, M., Pastore, E., Crawford, E., Plante, L., Al-Nabas, A., Morningstar, J., Kwok, G., Wilson, L., Donovan, E. and Ratzlan, J. (1964) J. Am. Chem. Soc., 86, 308.

2. DeGraw, J., Marsh, J., Acton, E., Crews, O., Mosher, C., Fujiwara, A. and Goodman, L. (1965) J. Org. Chem., 30, 3404.

3. Mead, J., Goldin, A., Kisliuk, R., Friedkin, M., Plante, L., Crawford, E. and Kwok, G. (1966) Cancer Res., 26, 2374.

4. Hakala, M. (1971) Cancer Res., 31, 813.

5. Mishra, L., Parmer, A., Mead, J., Knott, R., Taunton-Rigby, A. and Friedman, O. (1972) Proc. Am. Assoc. Cancer Res., 13, 76.

6. Nair, M. and Baugh, C. (1974) J. Med. Chem., 17, 223.

7. Kisliuk, R. and Gaumont, Y. (1970) in Chemistry and Biology of Pteridines, Iwai, K. et al. eds., International Academic, Ltd., Tokyo, pp. 357-364.

8. DeGraw, J., Kisliuk, R., Gaumont, Y. and Baugh, C. (1974) J. Med. Chem., 17, 470.

9. DeGraw, J. and Brown, V. (1976) J. Hetero. Chem., 13, 439.

X-RAY CRYSTALLOGRAPHY STUDIES OF THE STRUCTURE OF 5, 10-METHENYLTETRAHYDROFOLIC ACID

JUAN C. FONTECILLA-CAMPS and CHARLES E. BUGG
Comprehensive Cancer Center, Department of Microbiology and Institute of Dental Research, University of Alabama in Birmingham, University Station, Birmingham, Alabama 35294
CARROLL TEMPLE, JR., JERRY D. ROSE and JOHN A. MONTGOMERY
Department of Organic Chemistry Research, Kettering-Meyer Laboratory, Southern Research Institute, Birmingham, Alabama 35205.
ROY L. KISLIUK
Tufts University, School of Medicine, Boston, Massachusetts 02111

ABSTRACT

Two diastereomers of 5,10-methenyl-5,6,7,8-tetrahydrofolic acid were prepared, crystallized and examined by X-ray diffraction methods. For the natural diastereomer, the absolute configuration of atom C-6 in the reduced pyrazine ring is R, which corresponds to the S configuration of tetrahydrofolic acid.

INTRODUCTION

5,10-Methenyl-5,6,7,8-tetrahydrofolic acid [(5,10-CH-THF)$^+$] is an intermediate in the chemical and enzymic interconversions of 5- and 10-formyl-5,6,7,8-tetrahydrofolic acids (5-CHO-THF and 10-CHO-THF) and it results from the enzymic transformations of 5-formimino- and 5,10-methylene-5,6,7,8-tetrahydrofolic acids.[1] The methenyl derivative is also the cofactor in the formylation of glycinamide ribonucleotide by the transformylase (EC 2.1.2.2), an enzyme which apparently displays an unusual ability to utilize completely (5,10-CH-THF)$^+$ prepared from a racemic mixture of 10-CHO-THF.[2] In an effort to learn more about this unusual enzymic utilization of two diastereomers containing one identical (L-glutamate) and one dissimilar (C-6) asymmetric carbon atom, and to provide the first exact structural information on a tetrahydrofolic acid derivative, the preparation and X-ray analyses of crystals of (5,10-CH-THF)$^+$ were undertaken.

EXPERIMENTAL

THF, prepared by the chemical reduction of folic acid, was converted by successive treatment with formic and dilute hydrochloric acids to (±)-(5,10-CH-THF)$^+$Cl$^-$; $[\alpha]_D^{25}$ -8.8±0.8° (c 1.02% w/v, 12 $\underline{N}$

HCl). Reprecipitation of (+)-(5,10-CH-THF)$^+$ from 12 $\underline{N}$ HCl by
dilution to 6 $\underline{N}$ HCl gave a 70% recovery; $[\alpha]_D^{25}$ -12.2$\pm$0.4° (c 1.01%
w/v, 10 $\underline{N}$ HCl); λ_{max} in nm (ε x 10^{-3}): 1 $\underline{N}$ HCl — 286(12.4), 347(26.0).

Anal. Calcd for $C_{20}H_{22}ClN_7O_6 \cdot H_2O$ (mw 509.91): C, 47.11; H, 4.74;
Cl, 6.95; N, 19.23. Found: C, 47.33; H, 4.85; Cl, 7.20; H, 19.45.

The crystalline bromide hydrobromide salt of (5,10-CH-THF)$^+$ was
prepared for X-ray analysis from the chloride salt by dissolving it
in 48% (w/w) aqueous hydrobromic acid, which was then slowly equilibrated, by vapor diffusion, with a large excess of 29% (w/w) aqueous
hydrobromic acid. The crystals, which grew as large yellow plates,
are monoclinic, space group P2$_1$, with the cell parameters that are
listed in the first column of Table 1. Three-dimensional intensity
data were measured with an X-ray diffractometer. The crystal decomposed severely during data collection. Trial coordinates for the bromide
ions were readily obtained from Patterson maps, but subsequent Fourier
maps indicated that the remainder of the structure was considerably
disordered. Consequently, efforts to further characterize these
crystals were abandoned.

TABLE 1
CRYSTAL DATA FOR THE THREE PREPARATIONS OF (5,10-CH-THF)$^+$
Unit cell parameters were obtained by least-squares analysis of 2θ
values measured on a diffractometer

	(+)-(5,10-CH-THF)$^+$	(+)-(5,10-CH-THF)$^+$	(−)-(5,10-CH-THF)$^+$
Stoichiometry	?	$(C_{20}H_{23}N_7O_6)^{2+} \cdot$ 2Br$^-$ 2H$_2$O$\cdot$	$(C_{20}H_{23}N_7O_6)^{2+} \cdot$ 2Br$^-$ 2H$_2$O$\cdot$
Space Group	P2$_1$	P2$_1$	P2$_1$
a (Å)	12.718(1)	12.696(1)	12.459(1)
b (Å)	14.491(2)	14.487(2)	14.528(4)
c (Å)	6.982(1)	6.990(1)	7.006(2)
β (degrees)	100.83(1)	100.80(1)	96.06(2)

New samples of (5,10-CH-THF)$^+$ were prepared from material that
appears to be almost entirely the pure natural diastereomer (−)-5-CHO-
THF·Ca (calcium citrovorum). This material, obtained in a manner
similar to that used to prepare the original synthetic sample,[3] has an
$[\alpha]_D^{25}$ -25.2$\pm$0.4° (c 0.91% w/v, H$_2$O); λ_{max} in nm (ε x 10^{-3}): pH 7—286
(31.8); 0.1 $\underline{N}$ NaOH—282(31.0).

Anal. Calcd for $C_{20}H_{21}N_7O_7 \cdot 1.25$ Ca$\cdot 4H_2O$ (mw 593.6): C, 40.47;
H, 4.92; N, 16.52; Ca, 8.44; Ash(CaO), 11.81. Found: C, 40.85;
H, 4.78; N, 16.63; Ca, 8.51; Ash(CaO), 12.44.

Further recrystallization did not improve the optical rotation. This sample was compared to a commercial sample of (+)-5-CHO-THF[4] for biologic potency using Pediococcus cerevisiae and a broth dilution assay.[5] Three determinations made on each sample using separate weighings showed a relative potency of 1.95±0.16 (SD). In addition, the synthetic calcium citrovorum was at least twice as effective in the reversal of methotrexate toxicity in mice (Table 2).

A solution of this calcium citrovorum in 1 N HCl was allowed to stand for 1 hr before the resulting suspension was dissolved by the addition of 12 N HCl. Dilution with water gave a precipitate of (+)-(5,10-CH-THF)$^+$Cl$^-$·HCl; $[\alpha]_D^{25}$ + 11.4±0.8° (c 0.95% w/v, 12 N HCl) [lit. $[\alpha]_D^{23}$ + 46±3° (conc. and solvent not given)[1] and $[\alpha]_D^{23}$ + 68° (1 M HCl containing 1 M mercaptoethanol)[6]]; λ_{max} in nm (ε x 10^{-3}): 1 N HCl-286(12.1), 348(24.9).

Anal. Calcd for $C_{20}H_{22}ClN_7O_6 \cdot 0.9$ HCl·H$_2$O (mw 542.7): C, 44.26; H, 4.62; Cl, 12.41; N, 18.07. Found: C, 43.85; H, 4.80; Cl, 12.40; N, 18.04.

TABLE 2
COMPARISON OF L-(+)-5-CHO-THF[a] AND L-(-)-CF FOR REVERSAL OF METHOTREXATE TOXICITY IN NONTUMOR-BEARING BDF$_1$ MICE[b]

Dose (mg/kg)[c]	Survivors[d]	
	L-(-)-CF·Ca	L-(+)-5-CHO-THF·Ca
200	6/6	3/6
100	6/6	0/6
50	3/6	2/6
25	1/6	1/6
12.5	4/6	0/6

[a] Lederle Laboratories.
[b] A lethal dose (1000 mg/kg) of methotrexate was administered intra-peritoneally.
[c] This dose was administered subcutaneously at the time of the methotrexate dose.
[d] Mice were observed for 30 days postinjection.

The chloride hydrochloride was converted to the crystalline bromide hydrobromide suitable for X-ray analysis as described above for the mixture of diastereomers. To retard decomposition, crystals were sealed in glass capillaries for X-ray analysis. Crystal data are given in the second column of Table 1. Three-dimensional intensity data for 2162 independent reflections were used for the structural analysis. A complete trial structure was readily obtained by the heavy-atom method and was then refined by full-matrix least-squares. The current R index ($\Sigma ||Fo|-|Fc||/\Sigma |Fo|$) is 0.08; additional refinement is in progress, including the use of anomalous dispersion effects to confirm the absolute configuration. After the X-ray data were collected, the crystal was implanted in agar (in a Petri dish) containing medium,[5] ascorbic acid, and _Pediococcus cerevisiae_. After 24 hr at 37°C the appearance of bacterial growth was noted visually, providing evidence that this crystal contained the biologically active diastereomer.

The unnatural diastereomer of 5,10-CH_2-THF was prepared from (+)-5,10-CH_2-THF by the enzymatic depletion (thymidylate synthetase) of the natural diastereomer, (+)-5,10-CH_2-THF. This material was converted to (-)-(5,10-CH-THF)[+] by treatment with formic acid containing 2-mercaptoethanol. Treatment with dilute hydrochloric acid then converted this material to the chloride hydrochloride salt, which was purified by column chromatography. Crystals of the bromide hydrobromide salt were prepared by the same technique followed for the mixture of diastereomers and for the sample of (+)-(5,10-CH-THF)[+]. Crystals were sealed in glass capillaries for X-ray analysis. Crystal data are given in the third column of Table 1. X-ray intensity data were collected for 2358 independent reflections. The trial structure, which was readily obtained by the heavy-atom method, was refined by least-squares to R=0.06; additional refinement is in progress.

RESULTS AND DISCUSSION

The molecular structure of (+)-(5,10-CH-THF)[+], which appears to be the natural diastereomer, is shown in Figures 1(a) and 1(b). As can be seen from these drawings, the absolute configuration of atom C-6 in the reduced pyrazine ring is R, which corresponds to the S configuration of tetrahydrofolic acid. The molecular structure of (-)-(5,10-CH-THF)[+], which appears to be the unnatural diastereomer, is depicted in Figures 1(c) and 1(d). As expected, the major difference between this structure and that of (+)-(5,10-CH-THF)[+] is inversion at the C-6 position. As can be seen by comparing Figures 1(b) and 1(d), those portions of the molecules which include the pyrimidine, tetrahydro-pyrazine, imidazoline and benzene rings, plus the carbonyl groups, are nearly mirror images in the two structures. However, there is a fundamental difference in the conformations of the L-glutamate residues.

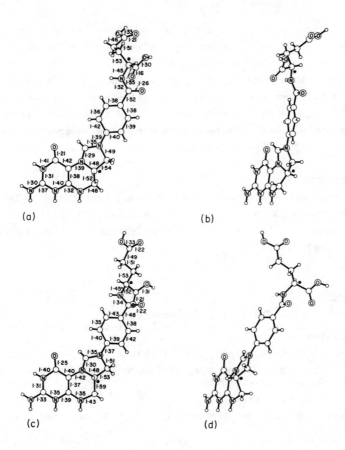

(a)

(b)

(c)

(d)

Fig. 1. Structures of the N-1-protonated derivatives of (+)-(5,10-CH-THF)$^+$ (a) and (b); and of (-)-(5,10-CH-THF)$^+$ (c) and (d). The absolute configurations were assigned by assuming that the glutamate residues have the L-configuration. Bond distances (Å) have estimated-standard-deviations of 0.02 Å. The asymmetric carbon atoms are designated by asterisks. This drawing was prepared by use of the computer program ORTEP.[7]

Examination of the bond distances in these two diastereomers (Figures 1(a) and 1(c)) indicates that there is a resonating conjugated system through the pyrimidine ring, the upper portion of the tetrahydropyrazine and imidazoline rings, and the benzene ring. This region is not completely planar, but all of the component atoms lie within 0.35 Å of a common plane. This near-planar arrangement may help explain why both diastereomers can serve as the cofactor for 5,10-methenyl THF:glycinamide ribonucleotide transformylase.

ACKNOWLEDGEMENTS

This research was supported by National Institutes of Health Research Grants CA-10914, CA-12159, CA-13148, CA-23141, DE-02670 and Contract Number N01-CM-43762. We wish to thank Dr. W. J. Suling for the bacterial assays and Dr. W. R. Laster for the toxicity reversal studies.

REFERENCES

1. Blakley, R.L. (1969) The Biochemistry of Folic Acid and Related Pteridines, American Elsevier Publishing Co., Inc., New York, pp. 1-569.

2. Warren, L. and Buchanan, J.M. (1957) J. Biol. Chem., 229, 613-640.

3. Cosulich, D.B., Smith, J.M.,Jr. and Broquist, H.P. (1952) J. Am. Chem. Soc., 74, 4215-5216.

4. Lederle Laboratories.

5. Sauberlich, H.E. and Baumann, C.A. (1948) J. Biol. Chem., 176, 165-173.

6. Ho, P.P.K. and Jones, L. (1967) Biochim. Biophys. Acta, 148, 622-628.

7. Johnson, C.K. (1965) ORTEP. Report ORNL-3794, Oak Ridge National Laboratory, Oak Ridge, Tennessee.

AUTOXIDATION OF 5-ALKYL-TETRAHYDROPTERIDINES
THE OXIDATION PRODUCT OF 5-METHYL-THF

JAAP A. JONGEJAN, H.I.X. MAGER and W. BERENDS
Biochemical and Biophysical Laboratory of the Technological University,
Julianalaan 67, Delft (The Netherlands)

INTRODUCTION

Oxidation of tetrahydropteridines in suitable media is known to produce the corresponding 7,8-dihydropteridines. When the hydrogen on N_5
of the starting pteridine is replaced by an alkylgroup, derivatives
are obtained in which the oxidative formation of the 5,6-double bond
is inhibited. Characterization of the oxidation products is then expected to give information on the course of the reaction with oxygen.

In 1967, Viscontini et. al.[1] described the oxidation of 5-methyl-
6,7-diphenyl-5,6,7,8-tetrahydropterin (1). A single product was
isolated, which they proposed to be a 4a-hydroxypterin (2a).

Based on the analogy of this model compound with the natural cofactor
5-methyl-tetrahydrofolic acid (3), Gapski et. al.[2] extended this
proposal, structure 4a, to a product obtained in the oxidation of
5-methyl-tetrahydrofolic acid.
This oxidation product is of interest, as it was identified as a major
excreted product of folic acid metabolism[3,4].
In both cases however, the oxidation products were shown to display a
remarkable stability to acidic and alkaline conditions, a stability
not to be expected for the proposed pseudo-base structures.

This prompted us to reinvestigate these proposals.

OXIDATION OF 5-METHYL-6,7-DIPHENYL-5,6,7,8-TETRAHYDROPTERIN

Synthesis of the 5-methyl-tetrahydropterin 1 was carried out by a route[5] involving the introduction of the methyl-substituent at the 5-aminogroup of the corresponding pyrimidine, thus ensuring the position of the methylgroup in the end product. Later on we replaced this synthesis by a less tedious route[6], which involves the direct hydroxymethylation of the parent tetrahydropterin.
Both routes were shown to lead to identical products.

Depending upon the conditions employed, the oxidation product could be obtained in yields up to 100%. It was identical with the compound described by Viscontini. Analytical and spectral data, combined with chemical degradation and derivatization, afforded some interesting clues regarding its structure[7]. Definite proof was obtained from X-ray crystallography on the acetyl-derivative by Van Koningsveld[8].

Contrary to the structure proposed by Viscontini, the oxidation product was found to be a pyrazino-s-triazine (2b), resulting from a rearrangement on peroxide level.

In order to study the mechanism of this rearrangement we carried out several labelling experiments. The oxygen atom incorporated at the former 4a-position was found to be derived exclusively from molecular oxygen. Performing the autoxidation in water enriched with heavy oxygen, no exchange was observed of the carbonyl oxygen originally present at the 4-position. In D_2O no incorporation of deuterium was detected at either the 6 or the 7-position, which proves that the corresponding 5,6-dihydropterin cannot be an intermediate. This was confirmed by the observation that oxidation of this 5-methyl-5,6-dihydropterin does not lead to the pyrazino-s-triazine rearrangement product.

As the speed of the autoxidation is drastically raised in going from neutral to alkaline media, we tried to establish which tautomeric form of the parent tetrahydropterin is most eagerly attacked by molecular oxygen. We found the reaction to proceed equally well with the derivatives 1,5,6 and 7.

$R = H$ **1**
$R = CH_3$ **5**

$R = H$ **6**
$R = CH_2\emptyset$ **7**

8

The 2,4-diaminopteridine **8** was examined only recently and preliminary
results show this compound to be relatively stable to air oxidation
in neutral and slightly alkaline media.

These results, combined with the fact that molecular oxygen is
incorporated at the 4a-position, indicate the following mechanism:

REARRANGEMENT OF RELATED 5-ALKYLTETRAHYDROPTERIDINES

The scope of this rearrangement was further investigated. Derivatives
9-31 were prepared by reductive hydroxymethylation and the 5-alkyl-
tetrahydropteridines were isolated and characterized as either the free
bases or their hydrochloric acid salts.
Autoxidation was then carried out in aquous alkaline medium (pH 13).

In all cases the corresponding pyrazino-s-triazine was the main product
isolated.

We concluded that the autoxidative rearrangement is rather insensitive
to substituent effects in the pyrazine part of the molecule. Bulky
substituents like the phenylgroups, distorting the tetrahydropyrazine-
ring, and the benzyl- and iso-propyl-groups on N_5, which might

shield the 4a-position, have little influence on the rearrangement.

	R_1	R_2	R_3	R_4		R_1	R_2	R_3	R_4
9,10	Me,Et	H	H	H	23,24	Me,Et	H	Me	Me
11	Benz	H	H	H	25	Benz	H	Me	Me
12,13	Me,Et	H	Me	Me	26	Me	Me	Ph	Ph*)
14,15	iPr,Benz	H	Me	Me	27,28	Me,Et	H	H	H
16,17	Me,Benz	H	Me	H	29	Benz	H	H	H
18,19	Me, Benz	H	H	Me	30	Et	H	Ph	Ph
20,21	Me	H	Ph,H	H,Ph	31	Me	H	—Bu—	

*) 1,4-dimethyl-5,6-diphenylpiperazin-2,3-dione was the major product.

For the identification of the rearrangement products the following
criteria were applied:
- The stoichiometry of the reaction, one mole of oxygen is taken up,
  no residual peroxides are detected,
- Mass-spectra show an m^+/e-increment of 14, corresponding to the
  incorporation of one O-atom and the loss of two H-atoms,
- PMR-spectra show the non-exchangeable protons in the pyrazine ring
  to be still present, the number of exchangeable protons is two
  less than in the starting pteridine,
- A most interesting feature is the occurrence of a one-proton singlet
  (δ 5.7 - 6.1 ppm, depending upon the substituents) in the PMR-
  spectrum of the products obtained after catalytic hydrogenation
  with the concomitant uptake of one mole of hydrogen.

The hydrogenated product obtained in the reduction of 2b was assigned
structure 2c on the basis of mass-spectral fragmentations.

OXIDATION OF 5-METHYL-TETRAHYDROFOLIC ACID DERIVATIVES

In order to prove whether the same rearrangement takes place in the case of the oxidation of 5-methyl-THF, we tried to apply the criteria mentioned above. However, as was pointed out by Gapski, the mass spectrum of the oxidation product does not show the molecular-ion, while the number of exchangeable protons in the PMR-spectrum is diffi- cult to estimate (4a.2H$_2$O requires 12, 4b.2H$_2$O requires 10 exchangeable protons). Elemental analysis shows figures which were accepted by Gapski to represent 4a, while we think them equally suited to represent the molecular formula of the pyrazino-s-triazine structure 4b. We solved these problems by studying the derivatives 32a,b:

$$32 \quad \xrightarrow[\substack{+O_2 \; -H_2O \\ \text{or: } +2H_2O_2 \\ -2H_2O}]{} \quad 33$$

$$\underline{a} \quad R= -N\langle \text{Me} \rangle \bigcirc \overset{\text{COOMe}}{\underset{\text{O H}}{C-N-CH}} \;\; \text{CH}_2\text{CH}_2\text{COOMe} \qquad \underline{b} \quad R= -N\langle \text{Me} \rangle \bigcirc \text{COOMe}$$

The amino- and carboxylic-protons of the side-chain were substituted by methylgroups to obtain a correct estimate of the number of exchangeable protons present in the oxidation products, without disturbing the character of the pteridine moiety. Both compounds were oxidized with the concomitant uptake of one mole of oxygen, products were isolated. The resulting esters were volatile enough to obtain their mass-spectra, displaying the molecular-ions expected for the pyrazino-s-triazine rearrangement products 33a,b.
PMR-spectra were in agreement with the spectra of the oxidized model compounds and were closely similar to the spectrum of the free acid of the 5-methyl-derivative published by Gapski. The integrated signals accounted for the loss of two protons.
From these arguments we concluded the oxidation products to be the pyrazino-s-triazine derivatives.

An initially disturbing observation was formed by the shift of the one-proton singlet in the spectra of the reduced derivatives. In the reduced oxidation product of the model 5,6-dimethyl-5,6,7,8-tetrahydro- pterin (18), this proton is displayed at 5.7 ppm. In the spectrum of the reduced 5-methyl-THF-oxidation product, published by Gapski, this proton is located at 5.5 ppm, as it is in the spectra of the reduced derivatives of 33a,b.Upon further reduction of these derivatives, 3 more moles of hydrogen can be introduced. As these compounds, now carrying a cyclohexane-sidechain, showed this proton to be located once again at 5.7 ppm, we contribute this upfield shift to a shielding effect of the benzene-nucleus, brought about by dimerization as described by Poe[9] for folic acid derivatives.

It should be noted that the UV-spectra of the oxidized compounds are likewise dominated by the strong absorption of the p-aminobenzoic acid chromophore, and yield little information regarding the pyrazino-s-triazine moiety. This was established by comparing the spectra of the compounds having a p-amino-benzoic acid side chain with those carrying a cyclohexane side chain (Details to be published).

CONCLUSION

The autoxidative rearrangement of 5-alkyl-tetrahydropteridines leading to pyrazino-s-triazine products, was shown to be a general reaction. Incorporation of molecular oxygen proves the occurrence of peroxy-intermediates. The same rearrangement was observed for 5,10-dimethyl-tetrahydro-folic and -pteroic acid. We conclude that this rearrangement takes place equally in the oxidation of 5-methyl-THF.

On the basis of these findings, the structure of the "5-methyl-dihydrofolic acid"-intermediate, isolated by Gapski from the hydrogen-peroxide oxidation of 3, and subsequently studied by Blair et. al.[10] and Deits et. al.[11], should be reconsidered. This compound might well have the 4a-hydroxy-structure rejected by Deits. The pyrazino-s-triazin structure of the 5-methyl-THF oxidation product provides an explanation for the observation that it is not metabolized by higher organisms.

REFERENCES
1. Viscontini, M. and Okada, T.(1967) Helv. Chim. Acta, 50, 1492.
2. Gapski, G.R., Whiteley, J.M. and Huennekens, F.M.,
   (1971) Biochemistry, 15, 2930.
3. Blair, J.A.(1975) in Chemistry and Biology of Pteridines,
   Pfleiderer, W. ed., de Gruyter, Berlin, N.Y., pp 373-405.
4. Barford, P.A. and Blair, J.A. Ibid, pp 413-427.
5. Viscontini, M. and Huwyler, S.(1965) Helv.Chim.Acta, 48, 764.
6. Matsuura, S. and Sugimoto, T.(1970) in Chemistry and Biology of
   Pteridines, Iwai, K. ed., Int.Acad.Print.,Tokyo, pp 35-42.
7. Jongejan, J.A., Mager, H.I.X. and Berends, W.(1975)Tetrahedron,31,
8. Van Koningsveld, H.(1975) Tetrahedron, 31, 541.   (533.
9. Poe, M. (1973) J.Biol.Chem., 248, 7025.
10. Blair, J.A.,Pearson, A.J. and Robb, A.J.(1975)J.C.S.Perkin II, 18.
11. Deits, T.L., Russel, A., Fujii, K. and Whiteley, J.M. in (1975)
    Chemistry and Biology of Pteridines, Pfleiderer, W. ed.,
    de Gruyter, Berlin, N.Y., pp 525-534.

ELECTROCHEMICAL PREPARATION OF TETRAHYDROFOLIC ACID
AND RELATED COMPOUNDS

SIANETTE KWEE

Institute of Medical Biochemistry, University of Aarhus,
DK-8000 Aarhus C, Denmark

HENNING LUND

Department of Organic Chemistry, University of Aarhus,
DK-8000 Aarhus C, Denmark

ABSTRACT

An electrochemical synthesis of 5,6,7,8-tetrahydrofolic acid (THF)
from folic acid (FA) has been developed. In the first step FA is reduced, via 5,8-dihydrofolic acid (5,8-DHF), to 7,8-DHF. Reduction of
the protonated 7,8-DHF cleaves C(9)-N(10), but reduction of the unprotonated compound at a more negative potential leads to THF in high
yield. The reduction is made at relatively low buffer concentration
which permits having a neutral pH in the bulk of the solution, but a
high pH at the electrode surface due to the electrogenerated base.

Besides the preparation of THF was studied the reduction of 5,10-
methenyl THF and 5,10-methylene THF.

INTRODUCTION

A polarographic investigation[1,2] of FA suggested that FA was reduced in the first step via 5,8-DHF to 7,8-DHF; in neutral or acidic
solution at a more negative potential the protonated 7,8-DHF was reduced to 6-methyl-7,8-dihydropterin, which at a slightly more negative potential was further reduced to 6-methyl-5,6,7,8-tetrahydro-
pterin. At higher pH a reduction of 7,8-DHF to THF was proposed. A
medium of high pH has certain disadvantages such as hydrolysis of the
compounds and a slow tautomerization of 5,8-DHF to 7,8-DHF.

A further investigation of these reactions could be of interest
for several reasons; a convenient synthesis of THF from FA might be
developed, and there might be found means (e.g. chiral electrodes[3])
to influence the distribution of the stereoisomers of THF in a desired
direction. It could possibly also be an attractive way for the preparation of 6-methylpterin.

Of analytical interest might be the electrochemical cleavage of the
C(9)-N(10) bond, which occurs under very mild conditions in the reduc-

tion of 7,8-DHF under slightly acidic to neutral conditions. As THF
is easily oxidized to 7,8-DHF a general method for the analysis of
the polyglutamyl side chain of THF might be developed.

Below is reported on an investigation of the electrochemical reduction of FA, of 5,10-methenyl THF, and of 5,10-methylene THF. The
reaction mechanism was investigated by means of classical polaro-
graphy, cyclic voltammetry and controlled potential reduction.

RESULTS AND DISCUSSION

The preparation of THF from FA is generally made by reduction with
an excess of $NaBH_4$; an electrochemical synthesis seems an attractive
alternative, since the work-up would be very simple. However, certain
problems had to be solved, before the method could be used.

One problem was that 7,8-DHF, an intermediate between FA and THF,
possesses the electrophor $-C(=Y)CHXR$, where Y is a heteroatom and X^-
a good leaving group. Such an electrophor[4] is under suitable conditions reduced to $-C(=Y)CH_2R + X^-$, which for 7,8-DHF means that the
bond $C(9)-N(10)$ is cleaved. This cleavage takes place, when the protonated 7,8-DHF is the reduced species.

The $N(5)-C(6)$ azomethine group is, as is the case for all azomethine groups[5], more easily reducible in the protonated form than in
the unprotonated one. Protonation is thus favourable for the uptake
of electrons, but it also makes the anilino group a better leaving
group. For unprotonated 7,8-DHF the leaving group would be a derivative of aniline anion, which is a strong base, but if N-10 is protonated, the leaving group is the much weaker base, a derivative of aniline. Protonation thus favours the cleavage.

A further complication arises from the fact, that not only the e-
quilibrium concentration of the protonated form in the equilibrium

$$7,8\text{-DHF} + H^+ \underset{k_{-1}}{\overset{k_1}{\rightleftharpoons}} 7,8\text{-DHFH}^+ \tag{1}$$

is of interest, but also the rate constant (k_1) of the protonation reaction. The reason is that the more easily reducible protonated form
is removed from the equilibrium by reduction, and at a given pH the
reactants will try to reestablish the equilibrium by protonation of
7,8-DHF. If k_1 is large, the protonated form may be the reduced species even some pH-units higher than the pK of the system.

At pH 8 the equilibrium of (1) is shifted well to the left, but the
rate of protonation is not negligible at high buffer concentration;

at pH higher than 8, hydrolysis becomes a complicating factor. The rate of protonation may be lowered by working at low temperatures and using a low concentration of buffer. As seen from the equation

$$RR'C=NR'' + 2e^- + 2H_2O \longrightarrow RR'CH-NHR + 2OH^- \qquad (2)$$

a base is created close to the electrode, and the electrochemical reduction thus takes place in surroundings which have a higher pH than that measured in the bulk of the solution. At relatively low buffer concentrations the pH-difference between the bulk and the electrode surface during electrolysis is sufficient to ensure, on the one hand that the preprotonation reaction (2) is sufficiently slow, and on the other hand that the bulk pH is sufficiently low to avoid serious problems with hydrolysis.

Under such conditions FA can be reduced to THF in good yield; direct UV-determination at 298 nm gave in different runs 85-100%, the same yields were found from the recovery of FA after reoxidation. The yield (98-99%) was also determined from the yield of 5,10-methenyl THF (λ 355 nm) and the concentration (0-1.5%) p-aminobenzoyl glutamic acid was determined by diazotization (Bratton-Marshal reagent).

5,10-Methenyl THF is a cyclic formamidine, an imidazoline, and it is as other formamidines reducible at the dropping mercury electrode (Table 1). The primary reduction product from a cyclic formamidine is an imidazolidine, which is not electrochemically reducible as such; a further reduction requires a ring opening (e.g. acid catalyzed) to an azomethine compound, a formimine derivative. The reactions may be formulated

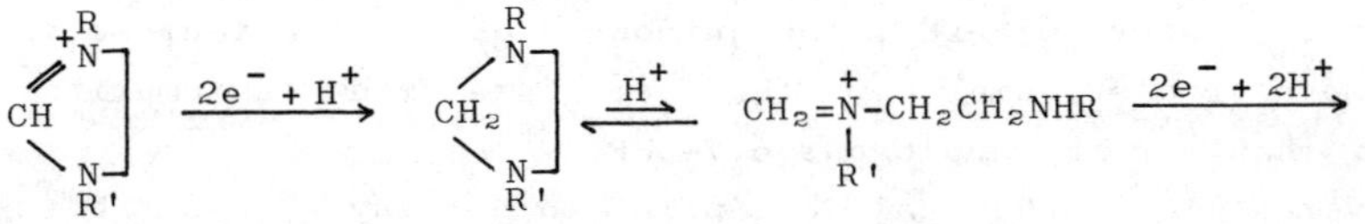

$$CH_3-NR'-CH_2CH_2-NHR$$

IV

(3)

The reaction is complicated by hydrolysis of I and III. In the presence of an excess of formic acid I (5,10-methenyl THF) is under suitable conditions found in a reasonable high concentration in equilibrium with the free diamine, $R'NHCH_2CH_2NHR$ (V), and the formyl derivative, $HCONR'CH_2CH_2NHR$ (VI). Of these (I, V and VI) only I is reducible, so I may thus be reduced electrochemically to II.

The further reduction is more difficult. In an equilibrium consisting of the diamine (V), formaldehyde, hydrated formaldehyde, the formimine derivative (III), III is present in a very low concentration. This would not be an insurmountable difficulty, compare e.g. the reductive alkylation of methylamine by cyclohexanone[6], if the formimino derivative was reduced at a potential sufficiently less negative than that of formaldehyde

$$\begin{matrix} R \\ \\ R' \end{matrix} \!\!\! >C=O \ + \ H_2NR'' \ \rightleftharpoons \ \begin{matrix} R \\ \\ R' \end{matrix} \!\!\! >C=NR'' \ + \ H_2O \tag{4}$$

Although a small prewave to the formaldehyde wave, presumably due to the azomethine compound (III), is visible on a polarogram of a mixture of THF and an excess of formaldehyde, it is too close to the large wave of formaldehyde to permit a selective reduction of III, even though the major part of formaldehyde is present as the unreducible hydrated form.

Although it has been possible to reduce N,N'-diphenylformamidine to the expected mixture of aniline and N-methylaniline, the right conditions for a high yield electrochemical synthesis of 5-methyl THF from THF and formaldehyde has not yet been found.

5-Methyl THF can be oxidized electrochemically and the oxidation product reduced again to 5-methyl THF as evidenced by the quasi-reversible oxidation-reduction couple observed on cyclic voltammetry of 5-methyl THF at a mercury electrode. Preparative oxidation of 5-methyl THF yields an unstable 5-methyl DHF of quinonoid structure, probably the 5-methyl-6,7-DHF. The quinonoid derivative tautomerizes into a more stable isomer, but the (acid catalyzed) tautomerization is slower than for the analogous 6,7-DHF.

Several electrochemical data point to 5-methyl-7,8-DHF being the electroactive species in slightly acid solution. The absence of an anodic wave seems to exclude a THF derivative with a double bond between $C(9)$ and $N(10)$, obtained by migration of the double bond in the DHF-derivative to an exocyclic position[7]. The presence of two reduction waves at pH 8 ($E_{\frac{1}{2}}^1 = -1.18$; $E_{\frac{1}{2}}^2 = -1.53$) points to a reductive cleavage of the $C(9)-N(10)$ bond during the first reduction and a reduction of the thus obtained 5,6-dimethyl-7,8-dihydropterin to the tetrahydropterin.

The observed reduction potentials are consistent with this interpretation, but the evidence is not conclusive. A 5,6-dihydroderiva-
tive could also produce two reduction waves, where the first one
would be a cleavage of a C-N bond and the second one the saturation
of an azomethine bond, but in that case the cleavage would involve
the $C(6)-N(5)$ bond with a resulting ring-opening.

On the basis of the above mentioned evidence the following reaction scheme is considered.

Under the assumption that the scheme is essentially correct,
further work is in progress along the lines of controlled oxidation
of 5-methyl THF to 5-methyl DHF, followed by reductive cleavage of
the $C(9)-N(10)$ bond with the aim of developing a general method for
the determination of the side chain in THF-derivatives.

TABLE 1

POLAROGRAPHIC HALF-WAVE POTENTIALS OF SOME DERIVATIVES OF FORMAMIDINE
V vs SCE; medium containing 40% alcohol

pH	N,N'-Diphenyl formamidine	N,N'-Diphenyl imidazoline	Imidazoline
4.7	-1.33	-1.15	
5.9	-1.35	-1.15	
7.5	-1.42	-1.15	-1.60
9.0	-1.55		-1.61

TABLE 2

VOLTAMMETRIC RESULTS OF SOME FOLIC ACID DERIVATIVES

Cathodic (E_{pc}) and anodic (E_{pa}) peak potentials (-V vs SCE) in cyclic voltammetry at a hanging drop mercury electrode, sweep rate 200 mVs^{-1}. Polarographic half-wave potentials ($E_{\frac{1}{2}}$) at a dropping mercury electrode.

pH	5,10-Methenyl THF E_{pc}	5-Methyl THF E_{pa}	E_{pc}	5-Methyl-6,7 DHF $E_{\frac{1}{2}}$	E_{pc}	5-Methyl-7,8 DHF $E_{\frac{1}{2}}(I)$	$E_{\frac{1}{2}}(II)$	$E_{pc}(I)$
6.0	1.67	0.17	0.27					
7.0	1.69	0.25	0.35					1.18
8.0	1.72 [1.17]^a	0.40	0.46	0.35		1.18^b	1.53	1.20
8.5		0.42	0.47		0.53			1.26
9.0	1.75 [1.19]^a	0.44	0.50	0.40				1.39
10.0		0.46	0.52					1.35

^{a} Small peak on second sweep, possibly due to 5-methylene THF.

^{b} After preparative reduction at this potential the catholyte had a wave at -1.55 V.

REFERENCES

1. Kretzschmar, K. and Jaenicke, W. (1971) Z. Naturforsch., 26b, 225-228.

2. Kretzschmar, K. and Jaenicke, W. (1971) Z. Naturforsch., 26b, 999-1002.

3. Miller, L. L. et al. (1975) J. Am. Chem. Soc., 97, 3549-3550.

4. Horner, L. and Lund, H. (1973) in Organic Electrochemistry, Baizer, M. M. ed., Marcel Dekker, New York, 731-779.

5. Lund, H. (1970) in The Chemistry of the Carbon-Nitrogen Double Bond, Patai, S. ed., Interscience Publishers, London, 505-564.

6. Lund, H. (1959) Acta Chem. Scand., 13, 249-267.

7. Deits, T. L. et al. (1975) Chemistry and Biology of Pteridines, Pfleiderer, W. ed., Walter de Gruiter, Berlin, 525-534.

OXIDATIVE AND REDUCTIVE CLEAVAGE OF FOLATES - A CRITICAL APPRAISAL

GARRY P. LEWIS AND PETER B. ROWE
Department of Child Health, University of Sydney, N.S.W. AUSTRALIA 2006

ABSTRACT

A critical analysis has been made of the C^9-N^{10} oxidative and reductive cleavage techniques used to analyse the chain lengths of folate polyglutamate derivatives. It was evident that the susceptibility to cleavage of this bond is dependent upon the state of reduction and the nature of any one carbon substitution. While this may not invalidate the reports of the properties of various tissue folates, such data should be viewed with some caution.

RESULTS AND DISCUSSION

The assumption has been generally made that oxidative and reductive cleavage of the C^9-N^{10} bond of folic acid derivatives results in the generation of a common family of p-aminobenzoyl-glutamate (pABG) derivatives varying only in the lengths of the γ-polyglutamyl side chains which are readily analysed[1,2]. Our studies indicate that this is not the case but that both techniques result in mixtures of N-substituted pABG, pABG as well as uncleaved folates.

Oxidation was carried out with potassium permanganate by a modification of the method originally described by Freed[3], using 2-mercaptoethanol to destroy excess permanganate and reducing the oxidation time to 30 sec. The reaction products were analysed on high performance anion exchange liquid chromatography (HPLC)[4] in conjunction with the Bratton-Marshall assay. Oxidation resulted in the effective cleavage of folic acid, dihydrofolic acid, tetrahydrofolic acid and 5-formyltetrahydrofolic acid to yield pABG. 5-Methyltetrahydrofolic acid was oxidised to 5-methyldihydrofolic acid while 5,10-methenyltetrahydrofolic acid and 10-formyltetrahydrofolic acid yielded 10-formylfolate which was stable. It was also demonstrated that pABG was sensitive to oxidation.

Of all the folate derivatives tested only folic acid and dihydrofolic acid were cleaved to pABG by the zinc-hydrochloric acid reduction method[5]. While tetrahydrofolic acid and 5-methyltetrahydrofolic acid were stable under fully reducing conditions, 5,10-methenyl-, 10-formyl- and 5-formyltetrahydrofolic acid yielded N-methyl-pABG. Most importantly the dominant mammalian tissue folate, 5-methyltetrahydrofolic acid was resistant to cleavage by either method.

The potential analytical problems resulting from the failure to

254

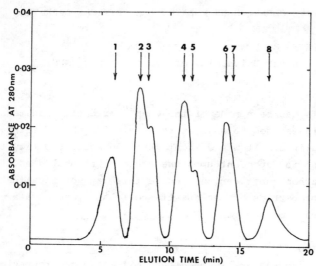

Fig. 1. HPLC elution profile of polyglutamate derivatives of pABG and 5-methyltetrahydrofolate containing two to five glutamate residues, previously subjected to oxidation. Markers are: 1,3,5,7 pABG containing two, three, four and five glutamate residues: 2,4,6,8, 5-methyltetrahydrofolate derivatives containing two, three, four and five glutamate residues.

cleave the C^9-N^{10} bond are illustrated in Fig 1. This shows the HPLC elution profile of a mixture of polyglutamate derivatives (containing from two to five glutamate residues) of pABG and 5-methyltetrahydrofolic acid previously subjected to oxidation. It is clear that significant errors could result from the assignment of polyglutamate chain lengths using either cleavage technique.

Acknowledgements. Supported by grants from the NH and MRC and the N.S.W. State Cancer Council.

References

1. Houlihan, C.M. and Scott, J.M. (1972) Biochem. Biophys. Res. Comm., 48, 1675-1681.

2. Baugh, C.M. Braverman, E. and Nair, M.G. (1974) Biochemistry, 13, 4952-4957.

3. Freed, M. (1966) in Methods of Vitamin Assay, 3rd ed., Interscience, New York, pp 236-239.

4. Lewis, G.P. and Rowe, P.B. (1978) Anal. Biochem. (in press).

5. Tyerman, M.J., Watson, J.R., Shane, B., Schutz, D.E. and Stokstad, E.L.R. (1977) Biochem. Biophys. Acta, 497, 234-240.

NEW HOMOFOLATE ANALOGS: ALTERATIONS IN THE BRIDGE REGION

M.G. NAIR, S.Y. CHEN, C.M. BAUGH, D. STRUMPF, Y. GAUMONT and R.L.
KISLIUK
University of South Alabama, Mobile, Alabama   36688; Tufts University,
Boston, Massachusetts   20111

ABSTRACT

Synthetic methods were developed for the unambiguous construction of
both 11-thiohomofolic acid 2 and 11-thiohomoaminopterin 3. Chemical
elaboration of the key intermediate 10 to the amino compound 6 was complicated because of the ability of compounds belonging to this series
(10, 11, 12) to undergo reverse Michael addition on treatment with
various nucleophiles, resulting in rearrangement. Detailed mechanistic
considerations of this rearrangement guided the successful synthesis of
both compounds 2 and 3, which were evaluated for their antifolate
activity using microorganisms. Studies were also done with dihydrofolate reductase and thymidylate synthetase.

INTRODUCTION

Homofolic acid 1 continues to be an interesting compound[1] due to its
diversified biological properties. 7,8-Dihydrohomofolic acid has been
shown to be an excellent substrate for *Lactobacillus casei* dihydrofolate
reductase and the resulting tetrahydro derivative an inhibitor of *Escherichia coli* thymidylate synthetase[2]. Catalytic hydrogenation of homofolic
acid results in the formation of a mixture of two diasteromers. These
isomers are able to carry one-carbon fragments at N^5 and N^{11} in the
form of a methylene bridge, and therefore, at least in theory, are
capable of taking part as pseudo-cofactors[3] in thymidylate biosynthesis.
Therefore, it was of interest to us to synthetize and evaluate homofolate analogs as potential substrates of dihydrofolate reductase[4], but
unable to function as pseudo-cofactors in thymidylate synthesis. These
compounds were therefore expected to interfere with tetrahydrofolate
utilization. As part of a continuing program aimed at developing such
analogs[5,6], the synthesis of 11-thiohomofolic acid was undertaken.

CHEMISTRY

The projected strategy required construction of amine 6 which on reacting with 4 and 5 would yield 30 and 31. By employing analogous
synthetic procedures previously developed in this laboratory, we hoped

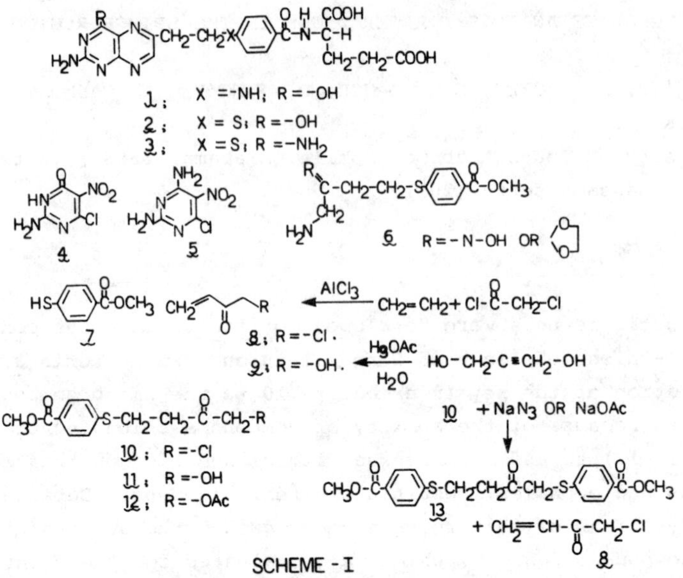

$$CH_2-CH_2-X \quad \overset{O}{\overset{\|}{C}}-\overset{H}{\overset{|}{N}}-\overset{COOH}{\underset{|}{\overset{|}{C}}}-H$$
$$\underset{CH_2-CH_2-COOH}{}$$

1; X = -NH; R = -OH
2; X = S; R = -OH
3; X = S; R = -NH_2

4

5

6   R = -N-OH OR

7

8; R = -Cl.
9; R = -OH.

$$CH_2=CH_2 + Cl-\overset{O}{\overset{\|}{C}}-CH_2-Cl$$ AlCl_3

$$HO-CH_2-C\equiv CH_2-OH$$ HgOAc / H_2O

$$CH_3O-\overset{O}{\overset{\|}{C}}-\langle\rangle-S-CH_2-CH_2-\overset{O}{\overset{\|}{C}}-CH_2-R$$

10; R = -Cl
11; R = -OH
12; R = -OAc

10 + NaN_3 OR NaOAc

$$CH_3O-\overset{O}{\overset{\|}{C}}-\langle\rangle-S-CH_2CH_2-\overset{O}{\overset{\|}{C}}-CH_2-S-\langle\rangle-\overset{O}{\overset{\|}{C}}-OCH_3$$
13

$$+ CH_2=CH-\overset{O}{\overset{\|}{C}}-CH_2-Cl$$
8

SCHEME - I

to convert 30 and 31 to their respective homopteroate analogs 39 and 40. Subsequent coupling of the homopteroates to glutamate by the solid phase technique was expected to yield the desired glutamate conjugates 2 and 3.

Theoretical considerations suggested to the possibility of a reverse Michael addition reaction which might take place on exposure of compounds belonging to the series 10 with either nucleophiles (X^-) or electrophiles (H^+). This is because the enolate generated in the system could easily collapse to a thermodynamically more stable enone 14 and a highly resonance stabilized thiophenolate anion. However, we decided to proceed with the synthesis according to this projected scheme with the hope that we might solve these problems if and when they arose. The required chloromethylketone 10 was prepared by nucleophilic addition of ρ-(carbomethoxy)thiophenol 7 with chloromethylvinylketone 8, which in turn was prepared from ethylene and chloroacetylchloride. Acetoxymethyl and hydroxymethyl vinyl ketones were prepared from 1,4-butynediol[8], which on reaction with 7, gave 12 and 11. Conversion of 11 to 10 was accomplished by thionylchloride.

The first realization of the occurrence of the retro Michael reactions took place when 10 was treated with excess sodium azide in an attempt to make the corresponding ketoazide. The main product, whose structure was subsequently established[7] as 13, was also the product of reaction between 10 and sodium acetate or equimolar amounts of

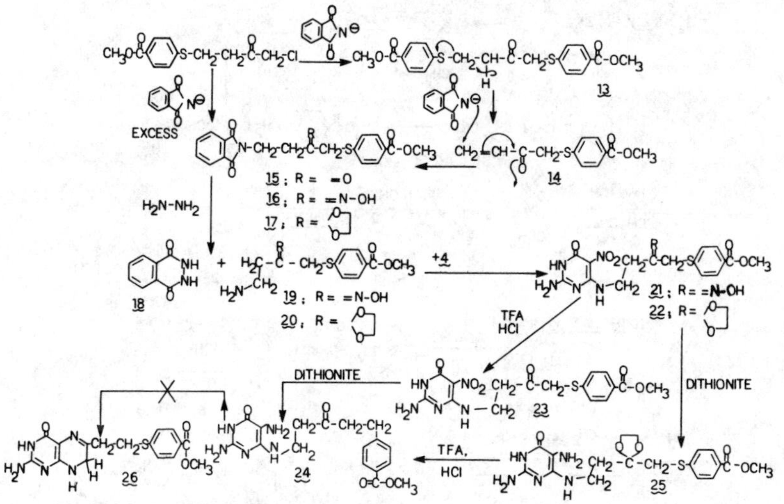

SCHEME II

potassium phthalimide. However, the use of two or more equivalents of potassium phthalimide in the above reaction gave a product whose spectral characteristics were consistant with the expected structure 29a. With this assumption, this compound was converted to the oxime which was then subjected to hydrazinolysis to obtain an amine which showed spectral characteristics expected of structure 6. Reaction of this amine with 4 and 5 gave the corresponding pyrimidine derivatives which were deprotected at the carbonyl function. Dithionite reduction of these compounds in aqueous DMF and subsequent cyclization oxidation techniques, which when applied to these compounds, failed to yield the pteridine derivatives. This failure to construct the pteridine ring prompted us to question the structure of the reaction product between 10 and potassium phthalimide, and consideration was given to alternate procedures to construct this homofolate framework. Attempts to make 47 with the aid of the mesyl intermediate 45 also failed.

Compound 11 (prepared from hydroxymethylvinyl ketone and 7) on treatment with 2,5,6-triamino-4-pyrimidinol under neutral conditions in DMF gave a mixture of products from which a pteridine with the desired sidechain could be isolated after hydrolysis and extensive chromatography in very poor yields. Permanganate oxidation of this material gave pteridine-6-carboxylic acid, establishing that the compound was the six isomer. Application of this technique to the preparation of the 4-amino derivative failed due to the formation of complex mixtures.

At this point we directed our attention to elucidation of the structure of the phthalimide reaction product of chloroketone 10. Examina-

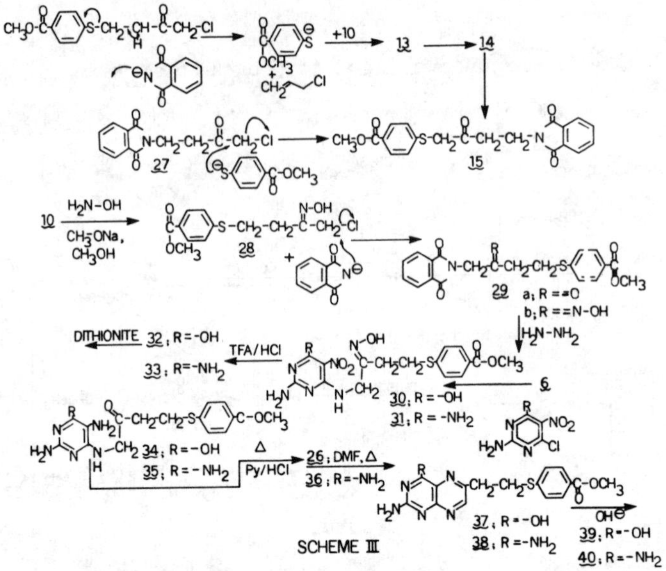

SCHEME III

tion of the mass spectral fragmentation pattern of the product revealed
that the compound did exhibit the unanticipated N-ethyl phthalimide
fragment corresponding to an m/e value of 174. Another interesting observation was that the mass spectrum did not exhibit an m/e value 195,
of the anticipated ρ-(carbomethoxy)-S-ethyl thiophenol fragment.
Coupled with the fact that the compound exhibited all the reactions of
a normal ketone and the NMR spectrum displayed the expected normal resonances of the methylene as a singlet, and the ethylene group as two
triplets the alternate structure 15 was considered for this product.
Therefore, an unambigious synthesis of this product was undertaken.
This was accomplished by conversion of authentic 27 prepared unambig-
iously from N-(3-carboxypropyl)phthalimide to 15 by reaction with ρ-
(carbomethoxy)thiophenol (Scheme III). Subsequently, the mechanism of
formation of 15 from 20 was elucidated in detail[7]. It became apparent
from these studies[7], that the initial formation of the enolate from 10
leads to the formation of 13. Due to the ease of formation of the
thermodynamically more stable 14 from 13, displacement reactions on 10
by a nucleophile should be carried out under conditions which avoid
enolate formation to get nonrearranged products. Therefore, the pyrimidine derivatives derived from 15 corresponded to structures 21-25
(Scheme II). The failure of formation of 26 from 24 was apparent based
on these mechanistic considerations. These considerations prompted us
to construct compound 28, which on reaction with potassium phthalimide
gave the desired 29a. The strategy was to prevent enolate formation by

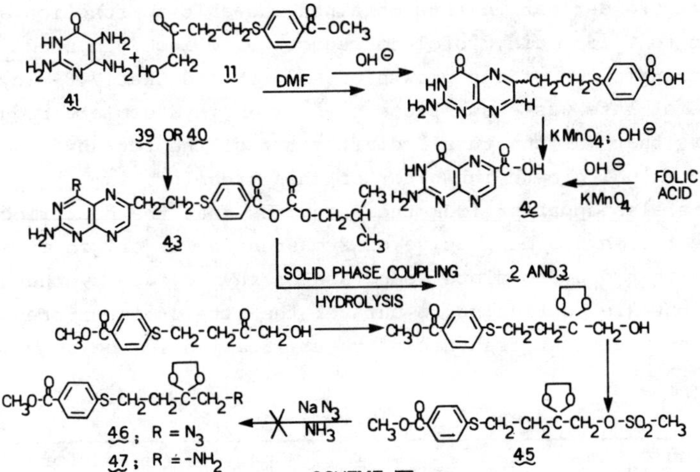

SCHEME IV

the selective protection of the carbonyl group prior to the displacement reaction[7]. Conversion of 29a to 39 and 40 was accomplished by a series of procedures involving deprotection of the carbonyl group with TFA/HCl, dithionite reduction of 34 and 35 in aqueous DMF and application of the simultaneous cyclization oxidative techniques on these reduction products to obtain 37 and 38. After hydrolysis to 39 and 40, these pteroate analogs were subjected to the solid phase coupling procedure for their elaboration to 2 and 3.

BIOLOGICAL EVALUATION

The biological responses of each organism towards various 11-thiohomopteroate derivatives are listed in Table I. Compound 2 did not inhibit the growth of either organism but the d,1-5,6,7,8-tetrahydro derivative obtained by catalytic reduction of 2 showed very powerful inhibition of the growth of S. faecium ($I_{50}=1.2 \times 10^{-9}$ g/ml) and L. casei ($I_{50}=8.3 \times 10^{-7}$ g/ml). Tetrahydro-11-thiohomofolic acid was not an inhibitor of L. casei thymidylate synthetase. The parent compound 2 was neither a substrate nor an inhibitor of L. casei dihydrofolate reductase. At the present time we do not know which of the diastereomers of tetrahydro-11-thiohomofolic acid contributes to this growth inhibition, nor has its mechanism been elucidated. As expected, 4-amino-4-deoxy-11-thiohomofolic acid 3 was a powerful inhibitor of the growth of both organisms ($I_{50}=2 \times 10^{-9}$ and 1×10^{-10} g/ml respectively).

An aqueous solution of the potassium salt of 2 was treated with sodium dithionite at room temperature and the reduction of 2 to 7,8-dihydro-11-thiohomofolic acid was monitored spectrally. The authentic

7,8-dihydro derivative thus obtained was able to function as a substrate to *L. casei* dihydrofolate reductase. Since compound 2 *per se* was not an inhibitor of the growth of *L. casei*; and that 7,8-dihydro-11-thiohomofolate was a substrate to *L. casei* dihydrofolate reductase, it appears that the "unnatural" diasteromer of the tetrahydro derivative is the actual growth inhibitor of this organism.

It is also apparent from these studies that the bacteriocidal effect of the tetrahydro derivative of 2 must have its origin at sites other than either dihydrofolate reductase or thymidylate synthetase. Investigations are continuing to unravel the site of interference of this compound against tetrahydrofolate utilization in the above organisms.

TABLE I

| Compound | | Conc: in mµg/ml for 50% inhibition | |
Number	Name	S. faecium	L. casei
2	11-thiohomofolic acid	>1600	>1600
3	11-thiohomoaminopterine	2.0	0.10
37	Methyl-11-thiohomopteroate	>1600	>1600
38	Methyl-4-amino-11-thio-homopteroate	16.0	400
39	11-thiohomopteroic acid	>1600	>1600
40	Methyl-11-thiohomopteroate	100	100
--	d,1,tetrahydro-11-thiohomofolic acid	1.2	830

ACKNOWLEDGEMENT

This investigation was supported by grants from the American Cancer Society (CH-53A to MGN) and National Institutes of Health (CA-10914 to RLK).

REFERENCES

1. DeGraw, J.I., J.P. Marsh, Jr., E.M. Acton, O.P. Crews, C.W. Mosher, A.M. Fujiwara and L. Goodman. *J. Org. Chem.* 30, 3404 (1965).

2. Goodman, L., J.I. DeGraw, R.L. Kisliuk, M. Friedkin, E.J. Pastore, E.J. Crawford, L.T. Plante, A. Nahas, J.F. Morningstar, Jr., G. Kwok, L. Wilson, E.F. Donovan and J. Ratzan. *J. Amer. Chem. Soc.* 86, 308 (1964).

3. Crusberg, T.C., R. Leary and R.L. Kisliuk. *J. Biol. Chem.* 245, 5292 (1970).

4. Nair, M.G. and P.T. Campbell. *J. Med. Chem.* 19, 825 (1976).

5. Hornbeak, H.R. and M.G. Nair. *Molecular Pharmacol.* 14, 299 (1978).

6. Nair, M.G., P.C. O'Neal, C.M. Baugh, R.L. Kisliuk, Y. Gaumont and M. Rodman. *J. Med. Chem.* 21, 673 (1978).

7. Chen, S.Y. and M.G. Nair. *J. Org. Chem.* 43, 000 (1978).

8. Arbuzov, Y.A. and A.M. Korolev. *Zh. Obshch. Khim.* 32, 3674 (1962).

AMIDES OF METHOTREXATE

JAMES R. PIPER AND JOHN A. MONTGOMERY

Kettering-Meyer Laboratory, Southern Research Institute, Birmingham, AL 35205 (U. S. A.)

ABSTRACT

Amides of methotrexate involving both the α- and γ-carboxyls of the glutamic acid moiety were prepared by alkylation of $\underline{N}$-[4-(methylamino)benzoyl]-L-α- and γ-glutamyl precursors with 6-(bromomethyl)-2,4-pteridinediamine. The compounds prepared were evaluated and compared with methotrexate with respect to ability to inhibit dihydrofolic reductase, cytotoxicity, and effect on L1210 murine leukemia.

INTRODUCTION

Methotrexate (MTX) has been used in the treatment of human cancer for over thirty years.[1] (Although still a mainstay in the treatment of acute leukemia, it is also used in the treatment of the head and neck and osteogenic sarcoma.) Response of human leukemias to MTX has been correlated with uptake, which occurs primarily via active transport.[2-5] Certain murine tumors deficient in this transport system are resistant to MTX but sensitive to other inhibitors of dihydrofolic reductase (DHFR) which enter cells by passive diffusion.[3,6] Acquired resistance in some leukemic cell lines has been shown to result from loss of the active transport mechanism.[4,7] These observations led us to attempt to prepare derivatives of MTX with altered transport characteristics but unaltered with respect to binding to DHFR. The finding that the γ-glutamate peptide congener $\underline{11}$ ($R_5 = Glu$), a significant metabolite of MTX in a number of mammalian tissues,[8-10] is equivalent to MTX as an inhibitor of DHFR from L1210 leukemia cells[9] led us to synthesize $\underline{11}$ ($R_5 = Glu$) and a number of other amides of MTX represented by structural types $\underline{11}$ and $\underline{12}$ for biologic evaluation.

MATERIALS AND METHODS

Syntheses

Previous work in this laboratory led to the development of an improved procedure for the preparation of MTX and analogs with varied side chains.[11] This procedure, which has been adapted to the production of kilogram quantities of high-purity

$$\underset{\textbf{1}}{\text{CbzN(CH}_3)\text{C}_6\text{H}_4\text{-COCl}} \xrightarrow[\text{H}_2\text{O-dioxan}]{\substack{\text{L-Glu 1-Bn ester} \\ (i\text{-Pr})_2\text{NEt}}} \underset{\textbf{2}}{\overset{\text{CH}_3}{\text{CbzNC}_6\text{H}_4\text{CONHCHCO}_2\text{CH}_2\text{C}_6\text{H}_5}}$$

Scheme with compounds:

1 → CbzN(CH₃)C₆H₄—COCl

2: CH₃ | CbzNC₆H₄CONHCHCO₂CH₂C₆H₅ ; (CH₂)₂CO₂H

5: CH₃ | CbzNC₆H₄CONHCHCO₂H ; (CH₂)₂CO₂CH₂C₆H₅

3: CH₃ | CbzNC₆H₄CONHCHCO₂CH₂C₆H₅ ; (CH₂)₂CONRR' (from 2, Et₃N, i-BuOCOCl, HNRR')

6: CH₃ | CbzNC₆H₄CONHCHCONHR ; (CH₂)₂CO₂CH₂C₆H₅

4: CH₃ | HNC₆H₄CONHCHCO₂H ; (CH₂)₂COR₅ (from 3, H₂, 5% Pd on C, dioxan)

7: CH₃ | HNC₆H₄CONHCHCOR₁ ; (CH₂)₂CO₂H

8: CH₃ | CbzNC₆H₄CONHCHCO₂CH₂C₆H₂(CH₃)₃-2,4,6 ; (CH₂)₂CONH₂

9: CH₃ | CbzNC₆H₄CONHCHCONH₂ ; (CH₂)₂CO₂H

10 → (pteridine) NH₂ / N / H₂N-N ... CH₂Br ·HBr

$$\xrightarrow[\substack{\text{Me}_2\text{NAc} \\ 4\text{-}5\text{ days} \\ \text{at }25°}]{\textbf{4 or 7}}$$

11: R₁ = OH   R₅ = NH₂, NHCH₃, N(CH₃)₂, NH(CH₂)₄CH₃, NHCH₂C₆H₅, Gly, Asp, Glu

12: R₅ = OH   R₁ = NH₂, Gly, Asp, Glu

MTX,[12, 13] involves the reaction of 6-(bromomethyl)-2,4-pteridinediamine hydro-bromide (10) with appropriate side-chain precursors. The process proved ideally suited for preparing the 11- and 12- types,[14] and the syntheses became principally exercises in unequivocal preparations of N-[4-(methylamino)benzoyl]-L-α- and γ-glutamyl precursors of structural types 4 and 7, which were readily achieved using adaptations of standard methods of peptide synthesis.

All but two of the protected side-chain precursors (types 3 and 6) were prepared by acylation of the appropriate amino compounds with the α- and γ-benzyl esters 2 and 5 using the mixed-anhydride method. Carboxyl groups of amino acids used in this coupling procedure were protected by benzyl groups. The protected precursor 8 was prepared from 1 and L-glutamine 2,4,6-trimethylbenzyl ester,[15] and 9 was prepared by ammonolysis of 2. The protective groupings of all precursors except 8 were removed by hydrogenolysis. Deprotection of 8 was effected by HBr.[15] The re-sulting 4- and 7- types were then treated with 10 to give the amides of MTX. In a typical procedure, the residue from evaporation of the hydrogenolysis solution was treated directly with 10. [The molar ratio of 10 to type 4 or 7 was 1:1.2. No base was required except for 4 ($R_5 = NH_2$)·HBr, which was treated with an equimolar amount of Et_3N prior to addition of 10.] Isolation of the products consisted simply of diluting the reaction solutions with water, adjusting the pH to 3.8, then washing the collected precipitates with water before drying in vacuo. In some instances, samples were reprecipitated from aqueous solutions of their sodium salts. Final products were obtained in high states of purity and free of MTX according to ele-mental analyses, spectral data (^{1}H NMR, UV, and field-desorption mass[16]), and analysis by high-pressure liquid chromatography.

Biological testing

Estimates of the binding affinities to DHFR for most of the amides prepared were obtained by a reported procedure.[17] Comparisons of the results with that produced by MTX are listed in Table 1. Data from cytotoxicity tests in the KB cell culture screens and the L1210 murine leukemia screen performed by standard methods[18] are also listed in Table 1.

Other investigators have studied these compounds with regard to transport and DHFR inhibition in murine tumor and normal cells[19] and human thymidylate synthe-tase.[20]

RESULTS

The comparative DHFR inhibition data shown in Table 1 would indicate the necessity of a free α-carboxyl, or a spatially equivalent free carboxyl, in MTX analogs for tight binding to the enzyme; whereas a free γ-carboxyl does not appear to be essential for binding. These results are in keeping with recently published X-ray crystallographic data on the MTX-DHFR complex.[21]

TABLE 1

BIOLOGICAL TEST RESULTS

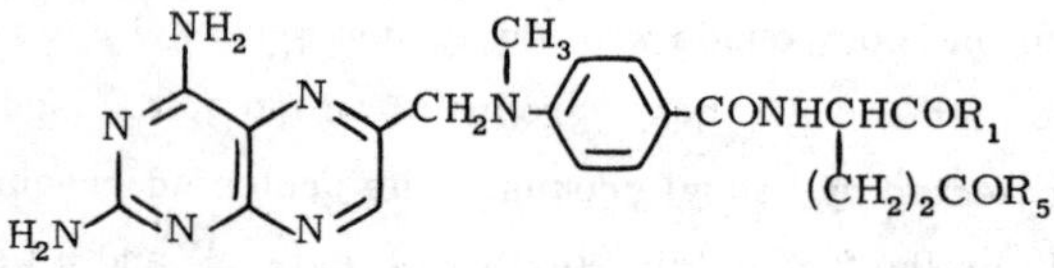

		DHFR Inhibition[a] (I_{50}[b]/I_{50} MTX[c])	Cytotoxicity (KB Cells) ED_{50}, $\mu g/ml$[d]	MTX Ratio	L1210 Optimal Dose (mg/kg),[d] qd 1-9	%ILS
R_1	R_5					
OH	OH	1	0.003	1	1.3	48
OH	NH_2	1.8	0.32	110	180	58
OH	$NHCH_3$	2.0	0.62	210	100	58
OH	$N(CH_3)_2$	2.2	0.86	290	50	44
OH	$NH(CH_2)_4CH_3$	2.1	2.8	930	200	55
OH	$NHCH_2C_6H_5$	—	< 1	—	100	33
OH	Gly	—	< 0.25	—	5	74
OH	Asp	0.7	1.4	470	5	65
OH	Glu	0.8	0.038	13	2.5	65
NH_2	OH	110	2.6	870	25	34
Gly	OH	—	2.8	930	50	41
Asp	OH	4.0	19	6300	25	47
Glu	OH	3.6	0.3	100	25	67

[a] Dihydrofolic reductase from commercial pigeon liver acetone powder.[17]
[b] Concentration of inhibitor required to inhibit the reduction of dihydrofolate to 50% of the control.
[c] I_{50} MTX in this system = 0.016 μM.
[d] See reference 18.

ACKNOWLEDGMENTS

This investigation was supported by the Division of Cancer Treatment, National Cancer Institute, National Institutes of Health, Department of Health, Education, and Welfare, Contract NO1-CM-43762.

REFERENCES

1. R. B. Livingston and S. K. Carter, "Single Agents in Cancer Chemotherapy," IFI/Plenum, New York, 1970, pp. 130-172.

2. J. R. Bertino and D. G. Johns, Ann. Rev. Med., 18, 27 (1967).

3. F. M. Sirotnak, D. M. Dorick, and D. M. Moccio, Cancer Treat. Rep., 60, 547 (1976).

4. R. C. Jackson, D. Niethammer, and F. M. Huennekens, Cancer Biochem. Biophys., 1, 151 (1975).

5. F. M. Huennekens and G. B. Henderson, "Chemistry and Biology of Pteridines," W. Pfeiderer, Ed., Walter de Gruyter, Berlin, 1976, pp. 179-196.

6. F. M. Sirotnak and R. C. Donsbach, Cancer Res., 36, 1151 (1976).

7. G. A. Fischer, Biochem. Pharmacol., 11, 1233 (1962).

8. M. G. Nair and C. M. Baugh, Biochemistry, 12, 3923 (1973).

9. S. A. Jacobs, R. H. Adamson, B. A. Chabner, C. J. Derr, and D. G. Johns, Biochem. Biophys. Res. Commun., 63, 692 (1975).

10. V. M. Whitehead, Cancer Res., 27, 408 (1977).

11. J. R. Piper and J. A. Montgomery, J. Org. Chem., 42, 208 (1977).

12. J. A. Ellard, U. S. Patent 4,080,325 (1978).

13. J. F. Gallelli and D. C. Chatterji, Cancer Treat. Rep., 62, 487 (1978).

14. Related amides have been prepared from MTX monoethyl esters by A. Rosowsky and C.-S. Yu, J. Med. Chem., 21, 170 (1978).

15. F. H. C. Stewart, Aust. J. Chem., 20, 365 (1967).

16. M. C. Kirk, W. C. Coburn, Jr., and J. R. Piper, Biomed. Mass Spectrom., 3, 245 (1976).

17. B. R. Baker, B.-T. Ho, and T. Nielson, J. Heterocycl. Chem., 1, 79 (1964).

18. R. I. Geran, N. H. Greenberg, M. M. Macdonald, A. M. Schumacher, and B. J. Abbott, Cancer Chemother. Rep., Part 3, 3 (no. 2) (1972).

19. F. M. Sirotnak, P. L. Chello, J. R. Piper, J. A. Montgomery, and J. I. DeGraw, Sixth International Symposium on the Chemistry and Biology of Pteridines, September 25–28, 1978, La Jolla, California.

20. Y.-C. Cheng, D. W. Szeto, B. J. Dolnick, A. Rosowsky, M. Chaykovsky, E. J. Modest, J. R. Piper, C. Temple, Jr., R. D. Elliott, J. D. Rose, and J. A. Montgomery, Sixth International Symposium on the Chemistry and Biology of Pteridines, September 25–28, 1978, La Jolla, California.

21. D. A. Matthews, R. A. Alden, J. T. Bolin, S. T. Freer, R. Hamlin, N. Xuong, J. Krauth, M. Poe, M. Williams, and K. Hoogsteen, Science, 197, 452 (1977).

ANTIFOLATE INHIBITORS OF THYMIDYLATE SYNTHETASE AS LIGANDS
FOR AFFINITY CHROMATOGRAPHY

LAURENCE T. PLANTE

Department of Biochemistry and Pharmacology, Tufts University School of Medicine,
Boston, Massachusetts, 02111, U.S.A.

ABSTRACT

Two inhibitors of thymidylate synthetase, N^α-[pteroyl-(tetra-γ-glutamyl)]lysine
and N^α-(5,8-bisdeazapteroyl)lysine were synthesized and coupled to Sepharose 4B-200
via the cyanogen bromide reaction. These matrices were useful in the purification of
L. casei thymidylate synthetase.

INTRODUCTION

Thymidylate synthetase catalyzes the reaction of methylenetetrahydrofolate with
dUMP to form dTMP and dihydrofolate[1]. The enzyme is usually purified by conventional
methods[2,3,4]. Chromatography utilizing derivatives of dUMP[5] and 5-FdUMP[6] attached
to Sepharose has been described. The bound enzyme was not displaced from either of
these columns by dUMP, indicating that they do not function as true affinity
matrices. Tetrahydromethotrexate aminoethyl Sepharose is reported to be useful in
the purification of this enzyme[7], but due to the instability of the ligand, the
column could be used only once. Methotrexate Sepharose has also been used in the
purification of human thymidylate synthetase[8].

In view of the high affinity of pteroylpolyglutamates[9,10,11] and 5,8-bisdeaza-10-
methylpteroylglutamate[12] for thymidylate synthetase, N^α-[pteroyl-(tetra-γ-glutamyl)]-
lysine (Fig. 1) and N^α-(5,8-bisdaza-10-methylpteroyl)lysine (Fig. 2) were prepared
and coupled to Sepharose 4B-200 via the cyanogen bromide reaction.

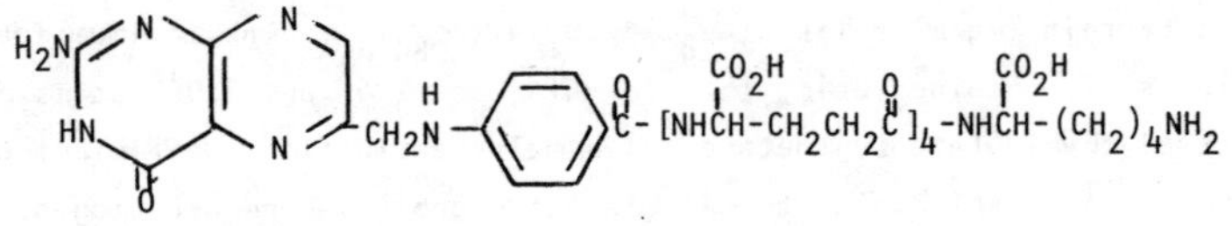

Fig. 1

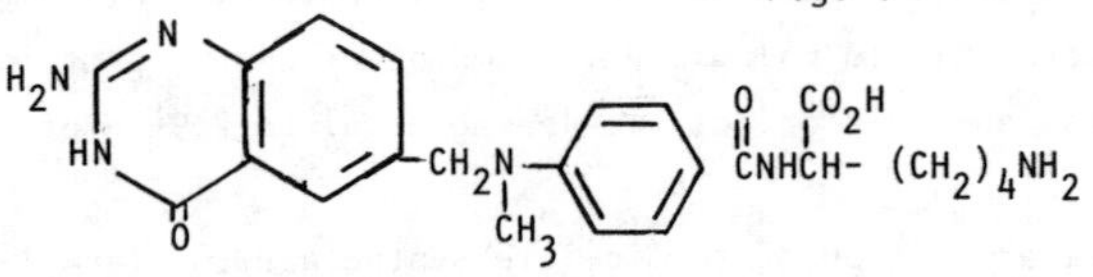

Fig. 2

MATERIALS AND METHODS

N^{α}-(tert.-Butyloxycarbonyl)-N^{ϵ}-(carbobenzoxy)-lysine resin ester was purchased
from Vega-Fox Biochemicals. Removal of the tert.-butyloxycarbonyl group with 50%
trifluoroacetic acid in methylene chloride, followed by four coupling cycles with
N-tert.-butyloxycarbonyl)-glutamic acid α benzyl ester as described[13] was followed
by coupling with N^{2}-acetyl-N^{10}-trifluoroacetylpteroyl isobutylcarbonic mixed anhydride. Cleavage from the resin was with anhydrous HBr in trifluoroacetic acid at
ambient temperature for five minutes. After evaporation of the trifluoroacetic acid
in vacuo the mixture was saponified with 100 ml 0.2 N sodium hydroxide (for 1 mmole
prep) at 100° (under Ar) for one hour. Filtration followed by adjustment of pH to
4 with HCl gave a precipitate of N^{α}-[pteroyltetra-(γ-glutamyl)]lysine. The R_f (N/10
ammonium bicarbonate on Whatman No. 1 paper, ascending) was 0.90, after purification
by gradient elution (0 to M ammonium bicarbonate) from DEAE cellulose. Amino acid
analysis of a hydrolysed sample indicated the presence of glutamic acid and lysine
in approximate ratio 4:1. This compound was coupled to cyanogen bromide activated
Sepharose as described[14], washed with water and stored at 3°.

5,8-Bisdeaza-10-methylpteroic acid was condensed with N^{ϵ}-(tert.-butyloxycarbonyl)-
lysine methyl ester via the mixed anhydride procedure. After saponification and
gradient elution from DEAE cellulose (0 to M) ammonium bicarbonate, N^{α}-(5,8-bisdeaza-
10-methylpteroyl)-N^{ϵ}-(tert.-butyloxycarbonyl)lysine showed λ_{max} = 300 nm, $\lambda_{225}/$
λ_{300} = 1.65, R_f = 0.78 (Eastman Chromagram, ethyl acetate:ethanol:acetic acid-2:1:1).
Following removal of the blocking group with 2N HCl at ambient temperature for one
hour, N^{α}-(5,8-bisdeaza-10-methylpteroyl)lysine was coupled to Sepharose 4B-200 containing a hydroxyhexylamido spacer via the cyanogen bromide reaction.

Extracts of Methotrexate resistant L. casei subjected to ribonuclease and deoxy-
ribonuclease digestion, ammonium sulfate precipitation and dialysis were prepared at
the New England Enzyme Center. The specific activity of thymidylate synthetase in
this crude extract was 4 units per mg protein. It was purified to 90 units per mg
protein by phosphocellulose chromatography[3]. One unit is defined as the amount of
enzyme required to synthesize 1 µmole dTMP per hour at 30°. Protein was determined
using the formula: protein (mg/ml = 1.45 (A_{280}) - 0.74 (A_{260})[15]. The maximum specific activities previously obtained using this formula were 216[2] and 220[16] units per
mg protein. L. casei thymidylate synthetase has a molar extinction coefficient of
108,000 at 280 nm[17]. Using this value to calculate the protein concentration of a
pure sample, the maximum specific activity is 350 units per mg protein. This higher
value was used in the present work only to calculate the amount of enzyme protein
absorbed to the affinity columns, one unit of activity being equal to 2.9 ng of
thymidylate synthetase.

The data of Table 1 show that absorption of thymidylate synthetase to pteroyl-
tetra (γ-glutamyl)lysine Sepharose requires dUMP. The absorption was most efficient
when 2-mercaptoethanol, CH_2O, and $MgCl_2$ were included in the loading solution

TABLE I

ABSORPTION AND ELUTION OF L. CASEI THYMIDYLATE SYNTHETASE FROM N^{α}-[PTEROYLTETRA-(γ-GLUTAMYL)]LYSINE SEPHAROSE.

Experiment	Absorption Buffer	Initial Spec. Activ.	Enzyme Units Added	Enzyme Units Eluted With Wash	Elution Buffer	Enzyme Units Eluted	% Recovery of Activ.	Spec. Activ.
1. No dUMP								
	3.5 ml Buffer 1	90	2100	5 ml Buffer 1 2100	-	-	100	90
2. Absorbed with dUMP, eluted by omitting dUMP								
	7.4 ml Buffer 2	90	970	12 ml Buffer 3 194	30 ml Buffer 4	557	70	177
3. Absorbed with dUMP, eluted with tetrahydrofolate								
	21 ml Buffer 5	90	1548	11 ml Buffer 6 0	16 ml Buffer 7	1209	77	158
4. Absorbed with dUMP, eluted with KCl								
	16 ml Buffer 5	90	1808	I 4 ml Buffer 5 0 II 9 ml Buffer 8 0 III 4 ml Buffer 9 0	13 ml Buffer 10	1780	98	213

Column size 0.6 cm by 8 cm; bed volume 2.3 ml; flow rate 1 ml/min; temp. 22°

Buffer 1 - 0.05 M KPO_4, 0.05 M KCl, pH 7.0
Buffer 2 - 0.05 M KPO_4, 0.01 M KCl, 4×10^{-5} M dUMP, pH 7.0
Buffer 3 - 0.05 M KPO_4, 4×10^{-5} M dUMP, pH 7.0
Buffer 4 - 0.05 M KPO_4, pH 7.0
Buffer 5 - 0.05 M Tris Cl, 0.001 M EDTA, 0.1 M 2-mercaptoethanol
 0.012 M CH_2O, 0.021 M $MgCl_2$, 4×10^{-5} M dUMP, pH 7.4.
Buffer 6 - 0.05 M Tris Cl, 0.001 M EDTA, 0.2 M 2-mercaptoethanol
Buffer 7 - 0.05 M Tris Cl, 0.001 M EDTA, 3×10^{-3} M tetrahydrofolate,
 0.2 M 2-mercaptoethanol, pH 7.4
Buffer 8 - same as Buffer 5 minus dUMP
Buffer 9 - 0.05 M Tris Cl, 0.001 M EDTA, pH 7.4
Buffer 10 - same as Buffer 9 plus 0.5 M KCl, pH 7.4

(buffer 5, exp. 3 and 4). Additional experiments showed that omission of $MgCl_2$ and CH_2O from buffer 5 leads to a decrease of 20% in the capacity of the matrix to absorb the enzyme. After absorption in buffer 5, the column could be washed without loss of activity even if dUMP were omitted (exp. 4). However, after absorption in phosphate buffer (exp. 2), omission of dUMP from the buffer caused enzyme elution. The enzyme

TABLE II

ABSORPTION AND ELUTION OF <u>L. CASEI</u> THYMIDYLATE SYNTHETASE FROM N^{α}-(5,8-BISDEAZA-10-METHYLPTEROYL)LYSINE HYDROXYHEXYLAMIDO SEPHAROSE.

Experi- ment	Absorp- tion Buffer	Initial Spec. Activ.	Enzyme Units Added	Enzyme Units Eluted With Wash	Elution Buffer	Enzyme Units Eluted	% Recov- very of Activ.	Spec. Activ.
1	6.0 mls Buffer 5	85	912	I 40 mls Buffer 5 446 II 40 mls Buffer 9 0	30 mls Buffer 10	384	82	140
2	12.5 mls Buffer 5	141	246	I 40 mls Buffer 5 0 II 40 mls Buffer 9 0	11 mls Buffer 10	99	40	121
3	44 mls Buffer 5	7.5	1006	I 100 mls Buffer 5 0 II 200 mls Buffer 9 0	I 30 mls Buffer 7 II 26 mls Buffer 10	0 351	35	47
4	7.1 mls Buffer 5	86	906	I 90 mls Buffer 5 0 II 45 mls Buffer 9 0	I 32 mls Buffer 7 II 123 mls Buffer 5 III 21 mls Buffer 10	0 0 350	39	110

Column size:
Experiments 1 and 2, 0.6 x 8 cms, 2.3 mls.
Experiment 3, 1.2 x 9 cms, 10 mls.
Experiment 4, 1.2 x 8 cms, 9 mls.

was eluted by tetrahydrofolate (Exp. 3) or by 0.5 M KCl (Exp. 4).

Elution with 0.5 M KCl proved to be most satisfactory since all of the activity was removed from the column and the specific activity corresponds to that of pure enzyme.

In Table II are shown the results of several experiments utilizing N^{α}-(5,8-bis-deaza-10-methylpteroyl)lysine as an affinity matrix for the purification of thymidylate synthetase. Tetrahydrofolate did not elute the enzyme (Table II, Exp. 3) from this column indicating it does not behave as a true affinity matrix. In separate experiments it was found that the N^{α}-pteroylpolyglutamyllysine column does not bind L. casei dihydrofolate reductase under the conditions of Experiments 1 and 2, Table 1, even when crude extracts were loaded. However, the N^{α}-5,8-bisdeaza-10-methylpteroyllysine column retained L. casei dihydrofolate reductase under these conditions, (Table II, Exp. 3). Prior removal of the reductase (Table II, Exp. 4) by phosphocellulose chromatography had no effect on elution by tetrahydrofolate. The second matrix may behave as a hydrophobic binder of thymidylate synthetase[7]. Both columns described have substantially higher capacity for the enzyme than matrices containing dUMP[5] or FdUMP[6], and they are stable to stripping with 0.1 N sodium hydroxide solution.

ACKNOWLEDGEMENTS

I wish to thank Ms Yvette Gaumont and Mr. Michael J. Beckage for the enzyme assays, and Drs. Edward J. Pastore and Roy L. Kisliuk for their kind encouragement during the course of this work. I thank the National Cancer Institute (CA 20539) for their support.

REFERENCES

1. M. Friedkin, Adv. Enzymol. 38, 235-292 (1973).

2. R.P. Leary and R.L. Kisliuk, Prep. Biochem. 1, 47-54 (1971).

3. J.H. Galivan, G.F. Maley and F. Maley, Biochemistry 14, 3338-3344 (1975).

4. J.A. Lyon, A.L. Pollard, R.B. Loeble and R.B. Dunlap, Cancer Biochem. Biophys. 1, 121-128 (1975).

5. P.V. Danenberg, R.J. Langenbach and C. Heidelberger, Biochem. Biophys. Res. Commun. 49, 1029-1033 (1972).

6. J.M. Whiteley, I. Jerkunica and T. Deits, Biochemistry 13, 2044-2050 (1974).

7. K. Slavik, W. Rode and V. Slavikova, Biochemistry 15, 4222-4227 (1976).

8. B.J. Dolnick and Y. Cheng, J. Biol. Chem. 252, 7697-7703 (1977).

9. R.L. Kisliuk, Y. Gaumont and C.M. Baugh, J. Biol. Chem. 249, 4100-4103 (1974).

10. M. Friedkin, L.T. Plante, E.J. Crawford and M. Crumm, J. Biol. Chem. 250, 5614-5621 (1975).

11. J.H. Galivan, F. Maley, and C.M. Baugh, Biochem. Biophys. Res. Commun. 71, 527-534 (1976).

12. O.D. Bird, J.W. Vaitkus, and J. Clarke, Mol. Pharm., 6, 573 (1970).

13. C.L. Krumdieck, and C.M. Baugh, Biochemistry 8, 1568-1572 (1969).

14. E.J. Pastore, L.T. Plante and R.L. Kisliuk, Methods Enzymol. 34B, 281-288 (1974).

15. E. Layne, Methods Enzymol. 3, 447-452 (1957).

16. N.V. Beaudette, N. Langerman, R.L. Kisliuk and Y. Gaumont, Arch. Biochem. Biophys. 179, 272-278 (1977).

17. R.P. Leary, N. Beaudette and R.L. Kisliuk, J.Biol.Chem. 250, 4864-4868 (1975).

18. A.J. Wahba and M. Friedkin, J. Biol. Chem. 237, 3794-3801 (1962).

NEW METHODS OF NEUTRAL ESTERIFICATION OF METHOTREXATE AND RELATED COMPOUNDS

ANDRE ROSOWSKY AND CHENG-SEIN YU

Sidney Farber Cancer Institute, Harvard Medical School, Boston, Mass. 02115 (U.S.A.)

ABSTRACT

Neutral esterification of methotrexate and related antifolates is accomplished readily by treatment with an alkyl or aralkyl halide and cesium carbonate in DMSO at room temperature. The resultant lipid-soluble ester derivatives show experimental antitumor activity that appears to be related to their capacity to act as prodrugs. Under appropriate conditions the cesium carbonate method can also be applied to the synthesis of esters of folic acid and 5-formyltetrahydrofolic acid (leucovorin).

INTRODUCTION

Lipid-soluble diesters of methotrexate (4-amino-4-deoxy-N[10]-methylpteroyl-L-glutamic acid, MTX) have been of interest for a number of years as potential prodrugs of this powerful folic acid antagonist. Einsenfeld and coworkers[1] briefly described the synthesis and some of the antitumor properties of MTX dimethyl ester in 1962. This was followed by a lapse of several years during which studies on MTX analogs were concerned mainly with the effect of changes in the pteridine ring or the C^9-N^{10} region of the molecule[2]. Then, in 1973, a series of MTX and 3',5'-dichloromethotrexate (DCM) esters was prepared independently in two laboratories[3,4] by acid-catalyzed esterification, and several of the diesters were evaluated as experimental antitumor agents[3,4]. More recently, these diesters have also received consideration as topical agents for the treatment of psoriasis[5].

Apart from their ability to function as lipophilic prodrugs, the diesters appear to have novel biological preperties of their own. Thus, MTX di-n-butyl ester[4] has been found to markedly inhibit [³H]-thymidine incorporation into DNA of cultured mouse and human leukemic cells[6], and evidence has been presented that this is a result of interference with uptake of the nucleoside from the growth medium[7]. On incubation in mouse serum in vitro, the di-n-butyl ester is converted rapidly to free MTX by esterase; however, in dog, monkey, and human serum, cleavage yields mainly the α- and γ-mono-n-butyl esters[8], which have been found to be almost as active as MTX as inhibitors of the enzyme dihydrofolate reductase[8,9].

We now report a new method of synthesis of MTX diesters which overcomes some of the inherent limitations associated with acid-catalyzed procedures[3,4]. This is a neutral esterification technique, involving reaction in DMSO with an alkyl or aralkyl halide in the presence of cesium carbonate. In addition to diesters of MTX

and other classical antifolates such as DCM and aminopterin (4-amino-4-deoxypteroyl-
L-glutamic acid, AMT), this procedure may be used to obtain diesters of folic acid
and 5-formyltetrahydrofolic acid (leucovorin). With very reactive species such as
2,6-dichlorobenzyl bromide, it is even possible to alkylate the disodium salts of
these compounds directly.

RESULTS AND DISCUSSION

In a typical experiment a suspension of MTX free acid (2.0 mmoles), cesium carbonate (4.0 mmoles), and 1-bromooctadecane (8.0 mmoles) in dry DMSO (50 ml) was
stirred at room temperature for 26 hours. After rotary evaporation (30 °C, vaccum
pump), the gummy residue was triturated with water, filtered, dried over P_2O_5, and
chromatographed on a silica gel column (40 g) using $CHCl_3$-MeOH mixtures ranging in
composition from 100:0 to 96:4. Pooling of TLC-homogeneous fractions and evaporation gave the heretofore undescribed MTX di-n-octadecyl ester (76% yield); mp 160-
168 °C; TLC: R_f 0.83 (silica gel, 3:1 $CHCl_3$-MeOH). Calcd. for $C_{56}H_{98}N_8O_5$: C,
70.10; H, 9.88; N, 11.68. Found : C, 70.05; H, 9.81; N, 11.60.

Other diesters of MTX that have been prepared in our laboratory are given in
Table 1. Primary halides appeared to be more reactive than secondary halides, and
bromides and iodides tended to be more reactive than chlorides. However, the
differences were not pronounced and it was possible in most instances to equalize
them by making small adjustments in the reaction time. The sterically hindered
cyclohexylmethyl derivative was isolated in only 17% yield, but this would presumably have been increased by lengthening the reaction time to 48 hrs as was done for
the other secondary halides. Allyl chloride gave only a 47% yield , but here again
a better yield would probably have been obtained by extending the reaction or using
allyl bromide. A number of aralkyl halides were also used successfully, and in the
benzyl series the chlorides were reactive enough to be used routinely in place of the
more expensive bromides. The reaction with benzyl chloride was found to also proceed satisfactorily with AMT and DCM. Several experimental variations were investigated, with no appreciable effect on yield. These included the addition of the
alkyl or aralkyl halide to pre-formed MTX dicesium salt, and the use of MTX disodium
salt in place of MTX free acid.

We were interested in examining whether sodium salts of MTX or AMT might be converted directly into esters if one used a sufficiently reactive alkyl or aralkyl halide. 2,6-Dichlorobenzyl bromide was considered a promising candidate for two reasons.
First, the electronegativity of the Cl atoms ought to enhance the reactivity of the
nearby benzylic carbon. Secondly, the presence of these ortho substituents ought
to favor nucleophilic attack on the benzylic carbon -- in other words, displacement
of the relatively bulky Br atom ought to provide steric relief. Our expectation
was rewarded when it was found that stirring MTX disodium salt with a stoichiometric

TABLE 1

SYNTHESIS OF DIALKYL AND BIS(ARALKYL) ESTERS OF METHOTREXATE VIA NEUTRAL ESTERIFI-CATION

Alkyl or aralkyl group	Halogen	Approx. reaction time, hours	% Yield	Mp, °C
1-Butyl	Br	24	75	153-155
1-Hexyl	I	18	69	155-157
1-Heptyl	I	18	63	150-152
1-Octyl	Br	24	84	131-134
1-Dodecyl	Br	24	74	128-130
1-Hexadecyl	Br	24	58	130-138
1-Octadecyl	Br	24	76	160-168
Cyclohexylmethyl	Br	24	17	159-161
2-Heptyl	Br	48	75	150-153
2-Dodecyl	Br	48	62	112-115
Allyl	Cl	24	47	146-154
Benzyl (MTX)	Cl	18	77	146-148
" (DCM)	Cl	18	74	194-198
" (AMT)	Cl	18	67	193-199
2,5-Dimethylbenzyl	Cl	24	70	135-137
3,4-Dimethylbenzyl	Cl	24	61	115-123
2,4,6-Trimethylbenzyl	Cl	24	49	147-155
4-Methoxybenzyl	Cl	24	60	112-114
6-Chloropiperonyl	Cl	24	61	130-138
3-Picolyl	Cl	24	33	115-125
2-Phenethyl	Br	18	75	116-125

amount of 2,6-dichlorobenzyl bromide in DMSO at room temperature for just 3 hrs, without added cesium carbonate and without excess alkylating agent, led to a 64% yield of MTX bis(2,6-dichlorobenzyl) ester; mp 175-180 °C; TLC: R_f 0.94 (silica gel, 3:1 $CHCl_3$-MeOH). Calcd. for $C_{34}H_{30}Cl_4N_8O_5$: C, 52.86; H, 3.92; Cl, 18.36; N, 14.51. Found : C, 52.46; H, 4.03; Cl, 18.34; N, 14.40.

In view of the ease with which MTX could be converted to diesters in the presence of cesium carbonate, we considered it worthwhile to investigate the esterification of folic acid, which has recently been reported[10] to give a pteridine ring-alkylated dimethyl ester on treatment with methyl iodide and potassium carbonate. We observed similarly that on reaction of folic acid with benzyl chloride and cesium carbonate in a 1:2:2 molar ratio in DMSO at room temperature for 48 hrs the principal product appears to be N^3-benzylfolic acid dibenzyl ester. In contrast, stirring folic acid disodium salt with two moles of 2,6-dichlorobenzyl bromide in DMSO (48 hrs, room temp) led to a 51% yield of a single product identified as folic acid bis(2,6-dichlorobenzyl) ester; mp 230 °C; TLC: R_f 0.56 (silica gel, 3:1 $CHCl_3$-MeOH). Calcd. for $C_{33}H_{27}Cl_4N_7O_6 \cdot 0.5H_2O$: C, 51.58; H, 3.67; Cl, 18.46; N, 12.76. Found : C, 51.35; H, 31.57; Cl, 19.01; N, 12.64. The lack of reaction of 2,6-dichlorobenzyl bromide at N^3 may be due to steric hindrance.

In order to further demonstrate the utility of the cesium carbonate method a number of esters of 5-formyltetrahydrofolate (leucovorin) were likewise prepared. Data on these heretofore unknown lipid-soluble leucovorin derivatives are given in Table 2. In contrast to the reaction of folic acid, there was no evidence of N^3 alkylation in leucovorin on treatment with benzyl chloride and cesium carbonate in a 1:2:2 molar ratio. The diminished N^3 reactivity in leucovorin relative to folic acid is perhaps attributable to the fact that the 5-formyl group can stabilize the OH-tautomeric form of the molecule, which thereby becomes resistant to ring alkylation. Once again, reaction with 2,6-dichlorobenzyl bromide was observed to occur with unusual ease as in the case of MTX and folic acid.

TABLE 2

SYNTHESIS OF DIALKYL AND BIS(ARALKYL) ESTERS OF LEUCOVORIN VIA NEUTRAL ESTERIFICATION

Alkyl or aralkyl group	Halogen	Approx. reaction time, hours	% Yield	Mp, °C
1-Hexyl	I	24	54	124-130
Benzyl	Cl	48	78	133-138
3,4-Dimethylbenzyl	Cl	48	30	136-143
2,4,6-Trimethylbenzyl	Cl	24	60	147-155
4-Methoxybenzyl	Cl	48	70	118-125
2,6-Dichlorobenzyl*	Br	4	67	155-162

*Reaction carried out on disodium salt

A number of the diesters reported in this paper have been tested for in vitro and in vivo biological activity. Against human lymphoblastic leukemia cells (CCRF-CEM line) in culture[11], all the alkyl esters up to the di-n-octyl were approximately equipotent on a molar basis (ID_{50} = 0.05-0.5 µM for the esters versus 0.02 µM for the parent acid). The longer-chain diesters showed a large drop in activity which probably reflects their poor water solubility. Against L1210 leukemia in the mouse[12], several of the diesters were as effective as MTX in prolonging the survival of treated animals. More importantly, when optimal doses were expressed as "MTX equivalents" -- i.e. the amount of MTX that would be released from the ester on complete hydrolysis -- the prodrug derivatives often showed a therapeutic advantage. Thus, whereas MTX bis(2,6-dichlorobenzyl) ester produced a 167% increase in lifespan (%ILS) at a MTX-equivalent dose of 12 mg/kg (q3d 1,4,7), MTX itself gave a 133% ILS at a dose of 60 mg/kg, i.e. a fivefold higher amount. At a dose of 15 mg/kg the % ILS with MTX was only 77%. Similar improved in vivo activity has been demonstrated in our laboratory with other aralkyl and long-chain alkyl diesters of MTX and DCM, and work on these promising compounds is continuing.

ACKNOWLEDGEMENT

This project was supported in part by Cancer Center Support Grant (Comprehensive) CA06516 from the National Cancer Institute. The authors acknowledge the help of Dr. Herbert Lazarus and Ms. Michelle Gorman in obtaining bioassay data, and are grateful to Drs. Emil Frei, III, and Edward J. Modest for their continued interest in this work.

REFERENCES

1. Eisenfeld, A. J., Mautner, H. G., and Welch, A. D. (1962) Proc. Am. Assoc. Cancer Res., 3, 316.

2. Mead, J. A. R. (1974) in "Antineoplastic and Immunosuppressive Agents," Sartorelli, A. C., and Johns, D. G., eds., Springer-Verlag, New York, Vol. 1, pp. 52-75.

3. Johns, D. G., Farquhar, D., Wolpert, M. K., Chabner, B. A., and Loo, T. L. (1973) Drug Metab. Dispos., 1, 580. Johns, D. G., Farquhar, D., Chabner, B. A., Wolpert, M. K., and Adamson, R. H. (1973) Experientia, 29, 1104. Loo, T. L., Johns, D. G., and Farquhar, D. (1973) Transplant. Proc., 5, 1161.

4. Rosowsky, A. (1973) J. Med. Chem., 16, 1190.

5. Weinstein, G. D., and McCullough, J. L. (1975) Arch. Dermatol., 111, 471. McCullough, J. L., Snyder, D. S., Weinstein, G. D., Friedland, A., and Stein, B. (1976) J. Invest. Dermatol., 66, 103. McCullough, J. L., Weinstein, G. D., and Hynes, J. B. (1977) J. Invest. Dermatol., 68, 362.

6. Curt, G. A., Tobias, J. S., Kramer, R. A., Rosowsky, A., Parker, L. M., and Tattersall, H. M. N. (1976) Biochem. Pharmacol., 25, 1943.

7. Beardsley, G. P., and Abelson, H. T. (1978) Proc. Am. Assoc. Cancer Res., 19, 45.

8. Rosowsky, A., Beardsley, G. P., Ensminger, W. D., Lazarus, H., and Yu, C.-S. (1978) J. Med. Chem., 21, 380.

9. Cheng, Y.-C., personal communication.

10. Temple, C., Jr., Kussner, C. L., and Montgomery, J. A. (1977) J. Heterocycl. Chem., 14, 885.

11. Foley, G. E., and Lazarus, H. (1967) Biochem. Pharmacol., 16, 659.

12. Geran, R. I., Greenberg, N. H., Macdonald, M. M., Schumacher, A. M., and Abbott, B. J. (1972) Cancer Chemother. Repts. Pt. 3, 6, 51.

SYNTHESIS OF DERIVATIVES OF TETRAHYDROFOLATE AS POTENTIAL MULTI-
SUBSTRATE AND PSEUDO COFACTOR INHIBITORS OF FOLATE ENZYMES

CARROLL TEMPLE, JR., ROBERT D. ELLIOTT, JERRY D. ROSE, AND
JOHN A. MONTGOMERY
Kettering-Meyer Laboratory, Southern Research Institute, Birmingham, AL 35205
(U. S. A.)

ABSTRACT

In the search for inhibitors of the folate enzymes, 5-, 10-, and 5,10-bridged
substituted derivative of 5,6,7,8-tetrahydrofolic acid (THF) were sought that are
either analogs of the covalent-linked substrate and cofactor or analogs of the cofactor alone. Several 5,10-bridged THF derivatives were prepared by treatment of
THF with phosgene, thiophosgene, and cyanogen bromide. Also, methods were
developed for the addition of isocyanates and isothiocyanates to THF to give 5-sub-
stituted derivatives, and for the reductive alkylation of THF with aldehydes to give
5-substituted and 5,10-disubstituted derivatives.

The six biologically active, one-carbon derivatives of 5,6,7,8-tetrahydrofolic
acid (THF) are interconverted by at least 15 enzymes. Although a considerable
amount of effort has been directed toward the investigation of these enzymes and the
reactions they catalyze, little of the work has been directed toward the identification
of inhibitors of these enzymes except for dihydrofolate reductase and thymidylate
synthetase. Important enzymes included GARP transformylase, AICRP transformylase, and thymidylate synthetase, which are involved in the function of tetrahydrofolate cofactors; and serine hydroxymethylase, 10-formyl-THF synthetase,
and 5,10-methylene-THF dehydrogenase, which are involved in the synthesis and
interconversions of tetrahydrofolate cofactors. The preparation and identification of
inhibitors of these folate enzymes might provide compounds useful for the treatment
of cancer.

In the search for inhibitors, 5-, 10-, and 5,10-bridged substituted derivatives of
THF were sought that are either analogs of the covalent-linked substrate and cofactor or analogs of the cofactor alone. The latter may not necessarily be the actual
inhibitor, but may be converted to the inhibitor by the formation of a covalent linkage with the substrate when both are bound to the enzyme.

$$HN-C(=O)...N(R_1)-CH_2N(R_2)-C_6H_4-CONHCH(CO_2H)CH_2CH_2CO_2H$$

(pteridine structure with H_2N, HN, R_1, R_2, CH_2N, phenyl, $CONHCH(CO_2H)CH_2CH_2CO_2H$)

2: $R_1 = R_2 = H$ (THF)

3: $R_1R_2 =$ CH_2

4: $R_1R_2 =$ CO

5: $R_1R_2 =$ CS

6: $R_1R_2 =$ $C=NH$

8: $R_1 = Me$, $R_2 = H$

9: $R_1 = R_2 = Me$

10: $R_1R_2 = CH_2CH_2$

11: $R_1 = CH_2Ph$, $R_2 = H$

12: $R_1 = (CH_2)_5OH$, $R_2 = H$

13: $R_1 = CH_2CO_2H$, $R_2 = H$

14: $R_1 = CH_2-$ (uracil ring) $=O$, $R_2 = H$

15: $R_1 = CONH_2$, $R_2 = H$

16: $R_1 = CONH(CH_2)_2Cl$, $R_2 = H$

17: $R_1 = CSNHEt$, $R_2 = H$

18: $R_1 = CSNHPh$, $R_2 = H$

The key intermediate, THF (**2**), is sensitive to air and light, undergoing auto-oxidation under acidic, neutral, and basic conditions.[1,2] Initially, our efforts were directed toward the preparation, isolation, and storage of solid **2**. Reduction of folic acid (**1**) in an aqueous, basic medium with an equal weight of NaBH$_4$[3] followed by precipitation of the product in the presence of ascorbic acid gave THF in 96% yield. This product, kept under a constant vacuum over P_2O_5 with protection from light, was used for the preparation of derivatives for a period of three to four weeks. Decomposition of THF was accompanied by a color change from creamy white to grey and eventually to brown. The grey discoloration appeared between one and two weeks, and as the intensity of the grey color increased, the amount of folic acid increased. Although THF prepared by this procedure contained boron impurities, these were usually removed during the preparation of derivatives (see below).

Although Slavik has reported that bridged analogs of 5,10-methylene-THF (**3**) were inactive as inhibitors of thymidylate synthetase,[4] further testing of these compounds was desired. Treatment of a suspension of THF in deoxygenated H_2O with a slow stream of phosgene for 1 hr gave **4**. Similarly, a solution of THF in aqueous NaOAc containing thiophosgene was stirred vigorously for 1.5 hr to give **5**. In the reaction of cyanogen bromide with an aqueous solution of THF at pH 6.5, the resulting crude **6** was purified by column chromatography on Sephadex (G-10).

The condensation of formaldehyde with THF to give the bridged N^5, N^{10}-methylene-THF (**3**) is well-documented. Kallen and Jencks have proposed that this reaction proceeded via the addition of formaldehyde to N-5 of THF to give $\underline{N}^5$-(hydroxymethyl)-THF, protonation and dehydration of the hydroxymethyl group of the latter to give the methylene iminium intermediate $[5\text{-}(CH_2=)\text{-}THF]^+$ ($\underline{7}$), and intramolecular nucleophilic attack by N-10 on the methylene carbon to give $\underline{3}$.[5] Since the reduction of $\underline{3}$ with hydride gave N^5-methyl-THF ($\underline{8}$) and apparently no $\underline{N}^{10}$-methyl-THF, this reaction is believed to involve $\underline{7}$ as an intermediate.[3]

In our laboratories the formation of 5-methyl-THF ($\underline{8}$) from THF, formaldehyde, and NaBH$_4$ under basic conditions gave a sample that was contaminated with a minor amount of a second compound (HPLC), which was not present in the sample resulting from NaBH$_3$CN reduction of 5,10-methenyl-THF chloride to give $\underline{8}$. This impurity, identified as 5,10-dimethyl-THF ($\underline{9}$), was the major product when THF was treated under acidic conditions with a five-fold excess of formaldehyde in the presence of NaBH$_3$CN. The formation of 5,10-methylene-THF ($\underline{3}$) from THF is inhibited by excess formaldehyde apparently because of the formation of 5,10-di(hydroxymethyl)-THF,[5] an intermediate that on reduction of both hydroxymethyl groups would give $\underline{9}$. A similar reaction sequence has been reported for the preparation of methyl 5,6,7,8-tetrahydro-5,10-dimethylpteroate.[6] In a related reaction, reductive alkylation at both N-5 and N-10 was observed on treatment of an aqueous solution of THF with 40% aqueous glyoxal solution and NaBH$_3$CN to give 5,10-ethylene-THF ($\underline{10}$),[7] which was purified by cellulose column chromatography.

Apparently the reductive alkylation of THF with an aromatic aldehyde has not been reported. Treatment of THF with benzaldehyde and reduction of the resulting adduct with NaBH$_4$, however, gave 5-benzyl-THF ($\underline{11}$). Similar conditions were used for the reaction of THF with 5-hydroxypentanal and 50% aqueous glyoxylic acid solution, respectively, to give 5-(5-hydroxypentyl)-THF ($\underline{12}$) and 5-(carboxymethyl)-THF ($\underline{13}$). In previous work, the condensation of THF with glyoxylic acid was shown to give the bridged adduct, $\underline{N}^5,\underline{N}^{10}$-(carboxymethylene)-THF.[8]

Although the alkylation of THF with 5-(chloromethyl)uracil gave 5-thyminyl-THF ($\underline{14}$), the preparation of $\underline{14}$ by treatment of a mixture of THF and 5-formyluracil with NaBH$_4$ in an aqueous medium was unsuccessful.[9] In contrast, $\underline{14}$ was prepared by the condensation of THF with 5-formyluracil in DMAC containing Linde 3A molecular sieve followed by treatment of the adduct with solid NaBH$_4$. Based on TLC data in which boron derivatives were detected with a spray of quinalizarin in H$_2$SO$_4$, this sample was complexed with either borohydrides or borates. The complex was disassociated by either elution of the sample from a silica gel column with 0.25 N HCl or by adjustment of a solution of the complex in 0.1 N HCl to pH 11.5 with Ca(OH)$_2$ followed by a readjustment to pH 3.8 to precipitate $\underline{14}$.

Another method for the preparation of analogs of the covalently-linked substrate and cofactor was provided by investigation of the addition of isocyanates and isothiocyanates to THF. Treatment of a deoxygenated solution of THF in aqueous NaOAc at room temperature with KCNO, 2-chloroethyl isocyanate, ethyl isothiocyanate, and phenyl isothiocyanate, respectively, gave good yields of **15**, **16**, **17**, and **18**. This method is currently being used to prepare similar types of compounds with long-chain carboxyalkyl groups in which the carboxy moiety might bind at the substrate site of the enzyme.

A combination of methods was used to ascertain the position of substitution in the THF molecule. The isolation of a product stable toward oxygen indicates that substitution occurred at N-5.[9] In contrast, THF and its 10-substituted derivatives are readily decomposed by oxygen. Also, nitrosation has been used to confirm the presence of an N-5 or an N-5,N-10-bridged substituent. This test is based on the observations that 5,10-methenyl-THF chloride was unreactive toward HNO_2, 5-formyl-THF consumed about an equivalent amount of HNO_2, and THF consumed an excess amount of HNO_2.[10] Presumably, the latter results from both nitrosation and oxidation of THF. Another method used to differentiate between N-5 and N-10 substituents was developed in our laboratory. Examination of the ^{1}H-NMR spectra in DMSO-d_6 showed that one pair of the phenylene protons of 10-acylfolic acids (7.6–7.7, 7.6–8.0 ppm) was considerably deshielded relative to one pair of the phenylene protons of folic acid (6.6, 7.7 ppm). Similarly, one pair of the phenylene protons of the bridged derivatives 4, 5, 6 and 5,10-methenyl-THF chloride (7.4–7.7, 7.8–7.9 ppm) in either DMSO-d_6 or D_2O was deshielded relative to THF (6.7, 7.7 ppm). In contrast, the chemical shifts of the phenylene protons of 5-formyl-THF, **8–12** and **14–18** (6.5–7.0, 7.5–7.9 ppm) were similar with those observed for THF, which provided support for the assignment of these compounds as 5-substituted THF derivatives.

Preliminary biological data indicated that none of these compounds were inhibitors of ten of the isolated folate enzymes.[11] In addition, no significant activity was observed when these compounds were tested against leukemia L1210 in mice.

ACKNOWLEDGMENTS

This investigation was supported by the Division of Cancer Treatment, National Cancer Institute, National Institutes of Health, Department of Health, Education, and Welfare, Contract NO1-CM-43762.

REFERENCES

1. Blair, J. A. and Pearson, A. J. (1974) J. Chem. Soc. Perkin Trans. II, 80–88.

2. Zakrzewski, S. F. (1966) J. Biol. Chem., 241, 2957–2961, 2962–2967.

3. Blair, J. A. and Saunders, K. J. (1971) Anal. Biochem., 41, 332–337.

4. Slavik, K. and Slavikova, V. (1969) Acta Univ. Carolinae, Med., Monogr., 37, 1–157.

5. Kallen, R. G. and Jencks, W. P. (1966) J. Biol. Chem., 241, 5851–5863.

6. Viscontini, M. and Bieri, J. (1972) Helv. Chim. Acta, 55, 21–31.

7. Bardos, T. J., Venkateswaran, P. S. and Kalman, T. I. (1968) 155th Am. Chem. Soc. Mtg., Abstract N64.

8. Ho, P. P. K., Scrimgeour, K. B. and Huennekens, F. M. (1960) J. Am. Chem. Soc., 82, 5957–5958.

9. Gupta, V. A. and Huennekens, F. M. (1967) Biochemistry, 6, 2168–2177.

10. Cosulich, D. B., Roth, B., Smith, J. M., Jr., Hultquist, M. E. and Parker, R. P. (1952) J. Am. Chem. Soc., 74, 3252–3263.

11. Mangum, J. H., unpublished results.

FOLATE ENZYMES IN MOUSE L-CELLS AS INFLUENCED BY AN EXTRA SUPPLY OF METHIONINE, FOLATE OR VITAMIN B12 IN THE CULTURE MEDIUM

Małgorzata Balińska and Barbara Grzelakowska-Sztabert

Department of Cellular Biochemistry, Nencki Institute of Experimental Biology, Polish Academy of Sciences, 02-093 Warsaw (Poland)

ABSTRACT

The effects of enriching the culture medium with methionine, folate or vitamin B12 on the activity in L-cells of seven folate-related enzymes and some dehydrogenases not involved in folate metabolism, are presented. Methionine was found to inhibit not only the activity of methionine synthetase which catalyse methylation of homocysteine to methionine, but also the activity of methylene-tetrahydrofolate reductase involved in the formation of methyl-tetrahydrofolate. In contrast, this amino acid stimulated the activity of serine hydroxymethyltransferase. The greatest effect of folate or vitamin B12 supplementation was found in the case of methionine synthetase and serine hydroxymethyltransferase.

INTRODUCTION

Regulation of the activity of key enzymes for interconversion of one carbon units within the folate pool by some amino acids or vitamin is fairly well documented in bacteria and fungi, but not in mammalian cells in culture except data for methionine synthetase[1-3] or dihydrofolate reductase[4]. Therefore, we checked the activity of seven folate-related enzymes in L-cells, after their prolonged cultivation in the presence of extra amounts of folate or of two compounds closely related to one carbon unit metabolism — vitamin B12 or methionine. To get more insight into the overall metabolism of cells grown under such conditions, we tested the values of their mitotic indices, measured the rate of incorporation of radioactive precursors into proteins and DNA, and determined the activity of some dehydrogenases, chosen as indicators of shugar metabolism.

MATERIALS AND METHODS

Growth of cells and preparations of extracts. Mouse L-cells were grown in Eagle medium as described previously[5]. In a number of experimental series, they were also grown in the above medium supplemented with extra amounts of methionine, folate or vitamin B12 (cyano form) at final concentrations of 2.2 x 10^{-3}M, 5 x 10^{-6}M and 7.7 x 10^{-6}M, respectively.

Approximately 48 hrs after subculturing, the cells were washed with PBS and harvested, as described elsewhere[3,5]. The pellet of cells was resuspended in an appropriate buffer, disrupted by sonication (3 times for 15 sec. in an MSE-ultrasonic), centrifuged at 20,000 g for 20 min and the supernatant was used for enzymatic assays.

Enzyme assays. The activity of the following enzymes was estimated by standard methods: dihydrofolate reductase (1.5.1.4)[5,6], serine hydroxymethyltransferase (2.1.2.1)[6], methylenetetrahydrofolate dehydrogenase (1.5.1.5)[6], formyltetrahydrofolate synthetase (6.3.4.3)[7], thymidylate synthetase (2.1.1.b)[8], vitamin B12 dependent methionine synthetase (2.1.1.13)[2], methylenetetrahydrofolate reductase (1.1.1.68)[9], lactate dehydrogenase (1.1.1.27)[10], glucose-6-phosphate dehydrogenase (1.1.1.49)[11] and isocitrate dehydrogenase (1.1.1.42)[12].

Protein content was determined by the method of Lowry et al.[13].

Incorporation experiments. For incorporation experiments, the cells washed out of the medium were suspended in PBS and incubated for 20 min. at 37°C with [^{14}C]leucine (1 μCi) or [^{3}H]thymidine (2 μCi). After incubation the cells were processed for estimation of protein and DNA contents[13,14] as well as for their radioactivity.

RESULTS

Effects of the extra supply of methionine, folate or vitamin B12 on the activity of folate-related enzymes in L-cells. As shown in Fig. 1, each of the compounds tested produced an increase in the activity of serine hydroxymethyltransferase; it was especially high in cells grown in the presence of extra amounts of methionine or vitamin B12 plus folate. Three other folate-related enzymes (Fig. 1) always exhibited lower activity in the cells grown in methionine-rich medium and higher activity in those grown in the media rich in folate and vitamin B12 (in comparison with the cells cultivated under the control conditions). Comparison of the relative changes in the activity of these enzymes shows that methionine synthetase is the enzyme which responds most to the components of the culture medium. Increase in the activity of methionine synthetase, under the influence of vitamin B12, was at least partly connected with the increase in its apoenzyme content, whereas the decrease in this enzyme activity, shown in cells grown in the presence of extra amounts of methionine, paralleled a decrease in the holoenzyme content only (Table 1).

Methionine and folate, when present in the incubation mixture, inhibited, to a greater or lesser degree, the activity of methionine synthetase, serine hydroxymethyltransferase and methylenetetrahydrofolate reductase (Fig. 2). Under the same experimental conditions, vitamin B12 affected neither the activity of serine hydroxymethyltransferase nor that of methylenetetrahydrofolate reductase but stimulated considerably the activity of methionine synthetase (Fig. 2).

None of the compounds used to supplement the culture medium had any evident effect on the activity, in L-cells, of dihydrofolate reductase, formyltetrahydrofolate synthetase or thymidylate synthetase.

Some metabolic aspects in L-cells of the extra supply of methionine, folate and vitamin B12. L-cells grown in all the enriched media incorporated radioactive leucine into acid-insoluble proteins more effectively (20-50 %) than those grown in the standard medium. On the other hand the rate of thymidine incorporation into DNA rose (by 60%) only in the cells grown in the medium enriched in folate plus vitamin B12. These data correspond to the biological observation that the cells grown either in the folate- or vitamin B12-rich media are characterized by the highest values of mitotic indices.

The activity of isocitrate and glucose-6-phosphate dehydrogenases did not change regardless of whether the cells were grown in the standard or the experimental media. Lactate dehydrogenase was the only enzyme whose activity was greater (by 50%) in cells grown in a methionine-rich medium.

In conclusion: in L-cells, under the influence of compounds used to enrich the medium, only the activity of the enzymes involved in the formation of folate derivatives indispensable for serine-glycine interconversion and methionine biosynthesis, was considerably affected. The stimulating effect of methionine and folate on serine

288

hydroxymethyltransferase seems to be a rather indirect one, in view
of their marginal effect on enzymic activity if present in the
incubation mixture. On the other hand, methionine and vitamin B12
seem to affect methionine synthetase directly partly in relation
to the proportional changes in the content of the apo- and holoform
of this enzyme.

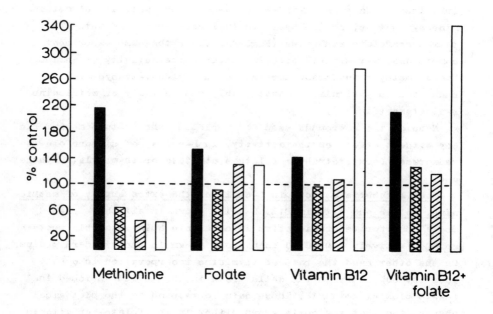

Fig. 1. Activity of serine hydroxymethyltransferase (■), methylenetetrahydrofolate dehydrogenase (⊗) and reductase (⊘), as well as
methionine synthetase (☐) in cells grown in the experimental media
containing extra amount of methionine, folate or vitamin B12.
    The activity is expressed as a percentage of that found in the
cells grown in the standard medium. The standard Eagle medium con-
tains methionine at 2×10^{-4}M, folate at 2.5×10^{-6}M and only traces
of vitamin B12 (10^{-11}M). In cells grown in the standard medium, the
specific activity of these enzymes, expressed as nmoles/mg protein/h
was as follows: serine hydroxymethyltransferase - 640, methylenetetrahydrofolate dehydrogenase - 105, methylenetetrahydrofolate
reductase - 0.25, methionine synthetase - 0.60.

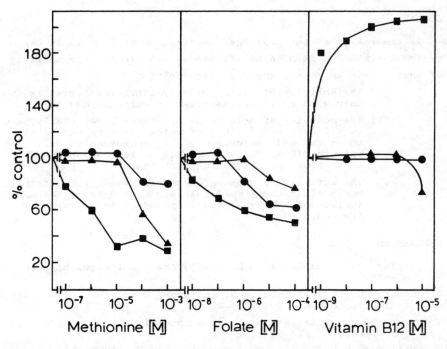

Fig. 2. Concentration effects of methionine, folate and vitamin B12,
when added to the incubation mixture, on the activity of serine
hydroxymethyltransferase (●), methylenetetrahydrofolate reductase
(▲) and methionine synthetase (■).

TABLE 1

HOLO- AND APOENZYME ACTIVITY OF METHIONINE SYNTHETASE IN L-CELLS
GROWN IN THE STANDARD AND IN THE EXPERIMENTAL MEDIA

Estimation of holo- and apoenzyme activity as described by Mangum
and North[15].

Medium	Activity (nmoles of methionine/mg protein/h)		
	Total	Holoenzyme	Apoenzyme
Standard	1.8	1.0	0.8
+ vitamin B12	5.0	1.2	3.8
+ methionine	0.8	0.2	0.6

SUMMARY

As the result of the prolonged cultivation of L-cells in Eagle medium enriched in methionine, folate or vitamin B12 the activity of some folate enzymes changes considerably:

(1) The activity of serine hydroxymethyltransferase is increased in the cells grown in enriched media.

(2) The activity of methionine synthetase, especially, and to a lesser extent that of methylenetetrahydrofolate reductase and dehydrogenase, is increased in cells from vitamin B12 or folate-enriched media and decreased in those from the methionine-rich one.

(3) The activity of dihydrofolate reductase, formyltetra-hydrofolate and thymidylate synthetase is not markedly influenced by any of the compounds used to supplement the medium.

REFERENCES

1. Taylor, R.T. and Hanna, M.L. (1975) Arch. Biochem. Biophys.,171, 507-520.

2. Kamely, D., Littlefield, J.W. and Erbe, R.W. (1973) Proc. Nat. Acad. Sci., U.S.A., 70, 2585-2589.

3. Grzelakowska-Sztabert, B. and Landman-Balińska, M. (1976) Biochem Soc. Trans., 4, 922-925.

4. Hillcoat, B.L., Swett, V. and Bertino, J.R. (1967) Biochim. Biophys. Acta, 293, 281-284.

5. Zielińska, Z.M., Grzelakowska-Sztabert, B., Koziorowska, J. and Manteuffel-Cymborowska, M. (1974) Int. J. Biochem., 5, 173-182.

6. Scrimgeour, K.G. and Huennekens, F.M. (1966) in Handbuch der Physiologisch und Pathologisch-Chemische Analyse, Springer Verlag, Berlin, 6B, 181-208.

7. Shejbal, J., Slavik, K. and Souček, J. (1962) Colln. Czech. Chem. Commun. Engl. Edn , 27, 1470-1475.

8. Roberts, D.W. (1966) Biochemistry, 5, 3546-3548.

9. Mudd, S.M., Uhlendorf, B.W., Freeman, J.M., Finkelstein, J.D. and Shih, V.E. (1972) Biochem. Biophys. Res. Commun., 46, 905-912.

10. Bergmeyer, H.U. and Bernt, E. (1974) in Methods of Enzymatic Analysis, Bergmeyer, H.U., ed., Verlag Chemie Weinheim, Academic Press, New York, London, Vol. 2, 574-583.

11. Löhr, G.W. and Waller, H.D. (1974) ibidem, 636-643.

12. Bernt, E. and Bergmeyer, H.U. (1974) ibidem, 624-631.

13. Lowry, O.H., Rosebrough, N.J., Farr, A.L. and Randall, K.J. (1951) J. Biol. Chem., 193, 265-275.

14. Burton, K. (1956) Biochem. J., 62, 315-323.

15. Mangum, J.K. and North, J.A. (1968) Biochem. Biophys. Res. Commun., 32, 105-110.

FOLATE SYNTHESIS IN NEUROSPORA CRASSA: CHANGES IN POLYGLUTAMATE LABELLING
ASSOCIATED WITH MEDIA COMPOSITION

EDWIN A. COSSINS and PATRICK Y. CHAN
Department of Botany, University of Alberta, Edmonton, Alberta, Canada, T6G 2E9

ABSTRACT

Neurospora crassa, wild type (FGSC 853) was cultured in a defined medium lacking
amino acids. By late exponential growth (22 h) the mycelium contained 0.86 ng
PteGlu equivalents mg dry wt.. This value was 1.7 ng when the medium contained
1 mM glycine but only 0.16 ng when 5 mM L-methionine was added. Tritiated p-aminobenzoate (p-ABA) was rapidly incorporated into the polyglutamyl folate pool of all
cultures. Glycine supplements increased this incorporation but L-methionine reduced
labelling by up to 90%. This latter inhibition was not observed in D-methionine-
supplemented cultures. In the absence of amino acid supplements the folates were
hexa- (ca 80%) and pentaglutamyl (ca 15%) derivatives. Glycine altered this distribution with the appearance of labelled heptaglutamates (ca 24%). In contrast,
L-methionine decreased hexaglutamate labelling but tritium was not detected in hepta-
or pentaglutamates. Methionine also inhibited incorporation of p-ABA into the
folates of a met-6 mutant which lacks folylpolyglutamate synthetase.

INTRODUCTION

There is growing evidence that glycine[1] and methionine[2] can modulate the folate
metabolism of Neurospora crassa. For example, glycine supplements increase the
levels of conjugated folate, elevate the specific activities of key folate-dependent
enzymes and stimulate flow of glycine carbon into typical products of C_1 metabolism[1].
In contrast, methionine reduces methylfolate synthesis by favoring the feedback
inhibition of $5,10-CH_2H_4PteGlu$ reductase by AdoMet[3]. In addition the activation of
cystathionine synthase by $5-CH_3H_4PteGlu_n$ is seen[2] as an important mechanism for
ensuring methionine synthesis when this amino acid is not available in the growth
medium. Clearly both glycine and methionine appear to modify polyglutamyl folate
concentrations in N. crassa. This possibility has now been examined in more detail
using the wild type and a methionine auxotroph lacking folylpolyglutamate synthetase.

MATERIALS AND METHODS

The Lindegren A, wild type (FGSC 853), an ethionine resistant mutant, eth-1
(FGSC 1212), a methionine auxotroph, met-6 (FGSC 1330) and a formate mutant, for
(FGSC 9) were maintained and cultured in defined media[1]. In some cases these media

Abbreviations: p-ABA = p-aminobenzoate; AdoMet = S-adenosylmethionine; Folates are
designated in accordance with IUPAC - IUB recommendations.

were supplemented with 1 mM glycine or with 1-5 mM L-methionine. At time intervals
samples of the growing mycelium were removed for folate analysis using *Lactobacillus
casei*[1]. In p-ABA feeding experiments, 20 μCi of [U-^{3}H]-p-ABA (0.1 μmole) were added
to each culture at spore inoculation. Extracted folates were either a) separated in
native form using DEAE-cellulose[4]; b) treated with conjugase[5] and then fractionated[6]
or c) oxidized to p-ABA-Glu$_n$ derivatives using permanganate[7]. Authentic p-ABAGlu$_5$
and p-ABAGlu$_7$ were kindly provided by Dr. Charles Baugh, Department of Biochemistry,
University of South Alabama. A p-ABA-requiring strain of *Saccharomyces cerevisiae*
was kindly supplied by Dr. John Scott, Trinity College, Dublin for biological synthesis of p-ABAGlu$_6$.

RESULTS AND DISCUSSION

After 22 h culture the wild type contained 0.86 ng PteGlu equivalents/mg dry wt.
of mycelium. Of this, 0.68 ng represented polyglutamyl folates. For cultures receiving 1 mM glycine the corresponding figures were 1.7 and 1.26 ng respectively.
Supplements of 1,3 and 5 mM L-methionine gave total folate levels of 0.42, 0.28 and
0.16 ng respectively. Growth of these cultures was not inhibited and polyglutamyl
derivatives represented 79-81% of each total. When [^{3}H]-p-ABA was supplied at spore
inoculation radioactivity accumulated in the mycelial folates as a function of growth
time. Glycine-supplemented cultures incorporated more ^{3}H (16,500 cpm/mg dry wt.)
than unsupplemented (14,000 cpm) or 5 mM L-methionine-supplemented (1,500 cpm)
cultures.

When folate extracts were chromatographed (Fig. 1) it was clear that ^{3}H entered
mono- and polyglutamyl folates. Glycine increased this incorporation, particular-
ily in the case of polyglutamyl folates (Fig. 1, fractions 90-110 and 120-140).
Other chromatographic analyses showed that 10-HCO- and 5-HCOH$_4$PteGlu were the
principal derivatives labelled with lesser amounts of ^{3}H (ca 40% of total) being
associated with methylfolates. The polyglutamyl chain lengths of these folates were
also examined after oxidation to p-ABAGlu$_n$ derivatives. Chromatography showed that
over 80% of polyglutamyl labelling was associated with hexaglutamates when mycelia
were grown on unsupplemented medium. The effect of various supplements on this
labelling pattern is summarized in Table 1. In all cases hexaglutamates were the
major forms labelled. However glycine gave labelling of a distinct heptaglutamate
peak. D-methionine did not alter polyglutamate labelling or total incorporation of
p-ABA. Labelling of mono-, di-, and triglutamates was too low to allow detection in
all of the extracts examined.

In other studies the glycine effect on folate labelling was examined in a formate-
requiring mutant (*for*, C-24, FGSC 9). This mutant lacks ability to cleave glycine
and is partially deficient in serine hydroxymethyltransferase[1]. Like the wild type,
this mutant incorporated [^{3}H]-p-ABA into folates and oxidation showed these to be

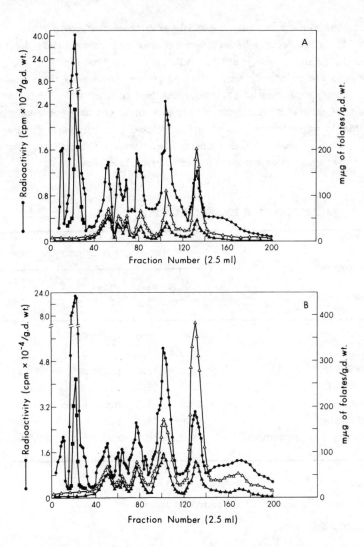

Fig. 1. DEAE-cellulose chromatography of labelled folates. Extracts were prepared after 22 h growth in (A) unsupplemented medium and (B) in media supplemented with 1 mM glycine. In both cases, 20 μCi of [U-³H]p-ABA were added at spore inoculation. Chromatography[4] was followed by conjugase treatment of individual fractions. Folates were assayed with *L. casei* before (▲) and after (Δ) such treatments. Radioactivities of native folates (●) and authentic [³H]p-ABA (■) were determined by scintillation counting.

principally hexaglutamates. Glycine supplements increased growth rates and folate labelling but heptaglutamates were not detected. Conceivably the latter have importance in glycine cleavage and it would be of some interest to examine the polyglutamate specificity of this enzyme. It is perhaps noteworthy that exogenous glycine stimulates the flow of [2-^{14}C]glycine into methionine[1] and that $CH_3H_4PteGlu_7$ activates the pathway of homocysteine synthesis in *N. crassa*. The cleavage reaction is inducible in many microorganisms[8] and it follows that exogenous glycine will enhance $CH_2H_4PteGlu$ production in such species. However the effectors for stimulating folate synthesis under·these conditions are still unknown.

TABLE 1

EFFECT OF MEDIA SUPPLEMENTS ON POLYGLUTAMYL CHAIN LENGTHS

Media supplement	^{3}H distribution in polyglutamates				
	Glu_5 %	Glu_6 %	Glu_7 %	Glu_n [a] %	$Total$ [b]
None	14.6	80.0	n.d.	5.6	12.2
1 mM glycine	n.d.[c]	56.0	24.0	20.0	18.5
1 mM L-methionine	n.d.	78.0	n.d.	22.0	4.1
5 mM L-methionine	n.d.	75.0	n.d.	25.0	2.0
1 mM D-methionine	13.0	80.3	n.d.	6.7	11.7
1 mM L-ethionine	1.6	78.4	n.d.	20.0	5.9
1 mM glycine + 1 mM L-methionine	9.2	84.0	n.d.	6.8	9.4

[a]Derivatives with 8 or more glutamyl residues.

[b]Total ^{3}H (cpmx10^{-3}/mg d. wt.) recovered in folates

[c]Labelling not detected.

As noted earlier, methionine supplements, by elevating AdoMet levels will curtail $CH_3H_4PteGlu_n$ production[2,3]. In further experiments (Table 2) both methionine and AdoMet accumulations were observed and these tended to increase with methionine supplementation of the medium. In the wild type these accumulations were accompanied by a progressive decrease in folate labelling. However there was no clear correlation in the two mutant strains. Both mutants contained more methionine and AdoMet than the wild type when methionine was either witheld (eth-1) or was growth limiting (met-6). In such cases folate labelling was less than 50% of the wild type. Additional methionine increased growth but folate labelling was lower on a dry wt of mycelium basis. In the eth-1 mutant this decrease included the polyglutamyl folates but these were lacking in met-6. The methionine mutant contained formyl and methyl monoglutamates, in agreement with earlier data[9]. Both types of folylmonoglutamates contained less ^{3}H as exogenous methionine was raised from 0.5 to 1.5 mM.

TABLE 2

METHIONINE SUPPLEMENTS AND FOLATE LABELLING: WILD TYPE, ETHIONINE RESISTANT AND MET-6 STRAINS.

Strain	L-methionine added	Total soluble pools (nmole/mg d.wt.)		Growth[a]	Folate labelling[b]
	(mM)	Methionine	AdoMet		
Wild type	none	0.13	1.4	137	14,000
	1	3.3	3.2	135	5,800
	3	7.5	5.8	140	3,400
	5	12.0	12.0	148	1,500
eth-resistant	none	7.7	3.2	100	4,100
	1	20.4	3.1	180	1,772
	3	32.0	6.3	200	1,100
	5	57.0	6.0	194	1,194
met-6	0.5	41	6.3	140	5,400
	1.0	47	6.0	183	1,900
	1.5	62	6.8	220	2,010
	3.0	90	12.0	180	2,800

[a]At 18 hr, expressed as mg d. wt/100 ml.

[b]Total ^{3}H incorporated into folate at 18 hr, expressed as cpm/mg d. wt.

The data for methionine-supplemented cultures cannot be interpreted solely on the basis of a feedback inhibition of $CH_2H_4PteGlu$ reductase. A single control of the reductase would lead instead, to an accumulation of formyl and unsubstituted folates. These folates, together with $CH_3H_4PteGlu_n$ derivatives, were present in much lower concentrations when growth occurred in the presence of exogenous L-methionine. Furthermore, the decrease in total folate pool size was as high as 80% in some cases which also argues against a selective regulation of those folates needed for the *de novo* synthesis of methionine. It should be emphasized that methionine, even at 5 mM, did not decrease growth so it is unlikely that the cultures were physiological-ly deficient in folates.

A possible explanation for these effects is that methionine or its metabolic products affected the production or turnover of folates not directly required for C_1 metabolism. Such derivatives could exist in a storage pool. If this suggestion is correct, folate turnover in unsupplemented and methionine-supplemented cultures should be significantly different. These possibilities are now being examined in the wild type and in methionine auxotrophs that lack polyglutamyl folates.

ACKNOWLEDGEMENTS

The authors thank Dr. Charles Baugh for kindly providing standard p-ABAGlu$_n$ derivatives. Dr. John Scott's helpful suggestions regarding biological synthesis of p-ABAGlu$_6$ are also acknowledged with thanks. The work was supported by a grant to the senior author from the National Research Council of Canada.

REFERENCES

1. Cossins, E.A., Chan, P.Y. and Combepine, G. (1976) Biochem. J. <u>160</u>, 305-314.

2. Selhub, J., Savin, M.A. Sakami, W., and Flavin, M. (1971)
    Proc. Nat. Acad. Sci. <u>68</u>, 312-314.

3. Burton, E.G., and Metzenberg, R.L. (1975)
    Arch. Biochem. Biophys. <u>168</u>, 219-229.

4. Chan, C., Shin, Y.S., and Stokstad, E.L.R. (1973) Can. J. Biochem. <u>51</u>, 1617-1623.

5. Roos, A.J., and Cossins, E.A. (1971) Biochem. J. <u>125</u>, 17-26.

6. Sotobayashi, H., Rosen, F. and Nichol, C.A. (1966) Biochemistry, <u>5</u>, 3878-3883.

7. Bassett, R., Weir, D.G. and Scott, J.M. (1976) J. Gen. Microbiol. <u>93</u>, 169-172.

8. Kikuchi, G. (1973) Mol.Cell. Biochemistry <u>1</u>, 169-187.

9. Selhub, J., Burton, E., and Sakami, W. (1969) Fed. Proc. <u>28</u>, 352.

FOLATE AND COBALAMIN INTERRELATIONSHIPS IN MOUSE LEUKEMIA L1210 CELLS

KATSUHIKO FUJII
Department of Biochemistry, Scripps Clinic & Research Foundation, La Jolla, CA 92037

ABSTRACT

The interrelationship between folates and cobalamins was investigated with mouse leukemia L1210 cells grown in a serum-free medium supplemented with albumin. Under these conditions, the cells grew well on folate, 5-methyltetrahydrofolate, or 5-formyltetrahydrofolate. In the absence of cobalamins, suppressed cell growth was observed only when 5-methyltetrahydrofolate was used as a folate source. This could be corrected fully by supplementation of the medium with 4 nM free cobalamin or 0.003 nM cobalamin bound to transcobalamin-II.

INTRODUCTION

Mammalian cells possess a cobalamin-dependent enzyme, 5-methyltetrahydrofolate: homocysteine methyltransferase (E.C. 2.1.1.13), which converts 5-methyltetrahydrofolate (the major serum folate) into tetrahydrofolate (Equation 1).

$$5\text{-Methyltetrahydrofolate} + \text{homocysteine} \longrightarrow \text{tetrahydrofolate} + \text{methionine} \quad (1)$$

Tetrahydrofolate is a cofactor for purine and pyrimidine biosynthesis and is essential for cell replication[1]. A second function of the enzyme is the formation of methionine. As a consequence of these two biosynthetic processes, cultured cells should require cobalamin if (a) methionine is replaced by homocysteine or (b) 5-methyltetrahydrofolate is used as the folate source.

It has been extremely difficult to demonstrate experimentally a clear-cut requirement for cobalamin in the replication of mammalian cells. This is due, primarily, to the fact that these cells are generally grown in the presence of whole serum. The amounts of endogenous cobalamins and their carrier protein, transcobalamin-II (TC-II) in serum are more than sufficient to support replication, and *added* cobalamin or TC-II thus has no demonstrable effect. This is in contrast to the readily demonstrated requirement for most other B-vitamins in the replication of eukaryotic cells or the requirement for cobalamin in the replication of certain bacterial cells. In these latter instances, no accessory proteins are required for uptake of the vitamins.

The present study was undertaken to define a set of experimental conditions under which an absolute requirement for cobalamin in the proliferation of mouse leukemia L1210 cells could be demonstrated *in vitro*. In the course of this investigation, the cobalamin requirement was found to be related to the form of folate supplied in the medium.

GROWTH OF CELLS

Mouse leukemia L1210 cells were adapted to grow and maintained routinely in a folic acid- and cyanocobalamin-free RPMI 1640 medium supplemented with bovine serum albumin (7 mg/ml) and 5-methyltetrahydrofolate (10 μM). Penicillin (100 units/ml) and streptomycin (50 μg/ml) were also present. This medium was developed via a series of experiments described in the following sections.

REPLACEMENT OF WHOLE SERUM BY SERUM ALBUMIN

The presence of 5-10% fetal calf serum or human serum in the medium is sufficient for optimal proliferation of L1210 cells, and the generation time of 11 to 12 hours is approximately equal to the cell division time *in vivo*[2]. Although multiple factors in the serum are required for growth of mammalian cells[3], it has been shown previously that certain cells can be cultured in serum albumin rather than whole serum[4]. For L1210 cells, optimal growth on albumin is achieved at a concentration of 7 mg/ml (Fig. 1).

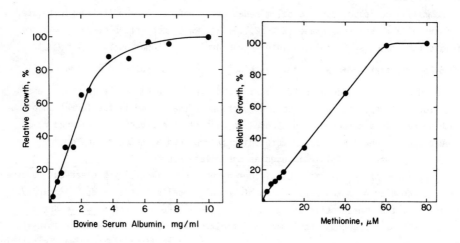

Fig. 1. Replacement of serum by bovine serum albumin.

Fig. 2. Requirement for methionine.

REQUIREMENT FOR METHIONINE AND FOLATE COMPOUNDS

To establish conditions under which the cobalamin requirement for cell replication was dependent on tetrahydrofolate formation and independent of methionine biosynthesis, the optimal concentration of this amino acid was determined (Fig. 2). Since growth was optimal at 6×10^{-5} M, the amount of methionine ordinarily supplied in RPMI 1640 medium (1×10^{-4} M) was sufficient. At this concentration of methionine, L1210 cells continued to proliferate if 5-formyltetrahydrofolate or folate was added to the medium (Fig. 3, upper curve). The generation time remained constant at 11 to 12 hours during more than 8 months of serial propagation of the cells in the presence or absence of cobalamins. In contrast, when 5-methyltetrahydrofolate was used as the folate source, cell division was gradually retarded in the absence of cobalamins·and, after 2 months of serial transfer, the generation time had increased to *ca.* 35 hours (Fig. 3, lowest curve).

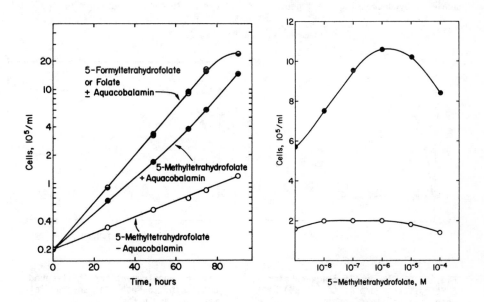

Fig. 3. (Left) Requirements for folate compounds and aquacobalamin. Lower curve, 5-methyltetrahydrofolate (10 μM) minus aquacobalamin (o——o); middle curve, ditto plus 10 nM aquacobalamin (●——●); upper curve, 5-formyltetrahydrofolate (1 μM) minus aquacobalamin (o——o) or plus 10 nM aquacobalamin (●——●). When folic acid (100 μM) was used, data similar to those for 5-formyltetrahydrofolate were obtained.

Fig. 4. (Right) Concentration dependence of 5-methyltetrahydrofolate in the presence and absence of aquacobalamin. Aquacobalamin, 10 nM (●——●); No aquacobalamin (o——o).

REQUIREMENT FOR AQUACOBALAMIN AND TRANSCOBALAMIN-II

The diminished cell replication with 5-methyltetrahydrofolate was corrected dramatically by the addition of aquacobalamin to the medium (Fig. 3, middle curve). Although the initial growth rate was slower than that with folate or 5-formyltetrahydrofolate, a nearly identical rate was achieved after a few divisions. Growth of the cells in the presence and absence of aquacobalamin is depicted in Fig. 4 as a function of the 5-methyltetrahydrofolate concentration. In the presence of aquacobalamin, optimal growth was obtained at 10^{-6} M 5-methyltetrahydrofolate.

The concentration dependence for aquacobalamin in supporting the growth of L1210 cells is shown in Fig. 5. Optimal growth was attained at 4 nM aquacobalamin; the concentration for half-maximal growth was 0.7 nM. Similar results were obtained with cyanocobalamin. In 3 days, replication in the presence of aquacobalamin was 6.3-fold greater than in its absence. Even more dramatic stimulation could be achieved by decreasing the inoculum density and prolonging the culture period.

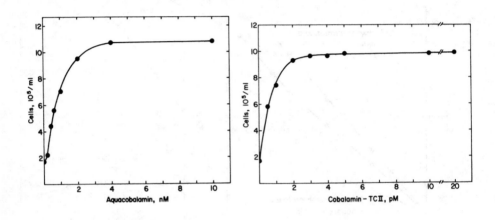

Fig. 5. Requirement for aquacobalamin. 5-Methyltetrahydrofolate (10 µM) was used as a folate source.

Fig. 6. Requirement for TC-II-bound cobalamin. 5-Methyltetrahydrofolate was used as in Fig. 5.

It was somewhat surprising to find that L1210 cells could utilize aquacobalamin in the apparent absence of TC-II, since uptake of the vitamin by mammalian cells is thought to be dependent upon this protein. To investigate this point, TC-II was purified from human serum via the procedure summarized in Table I. The 6000-fold purified preparation contained apo- and holo-TC-II in a ratio of 2:1, and its molecular weight was 39,000 (as judged by chromatography on Sephadex G-150). When this preparation was examined in an experiment similar to that shown in Fig. 5, maximal cell growth was achieved at a cobalamin-TC-II concentration of 0.003 nM (Fig. 6). The concentration for half-maximal growth was 0.0005 nM, or less than 1/1000 of that required when the free cobalamin is used.

TABLE I

PURIFICATION OF TRANSCOBALAMIN-II FROM POOLED HUMAN SERUM

Step	Volume	Protein	Cobalamin Content[a]		Cobalamin Binding Capacity[b]	
			Specific	Total	Specific	Total
	ml	*mg*	*ng/mg protein*	*ng*	*ng/mg protein*	*ng*
Human serum	2,470	188,000	0.0157	2,960	---	--
Supernatant of pH 5.4 treatment	2,590	183,000	0.0155	2,840	0.0102	1,860
First CM-cellulose	238	345	2.48	854	4.78	1,650
Second CM-cellulose	24	181	4.27	773	8.95	1,620
Sephadex G-150	21	17.2	33.0	567	62.2	1,070

[a] Cobalamin was assayed by a radioisotope dilution method[5].

[b] Unsaturated cobalamin-binding capacity was measured by the method of Puutula and Gräsbeck[6].

DISCUSSION

The present study has demonstrated that replacement of whole serum by albumin provides an ideal system for studying the biochemical interrelationship between cobalamin and folates in mouse leukemia L1210 cells. These cells can grow on 5-formyltetrahydrofolate, 5-methyltetrahydrofolate, and folate (each at different optimal concentrations). Growth is absolutely dependent upon the addition of cobalamin to the medium only when 5-methyltetrahydrofolate is used as the folate source. These results confirm that 5-methyltetrahydrofolate is converted into the coenzyme, tetrahydrofolate, via the cobalamin-dependent methyltetrahydrofolate:homocysteine methyltransferase. The present *in vitro* demonstration of the relationship between cobalamin and folates is consistent with the "methyl trap" hypothesis, which has been deduced mainly from *in vivo* considerations.

A requirement for cobalamin and TC-II, although small in magnitude, has also been reported for L5178Y cells[7]. In view of the present results, it seems likely that the growth medium used by these earlier investigators contained slightly less than the maximal amounts of TC-II and cobalamin needed for replication of L5178Y cells. Whole serum, even when dialyzed, ordinarily contains an excess of these components (see Table I), and it is necessary to use a reconstructed system in order to demonstrate an appreciable cobalamin or TC-II requirement.

Replacement of whole serum by albumin eliminates most, if not all, of the TC-II normally provided by the former. The high levels of free cobalamin (4 nM) required

302

for optimal growth of L1210 cells indicate that apo-TC-II is essentially absent from the albumin preparations, since the association constant[8] of TC-II for cobalamin is *ca.* 10^{11} M^{-1}. Transport of *free* cobalamin into the cells may have occurred via passive diffusion, pinocytosis of a protein-cobalamin complex (using an unspecified cobalamin binder with a relatively low affinity for free cobalamins), or induction of the synthesis of apo-TC-II by high levels of extracellular cobalamin.

ACKNOWLEDGMENTS

The author is indebted to Karin Vitols for advice in the preparation of the manuscript and to Mei Cheng for technical help. This work was supported by grants from the National Institutes of Health (CA 6522, CA 16600, and AM 07097) and from the American Cancer Society (CH-31). K.F. was a recipient of a fellowship from the California Division, American Cancer Society.

REFERENCES

1. Huennekens, F.M. (1968) in Biological Oxidations, Singer, T.P. ed., Interscience, New York, pp. 439-513.
2. Dixon, G.J., Dulmadge, E.A. and Schabel, F.M., Jr. (1966) Cancer Chemotherapy Rep., 50, 247-254.
3. Gospodarowicz, D. and Moran, J.S. (1976) Annu. Rev. Biochem., 45, 531-558.
4. Spieker-Polet, H. and Polet, H. (1976) J. Biol. Chem., 251, 987-992.
5. Ceska, M. and Lundkvist, U. (1971) Clin. Chim. Acta, 32, 339-354.
6. Puutula, L. and Gräsbeck, R. (1972) Biochim. Biophys. Acta, 263, 734-746.
7. Chello, P.L. and Bertino, J.R. (1973) Cancer Res., 33, 1898-1904
8. Hippe, E. and Olesen, H. (1971) Biochim. Biophys. Acta, 243, 83-89.

CULTURE CYCLE DEPENDENCE OF FOLATE DISTRIBUTION IN HUMAN CELLS

J.G. HILTON, B.A. COOPER, AND D.S. ROSENBLATT
Department of Physiology and Division of Haematology, Royal
Victoria Hospital; MRC Genetics Group and Department of Pediat-
rics, McGill University, Montreal, Quebec, Canada

INTRODUCTION

We have observed that human fibroblasts cultured <u>in vitro</u> accumulated folate and converted it to folate coenzymes, in both polyglutamate and monoglutamate forms[1]. The intracellular folate concentration in these cultured cells approached but did not equal or
exceed that of the PteGlu in the culture medium. PteGlu represented only a minority of the intracellular folate. The majority of
the intracellular folate is $5\text{-}CH_3\text{-}H_4PteGlu$ in both monoglutamate
and polyglutamate forms[2,3]. During folate deprivation, intracellular polyglutamates disappeared from the cell by first order
kinetics with a $T\frac{1}{2}$ of approximately 3.5 days. We have observed
that cells cultured in logarithmic growth accumulated more folate
than did cells cultured at confluence. We have also noted that a
small proportion of the folate associated with the cultured cells
after incubation with PteGlu entered a second incubation medium
rapidly, suggesting that there was a compartment of exchangeable
folate associated with the cells. This report describes some of
the characteristics of the exchangeable folate pool, and compares
the intracellular polyglutamate and monoglutamate folates in cells
exposed to PteGlu at different stages of the culture cycle.

MATERIALS AND METHODS

Human fibroblasts were cultured in Eagles minimum essential
medium with nonessential amino acids and the indicated concentrations of PteGlu[1,2,3]. Intracellular folate was fractionated on
Sephadex G-25 after extraction in 0.05M potassium phosphate, pH
9.2, followed by sonication, boiling, centrifugation, and filtration of the extract through Sephadex without freezing or storage.
All solutions contained 10 mM mercaptoethanol. Radioactivity was
determined with standard techniques utilizing internal standards,
and microbiological activity was determined with three standard
assay organisms: Lactobacillus casei, ATCC 7469, Steptococcus
fecalis, ATCC 8043, and Pediococcus cerevisiae, ATCC 8081. Cells
were counted in a Coulter counter, and protein was determined by
the method of Lowry[4].

RESULTS

When fibroblasts at confluence were incubated for 24 hours in [3]H (3',5'9) PteGlu, rinsed four times in situ with ice cold saline, and then incubated in fresh, folate-free medium at 37 deg., label was observed to enter the second incubation medium with a T$\frac{1}{2}$ of 5 min. Media obtained from cells incubated in different concentrations of PteGlu ranging from 1-50 uM, were pooled to provide sufficient radioactivity to allow fractionation of the exchangeable folate on Sephadex G-25 (Fig. 1). These folates consisted of polyglutamate folate (tubes 5-9), monoglutamate folate other than PteGlu (tubes 10-14) and PteGlu (tubes 17-23)[1]. The relationship between the concentration of PteGlu in which the cells were incubated, and the quantity of 'exchangeable folate' associated with the cells was complex, but could represent the sum of two hyperbolic curves saturating at 10^{-9}M and 10^{-5}M PteGlu. Exchangeable folate represented approximately 2% of the total folate associated with the cells.

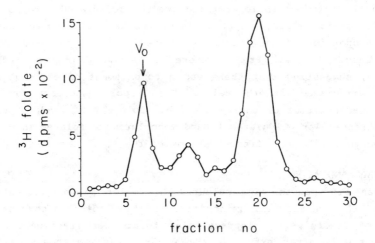

Fig. 1. Folate forms in 'exchangeable folate'. Second incubation medium was filtered through Sephadex G-25. Fractions appearing are polyglutamate folate, monoglutamate other than PteGlu, and PteGlu[1].

Fibroblasts were subcultured at low cell density into petri dishes, and at daily intervals replicates were exposed to 10^{-7}M [3]H PteGlu for 24 h. The non-exchangeable intracellular folate accumulated during 24 h at different days of the culture cycle was extracted, and fractionated on Sephadex G-25 (Fig. 2). It was apparent that as the cells entered logarithmic growth during the first days after subculture, the total quantity of folate accumulated over 24 h of incubation was greatest. Both polyglutamate and monoglutamate folate were greater after 24 h of incubation in cells in logarithmic growth than in confluent cells. PteGlu associated with the cells remained constant throughout the culture cycle.

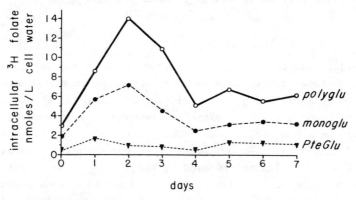

Fig. 2. Effect of the culture cycle on accumulation of folate over 24 h of incubation in 10^{-7}M PteGlu.

When fibroblasts in late logarithmic growth were incubated in different concentrations of PteGlu for 24 h, intracellular folate was proportional to the PteGlu concentration in which the cells were cultured. A similar relationship was observed with confluent cells grown in different concentrations of PteGlu. At all concentrations of PteGlu, logarithmic cells contained more folate than confluent cells. In cells grown in less than 10^{-7}M PteGlu, the ratio of polyglutamate:monoglutamate folate in the logarithmic cells was similar to that in confluent cells. (Table 1). In cells grown in higher PteGlu concentrations, the polyglutamate:monoglutamate ratio was significantly greater in confluent than in logarithmically growing cells (p = .004). In logarithmically growing cells, the proportion of intracellular folate which was polyglutamate was not altered by the PteGlu concentration in which the cells were cultured (r=.303, p = 0.2), whereas in confluent cells grown in more than 10^{-7}M PteGlu, the proportion of intracellular folate which was polyglutamate was greater than in similar cells grown in lower PteGlu concentrations (r = .872, p =.0004).

TABLE I

POLYGLUTAMATE:MONOGLUTAMATE RATIO IN FIBROBLASTS GROWN IN DIFFER-
ENT CONCENTRATIONS OF PTEGLU

PteGlu concentration in medium (M)

	4×10^{-5}	2×10^{-5}	4×10^{-6}	2×10^{-6}	5×10^{-7}	8×10^{-8}	1×10^{-8}	1×10^{-9}
confluent	6.76	9.45	8.99	5.91	3.14*	1.22	1.42	1.33
log-		3.22	2.06	1.44	1.47	1.59	1.15	2.56	2.01

* PteGlu concentration in medium (M) was 2.2×10^{-7}

DISCUSSION

These data indicate that a small proportion of the folate associated with human fibroblasts cultured in vitro in PteGlu was exchangeable with the medium after rinsing of the cells in situ with
cold saline, and that this folate is composed of PteGlu as well as
polyglutamate and monoglutamate folate other than PteGlu. Some of
the PteGlu in this fraction might have been loosely associated
with cell surfaces and not removed by the in situ rinses, but this
would be an improbable source for the non-PteGlu monoglutamates
and for the polyglutamate folates. The 'exchangeable' folate
represented only about 2% of the total folate associated with the
cells, and the non-PteGlu folates only about one half of this. It
was not possible to exclude leakage of intracellular contents into
the medium from damaged cells as a source of the non-PteGlu folates, although the reproducibility of the levels found, and the
relationship observed between PteGlu in the medium and 'exchangeable' folate concentration makes this improbable as the sole
source of this folate. The rate of entry of folate into a folate-
free second incubation medium exceeded considerably the rate of
diffusion reported for $5\text{-CH}_3\text{-H}_4\text{PteGlu}$[5],[6], and of polyglutamate
folate[5] from human erythrocyte ghosts.

If some of the folate associated with cells was exchangeable,
it suggests that non-exchangeable folate was different from exchangeable folate. One may postulate that this difference might
have been related to intracellular binding of folate, either by
enzymes, or by binders lacking enzyme activity. Such binding of
intracellular folate has been reported in liver cells[7],[8]. The
increased intracellular concentration of folate in growing fibroblasts incubated for 24 h in PteGlu over that seen in in confluent
cells, might be explained by increased intracellular folate bind-

ers in growing cells. Of the folate enzymes of fibroblasts which increase during logarithmic growth[9], dihydrofolate reductase might be considered a candidate for explaining the greater accumulation of intracellular folate by growing cells. The failure of intracellular PteGlu itself to increase in growing cells despite the increase in polyglutamate and other monoglutamate folate would suggest that dihydrofolate reductase might not be the only intracellular binder responsible.

The distribution of polyglutamate and monoglutamate (other than PteGlu) folate was relatively constant in most cells. In confluent cells at high external PteGlu concentrations, a larger proportion of intracellular folate was polyglutamate than in confluent cells at low external PteGlu concentrations or in logarithmic cells at all external PteGlu concentrations. We have observed that the lowest PteGlu concentration which supports optimal growth in fibroblasts in vitro is $5 \times 10^{-8}M$, and it was of interest that increased polyglutamate synthesis in confluent cells appeared to begin at about this concentration ($10^{-7}M$ and greater). It is possible that this additional polyglutamate synthesis represents storage of excess folate by the cell, whereas the proportion of polyglutamate observed in cells in logarithmic growth and in confluent cells grown in inadequate folate might represent the distribution of these folate coenzyme forms most effective for cell metabolism. In other studies, evidence of turnover of the polyglutamate pool of folate in these cells was observed[1].

SUMMARY

Human fibroblasts accumulated folates, including PteGlu, other monoglutamates, and polyglutamates. A small portion of this intracellular folate was rapidly exchangeable with the medium, and may have represented unbound intracellular folate which rapidly crossed the cell membrane. Even when incubated in PteGlu concentrations inadequate for growth, confluent cells accumulated both polyglutamates and monoglutamates after 24 hours. At higher PteGlu concentrations, the proportion of intracellular folate which was polyglutamate increased. In cells in logarithmic growth, this excess polyglutamate formation at high concentrations of PteGlu was not observed. At all PteGlu concentrations, the absolute level of intracellular folate was higher in logarithmic cells than in confluent cells.

ACKNOWLEDGEMENTS

We are grateful to S. Lue-Shing, N. Vera Matiaszuk and A. Pottier for technical assistant, to C.M. Baugh for his kind gift of PteGlu$_5$, to B. Stewart for assistance in preparation of the manuscript, and to the Medical Research Council of Canada for support through grant MT 802 and through the Genetics Group grant.

J.G. Hilton is in receipt of Studentships from the Collip Bequest to McGill University and the Conseil de la Recherche en Santé du Québec; B.A. Cooper is a Medical Research Associate of the Medical Research Council of Canada.

REFERENCES

1. Hilton, J.G., Cooper, B.A. and Rosenblatt, D.S.   Folate polyglutamate synthesis and turnover in cultured human fibroblasts. To be published.

2. Cooper, B.A. and Rosenblatt, D.S. (1976) Folate coenzyme forms in fibroblasts from patients deficient in 5,10 methylene tetrahydrofolate reductase, Biochemical Society Transactions 4, 921-922.

3. Rosenblatt, D.S. et al.   Folate distribution in cultured human cells: Studies on 5,10-CH2H4PteGlu reductase deficiency, to be published.

4. Lowry, O.H. et al. (1951)   Protein measurement with Folin phenol reagent, Journal of Biological Chemistry 193, 265-275.

5. Cooper, B.A. and Peyman, J. Folate leakage from human erythrocyte ghosts, to be published.

6. Branda, et al. (1978)   Folate-induced remission in aplastic anemia with familial defect of cellular uptake, N.E.J.M. 298, 469-475.

7. Zamierowski, M. and Wagner, C. (1974)   High molecular weight complexes of folic acid in mammalian tissues, Biochim. Biophys. Res. Comm. 60, 81-87.

8. Wagner, C. and Suzuki, N. (1978)   Purification and characterization of a folate binding protein from rat liver, Fed. Proc. 37, 1344.

9. Rosenblatt, D.S. and Erbe, R.W. (1973)   Reciprocal changes in the levels of functionally related folate enzymes during the culture cycle in human fibroblasts, Biochim. Biophys. Res. Comm. 54, 1627-1633.

10 Hoffman, R.M. and Erbe, R.W. (1974)   Regulation of folates in proliferating and quiescent human fibroblasts. Journal of Cell Biology 63, 141a.

FOLATE POLYGLUTAMATE AND FOLATE ENZYMES, INCLUDING A FOLYL POLYGLUTAMATE CLEAVAGE
ENZYME, AS BACTERIOPHAGE T4D BASEPLATE STRUCTURAL COMPONENTS

L.M. KOZLOFF, M. LUTE and L.K. CROSBY
Department of Microbiology and Immunology, University of Colorado Medical School,
Denver, Colorado 80262

ABSTRACT

The location of the 6 molecules of bacteriophage T4D-induced dihydropteroyl hexa-
glutamate on the hexagonal viral tail baseplate has been defined. The pteridine
portion lies under or near the T4D gene product 11 (gP11) and close to the tail plate
dihydrofolate reductase and thymidylate synthetase while the glutamate residues lie
under or near the attachment portion of the long tail fiber (gP34). These results
support the view that this viral-induced folic acid plays a role in linking together
the multicomponents of the viral baseplate and does not act as in its usual role as
a coenzyme. It has also been found that the viral-induced gP28 is involved in the
biosynthesis of the viral folate compound. This gene product has cleavage activity
on large folyl polyglutamate substrates containing 12-14 glutamate residues but not
on smaller folyl polyglutamates. This cleavage enzyme has also been shown to be a
structural component of the viral baseplate and to be located on the distal portion
of the baseplate central plug.

INTRODUCTION

We reported in 1965 that an unusual form of folic acid was a constituent of the
tail structure of the *Escherichia coli* T-even bacterial viruses[1]. Later analyses[2,3]
and reconstitution experiments[4,5] identified this compound as a dihydropteroyl hexa-
glutamate and showed that it was a constituent of viral tail baseplate. Recent
studies have dealt with three aspects of this problem. 1) What protein(s) bound
this folate to the tail structure? 2) How was the synthesis of this compound both
induced and regulated in the infected cells? 3) What role did this compound play
either in virus assembly or in DNA injection into the host cell? Work on these
problems led to the discovery in 1970 that the phage-induced dihydrofolate reductase[6]
was a baseplate component and in 1973 Mathews and his colleagues[7] reported that the
phage-induced thymidylate synthetase was also a viral component. These observations
led to a series of experiments confirming that both viral enzymes are tailplate
components. While the role of these two enzymes in either viral assembly or DNA
injection is not settled, it is known that the catalytic activities of these two
enzymes are not essential for them to fulfill their structural role. Attention has
centered on their exact location on the complex baseplate. This has been possible
because the variety of phage mutants available allows the use of structural probes

on both incomplete virus particles and viral substructures.

This paper deals briefly with the location of the dihydrofolate reductase and thymidylate synthetase[8,9], but is mainly concerned with location of the folate poly-glutamate on the baseplate and its biosynthesis in the infected cell. It has been found that the viral-induced gP28 is not only a specific enzyme for cleaving large folyl polyglutamates but also is a viral baseplate structural component.

MATERIALS AND METHODS

Standard methods for preparing and assaying bacteriophage stocks, various mutants and incomplete particles were used[2-6]. A method was devised to isolate the large folyl polyglutamates (containing ^{3}H-glutamate) which accumulate in *Escherichi coli* B infected with T4D 28am based on the procedures developed by Baugh *et al.*[10] and used also by Nakamura *et al.*[3] A method for measuring the release of ^{3}H-glu from this substrate was also developed using a modification of the radioactive assay described by Krumdieck *et al.*[11]

RESULTS

Location of the viral-induced folate, dihydrofolate reductase and thymidylate synthetase on the T4D tail baseplate. When the T4 morphogenetic sequence was worked out[12,13] it became possible to look at the specific location of the components of the viral folic acid on the baseplate using a variety of analytical probes. These results are summarized in Fig. 1. Fig. 2 is an amplification of the distal view of the baseplate structure taken from Crowther *et al.*[12] giving the location of some of the T4D gene products such as gP11, gP12 and gP9 on this structure. It has been found that the final baseplate is formed from a central plug (involving T4D gene products 29, 28, 26, 71, 27 and 5) and 6 "wedge-like" outer structures (involving T4D gene products 10, 11, 7, 8, 6, 53 and 25) while gP9 and gP12 are added later to the

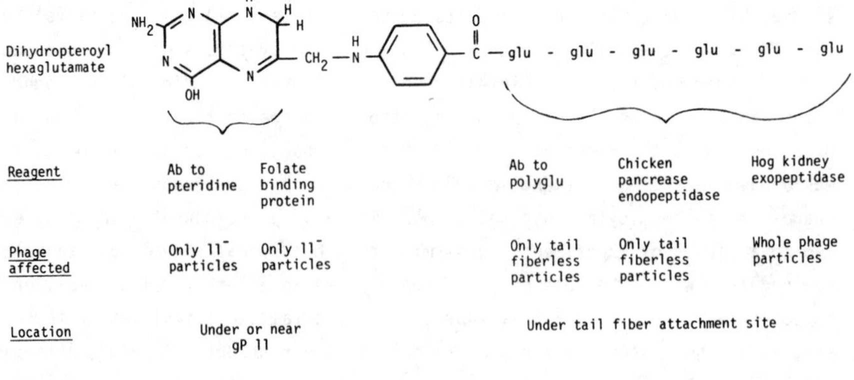

Reagent	Ab to pteridine	Folate binding protein	Ab to polyglu	Chicken pancrease endopeptidase	Hog kidney exopeptidase
Phage affected	Only 11⁻ particles	Only 11⁻ particles	Only tail fiberless particles	Only tail fiberless particles	Whole phage particles
Location		Under or near gP 11		Under tail fiber attachment site	

Fig. 1. Location of folate constituents on the baseplate of T4D bacteriophage.

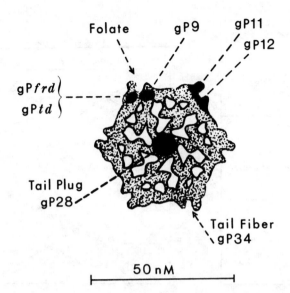

Fig. 2. Location of various baseplate components. These components are indicated on the hexagonal form of the baseplate. The diagram is from Crowther et al.[12] who originally located gP9, gP11, and gP12.

baseplate[13]. The locations of the folate components are indicated as well as some of the folate enzymes. While it has been known that the pteridine moiety was only exposed in 11⁻ particles, the exposure of the polyglutamate portion has only recently been observed in particles lacking the long tail fibers. Tail-fiberless particles cannot be activated by tail fibers in the presence of either antibody to polyglutamate or to highly purified γ-glutamyl endopeptidase from chicken pancreas. This unique location near the apex of the corners of the baseplate suggests that the polyglutamate portion plays a role in providing the flexible linkage between the long tail fiber and the baseplate.

Both the dihydrofolate reductase (frd) and thymidylate synthetase (td) of the tail baseplate are also located under or near gP11. It is known that they structurally interact, and that they are near the folate[11]. It has been proposed that a folate pteridine moiety is actually shared between or bound to both these enzymes.[9]

Function and location of T4D gP28. Early work showed that host cells infected with a T4D gene 28 amber mutant were deficient in pteroyl hexaglutamates. Analysis of the folyl polyglutamate compounds in these cells revealed that up to seven percent of the folate had accumulated as an unexpected large folyl polyglutamate containing possibly 12-14 glutamate residues[3]. Since cleavage enzymes are known to be necessary both for cleaving viral protein precursors and, in quite a different context, for cleaving folyl polyglutamate compounds the possibility was examined that the T4D gene 28 was a folyl polyglutamate cleavage enzyme. Initial biological results in crude extracts were encouraging[5], however no cleavage activity could be detected using substrates such as ^{14}C-labeled tri- or heptaglutamate compounds. Therefore, the large folyl polyglutamates from T4D 28am infected cells were labeled

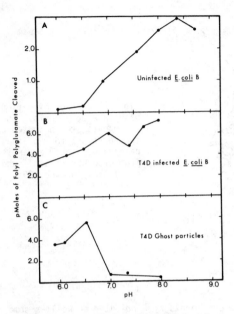

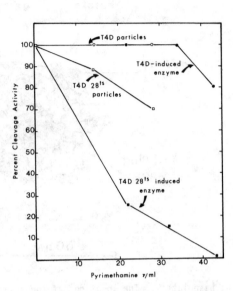

Fig. 3. Effect of pH on the folyl polyglutamate cleavage activity of (A)
extracts from uninfected *E. coli* B or
(B) T4D-infected *E. coli*; and (C)
highly purified T4D bacteriophage
ghost particles.

Fig. 4. Effect of pyrimethamine on the
folyl polyglutamate cleavage activity
of T4D and T4D 28ts ghost particles
and on the cleavage activity of the
enzymes induced by these phages in
E. coli B.

with ^{3}H-glu and isolated, and used as a substrate. At a substrate concentration of
only 2-3 x 10^{-7} M, enzymatic cleavage activity was found in extracts of both uninfected cells, T4D-infected cells and, surprisingly, in highly purified phage
particles. pH activity curves are shown in Fig. 3. Extracts of uninfected *E. coli* B
showed a single activity peak at about pH 8.4-8.5; cells infected with T4D had two
activity peaks, one at pH 8.0 or higher and an additional peak at pH 6.5-7.0. Phage
particles had only one peak of cleavage activity at pH 6.5. These results indicate
that T4D infection induced the formation of new enzyme with a pH optimum of 6.5 and
that this enzyme was incorporated into the phage structure.

A survey was made of the ability of various T4D amber mutants involved in baseplate assembly[13] to induce this acidic cleavage activity upon infection of the non-
permissive host cell. The T4D strains examined under restrictive conditions in
addition to wild-type were 10am, 29am, 26am, 27am, 51am, 28am and 28^{ts}; all induced
the formation of this enzyme except the two 28 mutants. The properties of T4D 28^{ts},
a phage temperature sensitive mutant, indicate that the gP28 was not only a cleavage
enzyme for folyl polyglutamates, but was also a viral baseplate constituent. For
example, it was found that changes in gP28 altered the heat lability of the virus
particle, the adsorption rate and the host range. These are all properties expected

of a baseplate protein. Further, it was found that T4D 28^{ts} phage plaque formation on *E. coli* B at 25° was inhibited by sulfadiazine and by pyrimethamine, a folate analogue, while wild-type T4D plaque formation was unaffected by both these compounds. The effect of pyrimethanime on the folyl polyglutamate cleavage activity of T4D wild-type particles and T4D-induced enzyme obtained from extracts as compared to these activities in T4D 28^{ts} system is shown in Fig. 4. The enzyme induced by the 28^{ts} virus in both particles and extracts was inhibited while the enzyme activity induced by wild-type phage was unaffected. In addition, it has been found that antiserum, prepared against highly purified baseplates, at a dilution of 1:150 inhibited 90% of the cleavage activity of T4D particles. A tentative location of the gP28 product on the central plug of the baseplate is shown in Fig. 2.

DISCUSSION AND SUMMARY

The relationship between folyl polyglutamate metabolism and T4 bacteriophage baseplate assembly is outlined on this page. There are a number of unexpected features which relate to viral-induced enzymes, baseplate components and the role of these elements in forming the complex baseplate. For example, the formation of dihydro-

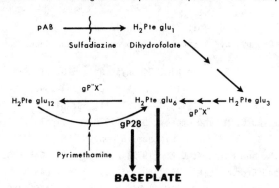

pteroyl hexaglutamate in infected cells is carefully regulated. Presumably host enzymes are used to form the tri-glutamate but some as yet unidentified viral-induced protein (gP"X") catalyzes the addition of more glutamates to the tri-glutamate to form the hexa-glutamate and possibly the same enzyme, in one or more steps, is responsible for the formation of the very large folyl polyglutamates. However, the genetic strategy of the viral genome includes the induction of a cleavage enzyme (gP28) which not only acts enzymatically on this large folyl polyglutamate, but also participates in forming the baseplate tail plug as a structural component. Even after assembly the enzymatic cleavage site is left exposed. It seems possible that this structural feature might offer some advantage to the virus particle in recognizing a pattern of carboxyl groups on the host cell surface.

It is also apparent that sulfa drugs and an inhibitor of the cleavage enzyme such as pyrimethamine will act together to lower the concentration of the hexa form and prevent baseplate assembly. Preliminary evidence indicates that the products of T4D genes 29 and 27, both structural components of the baseplate might also be responsible for the activities indicated as gP"X" in aiding the synthesis of the phage folate compound. These observations support the conclusion that this folate molecule plays a structural role in forming this part of the virus particle and does not participate in the catalytic events characteristic of those involved in either protein or DNA synthesis pathways. On the other hand, this non-enzymatic role for the folate does not rule out the possibility that the catalytic sites of the 3 folate enzymes are critical both for assembly or for DNA injection. In this connection, it should be emphasized that the baseplate is a "meta-stable" structure[13] which undergoes a radical change in conformation to form a central hole which permits the release of the viral DNA. These enzymes are likely elements for initiating these conformational changes.

ACKNOWLEDGEMENTS

This work was supported by Public Health Service Research Grant AI 06336 from the National Institute of Allergy and Infectious Diseases. We wish to thank Dr. Charles M. Baugh for the ^{14}C-labeled folates containing 3 glutamate residues and 7 glutamate residues, Dr. J. Burchall for the sample of pyrimethamine, and Dr. J. King for permission to use some of the material in Fig. 2.

REFERENCES

1. Kozloff, L.M. and Lute, M. (1965) J. Mol. Biol. 12, 780-792.
2. Kozloff, L.M., Lute, M., Crosby, L.K., Rao, N., Chapman, V.A. and DeLong, S.S. (1970) J. Virol. 5, 726-739.
3. Nakamura, K. and Kozloff, L.M. (1978) Biochim. Biophys. Acta 540, 313-319.
4. Kozloff, L.M., Lute, M. and Crosby, L.K. (1970) J. Virol. 6, 754-759.
5. Kozloff, L.M., Lute, M. and Baugh, C. (1973) J. Virol. 11, 637-641.
6. Kozloff, L.M., Verses, C., Lute, M. and Crosby, L.K. (1970) J. Virol. 7, 740-753.
7. Capco, G.R. and Mathews, C.K. (1973) Arch. Biochem. Biophys. 158, 736-743.
8. Mosher, R.A., DiRenzo, A.B. and Mathews, C.K. (1977) J. Virol. 23, 645-658.
9. Kozloff, L.M., Lute, M. and Crosby, L.K. (1977) J. Virol. 23, 637-644.
10. Baugh, C.M., Braverman, E. and Nair, M.G. (1974) Biochemistry 13, 4952-4957.
11. Krumdieck, C.L. and Baugh, C.M. (1970) Analy. Biochem. 35, 123-129.
12. Crowther, R.A., Lenk, E.V., Kikuchi, Y. and King, J. (1977) J. Mol. Biol. 116, 489-523.
13. Kikuchi, Y. and King, J. (1975) J. Mol. Biol. 99, 695-716.

THE METHYLTETRAHYDROFOLATE POOL IS SEPARATE FROM THE TETRAHYDROFOLATE POOL

J. PERRY, M. LUMB, J. VAN DER WESTHUYZEN, F. FERNANDES-COSTA, J. METZ AND
I. CHANARIN

M.R.C. Clinical Research Centre, Harrow, U.K. and South African Institute for
Medical Research, Johannesburg, South Africa

SUMMARY

$[G-^3H]5CH_3H_4PteGlu$ and $[2-^{14}C]H_4PteGlu$ were given intraperitoneally to the
normal fruit bat (<u>Rousettus aegypticus</u>). Both compounds were taken up rapidly
by the liver, but subsequent metabolism of each differed. Whereas $[2-^{14}C]H_4PteGlu$
was incorporated mainly into polyglutamyl folate, the greater proportion of
injected $[G-3H]H_5CH_3H_4PteGlu$ remained unconjugated, and its activity declined
steadily over 96 hours. Isotope uptake by the brain tissue was confined to
$[G-3H]5CH_3H_4PteGlu$ only. These results demonstrate the presence of two pools
of folate activity, not a single pool as previously supposed.

INTRODUCTION

The metabolism of folate coenzymes has previously been studied in the context
of a single pool of compounds where the biologically active forms are derived
from $H_4PteGlu$ and are metabolically interdependent. Nixon et al[1] indicated
that mammalian cells transferred over 80% of the methyl group of $5CH_3H_4PteGlu$
within 5 minutes of entry into the cell, and within an hour 80% of the
$H_4PteGlu$ had taken up a fresh methyl group. This study was undertaken to
determine the utilization of $[2-^{14}C]H_4PteGlu$ and $[G-3H]5CH_3H_4PteGlu$ given
simultaneously to mammals. The South African fruit bat was selected as
experimental animal as profound vitamin B_{12} deficiency can be produced readily
in this species.

MATERIALS AND METHODS

$[G-3H]5CH_3H_4PteGlu$ was prepared and purified from $[G-3H]5CHOH_4PteGlu$
(Amersham, 1·1 Ci/mmole) as previously described[2,3]. $[2-^{14}C]H_4PteGlu$ was
synthesized by Davis's technique[4] from $[2-14C]PteGlu$ (Amersham, 59 mCi/mmole) and
$5CH_3[2-^{14}C]H_4PteGlu$ via reduction of $[2-^{14}C]H_4PteGlu$ followed by conversion to
$[2-^{14}C]5,10,CHH_4PteGlu[5]$. Further reduction of this latter compound with $NaBH_4$
gave $5CH_3[2-^{14}C]H_4PteGlu$. The combined radiofolates were injected I.P., the
dose concentration being 0.4 μCi $[2-^{14}C]H_4PteGlu$ plus 1.8 μCi $[G-3H]5CH_3H_4PteGlu$,
and, for the rat experiments, 0.3 μCi $5CH_3[2-14C]H_4PteGlu$ plus 1.9 μCi
$[G-3H]5CH_3H_4PteGlu$. Tissues were prepared for radioactive counting, column
chromatography and microbiological assay by methods described fully elsewhere[6].

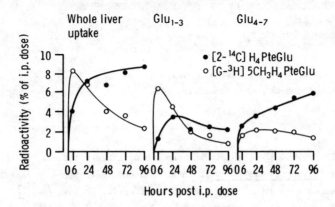

Fig. 1. The incorporation of [G-3H]5CH₃H₄PteGlu and [2-¹⁴C]H₄PteGlu into whole liver, and short and long chain folates.

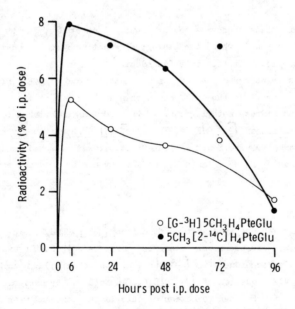

Fig. 2. The incorporation of [G-3H]5CH₃H₄PteGlu and 5CH₃[2-¹⁴C]H₄PteGlu into rat liver.

RESULTS

The incorporation of $[G-3H]5CH_3H_4PteGlu$ and $[2-^{14}C]H_4PteGlu$ into whole liver over the 96 hour period studied is shown in Fig. 1. The initial uptake of tritiated methyl folate was greater than that of $[2-^{14}C]H_4PteGlu$ being 8.4% of the dose given, compared with 4.2% for the $H_4PteGlu$ (p = <.0025). Methyl-folate activity then declines until at 96 hours the percentage dose retained by the liver is 2.46. The concentration of $H_4PteGlu$ increases, however, from its relatively low level of incorporation at 6 hours, rising to a maximum of 8.8% at 96 hours.

To determine whether this difference in incorporation was due to a mechanism such as an isotopic exchange of tritium which was not affecting the stability of the ^{14}C labelling, normal rats were injected I.P. with $[G-^3H]5CH_2$ $[2-^{14}C]H_4PteGlu$, and the incorporation of the double-labelled compound into liver followed during the same time period (Fig. 2). Both the ^{14}C and 3H activity followed the same pattern as that found for the tritium compound used in the bat experiments. The concentrations of both isotopes declined from a peak at 6 hours, showing that the decline in bat liver tritium activity was not due to isotopic variation but was a physiological process.

Column chromatography of bat liver extracts showed further differences between

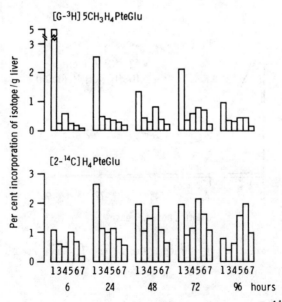

Fig. 3. Incorporation with time of $[G-3H]5CH_3H_4PteGlu$ and $[2-^{14}C]H_4PteGlu$ into folates of glutamyl chain length 1-7.

the two compounds (Fig. 3). Less of the 5CH$_3$H$_4$PteGlu was incorporated into the longer chain forms than H$_4$PteGlu and this monoglutamate activity declined with time. Polyglutamate formed from methylH$_4$folate remained almost constant with some progressive conversion up to 72 hours into penta-, hexa- and heptaglutamyl folates. This pattern of progressive incorporation with time of the isotope into longer chain forms was also seen with [2-14C]H$_4$PteGlu. Here, although the initial uptake was slower than that of [G-^{3}H]5CH$_3$H$_4$PteGlu the incorporation of isotope into polyglutamyl folates was more rapid, and monoglutamyl ^{14}C concentrations were always lower than those in the longer chain folates.

No ^{14}C activity could be detected in brain tissue homogenates (Fig. 4). Tritium uptake was lower in the liver, the maximum value being 0.5% of the dose 6 hours following injection. Chromatography of pooled brain extracts showed nearly all the radioactive material in the monoglutamate, although at 96 hours a small amount was detectable in triglutamyl folate.

The endogenous liver folate comprised mainly methyl and formyltetrahydrofolates in the conjugated form. No unsubstituted H$_4$PteGlu could be positively identified. Endogenous brain folate differed markedly from liver. The major peak was formyl monoglutamate. No polyglutamate with a chain length longer than 5 could be detected, and microbiological assay showed the polyglutamates were methylated folate only (Fig. 5).

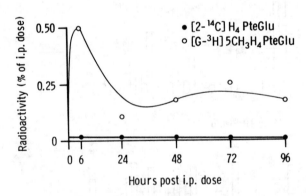

Fig. 4. The incorporation of [G-3H]5CH$_3$H$_4$PteGlu and [2-^{14}C]H$_4$PteGlu into brain.

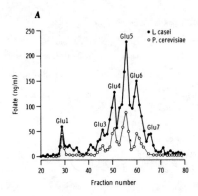
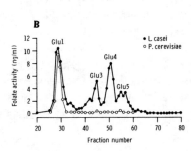

Fig. 5. Chromatographic separation on DE 52 cellulose of the endogenous folates of A) liver, B) brain.

DISCUSSION

There are significant differences in the way the 2 folate analogues are used by normal bats and there are significant differences between liver and brain. For many years it has been assumed that there is a single folate coenzyme pool transferring one-carbon units. Our data imply a methyl folate pool distinct from but presumably in equilibration with a tetrahydrofolate pool. In this respect the whole animal may behave differently from tissue cultures.

The difference in utilization of the two compounds is clearly shown when both liver and brain folate extracts are subjected to column chromatography. In liver, the greater proportion of $[G-^3H]5CH_3H_4PteGlu$ is not converted to polyglutamate, this being compatible with Spronk's[7] observation that methyl folate is not the preferred substrate for polyglutamate synthesis. A small proportion is conjugated, however, and persists in the liver over the 96 hour period. $[2-^{14}C]$ $H_4PteGlu$ is incorporated more slowly, but after 24 hours most of the ^{14}C activity is found in the long chain folates and as such is well retained.

Isotope incorporation into brain is compatible with what is known about choroid plexus transfer of folates[8]. Methyl folate can cross the blood—brain barrier[9] and this has been shown again here in bat brain. $2-^{14}C$ $H_4PteGlu$ apparently cannot enter C.S.F. as no ^{14}C activity was found, again confirming the independence of the two folate pools.

Although no estimates of folate excretion were done during this study our data are compatible with a greater catabolic rate for methylfolate than other analogues.

REFERENCES

1. Nixon, P.J. et al. (1973) J. Biol. Chem., 248, 5392-5396.
2. Perry, J. and Chanarin, I. (1973) Brit. Med. J., ii, 588-589.
3. Nixon, P.J. and Bertino, J.R. (1971) Anal. Biochem., 43, 162-172.
4. Davis, L. (1968) Anal. Biochem., 26, 459-460.
5. Rowe, P.B. (1968) Anal. Biochem., 22, 166-168.
6. Chanarin, I. et al. (1978) - To be published.
7. Spronk, A.M. (1974) Fed. Proc., 32, 471 A (abstract).
8. Spector, R. and Lorenzo, A.V. (1975) Science, 187, 540-542.
9. Chanarin, I. et al. (1974) Clin. Sci. Molec. Med., 46, 369-373.

MOLECULAR CLONING OF T4 PHAGE GENES CONTROLLING FOLATE METABOLISM

L. C. MEADE*, A. B. DIRENZO*, R. K. BESTWICK#, R. A. MOSHER*, AND C. K. MATHEWS#

*Department of Biochemistry, University of Arizona, Tucson, Arizona, and

#Department of Biochemistry and Biophysics, Oregon State University, Corvallis,

Oregon

ABSTRACT

Bacteriophage T4 is a large virus which encodes most of its own enzymes for DNA replication and DNA precursor biosynthesis. Two enzymes in the latter class, namely, dihydrofolate reductase and thymidylate synthetase, play additional roles, as yet undefined, as structural elements of the virion. This paper describes two approaches to learning more about the molecular properties of these enzymes and their biological roles. One approach involves studies of these enzymes by gel electrophoresis of labeled phage proteins, and the other involves molecular cloning of the genes coding for these enzymes.

INTRODUCTION

Bacteria infected by T-even phages, including T4, synthesize viral DNA at very high rates. In large part this is accomplished through production of virus-coded enzymes of DNA replication and DNA precursor biosynthesis. These and other factors make the T4 phage-infected bacterium an excellent system for studying the enzymology and regulation of DNA precursor biosynthesis. In turn this basic information might suggest new therapeutic approaches for the use of antimetabolites which interfere with deoxyribonucleotide production.

About ten per cent of the coding capacity of the T4 phage genome is used for production of enzymes of DNA precursor metabolism (Fig. 1). Some of these activities, such as those concerned with biosynthesis of the novel viral pyrimidine, 5-hydroxymethylcytosine, are unique to the infected cell. Others, including thymidylate synthetase and dihydrofolate reductase, augment pre-existing activities by the production of new, virus-coded enzyme molecules. Both of the latter enzymes participate in thymine nucleotide biosynthesis, as shown by physiological studies on phage mutants unable to synthesize one or the other enzyme[2]. In addition, both enzyme proteins are found in purified phage particles[3-7], evidently associated with the base-plate of the tail, which also contains a bound pteridine, dihydropteroylhexaglutamate[8].

This paper describes several approaches in our laboratory for quantitating these enzymes as structural proteins, assessing their apparent dual functions, understanding their molecular properties, and learning how the genes which encode them are expressed. One approach involves studying the synthesis, turnover, and virion

localization of dihydrofolate reductase by use of SDS-polyacrylamide gel electrophoresis and immunoprecipitation by a specific antibody. The other approach involves
amplification of the genes coding for these enzymes, using recombinant DNA methodology.

MATERIALS AND METHODS

Procedures for preparation of phage stocks, labeling of cells, purification and
assay of enzymes, and SDS-polyacrylamide slab gel electrophoresis and radioautography
were as described in previous publications from this laboratory[5,7,9].

Our approach to cloning the T4 genome used a plasmid, pBR322[10], as the cloning
vehicle. Phage DNA used in cloning was extracted from T4 dec8, a multiple mutant
which incorporates cytosine into its DNA instead of hydroxymethylcytosine, and hence
is subject to digestion by restriction endonucleases[11]. Further details of the
cloning experiments are given in Results.

RESULTS

Dihydrofolate reductase as a virion protein

Evidence supporting the idea that T4 dihydrofolate reductase is a structural protein includes the following: (1) enzyme activity can be detected in purified virion
preparations[3,7]; (2) the T4 frd gene, which codes for dihydrofolate reductase, determines a physical property of the virion, namely, heat lability[4,6]; and (3) antiserum
to homogeneous T4 dihydrofolate reductase binds to phage particles and inactivates
them, presumably by binding to the enzyme in situ[7,12]. Originally we sought to
identify and quantitate virion dihydrofolate reductase by SDS-polyacrylamide gel
electrophoresis of labeled phage proteins. We expected to see a band corresponding
to a molecular weight of 30,000, as reported for the T4 enzyme[9]. No such band was
seen, even when labeling was carried out only early in infection, when few if any
other structural proteins are being synthesized[7]. This could be because the enzyme
is present in minute amounts (fewer than five molecules per virion), or because it is
incorporated in a high-molecular-weight form, or as a lower-sized cleavage product,
or because a special class of late-synthesized enzyme molecules is used for viral
assembly. To evaluate these and other possibilities we prepared antiserum to homogeneous T4 dihydrofolate reductase and followed the synthesis and turnover of the
enzyme protein. The general approach was to label phage proteins with ^{14}C-amino
acids, extract the proteins and treat the extract with antibody, and to precipitate
the antigen-antibody complexes with goat anti-rabbit antibody. Labeled proteins in
the precipitate were then analyzed electrophoretically. Fig. 2 shows that only one
protein was specifically precipitated by this treatment and that this protein is not
present in extracts of cells infected with reductase-negative mutants. Surprisingly,
the migration rate of this band corresponds with a molecular weight of 22,000, considerably lower than that earlier determined for T4 dihydrofolate reductase and con-

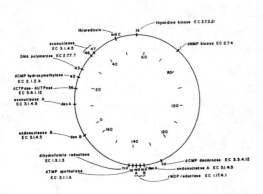

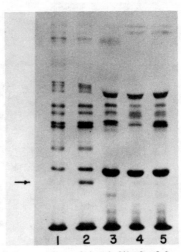

Fig. 1. Map positions on the T4 phage chromosome of genes controlling DNA precursor metabolism. The numbers in the interior represent distances in kilobase pairs from a reference point, the rllA/rllB cistron divide.

Fig. 2. Proteins reacting with T4 dihydrofolate reductase antiserum. 1, labeled T4D proteins plus serum from unimmunized rabbit; 2-5, reductase antiserum; 2, T4D proteins; 3, proteins from an amber frd mutant; 4, 5, proteins from deletion mutants affecting frd.

firmed in this study by other methods[13]. However, the purified enzyme migrates to the same position, as determined by staining of a non-radioactive gel, so it would appear that the enzyme protein has unusual physical properties.

Fig. 3 shows that the enzyme protein is synthesized only within the first ten minutes of infection, predominantly within the first five minutes. Moreover, the protein is not produced by cleavage from a higher-weight precursor, nor is it turned over or converted to a lower-molecular-weight form, as determined by a pulse-chase experiment. Therefore, several of the ideas advanced to explain our anomalous results must be discarded. However, the protein is undeniably present in T4 tails. Radioiodinated dihydrofolate reductase antiserum was prepared and incubated with phage tails. Radioactivity from the antiserum co-sedimented with T4 tails through a sucrose gradient, and binding was prevented by preincubation of the serum with purified T4 dihydrofolate reductase.

The baseplate of the tail consists of a central core, or hub, surrounded by six equivalent wedge-shaped subassemblies[14]. We prepared wedges and found that they bound to the anti-reductase antiserum, by the criteria mentioned above (Fig. 4). Thus, dihydrofolate reductase is a component of the wedge, and since there are six wedges per virion, it must be present at six or more molecules per virion. Our failure to detect the protein among the labeled components of purified tails may result from the fact that we labeled our proteins from two to six minutes after infection, whereas the bulk of the enzyme protein seems to be synthesized immediately after infection.

324

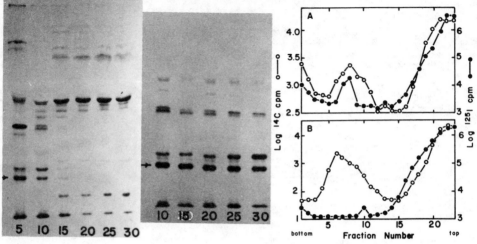

Fig. 3. A. Duration of synthesis of T4 dihydrofolate reductase. T4D-infected cultures were labeled for 5-minute intervals ending at the indicated times after infection, and analyzed as in Fig. 2. B. Absence of turnover of T4 dihydrofolate reductase. Cells were labeled from 2 to 6 minutes after infection and chased by a large excess of unlabeled amino acids. At each time aliquots were sampled and analyzed as in Fig. 2.

Fig. 4. Binding of T4 dihydrofolate reductase antibody to T4 tails. A. ^{125}I-labeled IgG was incubated with ^{14}C-labeled tails and the mixture was analyzed on a 5-20% sucrose gradient. B. Identical, except that the IgG was pre-incubated with purified dihydrofolate reductase. Same results were seen when wedges were used instead of tails.

Cloning T4 genes

It has been suggested[15] that virion dihydrofolate reductase undergoes a conformational change which accompanies the major structural transition undergone by the T4 baseplate as infection is being established; the same may be true for thymidylate synthetase. In order to study the roles of these proteins in this process and in the assembly of the baseplate, it would be desirable to be able to purify the enzymes in larger amounts than is possible with extracts of phage-infected cells prepared batchwise. Molecular cloning offers a suitable opportunity. Some of the plasmids in common use as cloning vectors are maintained in host cells at 20 to 30 copies per cell. If T4 genes cloned into such vectors were expressed, we might have at hand bacterial strains which could produce large amounts of particular phage gene products when grown in continuous culture, and hence could be used as sources for isolating these gene products. In addition, the application of rapid DNA sequencing methods to the inserted segments could yield much information about the structures of the proteins and the regulation of expression of the genes which encode them. Since the td gene, which codes for thymidylate synthetase, and the frd gene, which codes for dihydrofolate reductase, are adjacent on the T4 map (Fig. 1), one might hope to clone fragments containing both of these genes in a single insert.

Since T4 DNA contains glucosylated hydroxymethylcytosine instead of cytosine and hence cannot be degraded by restriction endonucleases, we used a multiple mutant of T4 which incorporates cytosine instead[11]. As a cloning vector we used the plasmid pBR322[10], a derivative of colE1, and for our initial cloning attempts we used the restriction enzyme PstI. The plasmid carries genes for resistance to tetracycline and to ampicillin, and there is a single PstI cleavage site, within the ampicillin resistance gene. Thus after ligation to a PstI digest of T4 DNA and transformation into a host E. coli strain bacteria which have taken up a plasmid (transformants) can be identified by their resistance to tetracycline. Those plasmids containing an inserted T4 DNA segment can be identified because they are resistant to tetracycline but sensitive to ampicillin. In addition the PstI site is close to the amp promoter, which favors the expression of any cloned genes. An additional technique was used to select specifically for any recombinant plasmids containing an active T4 td gene; we simply prepared a thymine auxotroph of our host strain, E. coli B834. The expression of the td gene within this strain would result in production of thymidylate synthetase and hence render the host strain thymine-independent.

Using Pl-EK1 conditions for containment, we incubated PstI-cleaved plasmid DNA with T4 DNA ligase and a PstI digest of cytosine-containing T4 DNA, which in turn contained about 30 discrete fragments. The ligation mixture was introduced into host bacteria by calcium-mediated transformation. Of the tetracycline-resistant colonies which arose, 23 were ampicillin-sensitive and were adjudged to have acquired an inserted T4 DNA segment. These modified plasmids were designated pLTR1, pLTR2,. . . . pLTR23, respectively. Of the 23, two were found to convert the thymine-requiring host to thymine independence, namely pLTR5 and pLTR7. These and the other plasmid-bearing strains were grown, extracted, and assayed for activity of thymidylate synthetase and dihydrofolate reductase. As shown in Table 1, both pLTR5 and pLTR7 pro-

TABLE 1

ENZYME ACTIVITIES OF PLASMID-BEARING E. COLI STRAINS

Cells were harvested for extraction in the mid-logarithmic phase of growth. Specific enzyme activities are recorded relative to an extract of T4D-infected E. coli B834 thy⁻.

E. coli strain	Dihydrofolate reductase	Thymidylate synthetase	E. coli strain	Dihydrofolate reductase	Thymidylate synthetase
T4D-infected B834	1.00	1.00	pLTR10	0.02	<0.01
B834T⁻	0.05	<0.01	pLTR12	0.05	0.21
B834T⁺	0.06	0.15	pLTR17	0.02	0.32
pBR322	0.08	<0.01	pLTR18	0.03	0.60
pLTR2	0.02	not tested	pLTR19	0.02	0.04
pLTR3	0.02	not tested	pLTR26	0.01	<0.01
pLTR5	0.13	1.56	pLTR27	0.13	<0.01
pLTR7	0.14	0.43	pLTR29	0.16	<0.01

duce elevated levels of thymidylate synthetase, comparable to what is seen in T4-infected cells. It seems virtually certain that this is the phage-coded, rather than the E. coli enzyme, because otherwise the host strains would have had to undergo two independent events -- transformation to tetracycline resistance and mutation to thymine independence -- the estimated frequency of these events occurring simultaneously is less than 10^{-11}. However, direct evidence regarding the origin of the new synthetase activity is now being sought.

Although some of the clones produce somewhat elevated levels of dihydrofolate reductase, none produces the enzyme in levels comparable to T4-infected cells. This could be because the T4 frd gene itself contains a PstI cleavage site, such that the intact frd gene could not be cloned by this approach. Currently we are preparing a new set of clones starting with an EcoRI digest of T4 DNA, and we shall ask whether any of these produce T4 dihydrofolate reductase at a high level.

SUMMARY

T4 Phage-coded dihydrofolate reductase. Using an antibody specific for this enzyme we were able to show that the protein is synthesized predominantly within the first five minutes of infection. The protein is not formed by cleavage from a high-molecular-weight precursor, nor is it turned over or converted to a smaller protein once formed. The enzyme protein is a component of the wedge substructure of the tail baseplate

Cloning T4 phage genes. A PstI restriction nuclease digest of cytosine-containing T4 DNA was ligated to PstI-cleaved plasmid pBR322 DNA. After transformation 23 plasmid-bearing clones were isolated which seem to contain inserted fragments of T4 DNA. Two of these seem to contain an active T4 td gene, i.e., they produce phage thymidylate synthetase at high levels.

ACKNOWLEDGEMENTS

Financial support for this work came from NIH Research Grant No. AI-15145. We thank Mr. Gerry Lasser and Mr. Philip Kroner for help with some of the experiments.

REFERENCES

1. Mathews, C. K. (1977) in Comprehensive Virology, Vol. 7, H. Fraenkel-Conrat and R. R. Wagner, eds., Plenum Press, New York, pp. 179-294.

2. Mathews, C. K. (1967) J. Virol. 1, 963-967.

3. Kozloff, L. M., Verses, C., Lute, M., and Crosby, L. K. (1970) J. Virol. 5, 740-753.

4. Mathews, C. K. (1971) J. Virol. 7, 531-533.

5. Capco, G. R. and Mathews, C. K. (1973) Arch. Biochem. Biophys. 158, 736-743.

6. Kozloff, L. M., Lute, M. and Crosby, L. K. (1977) J. Virol. 23, 637-644.

7. Mosher, R. A., DiRenzo, A. B. and Mathews, C. K. (1977) J. Virol. 23, 645-658.

8. Kozloff, L. M., Crosby, L. K., Rao, N., Chapman, V. A. and DeLong, S. S. (1970) J. Virol. 5, 726-739.

9. Erickson, J. S. and Mathews, C. K. (1970) Biochem.Biophys.Res.Comm. 43, 1164-1176.

FOLIC ACID METABOLISM IN MAN

ANNE E PHEASANT*, JOHN A BLAIR* and ROBERT N ALLAN†

*Department of Chemistry, University of Aston in Birmingham, UK

†General Hospital, Birmingham, UK

ABSTRACT

1. Two hospital patients receiving 60µg ^{14}C and ^{3}H labelled folic acid excreted only scission products in urine.

2. Three subjects receiving 5mg folic acid excreted predominantly 5-methyltetrahydrofolate (5MeTHF) and folic acid.

3. The ratio of folic acid:5MeTHF decreased in the presence of a malignancy.

INTRODUCTION

Past studies on the metabolism of folic acid using human volunteers have given rise to conflicting results[1-4]. The work presented here investigated the possibility that these differences reflect a dosage effect. Preliminary observations on the effect of malignant disease were also made.

METHODS

Five hospital patients, four suffering from terminal malignancies and one from hypertension with partial right hemiparesis, were given an oral dose of 2-[^{14}C], 3',5',9-[^{3}H] folic acid (60µg or 5mg folic acid). Urine was collected onto sodium ascorbate for periods of 0-6h, 6-12h and 12-24h after administration. Urine samples were sequentially chromatographed on DEAE-cellulose and Sephadex -G15[5]. Paper chromatography was performed on ethyl acetate extracts of the isolated ^{3}H metabolite using ethanol: butanol: ammonia: H_2O (10:10:1:4,V/V).

RESULTS AND DISCUSSION

Subjects receiving 60µg folic acid excreted 1.4% ^{14}C and 1.9% ^{3}H of the dose in 24h; those receiving 5mg folic acid 31.2% ^{14}C and 33.5% ^{3}H. DEAE-cellulose chromatography of the 0-6h urine samples showed that the radioactivity present in the urine from patients given the low dose separated almost completely into a ^{3}H only peak and a ^{14}C only peak indicating that the major urinary species were scission products. No folic acid was detected in the urine and little or no 5MeTHF. After the 5mg dose the major radioactive species in the

0-6h urine sample were folic acid and 5MeTHF.   Small quantities
of scission products were also detected.   The tritiated metabolite
observed co-chromatographed with p-acetamidobenzoyl-L-glutamate on
Sephadex-G15 and paper.   This scission product may be formed as a
metabolite after cleavage of the folate molecule in the gut
following biliary excretion (see previous communication).   It
elutes from DEAE-cellulose in a similar position to 10-formylfolate
and when using ^{3}H-folic acid only[1], the two metabolites may have been
confused.   The low recoveries of radioactivity in the urine after
the low dose probably indicate that this level is insufficient to
exceed the renal threshold value for the folates whereas the scission
products appear to have much lower renal threshold values, hence their
dominance of these urine samples.   This apparent variation in
urinary metabolites emphasises the importance of controlled dose
levels in this type of study.

In the case of those given 5mg folic acid the pattern of urinary
folates was compared with reference to the presence or absence of a
tumour.   A shift from folic acid in favour of 5MeTHF was observed
in the patients with malignancies.   Of the radioactivity excreted
by the control subject in 0-6h, 81% was folic acid and 10% was 5MeTHF
whereas the other subjects produced 62% folic acid, 27% 5MeTHF and
37% folic acid, 54% 5MeTHF.   When all 3 urine samples from the same
subject were studied, the pattern of metabolites remained constant
with time.   Thus, on the basis of these results, the presence of a
malignant tumour appears to cause a higher proportion of the folic
acid to be incorporated into the reduced folate pool.

REFERENCES

1.Chanarin, I. and McLean, A. (1967) Clin.Sci. 32 57-67.
2.Ratanasthien, K. (1975) PhD Thesis.   University of Aston in
  Birmingham.
3.Johns, D.G., et al.   (1961) J.Clin.Invest. 40 1684-1695.
4.Krumdieck, C.L., et al. (1978) Am.J.Clin.Nutr. 31 88-93.
5.Barford, P.A., et al. (1977) Biochem.J. 164 601-605.

PTERIDINE REGULATION OF UROPORPHYRINOGEN I SYNTHETASE ACTIVITY

WALTER N. PIPER, ROBERT B.L. van LIER AND DAVID M. HARDWICKE

Department of Pharmacology, University of California, School of Medicine, San

Francisco, California 94143

ABSTRACT

An activator has been obtained from purified uroporphyrinogen I synthetase pre-

parations by pretreatment of enzyme with 1 M KCl. This activator antagonized

[3]H-folic acid binding to a specific folate-binding protein, but failed to produce

growth of the folate requiring microorganism Lactobacillus casei (ATCC 7469) unless

pretreated with γ-glutamyl carboxypeptidase. The results indicate that a pteroyl-

polyglutamate is associated with uroporphyrinogen I synthetase, and may serve as a

coenzyme for this step of heme biosynthesis.

INTRODUCTION

The conversion of porphobilinogen (PBG) to uroporphyrinogen (uro) III is believed

to be mediated by two enzymes, uroporphyrinogen I synthetase and uroporphyrinogen III

cosynthetase .(Fig. 1). The presumed cosynthetase alone cannot form uroporphyrinogen.

However, its presence in uro I synthetase reactions enables the uro III isomer to be

formed. Published reports of increased PBG excretion during lead poisoning led us to

investigate the effect of $PbCl_2$ on uroporphyrinogen formation. Hemolysate uro I syn-

thetase was found to be inhibited by $PbCl_2$; whereas the hepatic enzyme was insensitive

to $PbCl_2$ unless dialyzed or purified[1]. The dialyzable protective factor was purified

from rat liver and characterized as a pteroylpolyglutamate derivative[2]. During

purification of rat hepatic uro I synthetase, it was discovered that the specific

activity decreased following a purification step employing DEAE cellulose-KCl gradi-

ents and ultrafiltration of the enzyme preparation. Aliquots of the ultrafiltrate

were found to restore the lost enzymatic activity. Studies were then conducted to

characterize the activator. The results of these studies are presented in this report.

330

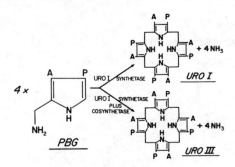

Fig. I   *Reaction scheme for uroporphyrinogen synthesis*

MATERIALS AND METHODS

Materials. Cultures of Lactobacillus casei (ATCC 7469) were purchased from the American Type Culture Collection, and the folate culture media and chick pancreas acetone powder were obtained from Difco. [3', 5' 9(n)-³H]-folic acid (63 Ci/mmole) was purchased from Amersham/Searle.

Animals. Sprague-Dawley rats (100-200 g) were purchased from Simonson Labs, Gilroy, California.

Uroporphyrinogen I synthetase purification. Enzyme was purified from rat liver as described previously[2], by employing heat treatment of hepatic cytosol (60° C for 5 min.), ammonium sulfate fractionation, DEAE cellulose chromatography with a 0-0.4 M KCl gradient, and Sephadex G-100 gel chromatography. Such enzyme preparations represented 1100-1200 fold purification from hepatic homogenates, and were stable for several weeks when stored at -20° C.

Uroporphyrinogen I synthetase assay. The activity of uro I synthetase was assayed by the method of Strand et al.[3]. Uroporphyrin was measured fluorometrically with an Aminco Bowman Spectrophotofluorometer with excitation and emission wavelengths of 405 nm and 595 nm, respectively.

Microbiological assay for folates. The microbiological assay for folate using L. casei was modified from the methods of Waters et al.[4] and Herbert[5].

Competitive protein binding assay for folates. The assay for folate by competitive protein binding was a modification of the method of Mortensen[6]. The extraction buffer step was omitted, and the reaction buffer was 0.1 M Tris-HCl, pH 9.3. The method of Rothenberg et al.[7] was used to purify the binding protein from milk. The standard was folic acid.

Preparation of γ-glutamyl carboxypeptidase (conjugase). Chick pancreas acetone powder was the enzyme source. Enzyme was isolated and endogenous folates removed by modifications of the methods of Bird et al.[8] and Mims and Laskowski[9].

Protein. The concentration of protein was determined by the method of Lowry et al.[10].

RESULTS

During purification of uro I synthetase from rat liver, it was observed that the specific activity usually decreased from 20-45 % after a step using DEAE cellulose chromatography and a 0-0.4 M KCl gradient, followed by ultrafiltration to concentrate enzyme fractions and to remove the KCl. Since we had previously discovered that a pteroylpolyglutamate protected against inhibition of uro I synthetase activity by $PbCl_2$ and also produced stimulation of uro I synthetase activity[2], we suspected that the ultrafilterable material might be a pteridine and proceeded to characterize it. The ultrafiltrate was collected, concentrated by lyophilization, dissolved in water, and aliquots tested for their effect on uro I synthetase activity after purification by DEAE cellulose chromatography using the KCl gradient. The ultrafiltrate was found to be an activator of uro I synthetase activity (Table 1).

TABLE I

Activation of Rat Hepatic Uroporphyrinogen Synthetase Activity by an Ultrafilterable Substance Released During Purification

Additions to Reaction Mixture[a]	Uro Synthetase Activity[b] (nmoles/mg protein/hr)
Enzyme	2.95 ± 0.04
Enzyme + Ultrafiltrate[c]	7.12 ± 0.12
Ultrafiltrate	0

[a]Enzyme Source: Rat hepatic uro I synthetase.

[b]Values represent the mean ± S.E.M for 3 determinations.

[c]Ultrafiltrate was obtained by concentration of enzyme (Amicon DM-5; 5000 molecular weight cut-off) following DEAE Cellulose chromatography using a 0-0.4 M KCl gradient.

TABLE 2

Loss of Uroporphyrinogen Synthetase Activity by Treatment of Enzyme with KCl and Restoration by a Dissociated Activator

Enzyme Treatment	Uro Synthetase Activity (nmoles/mg protein/hr)
Control[a]	2.72
KCl-Treated Enzyme[b]	0.30
Ultrafiltrate	0
KCl-Treated Enzyme + Ultrafiltrate	1.44

[a]Enzyme source: Rat hepatic uro I synthetase

[b]Enzyme was mixed in the presence of 1M KCl and 50 mM tris, pH 8 for 15 minutes at 5°C, followed by ultrafiltration with an Amicon DM-5 filter having a molecular weight cut-off of 5000

The ultrafiltrate did not contain any endogenous uro I synthetase activity, which indicates that enzymatic activation was not merely caused by additive quantities of enzyme.

Thus, it appeared as if salt treatment of enzyme preparations might provide a means of releasing activator for study. Therefore, aliquots of purified uro I synthetase (following Sephadex G-100 gel filtration) were subjected to treatment with 1 M KCl in 50 mM Tris-HCl buffer, pH 8 for 15 minutes at 5° C. KCl was removed from the enzyme by dialysis against 50 mM Tris-HCl, pH 8. The enzyme treated with KCl lost 90% of its activity, which could be restored to 53% of the control level by addition of the activator (Table 2).

In order to obtain evidence that the ultrafiltrate contained a pteroylglutamate, aliquots of ultrafiltrate were tested to determine whether they could produce growth of the folate-dependent microorganism L. casei (ATCC 7469) or could antagonize ^{3}H-folate-binding to a specific folate-binding protein. The ultrafiltrate failed to produce growth of the folate-dependent microorganism. However, ultrafiltrate was found to antagonize binding of ^{3}H-folic acid to the folate-binding protein as shown in Figure 2.

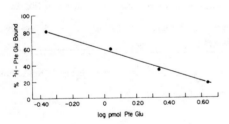

Fig. 2 **Assay of activator with a competitive protein-binding radioassay** (Values are expressed as pmol of pteroylmonoglutamate)

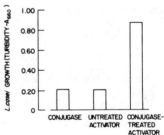

Fig. 3 Production of growth of the pteroylmonoglutamate-dependent microorganism Lactobacillus casei by pretreatment of the activator with γ-glutamyl carboxypeptidase (conjugase)

These observations indicated that the activator might be a pteroylglutamate. The folate-dependent microorganism L. casei (ATCC 7469) is known to be resistant to growth when pteroylpolyglutamates are used. However, no such discrimination between pteroylmono- or polyglutamates appears to occur in competitive protein binding radioassays employing ^{3}H-folic acid.

γ-Glutamyl carboxypeptidase enzyme preparations from chick pancreas were used in order to determine whether the folate present in the ultrafiltrate might be a pteroylpolyglutamate. Aliquots of ultrafiltrate were incubated with γ-glutamyl carboxypeptidase, boiled to inactivate the enzyme, and centrifuged. Supernatants were tested for their ability to produce growth of the folate-dependent microorganism L. casei (ATCC 7469). Treatment of ultrafiltrate with γ-glutamyl carboxypeptidase was found to produce growth of L. casei (ATCC 7469), as shown in Figure 3.

DISCUSSION

An activator of uro I synthetase is released from purified enzyme preparations following treatment with KCl. This substance antagonizes binding of ^{3}H-folic acid to a specific folate-binding protein, but fails to produce growth of the folate-dependent microorganism L. casei (ATCC 7469) unless pretreated with γ-glutamyl carboxypeptidase. These results indicate that the activator is a pteroylpolyglutamate derivative. Much additional work needs to be conducted in order to determine the role of pteridines in the regulation of uroporphyrinogen and heme synthesis. The chemical structure of the pteridine and the glutamate chain length must first be elucidated, and the kinetics of pteridine activation of uro I synthetase must be investigated. It is possible that this pteridine plays an important role in the formation of the correct physiologically active uroporphyrinogen III isomer. Recent work by Battersby et al.[11,12] and Scott et al.[13] has indicated that a C-1 transfer is involved in the mechanism of uroporphyrinogen III formation, which could be mediated by the pteroylpolyglutamate activator that we have recently discovered. Investigations are currently being conducted in order to answer these questions and elucidate how pteridines regulate uroporphyrinogen synthesis and the production of heme. Knowledge acquired on the mechanism of uroporphyrinogen synthesis will contribute to our understanding of lead poisoning and the genetic diseases characterized by alterations of heme biosynthesis, the porphyrias.

ACKNOWLEDGEMENTS

This research was supported by National Institutes of Health Grant ES-01343.

REFERENCES

1. Piper, W.N. and Tephly, T.R. (1974) Life Sci., 14, 873-876.

2. Piper, W.N. and van Lier, R.B.L. (1977) Mol. Pharmacol., 13, 1126-1135.

3. Strand, L.J., Meyer, U.A., Felsher, B.F., Redeker, A.G. and Marver, H.S. (1972) J. Clin. Invest., 51, 2530-2536.

4. Waters, A.H., Mollin, D.L., Pope, J. and Towler, T. (1961) J. Clin. Pathol., 14, 335-344.

5. Herbert, V. (1966) J. Clin. Pathol., 19, 12-16.

6. Mortensen, E. (1976) Clin. Chem., 22, 982-992.

7. Rothenberg, S.P., daCosta, M. and Rosenberg, Z. (1972) New England J. Med., 286, 1335-1339.

8. Bird, O.D., McGlohon, V.M. and Vaitkus, J.W. (1965) Anal. Biochem., 12, 18-35.

9. Mims, V. and Laskowski, M. (1945) J. Biol. Chem., 160, 493-503.

10. Lowry, O.H., Rosebrough, N.J., Farr, A.L. and Randall, R.J. (1951) J. Biol. Chem., 193, 265-275.

11. Battersby, A.R., McDonald, E. Williams, D.C. and Wurziger, H.K.W. (1977) J.C.S. Chem. Comm., 4, 113-115.

12. Battersby, A.R., Fookes, C.J.R., McDonald, E. and Meegan, M.J. (1978) J.C.S. Chem. Comm., 5, 185-186.

13. Scott, A.I., Ho, K.S., Kajiwara, M. and Takahashi, T. (1976) J. Am. Chem. Soc., 98, 1589-1591.

A STUDY OF THE MULTIPLE CHANGES INDUCED <u>IN VIVO</u>

IN EXPERIMENTAL ANIMALS BY INACTIVATION VITAMIN B_{12} USING NITROUS OXIDE

J.M. SCOTT, B. REED, B. McKENNA, P. McGING, S. McCANN, H. O'SULLIVAN, P. WILSON AND
D.G. WEIR

Departments of Biochemistry and Clinical Medicine, Trinity College, Dublin 2, Ireland

ABSTRACT

Nitrous oxide which is known to chemically oxidise vitamin B_{12} in the Co(I) state
has been used to inactivate cellular vitamin B_{12} <u>in vivo</u>. The <u>in vivo</u> biochemical
changes induced by such inactivation in animals include: (a) decreased ability to
metabolise 5-CH_3-H_4PteGlu; (b) increased urinary loss of 5-CH_3-H_4PteGlu; (c) abnormal dU suppression in bone marrow culture indicating impaired <u>de novo</u> pyrimidine biosynthesis, corrected by PteGlu and 5-CHO-H_4PteGlu but not corrected by 5-CH_3-H_4PteGlu
and partly corrected by cyanocobalamin; (d) decreased activity of methylmalonyl-CoA
mutase causing increased urinary excretion of methylmalonate and (e) decreased
fertility. Even after prolonged periods of exposure of mice to nitrous oxide for up
to six months no haematological, histological or neurological changes consistent
with human vitamin B_{12} deficiency were apparent. Similar studies with monkeys for
periods of up to two months showed the same results. These findings indicate that
nitrous oxide can be used to induce functional vitamin B_{12} deficiency with concomin-
ant biochemical changes in animals. However, unlike in humans where relatively short
periods of nitrous oxide exposure produced haematological changes, in animals it can
be concluded that megaloblastic changes occur much less readily, if at all.

INTRODUCTION

It is clear that the Co(I) form of vitamin B_{12} is susceptible to chemical
oxidation by nitrous oxide (N_2O)[1]. This gas has also been used to demonstrate <u>in
vitro</u> inactivation of purified vitamin B_{12} dependent enzymes such as dioldehydrate
and ethanolamine deaminase[2].

From as early as 1956 it has been clear that administration of N_2O for prolonged
periods to humans causes severe inhibition of the bone marrow[3]. Recently human subjects on N_2O treatment for up to one week have been shown to develop transient megaloblastic changes indicating that the mechanism of N_2O toxicity might be in its
ability to inhibit vitamin B_{12}[4]. The prospect of inducing functional deficiency of
vitamin B_{12} in animals in a controlled manner, has thus presented itself. In
addition the inability to induce haematological changes in any animal other than man
and to produce neurological changes in any animal other than monkeys and man, may be
resolved by the demonstration of functional vitamin B_{12} deficiency for definite
periods in such animal studies.

MATERIALS AND METHODS

Radiochemicals. Radioactive [methyl-^{3}H]thymidine ([^{3}H]TdR), (3',5',9(n)[^{3}H]PteGlu and [^{14}C]-5-CH$_3$-H$_4$PteGlu were all supplied by the Radiochemical Centre, Amersham, U.K.

Animals. Adult female Wistar rats (130-250g), adult female Laca mice (20-40g) were maintained in atmospheres of 20%:80% or 50%:50% O$_2$/N$_2$O for the time specified. Adult male monkeys (Cercopithecus nicritans) were kept in an atmosphere of 50%:50% O$_2$/N$_2$O for the time indicated.

Fertility studies. Nitrous oxide was shown to cause a 50% decrease in the fertility of Laca mice mated under 50% N$_2$O. This is in agreement with the findings of Kripke et al.[5] who demonstrated a decrease in spermatogenisis in male rats under N$_2$O.

Folate polyglutamate analysis[6,7]. We have been aware for some time that neither the oxidative or reductive cleavage techniques, cleave derivatives having a substitution at the 'N 10' position e.g. 10-CHO-PteGlu (Table 1). We have subsequently developed a modification which will deformylate these derivatives and can be used with either technique (Table 1). The acid step[7] cleaves 5-CH$_3$-H$_4$-PteGlu to PABGlu.

TABLE 1

A COMPARISON OF pABGlu FORMATION WITH OR WITHOUT THE ADDITION OF A DEFORMYLATION STEP BEFORE OXIDATIVE OR REDUCTIVE CLEAVAGE OF VARIOUS FOLATE DERIVATIVES.

Folate Derivative	% pABGlu after oxidative cleavage		% pABGlu after reductive cleavage	
	without deformylation	with deformylation	without deformylation	with deformylation
PteGlu	99%	98%	85%	86%
10-CHO-PteGlu	17%	99%	1.5%	87%
10-CHO-H$_2$PteGlu	1%	66%	1%	54%
pABGlu	81%	79%	78%	75%

Folate uptake studies were as previously described[6]

Identification of the liver monoglutamate was as before[8]

Methylmalonyl-CoA mutase loading studies were carried out as previously described[9]

dU suppresion was determined as described elsewhere[10]

RESULTS AND DISCUSSION

Folate uptake by mouse livers. Previous studies[11] had shown a decrease in liver uptake of [^{3}H] folate after N$_2$O treatment. These studies were extended and showed clear statistically significant decrease in folate polyglutamate biosynthesis after treatment with N$_2$O; mean ± S.D. for N$_2$O mice 0.24 ± 0.1 and for control mice 0.56 ± 0.24 (p < .001). Accompanying decreased liver uptake in N$_2$O treated animals was increased urinary loss. Similar studies using 5-[^{14}C]-CH$_3$-H$_4$PteGlu showed it to appear in the urine as what was identified[8,12] as its degradation product $5\text{-CH}_3\text{-H}_2\text{PteGlu}$ in increasing amounts, indicating that the compound had not been metabolised by removal of $[^{14}\text{C}]$ methyl group. Thus N_2O in some manner clearly decreases the ability of mouse liver to incorporate or to retain radioactive folate when compared to controls, when it is administered either as $[^3\text{H}]\text{PteGlu}$ or as $5[^{14}\text{C}]\text{-CH}_3\text{-H}_4\text{PteGlu}$.

Some experiments appeared to show increased accumulation of the $5\text{-CH}_3\text{-H}_4\text{PteGlu}$ as its monoglutamate in mouse liver[11] but this did not always happen and may be only a transient phenomenon related to exchange of extracellular radioactive monoglutamate with non-radioactive intracellular monoglutamate appearing to show elevation of a monoglutamate peak. In any event unlike the diminished total uptake, elevation of radioactive $5\text{-CH}_3\text{-H}_4\text{PteGlu}$ as a monoglutamate within the cell seems to be the exception rather than the rule. This folate polyglutamate analysis was carried out using a modification of the permangate oxidation cleavage method[6,7] which involved prior deformylation of any formyl folates present (Table 1).

These results indicate that N_2O by inactivating vitamin B_{12} decreases the ability of mouse liver to metabolise $5\text{-CH}_3\text{-H}_4\text{PteGlu}$ by the vitamin B_{12} dependent methionine synthetase and that this in turn, probably because the methylated form is an unsuitable substrate[13] decreases polyglutamate biosynthesis. As a further consequence there is decreased ability of the cells to retain newly incorporated folate with increased urinary loss. One must consider why a system has evolved where by the form of folate usually transported into the cell cannot be converted into a form which is retained without prior metabolism. It seems attractive to suggest that there is a purpose in this related to folate accumulation. It is possible that the rate of demethylation of $5\text{-CH}_3\text{-H}_4\text{PteGlu}$, controls the amount converted into polyglutamyl forms or that some type of metabolic trapping is involved resulting in cellular accumulation of folate.

De novo pyrimidine biosynthesis. The de novo synthesis of DNA thymine from dUMP involves methylation of deoxyuridylate (dUMP) to produce thymidylate (dTMP) and requires 5,10-methylenetetrahydrofolate $(5,10\text{-CH}_2\text{-H}_4\text{PteGlu})$[10]. Marrow cells in culture incorporate tritiated thymidine $([^3\text{H}]\text{TdR})$ into DNA by the salvage pathway and this incorporation can be suppressed by adding deoxyuridine (dU) to the culture medium to stimulate de novo thymidylate biosynthesis provided adequate $5,10\text{-CH}_2\text{-H}_4\text{PteGlu}$ is available. In folate deficient human[10] or rat[14] bone marrow the amount of suppression effected by the addition of dU is decreased and this reduction can be corrected by in vitro additions of PteGlu or $5\text{-CHO-H}_4\text{PteGlu}$ but is as expected unaffected by addition of vitamin B_{12}. In vitamin B_{12} deficient human bone marrow presumably because of the trapping of $5\text{-CH}_3\text{-H}_4\text{PteGlu}$[15] with consequent decreased availability of $5,10\text{-CH}_2\text{-H}_4\text{PteGlu}$ an abnormal dU suppression has also been found[10]. This was correctable by in vitro additions of PteGlu, $5\text{-CHO-H}_4\text{PteGlu}$ and vitamin B_{12} but not by addition of $5\text{-CH}_3\text{-H}_4\text{PteGlu}$. In contrast dU suppression studies in rats made vitamin B_{12} deficient by dietary restriction gave results similar to normals[16]. We

338

have found results comparable with those previously reported for vitamin B_{12} deficient human bone marrow (Fig. 1). The abnormal dU suppression is correctable by in vitro additions of PteGlu, 5-CHO-H_4PteGlu but not 5-CH_3-H_4PteGlu. Addition of cyanocobalamin caused partial correction probably due to increased production of methylcobalamin within the cell.

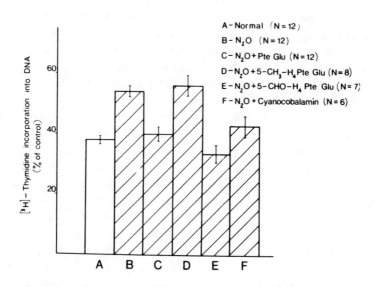

A - Normal (N = 12)
B - N_2O (N = 12)
C - N_2O + Pte Glu (N = 12)
D - N_2O + 5-CH_3-H_4Pte Glu (N = 8)
E - N_2O + 5-CHO-H_4 Pte Glu (N = 7)
F - N_2O + Cyanocobalamin (N = 6)

Fig. 1. Suppression of [^{3}H]TdR incorporation by a final concentration of 0.4 μM dU expressed as a percentage of control containing no dU ± (S.E.M.) from normal and N_2O treated rats. The effect of addition of PteGlu, 5-CH_3-H_4PteGlu, 5-CHO-H_4PteGlu and cyanocobalamin to the culture medium is also indicated.

Effect of N_2O treatment on methylmalonyl-CoA mutase. It is generally acknowledged that methionine synthetase involving the transfer of a methyl group proceeds via a Co(I) form of vitamin B_{12}[17]. More complex rearrangement reactions (e.g. methylmalonyl CoA mutase dioldehydrase, ethanolamine, deaminase) use the 5' deoxyadenosine form of the vitamin (coenzyme B_{12}) and their mechanism of action is unclear. Most of the evidence is against Co(I) being an intermediate[17]. Recently Corey et al.[18] have postulated a new mechanism for these types of reactions that does involve a Co(I) intermediate. Vitamin B_{12} deficient humans or animals are unable to metabolise propionate at the usual rate and excrete increased levels of methylmalonate in their urines. A function test based on intraperitoneal administration of propionate with quantitative urinary analysis of methylmalonate excretion can clearly differentiate vitamin B_{12} deficient animals from normals[9]. This test carried out on nitrous oxide treated animals showed them to have clearly elevated levels when compared to controls. These results would indicate that functionally this pathway is also imparied by N_2O treatment and makes it seem likely that a Co(I) intermediate is involved in the mechanism of methylmalonyl CoA mutase, if not all 5'deoxyadenosyl dependent enzymes. Another consequence of this result is that since both mechanisms of vitamin B_{12} dependent reaction are inhibited in vivo by N_2O the prospect of inducing vitamin B_{12} related neurological disorders by N_2O administration seems very likely.

Histological haematological and neurological studies. Vitamin B_{12} deficient humans develop haematologic and histologic changes quite rapidly and neurologic changes slowly. Vitamin B_{12} deficient monkeys while they did develop neurologic changes after five years on a vitamin B_{12} deficient diet showed no haematologic change[19]. Other species such as the rat, while they show vitamin B_{12} related biochemical abnormalities have never been found to show any of the morphological abnormalities associated with vitamin B_{12} deficiency in the human. In these animal studies the concern has always been present as to the possibility that the dietary deprivation was not complete enough or that rats or monkeys might obtain some vitamin B_{12} from their gut microflora. We have now kept mice under an atmosphere of 50% N_2O:50% O_2 for up to 8 months and have failed to observe any morphological change either haematological, gastrointestinal or neurological which could be considered related to vitamin B_{12} deficiency. Similar studies are in hand with monkeys who after two months N_2O treatment likewise show no change. In view of the report that a similar concentration of N_2O for 12 hour periods each day had in one week caused haematological changes in man[4], one must inevitably conclude that in mice or rats while biochemical abnormalities can be induced by either dietary control or by N_2O treatment, haematological, gastroenterological or neurological changes cannot be readily brought about.

The difficulty in inducing haematological changes in any animal other than man is clearly of great interest. Because of the great effectiveness of N_2O induction of haematological effects in man when compared to monkeys, rats of mice, one can now safely dispense with the usual explanations of the difference as being due to incomplete deficiency by dietary restriction or contribution of vitamin B_{12} by the animals microflora. It now appears quite clear that susceptibility exists in man which is markedly less or absent in other species. This difference is almost certainly centered around the interconversion of the following cofactors $5,10\text{-}CH_2\text{-}H_4PteGlu$, $5\text{-}CH_3\text{-}H_4PteGlu$, $H_4PteGlu$ and $5,10\text{-}CH_2\text{-}H_4PteGlu$. It appears to us that in the absence of vitamin B_{12} the critical factor is not only that $5\text{-}CH_3\text{-}H_4PteGlu$ is metabolically trapped as it clearly is[15] but really how rapidly other folate forms get cycled into that form from $5,10\text{-}CH_2\text{-}H_4PteGlu$. It is known that S-adensoylmethionine (SAM) prevents this conversion. If one extends the methyl trap hypothesis to include the concept that vitamin B_{12} deficiency the normal mechanism of stopping folate entering the

340

trap, namely the biosynthesis of SAM, which also cannot occur due to absence of vitamin B_{12} than all cellular folates would enter the trap in an unrestricted manner. Thus $5\text{-}CH_3\text{-}H_4PteGlu$ would act as a sink for all cellular folates the tap of which could not be turned off (due to inability to synthesise SAM) and the plug of which could not be opened due to inability to convert $5\text{-}CH_3\text{-}H_4PteGlu$ to $H_4PteGlu$. Perhaps animals other than man, in the absence of vitamin B_{12} retain better control over what enters this folate sink.

ACKNOWLEDGEMENTS

We would like to thank the Biomedical Trust and the Medical Research Council of Ireland who supported this work.

REFERENCES

1. Blackburn, R., Kyaw, M. and Swallow, A.J. (1977)   J. Amer. Chem. Soc. Farad. Trans. (i), 73, 250-255.

2. Schrauzer, G.N. and Stadlbauer, E.A. (1975)   Bio. inorg. Chem. 4, 185-198.

3. Lassen, H.C.A., Henrikson, E., Neukirch, F. and Kristensen, H.S. (1956) Lancet (i), 527-530.

4. Amess, J.A.L., Burman, J.F., Rees, J.M., Nancekievill, D.G. and Mollin, D.L. (1978) Lancet (ii), 339-342.

5. Kripke, B.J., Kelman, A.D., Shah, N.K., Balogh, K. and Handler, A.H. (1976) Anesthesiology 44, 104-113.

6. Houlihan, C.M. and Scott, J.M. (1972)   Biochem. Biophys. Res. Commun. 48, 1675-1681.

7. Bassett, R., Weir, D.G. and Scott, J.M. (1976)   J. Gen. Microbiol. 93, 169-172.

8. Brown, J.P., Davidson, G.E. and Scott, J.M. (1973)   J. Chromat. 79, 195-207.

9. Armstrong, B.K. (1967)   Br. J. Nutr. 21, 309.

10. Metz, J., Kelly, A., Swett, U.C., Waxman, S. and Herbert, V. (1968)   Brit. J. Haematol. 14, 575-592.

11. McGing, P., Reed, B., Weir, D.G. and Scott, J.M. (1978)   Biochem. Biophys. Res. Commun. (2), 82, 540-546.

12. Brown, J.P., Davidson, G.E. and Scott, J.M. (1973)   Biochim. Biophys. Acta 343, 78-88.

13. Lavoie, A., Tripp, E. and Hoffbrand, A.V. (1974)   Clin. Sci. Mol. Med. 47, 617-630.

14. Das, K.C. and Mohafty, D. (1978)   Proc. XVII Congress Int. Soc. Haematol. Paris 388.

15. Herbert, V. and Zalusky, R. (1962)   J. Clin. Invest. 41, 1263-1276.

16. Cheng, F.W., Shane, B. and Stokstad, E.L.R. (1975)   Brit. J. Haematol. 31, 323-336.

17. Barker, H. (1972)   Ann. Rev. Biochem. Eds. Snell, E.E., Boyer, P.D., Meister, A. & Sinseimer p.55. Ann. Rev. Inc. Palo Alto, Cal. U.S.A.

18. Corey, E.J., Cooper, N.J. and Green, M.L.N. (1977)   Proc. Nat. Acad. Sci. USA, 74, 811-815.

19. Agamanolis, D.P., Chester, E.M., Victor, M., Kark, J.A., Hines, J.D. and Harris, J.W. (1976)   Neurology 26, 905-914.

PTEROYLPOLYGLUTAMATE SYNTHESIS BY CORYNEBACTERIUM SP

BARRY SHANE[*]
Department of Biochemistry, The Johns Hopkins University School of
Hygiene and Public Health, Baltimore, Maryland 21205

TOM BRODY AND E.L. ROBERT STOKSTAD
Department of Nutritional Sciences, University of California, Berkeley,
California, 94720

Little is known about the substrate specificity or regulation of folylpolyglutamate synthetase, the enzyme(s) that catalyzes the addition
of glutamate moieties to the folate molecule. This report describes a
method for the identification of folates in Corynebacterium and some
preliminary experiments on the specificity of folylpolyglutamate synthetase in this organism. This organism was chosen as it has been reported to overproduce pteroyltriglutamate[1], which should make it a
good source of the enzyme and should simplify kinetic analyses with
different folate substrates.

METHODS

Identification of bacterial folates. Corynebacterium was cultured
aerobically at 37° for 3 days in medium containing [^{14}C]pABA. Polyglutamate chain lengths of bacterial and medium folates were determined by converting the folates to azo-dye derivatives and separating
the derivatives on polyacrylamide columns[2]. The azo-dye solutions were applied to short BioGel P2 columns (4x0.7cm) and desalted
by washing with 0.2N HCl. Under these conditions, the azo-dyes bound
tightly to the polyacrylamide. The dyes were eluted from the columns,
with some retardation, at pH7. Fractions containing the azo-dyes, as
measured by scintillation counting or by their absorbance at 540nm
(pH1), were adjusted to pH7 and chromatographed on BioGel P4 columns
(100x0.8cm). The columns were eluted with 0.1M Na phosphate buffer
PH7, containing 10mMEDTA.

Folylpolyglutamate synthetase assay. Enzyme extracts were prepared
by sonicating bacteria suspended in 20mM K phosphate buffer, pH7, for
20x15 sec. Cellular debris was removed by centrifugation and the
soluble fraction dialysed against 20mM K phosphate, pH7. Assay mix-

---

[*]
to whom correspondence should be addressed.

tures contained, in a total volume of 1ml, folate (100μM), KCl (200mM), MgCl$_2$ (10mM), ATP (5mM), tris buffer, pH9.5 (200mM, final pH9.2),mercaptoethanol (10mM), dithiothreitol (5mM),[^{14}C]glutamate (250μM; 2.5μCi), and enzyme extract. The mixtures were incubated under a N$_2$ or H$_2$ atmosphere at 37° for 2h, and the reactions were stopped by the addition of 1N HCl (1ml). Labelled folate compounds were converted to azo-dye derivatives and separated from [^{14}C]glutamate by chromatography on Bio-Gel P2.

RESULTS

In vivo synthesis of pteroylpolyglutamates. Fig. 1 shows the BioGel P4 elution profiles of the azodyes derived from labelled folates in Corynebacterium after culturing the bacteria in the presence of [^{14}C] pABA for three days. The major endogenous folate was a tetraglutamate while tri- and tetraglutamates, together with unmetabolized pABA, predominated in the medium. In the absence of added [^{14}C]pABA, similar folates were synthesized, as measured by the absorbance of the azo-dye derivatives. In this case the medium contained large amounts of pABA, indicating that Corynebacterium is also an overproducer of pABA. Individual folates were identified by chromatography of intact folates on DEAE cellulose, before and after γ-glutamylhydrolase

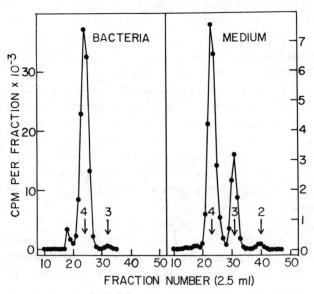

Fig. 1. BioGel P4 Separation of Corynebacterium folate derivatives.

treatment and by differential microbiological assay. The major
intracellular folates were 10-formyl-H_4PteGlu$_4$ and 10-formyl-PteGlu$_4$
with lesser amounts of 5-formyl-H_4PteGlu$_4$ and H_4PteGlu$_4$. 10-formyl-
PteGlu$_3$ and 10-formyl-PteGlu$_4$, together with pABAglu$_3$ and pABAglu$_4$,
predominated in the medium. No 5-methyl-H_4PteGlu$_n$ was detected.

In vitro synthesis of pteroylpolyglutamates. Table 1 shows the effect
of incubation conditions on the activity of folylpolyglutamate synthetase in Corynebacterium extracts. Enzyme activity was dependent
on folate and ATP, and was maximal at pH9.2 in tris buffer and at

TABLE 1

EFFECT OF INCUBATION CONDITIONS ON FOLYPOLYGLUTAMATE SYNTHETASE ACTIVITY

| Assay Mixture | Activity (pmol/h/mg protein) with | |
	H_4PteGlu	H_4PteGlu$_2$
Complete[a]	4027	39
- folate	2	2
- ATP	1	3
- KCl	7	1
- enzyme	0	0
- thiols	1450	–
5µM folate	444	2

[a] 100µM folate, 200mM KCl, 10mM MgCl$_2$, 250µM [^{14}C]glutamate, 10mM
mercaptoethanol, 5mM dithiothreitol, enzyme extract in tris buffer
pH 9.2, 5mMATP.

pH9.5-10 in glycine buffer. GTP and dATP were less effective substrates than ATP. K^+ stimulated the reaction maximally at 200mM.
Above this concentration it was inhibitory. Practically no
activity was detected in the absence of K^+. Activity was greatly reduced in the absence of thiols, almost certainly due to the instability
of H_4PteGlu under these conditions. H_4PteGlu was a much more effective
substrate than H_4PteGlu$_2$. In both cases only one glutamate moiety was
added to the molecule. At low H_4PteGlu concentrations (1µM), only the
diglutamate was formed. Attempts to increase the activity with
the diglutamate substrate, by varying the pH between 4 and 10, and
by varying the K^+ and substrate concentrations at the different pH
values, were unsuccessful.

Table 2 compares the effectiveness of various folate standards as
substrates for the enzyme and indicates the products formed. H_4PteGlu,
10-formyl-H_4PteGlu, and 5,10-methylene-H_4PteGlu were the most effective

monoglutamate substrates while 5-formyl-H_4PteGlu and H_2PteGlu exhibited lowered activities. With 100 µM substrate concentrations, the product

TABLE 2

SUBSTRATE SPECIFICITY OF FOLYPOLYGLUTAMATE SYNTHETASE

Substrate (100µM)	Specific Activity (pmol/h/mg)	Products
H_4PteGlu	4475	H_4PteGlu$_2$
H_4PteGlu$_2$	46	H_4PteGlu$_3$
H_4PteGlu$_3$	3	H_4PteGlu$_4$
5,10-methylene-H_4PteGlu	896	di- and triglutamates
5,10-methylene-H_4PteGlu$_2$	1448	tri- and tetraglutamates
5,10-methylene-H_4PteGlu$_3$	55	tetraglutamate
10-formyl-H_4PteGlu	2625	10-formyl-H_4PteGlu$_2$
10-formyl-H_4PteGlu$_2$	34	10-formyl-H_4PteGlu$_3$
10-formyl-H_4PteGlu$_3$	10	tetraglutamate
PteGlu	19	_[a]
PteGlu$_2$	10	-
H_2PteGlu	282	diglutamate
5-formyl-H_4PteGlu	701	-
pABAglu	1	-
pABA	0	-

[a] not determined

in each case was the diglutamate. Longer glutamate chain length products were only detected with the 5,10-methylene-H_4PteGlu substrate (fig. 2). At low folate concentrations (1-5µM), an identical pattern of products was observed. Tri- and tetraglutamate products were only formed with 5,10-methylene-H_4PteGlu as substrate.

H_4PteGlu and 10-formyl-H_4PteGlu di- and tri-glutamates were poor substrates for the enzyme and only a single glutamate moiety was added in each case. 5,10-methylene-H_4PteGlu di- and triglutamates were effective substrates and the diglutamate was converted to tri- and tetraglutamate products (fig. 2).

The values shown in table 2 are an approximate measure of the relative effectiveness of the different substrates. We have described procedures for the quantitative conversion of PteGlu$_n$, H_4PteGlu$_n$, and 10-formyl-H_4PteGlu$_n$ to azo-dye derivatives and their quantitative recovery from BioGel P2^2. However, the conversion of 5,10-methylene-

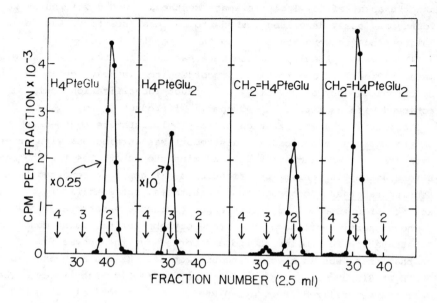

Fig. 2. BioGel P4 separation of synthetase products (100μM folate)

$H_4PteGlu_n$ to azo-dye derivatives was incomplete (approx. 20 per cent recovery). The values shown in Table 2 for the 5,10-methylene-$H_4PteGlu_n$ derivatives are underestimated. It should also be noted that the gluta-mate concentration used (250μM) was not saturating and that the folate concentration (100μM) may not have been saturating.

DISCUSSION

Although it has been reported that <u>Corynebacterium</u> overproduces pteroyltriglutamate[1], the major endogenous folates were tetraglutamate derivatives. Oxidized formyl tri- and tetraglutamate derivatives pre-dominated in the medium, presumably because of the aerobic culture con-ditions. The presence of large amounts of triglutamate in the medium but not in the bacteria suggests that triglutamates are more easily released by the bacterium than are tetraglutamates. Although this pref-erential release of shorter glutamate chain length folates is in keeping with previous studies on bacterial transport of folates[3], the mechanism of folate efflux in <u>Corynebacterium</u> is of interest, as this organism lacks the ability to transport PteGlu (unpublished data). It may, however, be possible that <u>Corynebacterium</u> will transport reduced folates.

The method described for the identification of pteroylpolyglutamates and the assay of folylpolyglutamate synthetase was developed as we found previously described methods to be unsatisfactory. Labile folate products were converted to the more stable azo-dye derivatives of $pABAglu_n$. These were easily separated from $[^{14}C]$gluta-mate on BioGel P2 and resolved, according to glutamate chain length, by chromatography on BioGel P4[2]. Product identification could be achieved with as little as 100 dpm $[^{14}C]$ product.

The initial characterization of folylpolyglutamate synthetase from Corynebacterium described in this report was carried out with crude extracts. It was necessary to determine the substrates for the enzyme before attempting enzyme purification as it has been reported that Neurospora crassa possesses two synthetases, one specific for $H_4PteGlu$ and the other specific for folate polyglutamate substrates[4].

The properties of the enzyme from Corynebacterium, using monoglutamate substrates, were similar to those reported for the enzyme from E. coli[5] in that there was an absolute requirement for K^+ and an energy source, and $H_4PteGlu$ and 10-formyl-$H_4PteGlu$ were effective substrates. The E. coli enzyme utilized 10-formyl-$H_4PteGlu$ more effectively than $H_4PteGlu$, and $H_2PteGlu$ and 5-formyl-$H_4PteGlu$ were not substrates. Products of the reaction in E. coli were identified as diglutamates and no longer gluta-mate chain length folates were detected. This observation may be due to using the wrong substrate as $H_4PteGlu_2$ and 10-formyl-$H_4PteGlu_2$ are poor substrates for the Corynebacterium enzyme while 5,10-methylene-$H_4PteGlu_2$ is an effective substrate. Preliminary results with enzyme from Lactobacillus casei and Streptococcus faecalis also suggest that 5,10-methylene-$H_4PteGlu_n$ are the most effective substrates (Shane, un-published data). This contrasts to the Chinese hamster ovary cell folypolyglutamate synthetase[6], which metabolizes $H_4PteGlu$ to poly-glutamate forms. In this case, $H_4PteGlu_2$ appears to be an effective substrate and K^+ is only slightly stimulatory.

ACKNOWLEDGEMENTS

This work was supported in parts by grants number CA-22717 and AM-08171 from the National Institutes of Health.

REFERENCES

1. Hutchins, B.L., Stokstad, E.L.R., Bohonos, N., Sloane, N.H. and Subba Row, Y. (1948) J. Am. Chem. Soc. 70-103.

2. Brody, T., Shane, B. and Stokstad, E.L.R. Anal. Biochem. (in press).

3. Shane, B. and Stokstad, E.L.R. (1976) J. Biol. Chem. 251, 3405-3410.

4. Sakami, W., Ritari, S.J., Black, C.W. and Rzepka, J. (1973) Fed. Proc. 32, 471.

5. Masurekar, M. and Brown, G.M. (1975) Biochemistry 14, 2424-2430.

6. Taylor, R.T. and Hanna, M.L. (1977) Arch. Biochem. Biophys. 181, 331-344.

FOLATE POLY-γ-GLUTAMYL DERIVATIVES AS COSUBSTRATES FOR CHICKEN LIVER AICAR TRANSFORMYLASE

JOSEPH E. BAGGOTT AND CARLOS L. KRUMDIECK

Department of Nutrition Sciences, University of Alabama, Birmingham

ABSTRACT

Hofstee's constants, Vm/Km, for the folyl poly- γ-glutamate cosubstrates N^{10}-formyltetra-hydropteroyl (glutamate)$_n$ (where n= 1,3,4,5,6, and 7) of the purine biosynthesis enzyme 10-formyl tetrahydrofolate : 5' phosphoribosyl-5-amino-4-imidazolecarboxamide formyltransferase have been determined. The preferred cosubstrate is the tetraglutamate. The regulatory implications of this finding are discussed.

INTRODUCTION

It is now well established that the folate cosubstrates occur and function in vivo as poly- γ-glutamyl derivatives of various chain lengths. The biochemical role of the polypeptide chain remains, however, largely unknown. For the past several years we have investigated the hypothesis that changes in the length of the poly-γ-glutamyl chain may play a role in the regulation of one-carbon metabolism. One mechanism by which this regulatory function could take place is by alteration of the enzyme-cosubstrate specificity mediated via changes in the length of the poly-γglutamyl chain[1]. A valuable method for examining enzyme-substrate specificity is to determine Hofstee's specificity constant[2], Vm/Km, which combines indicators of the two main events occuring during enzymatic catalysis: binding of the substrate (approximated by Km) and its subsequent chemical transformation (indicated by Vm). For any given folate-requiring enzyme this "efficiency-affinity" constant Vm/Km can be determined for all chain lengths of its corresponding folate cosubstrate to generate a specificity constant vs chain length profile. Such curve allows a direct comparison of the putative substrates even if, as is usually the case, they differ in both Vm's and Km's. The curve will go through a maximum with the enzyme's preferred cosubstrate. Furthermore, as demonstrated by Hofstee[2], the reaction rate will be proportional to Vm/Km when the concentration of substrate is low. Thus, for a folate requiring enzyme system, the flux of one carbon moieties through the reaction will be proportional to the Vm/Km of the folate cosubstrate present provided that it occurs at low concentration ([S] <Km). It must be noted here that, concerning the folate cosubstrates, the condition [S] <Km is most likely present in vivo. Figure 1 shows the specificity constant vs chain length profiles of three hypothetical folate-requiring enzymes. It is apparent that alterations in chain length would either increase or decrease the flux of one-carbon fragments through the reactions catalyzed by each enzyme. Perhaps more important, the flux through enzymatic reactions requiring the

same one-carbon substituent (for example formyl) could be independently regulated. It must be noted also that the figure represents only a theoretical situation in which the concentrations of all the various chain-length cosubstrates is the same. Since the various polyglutamates do not occur naturally in equimolar amounts, and since the actual rate of a reaction will be determined by the product of the proportionality constant Vm/Km times the concentration of the cosubstrate, ($v = \frac{Vm}{Km}$ [S]), it follows that changes in the concentration of preferred cosubstrates would produce large changes in flux, while similar changes in concentration of cosubstrates of low specificity would have much smaller effects. We report here experimentally generated Vm/Km vs chain length profiles that conform to the theoretical model.

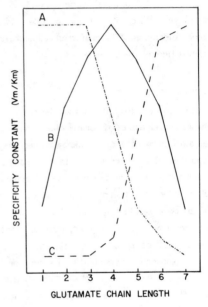

FIGURE 1.

Specificity constant vs chain length profile of three hypothetical folate-requiring enzymes.
See text.

RESULTS

We have recently completed the determination of Hofstee's specificity constants of the purine biosynthesis enzyme 10-formyl tetrahydrofolate : 5'-phosphoribosyl-5-amino-4-imidazole carboxamide formyltransferase (EC 2.1.2.3) for N^{10} formyl tetrahydro folate cosubstrates of varying poly-γ-glutamyl chain lengths. The enzyme (from now on refered to by its trival name AICAR transformylase) was purified approximately 400 fold from a homogenate of chicken liver. The activity of pteroylpoly-γ-glutamate hydrolase (conjugase) was determined during the purification to ascertain its removal since the co-purification of conjugase would greatly confound the kinetics of AICAR transformylase with the poly-γglutamyl cosubstrates. Fortunately the two activities were separated so that the specific activity of the purified AICAR transformylase was more than 100 times greater than that of conjugase.

The N^{10} formyl tetrahydropteroyl poly-γ-glutamates were synthesized from the corresponding pteroyl poly-γglutamates (obtained by solid phase synthesis[3]) by catalytic reduction and subsequent formylation to the (d, ℓ) N^5, N^{10} methenyl tetrahydro forms[4,5]. The latter were converted to the N^{10}formyl tetrahydropteroyl polyglutamates just prior to use by incubating at pH 7.4 in a mercaptoethanol containing buffer.

A new assay of AICAR transformylase based on the increase in optical density at 298 nm that follows conversion of the N^{10} formyltetrahydrofolate to tetrahydrofolate was developed and used throughout the study.

The kinetic parameters, K_m and V_m, for the folate cosubstrates N^{10} formyltetrahydropteroyl (glutamate)$_n$ where n=1,3,4,5,6 and 7, were determined at a saturating AICAR concentration. Since AICAR transformylase requires potassium ions for maximum activity, the kinetic parameters were determined at activating potassium ion concentration (25mM KCl) and at physiological potassium ion concentration (150mM KCl). The Km's were found to be 674, 1.65, 0.99, 2.56, 1.64 and 1.83 μM at 25mM KCl, and 353, 5.95, 1.07, 2.06, 1.95, and 3.13 μM at 150 mM KCl for n=1,3,4, 5,6 and 7 respectively. The relative Vm's were found to be 1.00, 0.157, 0.114, 0.130, 0.117 and 0.099 at 25mM KCl and 1.00, 0.867, 0.771, 0.545, 0.638 and 0.521 at 150mM KCl for n=1,3,4,5,6 and 7 respectively. The specificity constants Vm/Km were calculated and found to reach a maximum with the tetraglutamate cosubstrate at both concentrations of K^+ examined. At 150mM KCl the maximum was more pronounced. (Table I).

TABLE 1

RELATIVE SPECIFICITY CONSTANTS OF AICAR TRANSFORMYLASE

^{10}f H$_4$Pte(Glu)$_n$ *	Vm/Km	
n	25 mM KCl	150 mM KCl
1	1.0	1.0
3	64	52
4	78	250
5	34	93
6	48	120
7	36	59

*N^{10} formyltetrahydropteroyl (glutamate)$_n$.

Figure 2 shows the specificity constant vs chain length profile for AICAR transformylase at 150mM KCl. Also shown are the profiles of methionine synthetase (bovine brain), ketopantoate hydroxymethyl transferase (E. coli) and dihydrofolate reductase (human myelogenous leukemia cells) calculated from data of Coward et al[6]; Powers and Snell[7] and Coward et al[8]. All of these enzymes have increased specificity for the poly-γglutamate cosubstrates (when compared to

350

the monoglutamate) and the profiles are clearly qualitatively and quantitatively different. These differences could certainly allow for regulation of the flux of one carbon moieties through alterations in the chain length of the polyglutamate cosubstrates. It must be pointed out however that comparison of specificity profiles of various folate requiring enzymes ought to be made among enzymes from the same source if valid inferences about their role in regulation of one-carbon metabolism are to be drawn. It is evident that additional information on kinetic parameters of the pteroyl polyglutamates is sorely needed. It seems worth emphasizing again that these studies must be conducted with enzyme preparations that are essentially free of conjugase activity, otherwise, the differences between polyglutamates of various lengths would become obscured or disappear altogether.

FIGURE 2.

Specificity constant vs chain length profiles of AICAR trans-formylase, methionine synthetase, ketopantoate hydroxymethyl transferase and dihydrofolate reductase.

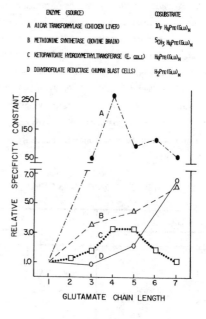

Metabolic regulation implies the modulation of reaction rates and it is agreed that this is achieved by control of the activities and concentrations of the enzymes. Rapid, short term regulation proceeds via changes in enzyme activity explained by the action of one or more of the following mechanisms:

i) substrate, product or end product inhibition or activation
ii) allosteric modification (activation or inhibition)
iii) covalent modification of the enzyme and
iv) modification of the enzyme by interactions with proteins or other macromolecules.

The data presented above suggests another mechanism for enzyme activity regulation, namely, the covalent modification of a cofactor (or cosubstrate). In folate metabolism the addition or deletion of γ-glutamyl residues around an optimal number would permit an almost "continuous" modification of the properties of the cofactor and consequently a rather fine regulation of enzyme activity. In keeping with the above we have reported alterations in the distribution of folates of different chain lengths resulting from experimental perturbations of the steady-state of one-carbon metabolism[9].

ACKNOWLEDGEMENTS

Support for this research was provided in part by P.H.S. Grant 1 T32 DE 07020-02, American Cancer Society Grant IN-66Q and P.H.S. Grant GM23453.

REFERENCES

1. Krumdieck, C.L., Cornwell, P.E., Thompson, R.W. and White, W.E. (1977) in Folic Acid, Biochemistry and Physiology in Relation to the Human Nutrition Requirement. Broquist, H.P. and Butterworth, Jr., C.E. eds. Natl. Acad. Scien., 25.

2. Hofstee, B.H.J. (1952) Science, 116, 329.

3. Krumdieck, C.L. and Baugh, C.M. (1969) Biochemistry, 8, 1568.

4. Hatefi, Y., Talbert, P.T., Osborn, M.J. and Huennekens, F.M. (1960) Biochemical Preparations, 7, 89.

5. Rowe, P.B. (1968) Anal. Biochem., 22, 166.

6. Coward, J.K., Chello, P.L., Cashmore, A.R. Parameswaran, K.N., DeAngelis, L.M. and Bertino, J.R. (1975) Biochemistry, 14, 1548.

7. Powers, S.G. and Snell, E.E. (1976) J. Biol. Chem. 251, 3786.

8. Coward, J.K., Parameswaran, K.N., Cashmore, A.R. and Bertino, J.R. (1974) Biochemistry, 13, 3899.

9. Thompson, R.W., Leichter, J., Cornwell, P.E. and Krumdieck, C.L. (1977) Am. J. Clin. Nutr., 30, 1583.

INTERACTION OF OXIDIZED AND REDUCED FOLATES WITH DIHYDROFOLATE REDUCTASE
FROM AMETHOPTERIN-RESISTANT LACTOBACILLUS CASEI

JANA M. BEDNAREK and R. BRUCE DUNLAP
Department of Chemistry, University of South Carolina, Columbia, South Carolina 29208

Dihydrofolate reductase catalyses the NADPH-dependent reduction of 7,8-dihydrofo-
late (H_2folate) to (-)-5,6,7,8-tetrahydrofolate ((-)H_4folate), which is subsequently
employed as a coenzyme in a wide variety of one carbon group transfer reactions. The
role of this enzyme as a metabolic target for a group of folate antagonists used in
the chemotherapy of cancers and certain other diseases is well established. The relative abundance of dihydrofolate reductase and its ease of isolation from amethopterin-
resistant sources coupled with its stability and low molecular weight (18,000 to
30,000) have made it a prime candidate for primary structure, chemical modification,
ligand binding, and X-ray crystallographic studies.

Dihydrofolate reductase isolated from amethopterin-resistant Lactobacillus casei
was shown to have a molecular weight of 18,300[1] and exhibited two forms (I and II),
which were resolved from one another by both gel electrophoresis and ion exchange
chromatography[2]. Further work showed that these two enzymic forms differed only by
the presence of an equimolar amount of tightly but noncovalently bound NADPH in form
II[2-4]. Our interests in the catalytic mechanism of the enzyme led to chemical modification studies of the enzyme which showed that a single tryptophyl residue was
necessary for both enzyme activity and the tight binding of NADPH[5]. Subsequently, in
collaboration with Dr. Freisheim's group at the University of Cincinnati, the complete amino acid sequence of the L. casei enzyme was determined[1]. Tryptophan-21 was
identified as a functional active site residue, and it was shown that the identity
and position of this residue was conserved in a number of dihydrofolate reductases
from other sources[6]. In an extension of our earlier work, the enzyme was shown to
form an electrophoretically stable binary complex with deamino-NADPH, but not with
acetylpyridine NADPH[7].

In earlier work, Otting and Huennekens[8] had shown that NADPH, amethopterin, and
the enzyme generate a ternary complex which is stable to gel electrophoresis. The
tightly bound ligands survive gel filtration chromatography but are dissociated from
the denatured enzyme. In addition, in the presence of amethopterin, the L. casei enzyme forms stable ternary complexes with deamino-NADPH, thio-NADPH, and acetylpyridine
NADPH but not with $NADP^{+}$[7]. We have also found that H_2folate and $NADP^+$ interact with
this enzyme to yield a tight ternary complex[7].

In light of these findings and our interests in identifying active site residues
and defining their roles in catalytic and binding phenomena associated with dihydrofolate reductase, we have investigated the interaction of the enzyme with folate,
amethopterin, H_2folate, and (-)H_4folate as monitored by gel electrophoresis, gel

filtration and carboxymethyl Sephadex chromatography, and absorbance and fluorescence spectroscopy.

Gel electrophoresis of dihydrofolate reductase incubated with up to a tenfold excess of folate, amethopterin, H_2folate, or $(-)-H_4$folate revealed a single band whose migration was identical to that of native enzyme alone. The fact that none of the folate analogue enzyme-binary complexes survived electrophoresis was confirmed in parallel experiments employing radioactive folate analogues. In each case, the radiolabeled folate migrated substantially faster than the protein. These results contrast sharply with those obtained with the NADPH-enzyme binary complex and the NADPH-amethopterin ternary complex, which were run as control samples.

Although the folate analogue-dihydrofolate reductase binary complexes were not stable when subjected to gel electrophoresis, they were observed to remain associated to varying degrees when isolated by gel filtration chromatography on Sephadex G-25 or Bio-gel P6 resins. Binding stoichiometries were evaluated using results of protein and enzyme assays coupled with scintillation counting data derived from the bound, radiolabeled ligand. By averaging the binding ratios (moles of folate analogue: moles of enzyme) determined across the peak from elution profiles obtained on Bio-gel P6 chromatography, the stoichiometries of several folate-enzyme binary complexes were calculated to be: folate: enzyme, 0.2:1; amethopterin: enzyme, 1:1; H_2folate: enzyme, 0.51:1; and $(-)-H_4$folate: enzyme, 0.97:1. The stability of these binary complexes was also evaluated by dialysis experiments.

Each of the binary complexes was characterized and could be identified by its distinctive absorption spectrum. For example, the amethopterin-enzyme complex yields an absorption spectrum with a peak at 283 nm, a shoulder at 287 nm (protein absorption), a shoulder at 310 nm, and a peak at 345 nm. The ratio of A_{283}/A_{345} was about 4.5. The absorbance spectrum of the H_2folate-enzyme complex is typified by a peak at 283 nm, a shoulder at 287 nm (enzyme), and a shoulder at 310 nm. The ratio of A_{282}/A_{310} varied from 3.38 to 2.56 as the stoichiometry of the complex increased from 0.45 to 0.76 moles of H_2folate bound per mole of enzyme.

The stability of several of the binary complexes was studied employing ion exchange chromatography. Chromatography of DEAE Sephadex resulted in the complete separation of the ligand from the enzyme. The enzyme-binary complexes of amethopterin and H_2folate were shown to survive chromatography on carboxymethyl Sephadex. As predicted on electrostatic grounds, these binary complexes eluted from carboxymethyl Sephadex resin substantially ahead of the free, native enzyme.

Interaction of the folate ligands with dihydrofolate reductase was also investigated by titration of protein fluorescence. The difference method of Kurganov[9] was employed to estimate the dissociation constants of the enzyme-folate analogue binary complexes as follows: enzyme: H_2folate, 2.56×10^{-6} M; enzyme: $(-)-H_4$folate, 1.28×10^{-6} M; and enzyme: amethopterin, 8×10^{-8} M.

These results indicate that H_2folate, $(-)-H_4$folate, and amethopterin interact with dihydrofolate reductase from amethopterin-resistant _L. casei_ to form binary complexes whose stoichiometry approaches 1:1 and whose dissociation constants are low. These findings are not only important in characterizing the ligand-enzyme interaction, but they find application in designing experiments on the identification and localization of residues involved in the active site of the enzyme.

ACKNOWLEDGEMENTS

Part of this research was supported by funds awarded to J. M. Bednarek from an American Cancer Society Institutional Grant to the University of South Carolina. R. B. Dunlap is the recipient of an American Cancer Society Faculty Research Award (FRA-144).

REFERENCES

1. Bitar, K. G., Blankenship, D. T., Walsh, K. A., Dunlap, R. B., Reddy, A. V. and Freisheim, J. H. (1977) FEBS Lett., 80, 119-122.

2. Dunlap, R. B., Gundersen, L. E. and Huennekens, F. M. (1971) Biochem. Biophys. Res. Commun., 42, 772-777.

3. Gundersen, L. E., Dunlap, R. B., Harding, N. G. L., Freisheim, J. H., Otting, F. and Huennekens, F. M. (1972) Biochemistry, 11, 1018-1023.

4. Huennekens, F. M., Dunlap, R. B., Freisheim, J. H., Gundersen, L. E., Harding, N. G. L., Levison, S. A. and Mell, G. P. (1971) Ann. N.Y. Acad. Sci., 186, 85-99.

5. Lui, J.-K. and Dunlap, R. B. (1974) Biochemistry, 13, 1807-1814.

6. Freisheim, J. H., Ericsson, L. H., Bitar, K. G., Dunlap, R. B. and Reddy, A. V. (1977) Arch. Biochem. Biophys., 180, 310-317.

7. Williams, T. J., Lee, T. K. and Dunlap, R. B. (1977) Arch. Biochem. Biophys., 181, 569-579.

8. Otting, F. and Huennekens, F. M. (1972) Arch. Biochem. Biophys., 152, 429-431.

9. Kurganov, B: I. Sugrobova, N. P. and Yakovlev, V. A. (1972) FEBS Lett., 19, 308-310.

THE AMINO TERMINAL SEQUENCE OF DIHYDROFOLATE REDUCTASE FROM *E. COLI* K12 STRAINS MB 3746 AND MB 3747

CARL D. BENNETT, JOHN A. RODKEY, MARTIN POE*, JOSEPH K. WU* AND
KARST HOOGSTEEN*
Merck Sharp & Dohme Research Laboratories, West Point, Pa. 19486
and *Merck Institute for Therapeutic Research, Rahway, N.J. 07065

One useful approach to insight into the role of the various structural features on DHFR (dihydrofolate reductase or 5,6,7,8-tetrahydrofolate:NADP$^+$ oxidoreductase E.C.1.5.1.3) as revealed from its crystal structure[1] is to examine the properties of closely related enzymes that exhibit small, known differences in their primary sequence. The DHFR sequences published to date on bacterial DHFRs as purified from *Escherichia coli* MB 1428[2,3], *E. coli* RT-500[4], *Streptococcus faecium*[5] and *Lactobaccillus casei*[6] have shown a high degree of homology between the primary sequences of these enzymes. We present here data on the amino terminal portion of the primary sequence of the DHFR isolated from each of two trimethoprim-resistant strains of *E. coli* K12, strains MB 3746 and MB 3747, which were discovered by Breeze *et al*[7].

The DHFR from *E. coli* MB 3746 and MB 3747 were isolated and purified as described by Poe *et al*[8]. The protein (200 nanomoles of 3746 and 150 nanomoles of 3747) was reduced and alkylated with sodium iodoacetate[3] and dialyzed to remove the reagents. After lyophilization, the protein was taken up to 450 µl of trifluoroacetic acid and placed in the spinning cup of a Beckman 890C sequencer. The program used was the Beckman Fast Protein Program. Resultant PTH amino acids were quantitated by GC and HPLC[9]. The repetitive yield was 96.1% for 3746 and 94.1% for 3747. The first 42 residues of each protein were identified, as shown in Table I. The protein from 3746 was further sequenced through residue 54, except that residues 47, 49 and 53 were not identified. These 9 additional residues were also identical to the corresponding residues in the protein from MB 1428.

Presented in Table I is the amino terminal sequence of *E. coli* MB 3746 in the usual one-letter code. This is identical to the 42 amino terminal residues of the primary sequence of *E. coli* MB 1428 DHFR[3], and differs from the corresponding portion of *E. coli* RT-500 DHFR at position 37 where the RT-500 enzyme has aspartate instead of asparagine. The amino terminal sequence of MB 3747 DHFR differs from that of MB 3746 DHFR only in that residue 20 is isoleucine, replacing

TABLE I

	10	20	30

M I S L I A A L A V D R V I G M E N A M P W N L P A D L A W

	40	50

F K R N T L N K P V I M G R H T X E X I G R X L

Amino terminal sequence of *E. coli* MB 3746 DHFR.

---

methionine. Thus all four *E. coli* strains have amino terminal sequences up to residue 42 that differ by at most one residue. These changes can all be related by single base changes in the DNA coding for this protein. The homologies between *S. faecium* DHFR and *E. coli* DHFR noted by Gleisner *et al*[5] and between *L. casei* DHFR and *E. coli* DHFR by Bitar *et al*[6] apply, at least for the amino terminal quarter of the proteins, to all four *E. coli* reductases.

The 3746 and 3747 reductases are closely related to one another and to the dihydrofolate reductase from *E. coli* MB 1428[8]. They both exhibit an apparent molecular weight of 17,500 with almost identical amino acid compositions. The turnover numbers in moles of dihydrofolate reduced per minute per mole enzyme at pH 7.2 and 25° are 630 and 740 for the 3746 and 3747 enzymes, respectively; the K_M values for dihydrofolate are 1.6 and 7.3 µM and the inhibition constants for trimethoprim are 1.1 and 11 nM, respectively. The pH at which maximal enzyme activity is observed is 8.0 and below 6.4 for the two enzymes. The 3747 reductase is thus like mammalian reductase in two respects: a lowered affinity for trimethoprim and maximal activity well below neutral pH. The pmr spectra at 300 MHz of the binary methotrexate complexes of the 1428,3746 and 3747 reductases are similar.

The residues proposed to be homologous to residue 20 of *E. coli* DHFR are leucine 19 in *L. casei* DHFR[6] and leucine 20 in *S. faecium* DHFR[5]. The sidechain of this residue in the ternary complex of *l. casei* DHFR with NADPH and methotrexate forms part of the boundary of the hydrophobic pocket for the nicotinamide ring[10]. It is unlikely that the substitution of methionine for leucine would substantially affect this hydrophobic pocket. Asparagine 37 in the crystal structure of both complexes of DHFR[1,10] is remote from both the methotrexate and NADPH sites. Thus, it seems unlikely that the differences in the biochemical properties of the four *E. coli* reductases can be accounted for by the differences between their first 42 amino terminal residues.

REFERENCES

1. Matthews, D.A., Alden, R.A., Bolin, J.T., Freer, S.A., Hamlin, R.,
    Xuong, N., Kraut, J., Poe, M., Williams, M.N. and Hoogsteen, K.
    (1977) Science, 197, 452-455.

2. Bennett, C.D. (1974) Nature, 248, 67-68.

3. Bennett, C.D., Rodkey, J.A., Sondey, J.M. and Hirschmann, R.F.
    (1978) Biochemistry, 17, 1328-1337.

4. Stone, D., Phillips, A.W. and Burchall, J.J. (1977) Europ. J.
    Biochem., 72, 613-624.

5. Gleisner, J.M., Peterson, D.L. and Blakley, R.L. (1974) Proc.
    Natl. Acad. Sci. U.S.A., 71, 3001-3005.

6. Bitar, K.G., Blankenship, D.T., Walsh, K.A., Dunlap, R.B.,
    Reddy, A.V. and Freisheim, J.H. (1977) FEBS Letters, 80, 119-122.

7. Breeze, A.S., Sims, P. and Stacey, K.A. (1975) Genet. Res.,
    Cambridge, 25, 207-214.

8. Poe, M., Breeze, A.S., Wu, J.K., Short, C.R. and Hoogsteen, K.
    (1978) J. Biol. Chem., in press.

9. Rodkey, J.A. and Bennett, C.D. (1976) Biochem. Biophys. Res. Commun.
    72, 1407-1413.

10. Matthews, D.A., Alden, R.A., Bolin, J.T., Filman, D.J., Freer, S.T.,
    Hamlin, R., Hol, W.G.J., Kisliuk, R.L., Pastore, E.J., Plante, L.T.,
    Xuong, N. and Kraut, J. (1978) J. Biol. Chem., in press.

Kisliuk/Brown, eds. Chemistry and Biology of Pteridines

361

MULTIPLE FORMS OF DIHYDROFOLATE REDUCTASE

DAVID P. BACCANARI and JAMES J. BURCHALL
Department of Microbiology, Wellcome Research Laboratories, Research Triangle Park,
North Carolina, U.S.A.   27709

INTRODUCTION

Multiple forms of dihydrofolate reductases are commonly observed on electrophoresis and column chromatography. However, the causes of these multiplicities may
or may not be understood. Early examples include the isolation of both the free
enzyme and a naturally occurring, stable, enzyme-NADPH binary complex (which is
apparently a major intracellular enzyme form) from chicken liver[1], L. casei[2], and
L1210 cells[3]. The current method of purifying reductases by affinity chromatography
and elution with folate or dihydrofolate can result in the generation of stable
enzyme-folate or enzyme-dihydrofolate binary complexes as additional enzyme
forms[4,5,6]. Another type of enzyme-"ligand" interaction which has caused reductase
multiplicity is the binding of the LM4 mouse lymphoma enzyme with the bromophenol
blue tracking dye used in electrophoresis[7]. Some of the multiplicity observed with
the enzyme is due to genetically different forms. S. faecium var. durans A contains
two reductases; one is specific for dihydrofolate whereas the other can utilize both
dihydrofolate and folate as substrates[8,9]. Phage infected E. coli synthesize both
the viral coded and the normal bacterial enzyme[10]. More recently, it was shown that
there are several distinct types of E. coli which contain extrachromasomal R-factors
and can produce both the normal trimethoprim sensitive chromosomal enzyme and novel
trimethoprim resistant R-factor enzymes[11,12,13].

There are a number of other cases where the occurrence of polymorphism is well
documented, but its cause is unknown. Hängii and Littlefield[14,15] performed a detailed physical and kinetic analysis of the two electrophoretically different forms
of dihydrofolate reductase present in a Methotrexate resistant line of hamster kidney
cells. Both forms have identical properties and tryptic maps, and both are found
(though not overproduced) in the Methotrexate sensitive parent cell line. Chicken
liver dihydrofolate reductase, purified by affinity chromatography, exhibits four
enzyme species on isoelectric focusing[6]. The major enzyme forms are the free enzyme
and the enzyme-dihydrofolate complex, but the nature of the other forms is not known.
A similar situation may exist with the bovine liver enzyme[5,16]. It is postulated
that 5-25% of the enzyme species seen on electrofocusing may represent deamidation
products[5]. The "minor" forms have identical specific activity, molecular weight and
amino acid compositions as the native enzyme[16]. Several different types of multiplicities have been observed with the enzyme from D. pneumoniae. The wild-type enzyme has a molecular weight of 20,000, however some Methotrexate-resistant mutants

362

produce both the normal size enzyme and an aggregated enzyme form[17]. Other mutants
are markedly labile during storage, and novel enzyme forms are seen on DEAE-chromato-
graphy[18]. The physical basis for these observations is unknown.

In addition to the above specific examples, there exists a large body of literature (reviewed by Blakley[19]) pertaining to modification of reductases by salts, urea
and sulfhydryl reagents. These reactions could be related to the occurrence of
multiple enzyme forms. As a particular case, we have examined the dihydrofolate reductase from E. coli RT500 and observed numerous molecular forms. This study shows
that all but two of the species are attributed, either directly or indirectly, to
sulfhydryl modification. The remaining two species are shown to be genetically
different isozymes with different physical and kinetic properties.

RESULTS AND DISCUSSION

Enzyme purification. Purification of large amounts (gram quantities) of dihydrofolate reductase to homogeneity in the absence of sulfhydryl reagents results in a
variety of multiple enzyme forms on gel filtration and electrophoresis[20]. The enzyme
has a molecular weight of 18,000 by Sephadex chromatography, however after storage
and rechromatography, a high molecular weight form comprising about 20% of the total
protein is observed. The conversion of monomer to aggregate can be rapid (up to 10%
in 17 hr at 5°), but incubation of the aggregate in 10 mM DTT results in reconver-
sion to the monomer. Therefore, there is a DTT reversible monomer → aggregate association of the E. coli enzyme. Preparative electrophoresis of the DTT treated enzyme
shows at least seven enzyme species (Fig. 1).

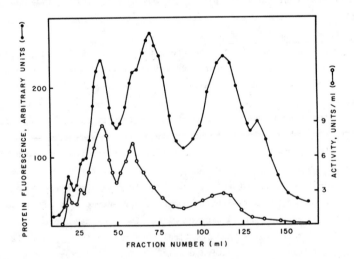

Fig. 1. Preparative electrophoresis of dihydrofolate reductase purified in the absence of DTT. The rapidly migrating enzyme species elute in the early fractions.

Although the elution profile is complex, two major classes of enzyme are apparent when the ratios of enzymic activity to protein fluorescence are considered. Those enzymes eluting before fraction 65 have a high ratio (S.A.) whereas the latter fractions have a low ratio. Thus, there may be as few as two forms of dihydrofolate reductase from which all the other species are generated. Since DTT was already shown to disrupt the aggregated enzyme species, the effect of having DTT present throughout the entire purification was examined. The enzyme was also purified more rapidly and in smaller amounts[21]. Under these conditions, only one enzymic species was observed on gel filtration, and electrophoresis of the enzyme showed two closely migrating protein bands (called form 1 and form 2). When the preparation was analyzed by preparative electrophoresis the pattern shown in Figure 2 was observed. Therefore, all

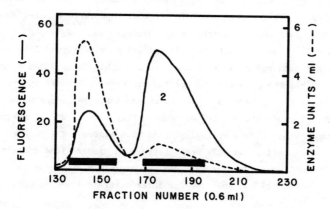

Fig. 2. Preparative electrophoresis of dihydrofolate reductase purified in the presence of DTT.

but two of the enzyme species seen in Figure 1 were generated during purification of the enzyme in the absence of a sulfhydryl protecting reagent.

Forms 1 and 2 are not interconvertible. Both forms 1 and 2 were observed on electrophoresis of crude cell extracts. They were also observed in extracts of (1) cloned cells harvested in early log, late log or stationary phase; (2) cells disrupted by sonication or French press; (3) cells grown in minimal or rich media; (4) cells grown in the presence of a subinhibitory level of trimethoprim. No interconversion between purified forms 1 and 2 was observed after 6-week storage pH 7, 24 hr at pH 2 or pH 10. Ultraviolet absorption spectra indicate the enzymes are free of 360 nm absorbing ligands (NADPH, dihydrofolate or folate).

Kinetic properties. The pH-activity profiles of forms 1 and 2 are strikingly different. Form 1 has a double pH optimum with similar enzymic activities at pH 4 and 7. Form 2 has no pH optimum. Its enzymic activity increases as the pH is decreased from 9 to 4. At pH 7 the turnover number of form 1 is about 15-fold greater than form 2; at pH 4 both forms have nearly equal turnover numbers (Table 1). The kinetic properties of forms 1 and 2 determined at pH 7 are also shown in Table 1.

The enzymes differ in their Km for dihydrofolate and Ki for trimethoprim (TMP) and pyrimethamine (PYR).

TABLE 1

KINETIC PROPERTIES OF FORMS 1 AND 2

	Apparent K_m (µM)		Apparent K_i (nM)		Turnover Number	
	FH_2	NADPH	TMP	PYR	pH 7	pH 4
FORM 1	8.9 ± 2.1	4.4 ± 1.0	1.3	200	1800	1107
FORM 2	0.65 ± 0.1	2.3 ± 0.5	106	1060	126	1155

Generation of other forms. Both forms 1 and 2 contain 2 moles sulfhydryl/mole enzyme and are stable in the presence of DTT. However, storage or heating in the absence of DTT results in the generation of two new electrophoretic species which have molecular weights of 18000, no detectable sulfhydryls, and are converted back to forms 1 and 2 by DTT. Thus, some of the multiplicity seen if Figure 1 is due to forms 1 and 2 and their oxidized counterparts called reducible forms 3 and 4, respectively. Prolonged heating or storage generates proteins with electrophoretic mobilities similar to reducible forms 3 and 4 but which cannot be converted back to forms 1 and 2 by DTT. These proteins, called nonreducible forms 3 and 4, are monomers and may represent higher enzyme sulfhydryl oxidation states. The high molecular weight aggregated enzyme species has only been observed in preparations containing nonreducible forms 3 and 4, and the aggregate can be completely disrupted to nonreducible forms 3 and 4 by DTT[21]. These complex interconversions are summarized in Figure 3.

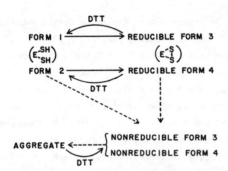

Fig. 3. Interconversion scheme for various forms of dihydrofolate reductase. Likely, but unproven, reactions shown by dashed arrows.

Trimethoprim binding. It was previously shown that there were two trimethoprim binding species of E. coli dihydrofolate reductase[22]. The two species, present in equal proportions, possessed one binding site per mole and had trimethoprim K_D values of 14 and 1400 nM respectively. Formation of the ternary complex with NADPH resulted in a single species with a trimethoprim K_D of 1.9 nM and interconversion of the two

species. Similar equilibrium dialysis experiments were repeated with pure forms 1
and 2. Form 1 has binary and ternary K_D values of 15 nM and 0.09 nM, respectively,
whereas the values for form 2 are 1000 nM and 4 nM, respectively. In each case,
there is 1 mole of ligand binding site/mole enzyme. These data are in agreement with
the kinetic determinations (Table 1) which also show that form 2 has a lower affinity
for trimethoprim than form 1. Although there is strong cooperativity upon binding
with NADPH, each species has a distinctly different ternary complex, and they are not
interconverted through the ternary complex.

    Structural studies. Antibodies, because of their sensitivity and high specifi-
city, are often used as structural probes among related proteins, and the degree of
cross reactivity is a function of the similarity of their 1°, 2° and 3° structures.
Rabbit antibody prepared against form 1 shows a strong cross reactivity with form
2. The 50% inhibitory titers (41 µL for form 1 and 68 µL for form 2) are within
experimental error. For example, the titer for the E. coli K12 enzyme is 70 µL,
whereas the more distantly related gonococcal and B. fragilis enzymes have titers of
780 and >1000 µL, respectively. The rat liver enzyme does not cross-react at all.

    Tryptic mapping of forms 1 and 2 gives even more conclusive evidence that they
have similar, but not identical, primary structures (Fig. 4). Form 2 has two yellow
ninhydrin fragments (Y), whereas form 1 has only one. Another form 1 fragment
(heavily shaded) is transposed to the hatched non-yellow fragment in the form 2 map.
t is likely that these peptides are a functional part of the active site, and their
modification leads to the markedly different kinetic properties of the isozymes.

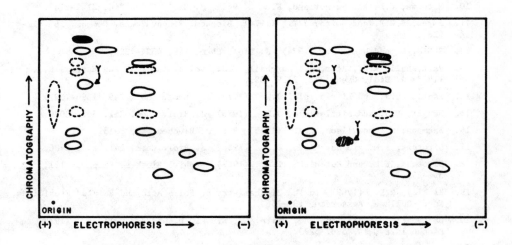

Fig. 4. Tryptic maps of form 1 (left panel) and form 2 (right panel) dihydrofolate
reductase. The light staining peptides are shown with dashed borders. Those fragments unique to form 2 are hatched; the fragment found only in form 1 is filled.

SUMMARY

Two species of E. coli dihydrofolate reductase (forms 1 and 2) are classified as genetically independent isozymes because of their differences in primary structure. Although they have distinct physical and kinetic properties, their physiological role is as yet unknown. A number of other enzyme species can be generated from forms 1 and 2 via sulfhydryl oxidations. Similar interconversion mechanisms should be considered in future examinations of the multiplicities observed with other bacterial and mammalian dihydrofolate reductases.

REFERENCES

1. Huennekens, F.M., Dunlap, R.B., Freisheim, J.H., Gundersen, L.E., Harding, N.G., Levison, S.A. and Mell G.P. (1971) Ann. N.Y. Acad. Sci. 186, 85-99.

2. Dunlap, R.B., Gundersen, L.E. and Huennekens, F.M. (1971) Biochem. Biophys. Res. Commun. 42, 772-777.

3. Perkins, J.P., Hillcoat, B.L. and Bertino, J.R. (1967) J. Biol. Chem. 242, 4771-4776.

4. Pastore, E.J., Plante, L.T. and Kisliuk, R.L. (1974) Methods Enzymol. 34B, 281-288.

5. Kaufman, B.T. and Kemerer, V.F. (1976) Arch. Biochem. Biophys. 172, 289-300.

6. Kaufman, B.T. and Kemerer, V.F. (1977) Arch. Biochem. Biophys. 179, 420-431.

7. Hiebert, M., Gauldie, J. and Hillcoat, B.L. (1972) Anal. Biochem. 46, 433-437.

8. Nixon, P.F. and Blakley, R.L. (1968) J. Biol. Chem. 243, 4722-4731.

9. Albrecht, A., Pearce, F.K., Suling, W.J. and Hutchison, D.J. (1969) Biochemistry, 8, 960-967.

10. Mathews, C.K. and Sutherland, K.E. (1965) J. Biol. Chem. 240, 2142-2147.

11. Amyes, S.G.B. and Smith, J.T. (1974) Biochem. Biophys. Res. Commun. 58, 412-418.

12. Sköld, O. and Widh. A. (1974) J. Biol. Chem. 249, 4324-4325.

13. Pattishall, K.H., Acar, J., Burchall, J.J., Goldstein, F.W. and Harvey, R.J. (1977) J. Biol. Chem. 252, 2319-2323.

14. Hängii, U.J. and Littlefield, J.W. (1974) J. Biol. Chem. 249, 1390-1397.

15. Hängii, U.J. and Littlefield, J.W. (1976) J. Biol. Chem. 251, 3075-3080.

16. Baumann, H. and Wilson, K.J. (1975) Eur. J. Biochem. 60, 9-15.

17. Sirotnak, F.M. and Hutchison, D.J. (1966) J. Biol. Chem. 241, 2900-2906.

18. Sirotnak, F.M. and Hutchison, D.J. (1967) Archiv. Biochem. Biophys. 121, 352-357.

19. Blakley, R.L. (1969) in The Biochemistry of Folic Acid and Related Pteridines, North-Holland, Amsterdam, 139-156.

20. Baccanari, D., Phillips, A., Smith, S., Sinski, D. and Burchall, J. (1975) Biochemistry, 14, 5267-5273.

21. Baccanari, D.P., Averett, D., Briggs, C. and Burchall, J. (1977) Biochemistry, 16, 3566-3572.

22. Pattishall, K., Burchall, J. and Harvey, R.J. (1976) J. Biol. Chem. 251, 7011-7020.

367

INVESTIGATION OF THE 5-FLUORODEOXYURIDYLATE: 5,10-METHYLENETETRAHYDRO-
FOLATE: THYMIDYLATE SYNTHETASE TERNARY COMPLEX BY ^{19}F NMR SPECTROSCOPY

R. A. BYRD, W. H. DAWSON, P. D. ELLIS, and R. B. DUNLAP
Department of Chemistry, University of South Carolina, Columbia, South Carolina 29208

Thymidylate synthetase mediates the 5,10-methylenetetrahydrofolate ($5,10\text{-}CH_2H_4$fo-
late)-dependent conversion of 2'-deoxyuridylate (dUMP) to form thymidylate and
7,8-dihydrofolate. Model studies of this reaction suggest that the initial step in
the catalytic mechanism is the attack of an active site nucleophile on carbon 6 of
the pyrimidine ring[1]. The carbanion generated in this process is then envisioned to
attack $5,10\text{-}CH_2H_4$folate or its cationic imine form to yield a transitory ternary complex (1a). Chemical modification of thymidylate synthetase with numerous sulfhydryl

1a, X = H

1b, X = F

R = 5'-phospho-2'-deoxyribose

group reagents has provided evidence supporting the role of a cysteine residue as a
catalytic nucleophile[1-3]. Interest in the initial steps of the catalytic mechanism
has been enlivened by the discovery that 5-fluorodeoxyuridylate (FdUMP), a potent inhibitor of thymidylate synthetase, interacts with the enzyme and $5,10\text{-}CH_2H_4$folate to
form stable, covalent ternary complexes whose proposed structure is 1b[1]. It is postulated that the enzyme functions with FdUMP in the initial stages of catalysis in a
manner quite analogous to its action with dUMP. The stability of the inhibitor-
cofactor-enzyme complexes compared with the transitory nature of the $dUMP\text{-}5,10\text{-}CH_2H_4$
folate-enzyme complex can be appreciated in terms of the tendency for the next stage
of the reaction to occur: proton abstraction from carbon 5 of the pyrimidyl ring of
the substrate-cofactor-enzyme transitory complexes should be facile while cleavage of
the C-F bond in the inhibitory ternary complex and removal of F^+ is highly unfavorable.

Using the understanding of the mechanism of action of thymidylate synthetase and
its inhibition by substituted pyrimidine nucleotides as a primary objective, a major
thrust of these laboratories has involved the physical and chemical characterization
of the formation and structure of the $FdUMP\text{-}5,10\text{-}CH_2H_4$folate-enzyme ternary complexes[3]. These investigations have employed gel electrophoresis, ion exchange chromatography, and radiolabeling techniques in the identification, separation, and determination of stoichiometry of the ternary complexes[4-5]. Further characterization of
the ternary complexes was performed with absorbance, circular dichroic, and fluorescence methods[6]. Our investigations have provided evidence for an average of 1.7

active sites per enzyme dimer and have shown that modification of catalytic sulfhydryl groups is correlated directly with the loss in both enzyme activity and the extent of ternary complex formation[3].

In order to understand the catalytic mechanism in more detail and, in particular, to elucidate the initial steps more fully, we have investigated the structure of the ternary complex by ^{19}F nmr[7-8]. When the binding of FdUMP in the native ternary complex was studied with ^{19}F nmr, a 12.4 ppm chemical shift of the 5-fluoro substituent towards increased shielding was observed. Using comparable analyses of model compounds (5-fluoro-6-methoxy-5,6-dihydrouracil and 5-fluoro-6-methoxy-5-methyl-5,6-dihydrouracil), it is possible to interpret the latter chemical shift as reflecting the result of attack by an enzyme-bound nucleophile at carbon 6 of the pyrimidinyl ring followed by the attachment of the methylene group of 5,10-CH$_2$H$_4$folate at carbon-5 of FdUMP. Verification of this interpretation was obtained indirectly by loss of H-F coupling (unresolved) and directly by observing a ^{13}C-^{19}F coupling constant when ternary complex was formed using cofactor prepared with dideuteroformaldehyde and ^{13}C-(90% enriched)-dideuteroformaldehyde, respectively. For example, comparison of the ^{19}F nmr spectrum of ternary complex containing 5,10-CD$_2$H$_4$folate with the spectrum obtained with the isotopically normal species indicated a decreased linewidth for the former system, which, in turn, readily demonstrated that the alkyl substituent at carbon 5 of the pyrimidine is the methylene group of the cofactor. Further, the experimentally determined magnitude for J_{HF} suggested that the methylene group in the native ternary complex is motionally restricted, a result which is consistent with the specific orientation in which reacting groups are expected to be held at the enzymic active site.

The ^{19}F nmr spectrum obtained from ternary complex following denaturation in the presence of 1% sodium dodecyl sulfate exhibited a single resonance with a chemical shift of 1.9 ppm shielded with respect to free FdUMP; this result agrees very well with the ^{19}F chemical shift reported by Santi et al.[9] for an FdUMP-containing peptide recovered from a Pronase digestion of ternary complex. Sharpening of the ^{19}F resonance upon denaturation occurred in concurrence with the greater mobility of the denatured ternary complex. However, in light of the 10.5 ppm shift of the ^{19}F resonance toward deshielding following denaturation of the ternary complex and the similarity of the position of the resulting resonance to that of free FdUMP, it was necessary to confirm that the methylene group was still attached at carbon 5 of the pyrimidine ring. Measurement of a carbon-fluorine spin-spin coupling constant, geminal J_{CF}, through linewidth studies of ^{19}F nmr spectra of ternary complexes containing either 5,10-CD$_2$H$_4$folate or 5,10-^{13}CD$_2$H$_4$folate in both the native and denatured states gave similar values, thus indicating that with the denatured enzyme the ternary complex remains intact.

In attempting to account for the shift observed on denaturation of the ternary complex, the possible effects of conformational change in the pyrimidine ring were considered. The carbonyl groups of 5,6-dihydrouracil derivatives are known to possess trigonal geometry which imparts a half-chair conformation to this portion of the ring[10], such that the substituents at the 5 and 6 positions are staggered relative to one another, as found in substituted cyclohexanes. A structure of this geometry could be envisioned to undergo a simple ring inversion which corresponds to a rotation about the 5,6-carbon-carbon bond and which interchanges the relative axial and equitorial positions of the substituents. The two isomers of the pyrimidine ring in the ternary complex which would correspond to such a conformational change are shown below in a configuration in which the methylene group of the cofactor and the sulfhydryl group of the enzyme are _trans_ to one another.

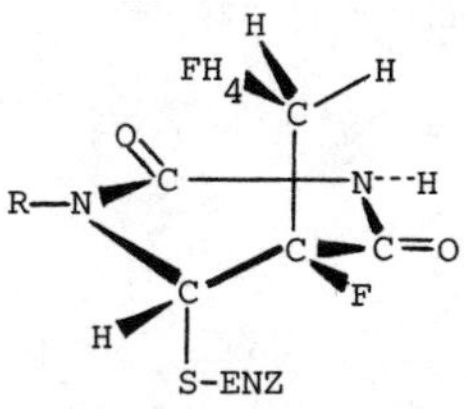

Native Ternary Complex 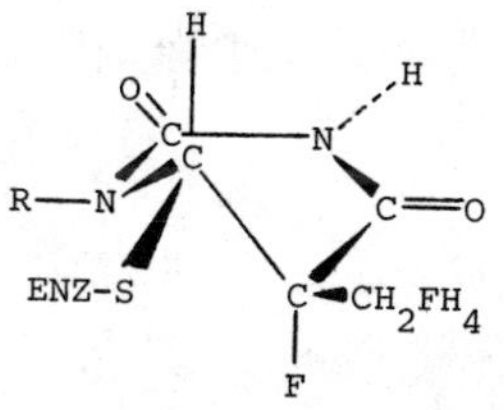   Denatured Ternary Complex

R = 2'-deoxyribosyl 5'-phosphate

Indirect measurement of the ^{1}H-^{19}F coupling constants to both the CH_2 of cofactor and H_6 of the pyrimidine ring (using deuterium differencing) and application of the Karplus-type relationship enabled a detailed representation of the relative spatial orientations of the groups on the pyrimidine 5,6-bond to be derived. In native ternary complex one proton of the methylene group of 5,10-methylenetetrahydrofolate is _trans_ to the fluorine while the other is _gauche_. The proton at C-6 of the nucleotide and the fluorine are in a _pseudo-trans_-diequatorial relationship (ie. the cysteine and the methylene group must be _trans_-diaxial). Denaturation alters this arrangement such that the fluorine and the C-6 proton are _trans_-diaxial. The details of these investigations are currently _in press_[8].

ACKNOWLEDGEMENTS

This research was supported by National Institutes of Health grants CA15645 and CA12842 from the National Cancer Institute. Support by the American Cancer Society through a Faculty Research Award (FRA-144) to R. B. Dunlap and the Alfred P. Sloan Fellowship to P. D. Ellis is greatly appreciated.

REFERENCES

1. Danenberg, P. V. (1977) Biochim. Biophys. Acta, 473, 73-92.
2. Dunlap, R. B., Harding, N. G. L. and Huennekens (1971) Biochemistry, 10, 88-97.

3. Plese, P. C. and Dunlap, R. B. (1977) J. Biol. Chem., 252, 6139-6144.

4. Aull, J. L., Lyon, J. A. and Dunlap, R. B. (1974) Microchem. J., 19, 210-218.

5. Aull, J. L., Lyon, J. A. and Dunlap, R. B. (1974) Arch. Biochem. Biophys., 165, 805-808.

6. Donato, H., Aull, J. L., Lyon, J. A., Reinsch, J. W. and Dunlap, R. B. (1976) J. Biol. Chem., 251, 1303-1310.

7. Byrd, R. A., Dawson, W. H., Ellis, P. D. and Dunlap, R. B. (1977) J. Am. Chem. Soc., 99, 6139-6141.

8. Byrd, R. A., Dawson, W. H., Ellis, P. D. and Dunlap, R. B., J. Am. Chem. Soc., in press.

9. Santi, D. V., Pogolotti, A. L., James, T. L., Wataya, Y., Ivanetich, K. M. and Lam, S. L. (1976) in Biochemistry Involving Carbon-Fluorine Bonds, Filler, R., ed., American Chemical Society, Washington, D.C., pp. 63-66.

10. James, M. N. G. and Matsushima, M. (1976) Acta Cryst., B32, 957.

Kisliuk/Brown, eds. Chemistry and Biology of Pteridines

PURIFICATION OF GLYCINEAMIDE RIBONUCLEOTIDE TRANSFORMYLASE*

C.A. Caperelli†, G. Chettur, L. Lin-Kosley, and S.J. Benkovic
Department of Chemistry, The Pennsylvania State University, University Park, PA 16802

INTRODUCTION

Glycineamide ribonucleotide transformylase (5,10-methenyltetrahydrofolate: 2-amino-N-ribosylacetamide-5'-phosphate formyltransferase, EC 2.1.2.2), an enzyme of the purine biosynthetic pathway which utilizes 5,10-methenyltetrahydrofolate as cofactor for the transfer of a one-carbon unit at the formate level of oxidation (Eq.1),

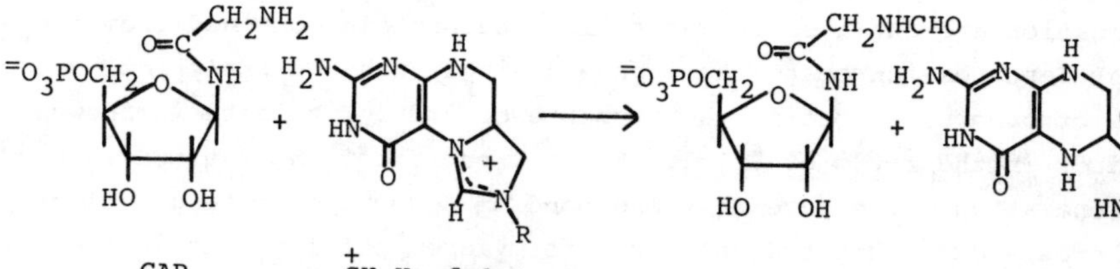
GAR
$\overset{+}{C}H$-H_4-folate
FGAR
H_4-folate
R = p-aminobenzoyl glutamate

(Eq.1)

has been purified 240-fold from chicken liver.[1] Purification of the GAR-transformylase resulted in concommitant enrichment of 10-formyltetrahydrofolate synthetase, 5,10-methenyltetrahydrofolate cyclohydrolase, and 5,10-methylenetetrahydrofolate dehydrogenase. A modified purification resulted in enrichment of two additional folate activities, 5-aminoimidazolecarboxamide ribonucleotide transformylase and serine transhydroxymethylase. A discussion of the properties of the transformylase and the possible in vivo association of the folate enzymes with the transformylase are described herein.

STEREOCHEMISTRY AND STOICHIOMETRY OF 5,10-METHENYLTETRAHYDROFOLATE UTILIZATION BY GAR-TRANSFORMYLASE

The stereochemical and stoichiometric experiments were performed with chemically prepared (±)-L-$^{14}\overset{+}{C}H$-H_4-folate[2] and with (+)-L-$^{14}\overset{+}{C}H$-H_4-folate derived from enzymatically prepared[3] (-)-L-H_4-folate. The stereochemical reactions were run with an excess of substrate and

*Abbreviated as GAR-transformylase.
†Postdoctoral Fellow of the Damon Runyon-Walter Winchell Cancer Fund, 4/1/76-3/31/78.

either the chemically or enzymatically prepared cofactor as the
limiting reagent. The reaction solutions were chromatographed on
QAE-Sephadex to separate radiolabeled product from any excess radiolabeled cofactor. Identification of ^{14}C-FGAR was made by an assay for
sugar and by its co-elution with authentic FGAR by paper chromatography. For the determination of stoichiometry, an aliquot of the
reaction was assayed for H_4-folate[4] and this was compared to the
production of ^{14}C-FGAR isolated by ion-exchange chromatography.

RESULTS AND DISCUSSION
Enzyme Purification

The purification of GAR transformylase is summarized in Table I.
The ratios of specific activities for the four folate enzymes,
designated A, B, C and D, during the course of transformylase purification are outlined in Table II. The protein obtained from the
GAR-Sepharose chromatography gave a single band on analytical gel
electrophoresis, but in the presence of dodecyl sulfate it showed two
bands in the ratio of 1.7:1. Further purification resulted in a
preparation which gave only one band on dodecyl sulfate gel electrophoresis and exhibited only transformylase activity. As in the case
of the B, C and D activities isolated from sheep[5] and porcine[6] liver
and from yeast[7], a single trifunctional protein, designated formyl-
methenyl-methylenetetrahydrofolate synthetase (combined), appears to
be responsible for these three catalytic activities.

Sucrose density gradient ultracentrifugation[8] indicated a
molecular weight of 100,000 for the transformylase and 160,000 for
the trifunctional protein. Molecular weights of 201,000; 218,000;
and 150,000 have been reported for the trifunctional protein from
sheep liver[5], porcine liver[6] and yeast[7], respectively. Subunit molecular weights were estimated from dodecyl sulfate gel electrophoresis[9]
as 63,000 for transformylase and 83,000 for the trifunctional protein,
consistent with homodimeric structures.

The modified purification procedure resulted in a preparation
which exhibited four bands on dodecyl sulfate gel electrophoresis and
the additional two folate activities, 5-aminoimidazolecarboxamide
ribonucleotide transformylase and serine transhydroxymethylase, after
GAR-Sepharose chromatography. Omission of the Sephadex G-100
chromatography, which resulted in the appearance of these additional
activities, suggests that they are more loosely associated with the
transformylase than is the trifunctional protein.

TABLE I

PURIFICATION OF GAR TRANSFORMYLASE

Purification Step		Vol. (ml)	Units[a]	Units/mg	Purification
1.	Homogenate supernatant	400	87.5	0.0032	1.0
2.	Protamine sulfate supernatant	500	88.5	0.0065	2.0
3.	Ammonium sulfate 40-55%	250	81.5	0.0113	3.5
4.	Bio-Gel HTP	55	61.1	0.0417	13.0
5.	Sephadex G-100[b]	110	30.1	0.0465	14.3
6.	Bio-Gel HTP (MgATP)[c]	40	22.2	0.0981	31.0
7.	GAR-Sepharose[d]	2	0.63	0.7616	238.0
6a.	DEAE-Cellulose[e]	4	3.59	0.146	45.0
7a.	GAR-Sepharose[f]	8	0.088	1.294	404.0

[a]Units are expressed as micromoles per minute.

[b]Approximately 50% of the total protein was removed by this step. The specific activity (hence, the yield) is low due to high phosphate inhibition of the transformylase assay.[10]

[c]75% of the G-100 fraction was applied to the HTP column, hence the yield of this column is 98%.

[d]A small portion of the HTP fraction was chromatographed on GAR-Sepharose.

[e]25% of the G-100 fraction was chromatographed on DEAE-Cellulose.

[f]A small portion of the DEAE-Cellulose fraction was applied to the GAR-Sepharose.

Stereochemistry and Stoichiometry of 5,10-Methenyltetrahydrofolate Utilization by GAR Transformylase

Even after prolonged incubation, GAR-transformylase used only half of the diastereomeric mixture which comprises the chemically prepared cofactor, in contrast to an earlier report.[11] Isolation and recycling of the remaining ^{14}CH-H_4-folate yielded no further conversion of GAR to ^{14}C-FGAR as depicted in Figure 1. Complete utilization of $(+)$-L^{14}CH-H_4-folate is also shown. Comparison of the amount of ^{14}C-FGAR formed in the reaction to the amount of H_4-folate produced showed a ratio of 1.2:1.0 indicating that one FGAR is produced for each CH-H_4-folate utilized.

374

Viability of Associated Activities for Providing 5,10-Methenyltetrahydrofolate

In order to test whether the trifunctional protein could provide a source of $5,10\text{-}\overset{+}{CH}\text{-}H_4$-folate for the transformylase, a series of reactions were run in the presence of GAR employing the substrates for the trifunctional protein, as depicted in Equation 2, and analyzed for the production of FGAR.

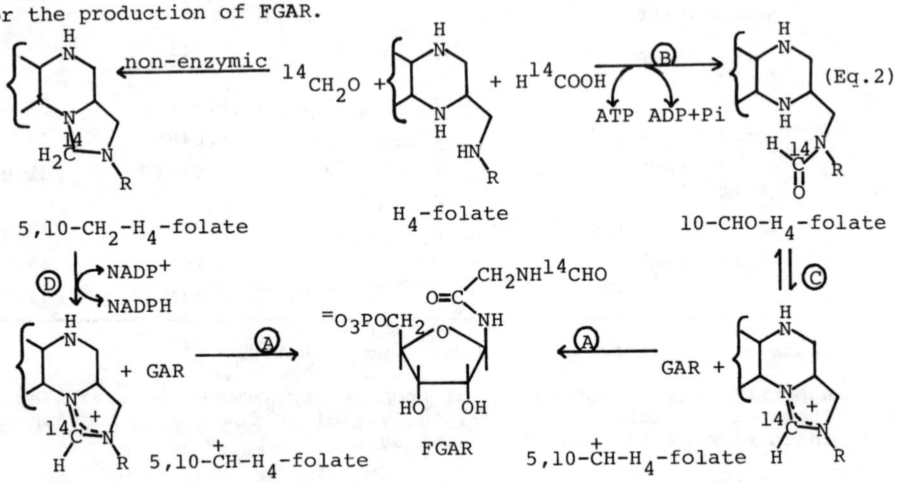

$$\text{(Eq.2)}$$

5,10-CH$_2$-H$_4$-folate   H$_4$-folate   10-CHO-H$_4$-folate

+ GAR   FGAR   GAR +

$5,10\text{-}\overset{+}{CH}\text{-}H_4$-folate $5,10\text{-}\overset{+}{CH}\text{-}H_4$-folate

Figure 2 depicts the results obtained through the use of 10-formylsynthetase and cyclohydrolase (B and C) and the dehydrogenase (non-enzymic and D), in addition to the elution profile for the reaction commencing with GAR and $^{14}\overset{+}{CH}\text{-}H_4$-folate and a control where GAR was omitted. These results indicate that ^{14}C-FGAR and, by inference, $^{14}\overset{+}{CH}\text{-}H_4$-folate could be produced by the trifunctional protein and may reflect a metabolically advantageous in vivo association of these two proteins.

SUMMARY

GAR transformylase has been purified 240-fold from chicken liver along with formyl-methenyl-methylenetetrahydrofolate synthetase (combined). The transformylase has been shown to be specific for the $(+)\text{-L-}\overset{+}{CH}\text{-}H_4$-folate and produces one mole of product per mole of cofactor utilized. The ability of the trifunctional protein to produce cofactor for the transformylase suggests a possible in vivo association of these enzymes which catalyze $\overset{+}{CH}\text{-}H_4$-folate synthesis and require this cofactor for a one carbon unit transfer, thus offering a solution for the efficient utilization of the hydrolytically labile $\overset{+}{CH}\text{-}H_4$-folate.

TABLE II

SPECIFIC ACTIVITY RATIOS FOR THE FOLATE ACTIVITIES

Purification Step		Specific Activity Ratios[a]		
		B/A	C/A	D/A
1.	Homogenate supernatant	9.2	6.7	2.1
2.	Protamine sulfate supernatant	8.6	3.9	2.6
3.	Ammonium sulfate 40-55%	16.2[b]	4.8	2.6
4.	Bio-Gel HTP	9.0	3.7	2.4
5.	Sephadex G-100	19.9[b]	4.9	2.2
6.	Bio-Gel HTP (MgATP)	6.4	3.6	2.1
7.	GAR-Sepharose	0.84	1.04	1.03
6a.	DEAE-Cellulose	0.26	0.48	0.12
7a.	GAR-Sepharose	0	0	0

[a]The four folate activities are: A, glycineamide ribonucleotide trans-formylase; B, 10-formyltetrahydrofolate synthetase; C, 5,10-methenyl-tetrahydrofolate cyclohydrolase; and D, 5,10-methylenetetrahydro-folate dehydrogenase.

[b]10-formyltetrahydrofolate synthetase activity is enhanced by NH_4^+ and K^+.[12]

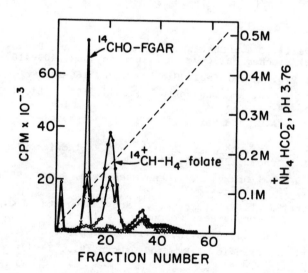

Fig. 1. Elution profiles for stereochemical experiments. GAR + (±)-L-^{14}CH-H_4-folate, (–•—•–); recycling of remaining (±)-L-^{14}CH-H_4-folate, (–o—o–); and GAR + (+)-L-^{14}CH-H_4-folate, (–x—x–).

376

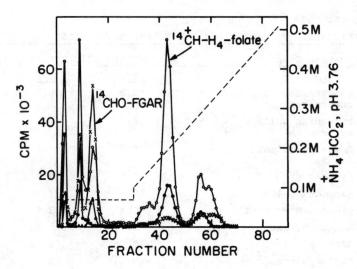

Fig. 2. Elution profiles for flow-through experiments. GAR + $^{14}CH-$
H_4-folate, (-o—o-); $H^{14}COOH + H_4$-folate, (-x-x-); $^{14}CH_2O + H_4$-folate,
(-▲-▲-); and control, $^{14}CH-H_4$-folate, GAR omitted (-●-●-).

ACKNOWLEDGEMENT

This work was supported by a grant from the Public Health
Service (GM 24129).

REFERENCES

1. Caperelli, C.A., Chettur, G., Lin, L.Y., and Benkovic, S.J.
    (1978) Biochem. Biophys. Res. Commun., 82, 403-410.

2. Rowe, P.B. (1968) Anal. Biochem., 22, 166-168.

3. Mathews, C.K. and Huennekens, F.M. (1960) J. Biol. Chem., 235,
    3304-3308.

4. Bratton. A.C. and Marshall, E.K. (1939) J. Biol. Chem., 128,
    537-550.

5. Paukert, J.L., Straus, L. D'A., and Rabinowitz, J.C. (1976)
    J. Biol. Chem., 25, 5104-5111.

6. Tan, L.U.L., Drury, E.J., and MacKenzie, R.E. (1977) J. Biol.
    Chem., 252, 1117-1122.

7. Paukert, J.L., Williams, G.R., and Rabinowitz, J.C. (1977)
    Biochem. Biophys, Res. Commun., 77, 147-154.

8. Martin, R.C. and Ames, B.N. (1961) J. Biol. Chem., 236, 1372-1379.

9. Weber, K., Pringle, J.R., and Osborn, M.J. (1972) Methods in
    Enzymol, 26, 3-27.

10. Lin, L.Y. (1978) Ph.D. Thesis, The Pennsylvania State University.

11. Warren, L. and Buchanan, J.M. (1957) J. Biol. Chem., 229, 613-625.

12. Himes, R.H. and Harmony, J.A.K. (1973), CRC Crit. Rev. in Biochem,
    501-535.

HUMAN THYMIDYLATE SYNTHETASE:

ACTIONS OF FOLATE AND METHOTREXATE ANALOGS

YUNG-CHI CHENG, DANIEL W. SZETO AND BRUCE J. DOLNICK

Department of Experimental Therapeutics, Roswell Park Memorial Institute, New York
State Department of.Health, Buffalo, New York 14263

ANDRE ROSOWSKY, CHENG-SEIN YU AND E.J. MODEST

Division of Medicinal Chemistry and Pharmacology, Sidney Farber Cancer Institute,
Harvard Medical School, Boston, Massachusetts 02115

J.R. PIPER, C. TEMPLE, JR., R.D. ELLIOTT, J.D. ROSE AND J.A. MONTGOMERY

Kettering-Meyer Laboratory, Southern Research Institute, Birmingham, Alabama 35205

INTRODUCTION

Thymidylate synthetase (E.C.2.1.1.b), an enzyme which catalyzes the de novo
biosynthesis of TMP, has been considered as an important target for cancer chemotherapy[1]. We have recently purified and characterized this enzyme derived from the
peripheral blast cells of several acute leukemic patients[2]. The properties of TMP
synthetase derived from different individuals appear to be the same with respect to their
physical and kinetic properties. On the other hand, thymidylate synthetase derived from
other sources[3,4,5] showed several qualitative differences. This paper summarizes the
studies of the effects of various folate and MTX analogs on human thymidylate synthetase
activity. These studies may serve as the basis for designing and synthesizing new folate
analogs which express inhibitory actions on TMP synthetase.

MATERIALS AND METHODS

Chemicals. MTX and folate analogs were prepared as described[2,6-12]. All other
chemicals were of reagent grade.

Enzyme Preparation and Assay. Thymidylate synthetase was purified from blast cells
of patients with acute myelocytic leukemia as described by Dolnick and Cheng[1]. The
enzyme was assayed by the tritium release procedure of Roberts[13] as described[2,6,7].
Ki determination and multiple inhibitor studies were performed as described[2,6].

RESULTS

I. Kinetic Evidence Supporting the Hypothesis that Two Types of Folate Binding
Sites Occur on Human Thymidylate Synthetase.

1. Methotrexate (MTX) is a non-competitive and 10-methylfolate (10-CH_3-
Pte-Glu) is a competitive inhibitor with respect to the natural substrate
5,10-CH_2-H_4PteGlu.

2. Multiple inhibitor studies indicate that neither MTX nor $10\text{-}CH_3\text{-}PteGlu$ could antagonize the action of one another on human thymidylate synthetase.

3. Dihydrofolate ($H_2PteGlu$), a non-competitive inhibitor for thymidylate synthetase with respect to $5,10\text{-}CH_2\text{-}H_4PteGlu$, competes with MTX, but does not antagonize the action of $10\text{-}CH_3\text{-}PteGlu$. This data suggests that $10\text{-}CH_3\text{-}PteGlu$ and MTX can bind to the enzyme simultaneously without interfering with each other's action.

II. The Kinetic Values of Polyglutamate vs. Monoglutamate Derivatives of $5,10\text{-}CH_2\text{-}$Pte for Thymidylate Synthetase.

Substrate	Vmax	Km (μM)
$5,10\text{-}CH_2\text{-}H_4PteGlu$	100%	31 ± 8.3
$5,10\text{-}CH_2\text{-}H_4Pte(Glu)_5$	200%	2.2 ± 0.1

The polyglutamate residue is shown to enhance the substrate binding affinity by an approximately 14-fold decrease in Km value and by a 2-fold increase in turnover rate.

III. Inhibition of TMPS by Various Folate Analogs

Inhibition studies were conducted with folate analogs having either a 4-amino or 4-hydroxyl group, a methyl, formyl or no substitution at the N-10 position, and at various stages of reduction of the pteridine ring. Some of the results are shown in Table 1.

TABLE 1

Compound	K_i (μM)	Variable Substrate			
		$5,10\text{-}CH_2\text{-}H_4PteGlu$		$5,10\text{-}CH_2\text{-}H_4Pte(Glu)_5$	
		Inhibition[a]		K_i (μM)	Inhibition
PteGlu	4×10^1	C		------	------
$10\text{-}CH_3\text{-}PteGlu$	1	C		1.2	C
Methotrexate	2.8×10^1	N.C.		1.7×10^1	N.C.
Aminopterin	2.9×10^2	N.C.		------	------
$Pte(Glu)_5$	$2^{[b]}$, $13^{[c]}$	N.C.		------	------
$H_2Pte(Glu)_5$	------	----		6	N.C.
$5,8\text{-}Dideaza\text{-}10\text{-}CH_3$ $PteGlu^{[d]}$	$0.11^{[b]}$, $0.21^{[c]}$	N.C.		------	------
$5,8\text{-}DideazaPteGlu^{[d]}$	0.78	N.C.		------	------

The experimental details are described in reference #6.

[a] C stands for a competitive inhibitor; N.C. stands for a non-competitive inhibitor.

[b] K_i slope.

[c] K_i intercept.

[d] D. Szeto and Y.C. Cheng, "unpublished data."

Substitution of the 4-hydroxyl by a 4-amino group in the folate molecule not only increased the K_i value about one order of magnitude but also changed the mode of inhibition from competitive to non-competitive with respect to $5,10\text{-}CH_2\text{-}H_4PteGlu$. This effect was observed regardless of whether a 10-methyl group is present. Reduction of the pteridine ring to the dihydro level could also change the type of inhibition; this was exemplified by PteGlu and $H_2PteGlu$. However, the reduction of $10\text{-}CH_3\text{-}PteGlu$ to $10\text{-}CH_3\text{-}H_2PteGlu$ did not result in the change of a competitive to a non-competitive type of inhibition. 5,8-DideazaPteGlu and $5,8\text{-dideaza-}10\text{-}CH_3\text{-}PteGlu$ had K_i values approximately one order of magnitude lower than their parent compounds, PteGlu and $10\text{-}CH_3\text{-}PteGlu$. $5,8\text{-Dideaza-}10\text{-}CH_3\text{-}PteGlu$ was found to have inhibitory effects on the growth of HeLa cells in culture even at the concentration of $0.5\,\mu M$.

IV. Inhibition of TMPS by Positional Isomers and MTX Homologs.

The glutamyl moiety of MTX is essential for binding. Substitution of the glutamyl moiety by various amino acids, such as β-aminoglutaric acid, α-aminoadipic acid and α-aminopimelic acid, had little effect on binding affinity. The data presented in Table 2 suggest that the absolute requirement for binding is the presence of a free carboxyl group in the approximate vicinity of the α-carboxyl of the glutamate side chain.

V. Inhibition of TMPS by Esters and Amides of MTX.

The importance of a free α-carboxyl group on the glutamate moiety was demonstrated by the drastic loss of inhibitory activity on esterification or amidation of the α-carboxyl group (Table 2). A 4- to 5-fold decrease in binding affinity was observed with MTX α-monoamide and MTX α-monobutyl ester (data not shown). However, derivatization of the γ-carboxylate of the glutamate side chain resulted in little change in binding affinity.

VI. Inhibition of TMPS by Peptide Derivatives of MTX.

Attachment of a free aspartate or glutamate residue to the γ-carboxyl group of MTX via a peptide bond increased the binding affinity of MTX to the enzyme by 5-fold and 8-fold (Table 2), respectively. In contrast, the α-glutamyl derivative of MTX gave the same level of inhibition as MTX. Conjugation of diethyl glutamate at the α-carboxyl of MTX resulted in a drastic loss of activity. On the other hand, conjugation of diethyl glutamate at the γ-carboxyl group resulted in a small loss of binding affinity.

TABLE 2

(continued)

R_1	R_2	TMP Synthetase K_i (μM)
-OH	-OH	30
$-OC_4H_9$	-OH	220
-OH	$-OC_4H_9\text{-}\underline{n}$	40
$-OC_2H_5$	$-OC_2H_5$	200
-Glu	-OH	30
-Asp	-OH	68
-diethyl Glu	-OH	450
-OH	-Glu	4
-OH	-Asp	6
-OH	-diethyl Glu	67
-diethyl Glu	-diethyl Glu	940

$*$ K_i determinations are described in reference #7.

CONCLUSION

1. For both site A and site B, increasing the number of glutamyl residues on folate or MTX derivatives increases their binding affinities.

2. Substitution of hydrogen for a methyl group in N^{10} position of folate or aminopterin enhances binding to both site A and site B.

3. For MTX analogs:
   a. The glutamyl moiety of MTX is essential for binding.
   b. A free α-carboxyl group on the glutamyl moiety or a free carboxyl group in that vicinity is essential for binding.
   c. Conjugation of aspartyl group at γ-carboxyl of MTX also enhances binding.
   d. Reduction of MTX to H_2MTX increases inhibitory potency by 6-fold and further reduction to H_4MTX increases potency an additional 1.4-fold.

4. Modification of the pteridine ring of PteGlu by replacing the nitrogen in N^5 and N^8 positions with carbon increases the binding by approximately one order of magnitude.

Based on the data obtained, a few interesting compounds can be postulated as potential inhibitors of thymidylate synthetase. For instance, γ-glycine MTX, a peptide derivative, is a candidate which may have a high affinity for thymidylate synthetase while being resistant to conjugase activity. Recently, this compound has been synthesized by Montgomery and co-workers. Biological testing with regard to transport and conjugase resistance is being conducted in their laboratory.

ACKNOWLEDGEMENT

This work was supported in part by Research Project Grants CA-14078 and CA-18499, by Cancer Center Grant CA-06516 and by Contract No. 1-CM43762 all from the National Cancer Institute, and by Grant CH-23 and CH-29 from the American Cancer Society.

REFERENCES

1. Danenberg, P.V. (1977) Biochim. Biophys. Acta, 473, 73.

2. Dolnick, B.J. and Cheng, Y-C. (1977) J. Biol. Chem. 251, 7697.

3. Greenberg, D.M., Nath, R. and Humphreys, G.K. (1961) J. Biol. Chem. 236, 2271.

4. Fridland, A., Langenbach, R.J. and Heidelberg, C. (1971) J. Biol. Chem., 246, 7110.

5. Gupta, V.S. and Meldrum, J.B. (1972) Can. J. Biochem., 50, 352.

6. Dolnick, B.J. and Cheng, Y-C. (1978) J. Biol. Chem., 253, 3563.

7. Szeto, D.W. "et. al." (1978) Biochemical Pharmacology, submitted.

8. Rosowsky, A. (1973) J. Med. Chem., 16, 1190.

9. Rosowsky, A. (1975) Abstracts of Papers, 25th IUPAC Congress, Jerusalem, Israel, July 6-11, pp. 228.

10. Rosowsky, A., Ensminger, W.D., Lazarus, H. and Yu, C.-S. (1977) J. Med. Chem., 20, 925.

11. Rosowsky, A. and Yu, C.-S., (1978) J. Med. Chem., 21, 170.

12. Montgomery, J.A., "et. al." "unpublished data."

13. Roberts, D. (1966) Biochemistry, 5, 3546.

NMR STUDIES OF ^{13}C LABELED DIHYDROFOLATE REDUCTASE

LENNIE COCCO, RAYMOND L. BLAKLEY, ROBERT E. LONDON[*], JOHN P. GROFF, THOMAS E. WALKER[*]
AND NICHOLAS A. MATWIYOFF[*]
Department of Biochemistry, University of Iowa, Iowa City, Iowa 52242
Los Alamos Scientific Laboratory, University of California, Los Alamos, New
Mexico 87545 (*)

ABSTRACT

Results of ^{13}C NMR studies of dihydrofolate reductase containing ^{13}C labeled
arginine, methionine or tryptophan are discussed. Several spin-labeled ligands
have been used to indicate residues in the proximity of the binding site.

INTRODUCTION

Dihydrofolate reductase (DHFR), is the target in cancer chemotherapy of almost
irreversible inhibition by the substrate analog methotrexate (MTX). Studies
of the enzyme from both mammalian and bacterial sources have revealed important
information concerning the structure and mechanism of this enzyme.

A relatively new technique for the study of protein structure, involving the use
of NMR to monitor specifically labeled amino acids of the protein, has been used
as part of our continuing study of DHFR.[1-5] Isoenzyme II has been purified from
Streptococcus faecium var. Durans strain A grown on medium containing ^{13}C labeled
Arg, Met or Trp. ^{13}C NMR spectra of the labeled enzymes, alone and in complexes
with ligands, provide information about the molecular motions of the amino acids
involved and of the overall protein structure.

MATERIALS AND METHODS

The enzymes were isolated from *S. faecium var. Durans* strain A grown on a medium
containing [*guanidino*-^{13}C]arginine or [*methyl*-^{13}C]methionine or [γ-^{13}C]tryptophan by
published procedures[1,2]. The various spin labeled ligands were prepared as described
in ref. 6 (compound I) and ref. 7 (compounds II - V).

The ^{13}C NMR spectra were obtained with a Varian XL-100-15 at 25.2 MHz in the
Fourier transform mode. The enzyme was at a concentration of 0.6 to 1.0 mM in
50 mM potassium phosphate buffer, pH 7.3, containing 0.5 M KCl. The arginine enzyme samples were in 99% D_2O buffer while the methionine and the tryptophan enzyme
samples were in buffer containing 10% D_2O. Ligand concentrations were such that
the enzyme was more than 95% saturated.

RESULTS AND DISCUSSION

Fig. 1 shows that up to six guanidino ^{13}C resonances spanning 1.2 ppm have been resolved for the eight Arg. residues, seven methyl ^{13}C resonances spanning 3 ppm have been resolved for the seven Met residues and four indole ^{13}C resonances spanning 5.4 ppm have been resolved for the four Trp residues of the enzyme. The ^{13}C NMR spectra mostly exhibit narrow resonances, and information obtained from the spectra, such as the chemical shifts and spin-lattice relaxation times (T_1), can be interpreted in terms of the conformational states of the enzyme and the interactions of the ^{13}C labeled residues with bound ligands.

Spectra of the [^{13}C]Arg-labeled DHFR indicate two classes of Arg residues. T_1 studies in D_2O and in H_2O provide evidence that residues of the first class (5 of 8 Arg) have a significant degree of internal motion and are probably accessible to solvent. The remaining 3 arginines exhibit shorter T_1 values which vary inversely with temperature, and smaller values for the nuclear Overhauser enhancement (NOE). This indicates that the internal motion of these residues is slow relative to the overall rotational motion of the protein and is consistent with relative inaccessibility to solvent. Chemical shift data of ligand complexes suggest assignment of the furthest upfield peak to Arg-44 and changes produced by pteridine binding may be due to COOH interactions with Arg-32 and 58.[1,3]

Spectra of the Met-labeled enzyme and simulation of the spectra of several complexes gave linewidth, NOE and T_1 values. These indicated that in addition to rapid rotation of the methyl group about its axis, rotation occurs about the CH_2-S bond but the methyl group oscillates through a relatively narrow angular range ($\sim$90° and $\sim$180°). The large downfield shift of one Met resonance (at least 1.7 ppm) upon binding of NADP$^+$ is probably due to a combination of the nicotinamide ring currents and a proposed charge transfer between the nicotinamide ring and the Met sulfur. From preliminary studies on carboxymethylated DHFR, tentative assignment of two resonances shifted upfield by MTX binding have been made to Met-28 and Met-50 in the *S. faecium* sequence.

In the spectrum of the Trp-labeled enzyme there are two unusual resonances: One broadened and showing a large upfield shift and the other a double resonance. Each corresponds to one of the four labeled residues. The effects of temperature on the chemical shift and linewidth of these unusual resonances confirms that each corresponds to a residue undergoing slow exchange between alternative stable conformations[6]. These conformational transitions of the Trp residues may involve a large part of the DHFR. The sharpening of the upfield shifted resonance in the presence of several ligands (Fig. 1 and ref. 5) is consistent with the exchange process and suggests that they lock the residues (and possibly the enzyme) into one conformation. Since chemical modification of Trp 21 inactivates the *L. casei* DHFR[8] and this residue is conserved in all reductase sequences investigated, this residue

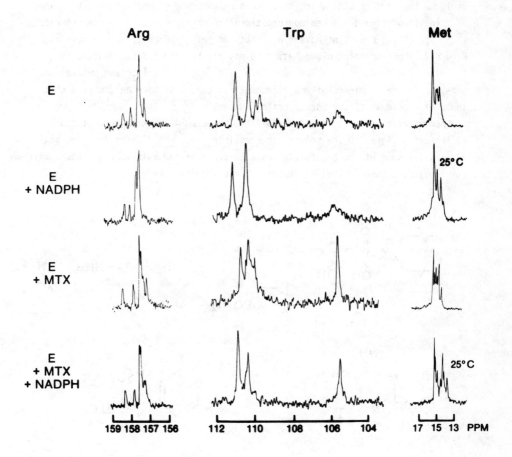

Figure 1. ^{13}C NMR spectra of dihydrofolate reductase containing [*guanidino*-^{13}C]-Arg, [γ-^{13}C]Trp or [*methyl*-^{13}C]Met, alone and in complexes with ligands. Spectra obtained as described in methods at 15°C except where noted. Note peak intensities are not comparable between different labels.

appears to be at the active site. One of the resonances changed by ligand binding therefore probably corresponds to Trp 21.

The changes in chemical shifts induced by ligands in the resonances of Met-, Arg- and Trp-labeled enzyme (Fig. 1) may be interpreted in two ways. They could result from direct interaction of the ligand with the respective residues, or they could be indirect effects which occur when neighboring side chains are rearranged as a result of ligand-induced conformational transitions. In order to separate these effects we have synthesized a variety of spin-labeled ligands, shown in Figure 2. Corresponding diamagnetic ligands can be produced by reduction of the nitroxide group with sodium ascorbate. The chemical shifts and relaxation behavior in the complexes of the diamagnetic ligands can then be compared with those of complexes of the paramagnetic ligands.

Spectra of compound I complexed to Arg-labeled DHFR demonstrate that those resonances assigned to the solvent inaccessible class are distant from the active site, while some of the accessible residues are near the spin label. This confirms our conclusion based on relaxation and chemical shift data.

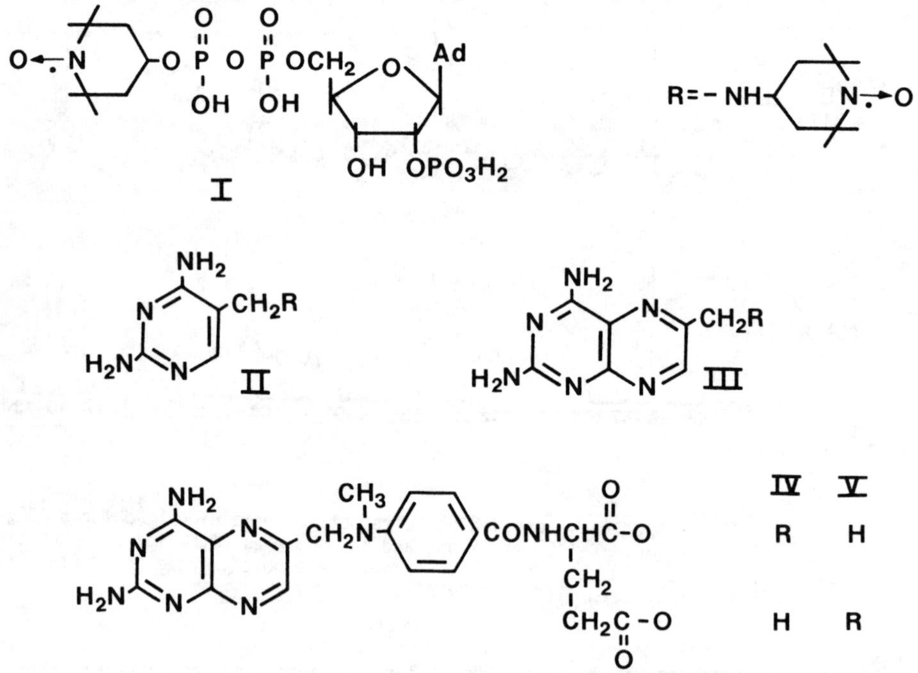

Figure 2. Structures of the spin-labeled ligands.

Although the resolution of the various resonances in the spectra in Figure 3 is incomplete, some important conclusions can be reached. Firstly, those resonances whose chemical shifts are clearly changed by ligand binding, so that they lie outside the shift range for resonances of the uncomplexed enzyme, are all strongly relaxed by the paramagnetic ligand. The data suggest that the marked, ligand-induced chemical shift changes are direct effects. Other prominent resonance peaks which appear in the diamagnetic spectrum of the complexes but not in that of the uncomplexed enzyme, are also strongly relaxed in the spectrum of the paramagnetic complex, so that these marked spectral changes are probably also due to direct effects.

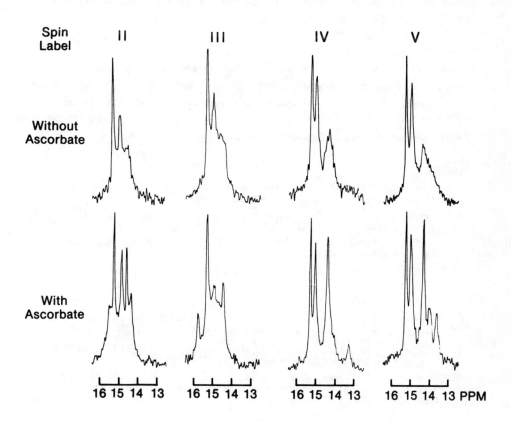

Figure 3. ^{13}C NMR spectra of ternary complexes of Met-labeled DHFR ($\sim$ 1 mM), NADPH ($\sim$ 1.5 mM) and spin-labeled ligands ($\sim$ 1 mM) II-V, in the presence and absence of ascrobate at 15°C.

Surprisingly, all four spin-labeled antifolates increased the relaxation of two or more Met residues, despite the varying lengths of the spin-labeled sidechain. Met-28 and Met-50 of the *S. faecium* DHFR correspond in *Escherichia coli* DHFR to Leu-28 and Ile-50 which form a hydrophobic pocket in which the aromatic ring of the p-aminobenzoyl moiety of MTX binds[9]. It is likely, therefore, that these residues contribute resonances that are shifted in the diagmagnetic complexes and relaxed in the paramagnetic ones, especially in the case of ligands II and III. Since Met-5 of the *S. faecium* reductase corresponds to Ile-5 of the *E. coli* enzyme which is in Van der Waals contact with the pteridine ring of bound MTX[9], it probably contributes a resonance which is also relaxed. The 3 or 4 resonances relaxed by ligands IV and V may include those of Met-5, -28 and -50, if the glutamic acid amide sidechain adopts a configuration that brings the spin label within 10-15 Å of C^ε of these sidechains.

ACKNOWLEDGEMENTS

We thank Drs. G. R. Buettner and L. W. Oberley for assistance with epr measurements, W. E. Wageman for assistance with NMR work, and G. S. Mellville, G. Thorgaard and A. W. Roetker for technical assistance. This work was supported in part by US PHS Research Grants CA 13840 from the National Cancer Institute and 1P07 RR 00962 (NAM) from the Division of Research Resources.

REFERENCES

1. Cocco, L., Blakley, R. L., Walker, T. E., London, R. E. and Matwiyoff, N. A. (1977), Biochem. Biophys. Res. Comm. 76, 183-188.

2. Blakley, R. L., Cocco, L., London, R. E., Walker, T. E. and Matwiyoff, N. A. (1978), Biochemistry 17, 2284-2293.

3. Cocco, L., Blakley, R. L., Walker, T. E., London, R. E. and Matwiyoff, N. A. (1978), Biochemistry (in press).

4. London, R. E., Groff, J. P. and Blakley, R. L., Science (submitted for publication).

5. Groff, J. P., London, R. E. and Blakley, R. L., (manuscript in preparation).

6. Cocco, L. and Blakley, R. L., (manuscript in preparation).

7. Blakley, R. L., Piper, J. R. and Montgomery, J. A. (manuscript in preparation).

8. Freisheim, J. H., Ericsson, L. H., Bitar, K. G., Dunlap, R. B., and Reddy, A. V. (1977) Arch. Biochem. Biophys. 180, 310-

9. Matthews, D. A., Alden, R. A., Bolin, J. T., Freer, S. T., Hamlin, R., Xuong, N., Kraut, J., Poe, M., Williams, M. and Hoogsteen, K. (1977) Science 197, 452-453.

THE METHYLENETETRAHYDROFOLATE-DEPENDENT BIOSYNTHESIS OF RIBOTHYMIDINE IN THE TRANSFER-RNA OF *STREPTOCOCCUS FAECALIS*

ANN S. DELK, DAVID P. NAGLE, JR., AND JESSE C. RABINOWITZ
Department of Biochemistry, University of California, Berkeley, CA 94720

ABSTRACT

The methyl carbon of ribothymidine in the tRNA of *Streptococcus faecalis* and *Bacillus subtilis* is derived from 5,10-methylenetetrahydrofolate, not *S*-adenosylmethionine[1]. We have purified to homogeneity the enzyme responsible for this novel reaction in *S. faecalis* and shown that, unlike thymidylate synthetase, the ribothymidine enzyme apparently utilizes flavin in reducing the one-carbon unit, with the third hydrogen of the methyl moiety derived, either directly or indirectly, from solvent.

INTRODUCTION

During an investigation of the role of folate in the initiation of protein synthesis in *Streptococcus faecalis*[2], we observed that although the methylated residue ribothymidine is present in loop IV of the tRNA of cells grown in the presence of folate, an unmodified uridine is found in its place in folate-free cells[2,3]. Since *in vivo* labeling experiments revealed that the methyl carbon of this residue can be derived from formate, but not methionine, we speculated that a one-carbon folate derivative is involved in a novel RNA methylation[4]. Similar results were obtained with *Bacillus subtilis* and *Bacillus cereus*[5].

Using crude enzyme preparations, we showed that 5,10-methylenetetrahydrofolate is used *in vitro* as the one-carbon donor[1]. The reaction thus appears analogous to the thymidylate synthetase-catalyzed methylation of deoxyuridylate[6]. However, unlike thymidylate synthetase, which uses methylenetetrahydrofolate as the source of both the one-carbon unit and the two electrons and hydrogen (from position 6) necessary for the reduction of the methylene carbon of the folate cofactor to the methyl carbon of the modified residue[6], the ribothymidine enzyme appeared to employ a different mechanism for this reduction. Specifically, we observed a requirement *in vitro* for reduced flavin and no incorporation of label from [6-^{3}H]tetrahydrofolate into ribothymidine *in vitro* or *in vivo*[1].

We have refined the assay, overcoming the need for boiled extract observed previously[1], and purified the ribothymidine enzyme from *S. faecalis* to homogeneity in an effort to elucidate the mechanism of this novel reaction and its relationship to that of thymidylate biosynthesis.

MATERIALS AND METHODS

Procedures were similar to those described[1]. The purification of the enzyme and details of the methodology will be reported elsewhere.

Standard assays[1], based on release of tritium from [*pyrimidyl*-5-^{3}H]-tRNA(UΨC), were performed under the following conditions: 40 mM Na-Bicine, pH 9.5; 40 mM Tris-HCl, pH 7.5; 180 mM NH_4Cl; 5 mM Na-EDTA; 100 mM 2-mercaptoethanol; 4 mM NADPH, 10 mM NADH, 0.25 mM FAD; 4 mM (*dl*)-L-5,10-methylenetetrahydrofolate; 10 μM [^{3}H]tRNA(UΨC); < 3 x 10^{-5} μmol/min of enzyme activity; 0.100 ml, 37°C, N_2 atmosphere, 15 min.

RESULTS

The purification of the enzyme is illustrated in Table I and Figure 1.

TABLE I

PURIFICATION OF ENZYME

Fraction	Spec. Act.[a]
1. S13	0.07
2. DEAE-cell.	1.14
3. P-cell.	34.60
4. tRNA-Seph.	84.00

[a] μmol/min/mg x 10^3

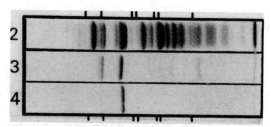

Fig. 1. SDS-polyacrylamide gel electrophoresis of samples described in Table I. Hash marks: Φ29 proteins of, left to right, M_r x 10^{-3} = 80, 70, 54, 48, 40, 36, 28.

The protein was >95% pure after tRNA-Sepharose chromatography. Trace contaminants could be removed by hydroxylapatite chromatography.

Chromatography on Sephadex G-150 showed the native enzyme to be of M_r ≈115,000; denaturing gels (Fig. 1) revealed a protein of M_r ≈ 58,000.

FAD, EDTA, mercaptoethanol, and glycerol were required after DEAE-cellulose chromatography to stabilize the enzyme. Even under these conditions, activity is gradually and, at present, irreversibly lost.

The enzyme is specific for tRNA(UΨC), with no enzymatic release of tritium observed from [^{3}H]tRNA(TΨC). Base analyses[1] of tRNA(UΨC) after incubation with the enzyme demonstrate that ribothymidine is made and that the amount of ribothymidine synthesized is approximately equal to the amount of tritium released. Complete conversion of tRNA(UΨC) to tRNA(TΨC) can be obtained *in vitro*. The K_m for tRNA(UΨC) is 2.5 μM.

Pure enzyme uses 5,10-methylenetetrahydrofolate as the one-carbon donor. 5-Methyltetrahydrofolate stimulates little or no tritium release and results in no ribothymidine formation. A small amount of tritium is released from [³H]tRNA(UΨC) in the absence of any folate cofactor. The K_m for (dl)-L-5,10-methylenetetrahydrofolate is approximately 1 mM.

As illustrated in Figure 2, pure enzyme requires reduced flavin *in vitro*. $FADH_2$, routinely generated nonenzymatically *in situ* from FAD and NAD(P)H, is superior to $FMNH_2$ and reduced riboflavin (not shown).

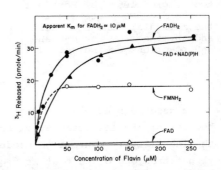

Fig. 2. Requirement for reduced flavin. Conditions as in text, except as follows: ●, $FADH_2$; ▲, FAD plus 4 mM NADPH and 10 mM NADH; o, $FMNH_2$; Δ, FAD with no NADPH or NADH.

Essentially no label was incorporated into ribothymidine from methylene-[6-³H]tetrahydrofolate, prepared by incubation of [6-³H]tetrahydrofolate* with unlabeled formaldehyde. However, ¹⁴C was incorporated from [¹⁴C]methylene-[6-³H]tetrahydrofolate, made with [¹⁴C]formaldehyde. The amount of ³H found with ribothymidine was < 3% of theoretical and the label appeared to come from degraded [³H]tetrahydrofolate. No label from [6,7-³H]tetrahydrofolate was incorporated into ribothymidine.

When the reaction was carried out in tritiated water, label was incorporated into ribothymidine, but at low efficiency (≈ 10% theoretical). Therefore, incorporation of hydrogen from solvent was examined by carrying out the reaction in deuterated solvent (containing about 87% deuterium oxide and 12% glycerol, v/v). The tRNA was hydrolyzed in acid; the bases were converted to trimethylsilyl derivatives and analyzed by gas chromatography-mass spectrometry**. A sample of tRNA containing ribothymidine synthesized *in vivo* in ordinary water was used as a control.

The derivative of thymine from the control showed the expected molecular ion of mass 270 (Fig. 3b). Approximately 65% of the molecular ions from the deuterium sample were shifted one mass unit to 271. The uracil derivatives from both samples displayed a molecular ion of mass 256.

---

*1.2 Ci/mmol, prepared and generously donated by A.L. Pogolotti and D.V. Santi and used without dilution with unlabeled tetrahydrofolate.

**A.S. Delk, D.P. Nagle, Jr., J.C. Rabinowitz, K. Straub, and A.L. Burlingame, manuscript in preparation.

Fig. 3. GC/MS analyses of di-
(trimethylsilyl) derivatives
of bases from tRNA containing
ribothymidine synthesized *in
vitro* in deuterium oxide (D_2O)
and *in vivo* in ordinary water
(H_2O). a) Portions of the
two GC profiles. b) Portions
of the four MS plots showing
the molecular ions of uracil
and thymine from the H_2O and
D_2O reactions as indicated.

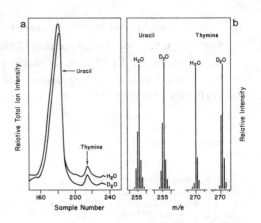

We have been unable to identify the folate product of the reaction
because of the low activity of the pure enzyme (<0.1 µmol/min/mg) and
the inability to convert to product a significant quantity of the methylenetetrahydrofolate that is required for the *in vitro* reaction.

DISCUSSION

The enzyme responsible for ribothymidine formation in *S. faecalis* tRNA
has been purified to homogeneity and shown to have an M_r of about
115,000 and two subunits of M_r about 58,000 (Fig. 1).

As data obtained with crude enzyme had indicated[1], the enzyme is
specific for tRNA(UΨC) lacking ribothymidine and utilizes 5,10-methyl-
enetetrahydrofolate as the one-carbon donor.

The *in vitro* reaction is dependent upon reduced flavin, with a preference for $FADH_2$ (Fig. 2). Stimulation of activity by NADPH and NADH and
by other reducing systems, including clostridial ferredoxin, spinach
NADP oxidoreductase and *Escherichia coli* thioredoxin reductase, appears to
result from the abilities of these compounds to reduce free flavin in
the enzyme buffer, rather than to interact directly with the enzyme.

Essentially no incorporation of tritium from the 6 position of tetrahydrofolate into ribothymidine was observed. These data suggested that,
unless an unusually large isotope effect is involved, ribothymidine formation, unlike deoxythymidylate biosynthesis, does not involve the
transfer of hydrogen from C-6 of the folate cofactor to the one-carbon
unit. Transfer of hydrogen from C-7 also appeared to be excluded.

The small amount of incorporation of label into ribothymidine from
tritiated water suggested that the third hydrogen might be derived from
solvent. Synthesis of ribothymidine in solvent containing deuterium
oxide, followed by mass spectrometry of the trimethylsilyl derivative

of thymine, revealed a shift in mass of about 65% of the molecular ions from 270 to 271, demonstrating the incorporation of deuterium (Fig. 3). The failure of all thymine residues to acquire deuterium is consistent with the presence of hydrogen from residual water and exchangeable positions on glycerol and a deuterium isotope effect. Since the uracil derivative showed no incorporation of deuterium, it is concluded that the deuterium in thymine is in the methyl moiety and not at C-6, the only other hydrogen-containing position on the derivatized base.

These data show that the third hydrogen of the methyl moiety of ribothymidine is derived from solvent, but do not distinguish between direct transfer and indirect transfer *via* an exchangeable position on the enzyme or on the reducing cofactor. This mechanism is in contrast to that involved in thymidylate biosynthesis where the third hydrogen is derived from C-6 of methylenetetrahydrofolate.

The reducing agent involved directly in ribothymidine formation remains to be established. Technical difficulties have prevented the direct analysis of the folate product of the reaction. Due to a substantial difference in the K_m values for tRNA(UΨC) and methylenetetrahydrofolate, the reaction is usually carried out with a large excess of methylenetetrahydrofolate relative to tRNA and the amount of folate product synthesized is small relative to the amount of folate substrate present. The slow turnover of the enzyme (10 mol product/min/mol enzyme) and the nonenzymatic dissociation of the folate substrate into formaldehyde and tetrahydrofolate have hampered experiments designed to overcome this difficulty. Thus, it has not been possible to determine if tetrahydrofolate or dihydrofolate is the product.

The specific requirement for reduced flavin, rather than any low potential reducing agent, implies that flavin is uniquely involved in the reaction. In addition, the enzyme is stabilized by FAD, suggesting that the enzyme may be a flavoprotein. We have been unable to examine pure enzyme for flavin because active enzyme could not be prepared in the absence of added flavin.

The capacity in which added $FADH_2$ participates in the reaction is unclear. The observed K_m for $FADH_2$ ($\simeq 10 \, \mu M$) is large relative to other flavin-utilizing enzymes, which suggests that exogenous $FADH_2$ could be serving in a nonphysiological manner to regenerate reduced enzyme. We have considered that a specific enzyme serves this function *in vivo*, but have been unable to obtain evidence to support this theory. We calculate that the turnover number of the enzyme in crude extracts is about equal to that of pure enzyme, suggesting that either there is no reductase or it is inactive in our *in vitro* system. The activity observed *in vitro* could account for complete tRNA modification *in vivo*.

In view of our findings, we propose that the formation of ribothymidine in the tRNA of *S. faecalis* occurs *via* the following reaction:

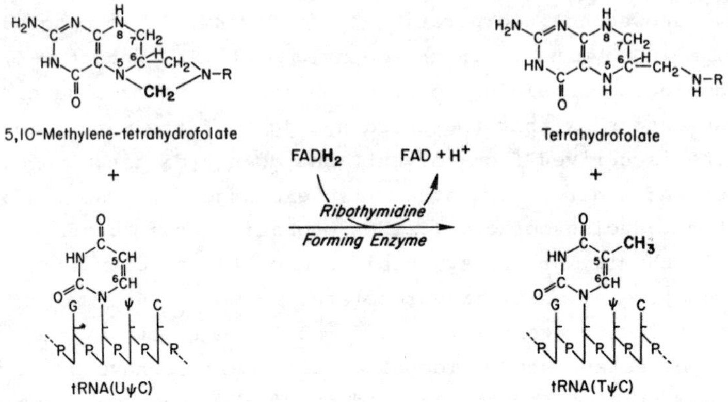

5,10-Methylene-tetrahydrofolate

Tetrahydrofolate

tRNA(UψC)

tRNA(TψC)

The acquisition of the third hydrogen from solvent does not preclude the oxidation of tetrahydrofolate; thus, the identity of the folate product remains to be established. However, the specific — and apparently absolute — requirement for reduced flavin *in vitro* suggests that flavin, not tetrahydrofolate, is the reducing agent, with hydrogen derived from solvent either directly or *via* the rapidly exchangeable N-1 or N-5 position of exogenous $FADH_2$ or enzyme-bound flavin or perhaps *via* another prosthetic group or amino acid residue on the enzyme.

ACKNOWLEDGEMENTS

This work was supported by grants from NIH, the Cystic Fibrosis Foundation and the American Cancer Society. We are grateful to Edna Kearney, Bill Kenney, Dan Santi, and Linda D'Ari for helpful discussions and to Susan Brown for patient typing, and indebted to Ken Straub and Al Burlingame for the mass spectrometry, funded by a grant from NIH to A.B.

REFERENCES

1. Delk, A.S., Romeo, J.M., Nagle, D.P., Jr., and Rabinowitz, J.C. (1976) J. Biol. Chem., 251, 7649-7656.
2. Samuel, C.E., and Rabinowitz, J.C. (1974) J. Biol. Chem., 249, 1198-1206.
3. Delk, A.S., and Rabinowitz, J.C. (1974) Nature, 252, 106-109.
4. Delk, A.S., and Rabinowitz, J.C. (1975) Proc. Nat. Acad. Sci. USA, 72, 528-530.
5. Romeo, J.M., Delk, A.S., and Rabinowitz, J.C. (1974) Biochem. Biophys. Res. Commun., 61, 1256-1261.
6. Friedkin, M. (1973) Adv. in Enzymol., 38, 235-292.

PROPERTIES OF DIHYDROFOLATE REDUCTASE FROM A METHOTREXATE RESISTANT SUBLINE OF HUMAN KB CELLS AND ITS INTERACTION WITH POLYGLUTAMATES *

BARBARA A. DOMIN, YUNG-CHI CHENG‡ AND MAIRE T. HAKALA
Department of Experimental Therapeutics, Grace Cancer Drug Center, Roswell Park
Memorial Institute, New York State Department of Health, Buffalo, New York 14263

ABSTRACT

Dihydrofolate reductase was obtained from a methotrexate resistant subline of human KB cells which had high levels of the enzyme. It was purified by ammonium sulfate fractionation and affinity chromatography on MTX-Sepharose.

Using $H_2PteGlu$ as the substrate at pH 7.5 the purified enzyme was activated by KCl with an optimum at 150 mM. Two pH optima were observed, one at pH 4-5 and one at pH 7.2 to pH 8.2. The activation energy was 9.64 Kcal/mole at pH 7.5. Chromatography on G-75 Sephadex revealed a molecular weight of $18,000 \pm 10\%$. The isoelectric point was 7.5 in contrast to the enzyme from mouse Sarcoma 180/MTX cells which had an isoelectric point of 8.6.

Titration with methotrexate, at pH 7.5 and 37°C in the presence of 150 mM KCl, showed that the KB/MTX enzyme has a turnover number of 1,300 min.$^{-1}$ while that of mouse enzyme was 415 min.$^{-1}$. The K_i for methotrexate was 4×10^{-11}M for KB/MTX and 1.4×10^{-10}M for the mouse enzyme. For the KB/MTX enzyme, the K_m of $H_2PteGlu$ at pH 7.5 and 37°C was 0.67 μM, the K_m for NADPH was 11.1 μM. $H_2PteGlu_5$ could serve as the substrate for the purified enzyme from KB/MTX cells with a Km of 0.58 μM and gave a Vmax of 91% of that when $H_2PteGlu$ was used as the substrate.

Using 2.56 m units of enzyme at pH 7.5, $PteGlu_5$ at 11.5 μM showed no substrate activity. It was found to be a competitive inhibitor of the reduction of both $H_2PteGlu$ and $H_2PteGlu_5$. The K_I (5.0×10^{-8}M) was the same value when either $H_2PteGlu$ or $H_2PteGlu_5$ was the substrate. $H_4PteGlu_5$ did not inhibit $H_2PteGlu$ reduction even at 17 μM.

INTRODUCTION

Dihydrofolate reductase (E.C.1.5.1.3) which catalyzes the reduction of dihydrofolate to tetrahydrofolate in the presence of NADPH is a central enzyme in folate metabolism in that

* This work was supported in part by NIH, USPHS Grants CA-14078, CA-18499 and CA-04175 and American Cancer Society Grant CH29.

‡ Scholar of the American Leukemia Society and to whom reprint requests should be addressed.

† Abbreviations used are: $H_4PteGlu_5$, ±-L-5,6,7,8 tetrahydrofolate pentaglutamate; $H_2PteGlu_5$, 7,8-dihydrofolate pentaglutamate; $H_2PteGlu$, 7,8-dihydrofolate; PteGlu, pteroylglutamic acid; $PteGlu_5$, pteroyl pentaglutamate; MTX, methotrexate; ALL, acute lymphocytic leukemia; AML, acute myelocytic leukemia.

it regenerates tetrahydrofolate from the dihydrofolate product of the thymidylate synthetase reaction. Although many studies on purified dihydrofolate reductases from bacterial and mammalian sources have been done[1], limited information about the human enzyme is available[2-5]. More information on the properties of the human reductase would help to elucidate its central role in human folate metabolism especially with regard to the role of polyglutamates. With this in mind, we have investigated the properties of purified dihydrofolate reductase from a cultured methotrexate resistant subline of human KB cells.

MATERIALS AND METHODS

Folic Acid[†], methotrexate and their derivatives were prepared by the procedures as described previously[5-9]. $H_2PteGlu_5$ was further purified by passage thru Sephadex G-25 with deionized water containing 50 mM dithiothreitol. The Methotrexate-Sepharose affinity gel was generously provided by Dr. David Bacchanari of Wellcome Research Laboratories.

Enzyme Assay. Enzyme activity was determined at 37°C spectrophotometrically by measuring the decrease in absorbance at 340 nm which accompanies the reduction of dihydrofolate to tetrahydrofolate and the oxidation of NADPH to NADP. A unit of enzyme activity is defined as the conversion of 1 μmole of substrate/min. The standard assay mixture contained 50 mM potassium phosphate pH 7.5 buffer, 150 mM KCl, 10 mM mercaptoethanol, 100 μM NADPH, and 20 μM $H_2PteGlu$ in a final volume of 1.0 ml. The reaction was started by the addition of $H_2PteGlu$.

Cells. The maintenance, preparation, and harvesting of mouse Sarcoma 180 AT/3000 cells were performed as previously described[10]. The subline of human KB cells, 7400-fold resistant to methotrexate, with a 40-70 fold elevation of dihydrofolate reductase, was maintained in RPMI-1640 medium containing 50 μM MTX, 30 μM dThd, and 2 μM folic acid. In order to remove the bound MTX, two weeks before harvesting the cells were transferred and maintained in medium supplemented by 100 μM hypoxanthine, 30 μM dThd, 100 μM glycine and containing no MTX or folic acid. Harvesting was carried out as described for the Sarcoma 180 AT/3000 cells.

Enzyme Purification. Cell pellets were suspended in 4 volumes of 0.01 M Tris-Cl buffer pH 7.5 containing 1.5 mM $MgCl_2$ and 3 mM dithiothreitol. They were frozen and thawed 3 times and sonicated with 3-15 sec. bursts. KCl was added to a final concentration of 0.15 M and the sonicate was centrifuged. The supernatant was fractionated with solid ammonium sulfate, the 55% to 90% saturation fraction was collected, redissolved in 0.01 M Tris-Cl buffer pH 7.5 containing 10% glycerol and 2 mM dithiothreitol and dialyzed overnight at 4°C. The sample was diluted with 3 volumes of the above buffer and applied to a MTX-Sepharose affinity column, 1 x 4 cm, which was equilibrated with the same buffer. The column was run at room temperature. All buffers contained 10% glycerol and 2 mM dithiothreitol. Extraneous protein was removed during the loading of enzyme and with the change to 0.5 M Tris Cl pH 8.5 buffer. The enzyme eluted as a single peak midway through the linear $H_2PteGlu$ gradient (0 to 100 μM in 0.5 M Tris Cl, pH 8.5) with a recovery of 100%. For removal of salt and excess $H_2PteGlu$, purified enzyme was passed through a Sephadex G-25 column and eluted with 0.01 M Tris Cl, pH 7.5, containing 10% glycerol and 2 mM dithiothreitol. Recovery was usually 70%. The Sephadex G-25 preparation was used as the pure enzyme for all studies.

Isoelectric Focusing. Isoelectric focusing was run for 24 hours at 800 volts in a 110 ml LKB electrofocusing column according to the procedure of Haglund[11].

RESULTS

General Properties. Enzyme activity steadily increases with increasing KCl, reaching a maximum of 1.6 fold at 0.15 M. The activity decreases sharply with higher concentrations of KCl, until control values are reached. No inhibition below control activity is seen up to 0.4 M KCl. This activation profile is consistent with data obtained for other mammalian enzymes. At 37°C in the presence of 150 mM KCl with $H_2PteGlu$ as substrate, enzyme activity is maximal at the lowest pH measured, (5.4) and decreases to pH 7 where a second broad optimum occurs between pH 7.2 and 8.2.

The molecular weight of the purified enzyme as determined by Sephadex G-75 chromatography was 18,000. An Arrhenious plot with $H_2PteGlu$ as substrate at pH 7.5 in the presence of 150 mM KCl showed linearity over the temperature range used, 28°C to 42°C with an activation energy of 9.64 Kcal/mole.

Isofocusing of Sephadex G-25 purified enzyme from KB/MTX cells showed a single enzyme species with an isoelectric point of 7.5. When this enzyme preparation was preincubated with 100 μM NADPH, the same profile was observed. The enzyme preparation from the affinity column which was in the presence of $H_2PteGlu$ also gave the same isofocusing profile. In comparison, isofocusing of purified enzyme from the mouse S180 AT/3000 cell line (12,13) demonstrated a single species of enzyme with a higher isoelectric point of 8.6. This suggests a basic structural difference between the mouse S180 AT/3000 and human KB/MTX enzymes.

Michaelis Constants for $H_2PteGlu$ and NADPH. Initial velocity studies were performed by varying the concentration of one substrate while keeping the concentration of the second substrate constant. The Km of NADPH was determined to be 11.1 μM in the presence of 2.7 μM $H_2PteGlu$. In the presence of 100 μM NADPH the Km of $H_2PteGlu$ was determined to be 0.67 μM.

Interaction with Methotrexate. The interaction at 37°C, pH 7.5, 150 mM KCl, of purified dihydrofolate reductase from KB/MTX and S180 AT/3000 cells with methotrexate was studied by means of the Ackerman and Potter[14] plot using the methods developed by Cha[15,16]. A preincubation time of 15 min. was found to be sufficient for equilibration between enzyme and methotrexate. Both plots demonstrate the tight binding characteristics of methotrexate. The enzyme intercept vs. methotrexate concentration reveals a methotrexate binding site concentration of 45 nM for human and 150 nM for mouse enzyme in our experiment. The replot of the v intercept vs. methotrexate concentration yields a slope or turnover number of 1300 min.$^{-1}$ for human and 415 min.$^{-1}$ for mouse enzyme for each MTX binding site. When the same data was plotted as: $\frac{v_o}{v_i}$ vs. MTX concentration, the I_{50} values for different enzyme concentrations could be estimated and the K_i calculated according to the equation developed by Cha[15]: $I_{50} = 1/2$ Et $+ K_i$. These were .04 ± .01 nM for KB/MTX enzyme and .14 ± .01 mM for S180 AT/3000 enzyme.

Several methotrexate analogs were tested for inhibition of the purified enzyme from KB/MTX cells in comparison with methotrexate. Esterification and amidation of the α-carboxyl group and the addition of a glutamate moiety to this group decreased the binding affinity more than three hundred fold. In contrast, no drastic change in the inhibition was observed when these modifications were at the γ carboxyl group. Thus, the α-carboxyl group seems essential for tight binding behavior[17].

Interaction with Polyglutamates. Enzyme activity was measured at 37°C, pH 7.5, in the presence of 150 mM KCl using $H_2PteGlu_5$ as a substrate. The Km was found to be 0.58 μM and Vmax was 91% of that when $H_2PteGlu$ was used as the substrate. $PteGlu_5$ did not show substrate activity at concentrations of 4.6 or 11.5 μM at pH 7.5, but it inhibited the reduction of both $H_2PteGlu$ and $H_2PteGlu_5$. $H_4PteGlu_5$ showed no inhibition of $H_2PteGlu$ reduction even at 17 μM. The type of inhibition by $PteGlu_5$ was investigated further and was found to be competitive both with $H_2PteGlu$ and $H_2PteGlu_5$. The K_i was determined to be 5.0×10^{-8}M for $PteGlu_5$ with either $H_2PteGlu$ or $H_2PteGlu_5$ as substrate.

SUMMARY

In many of its physical properties such as molecular weight, pH profile, and activation by KCl, the purified enzyme from human KB/MTX cells resembles other mammalian enzymes such as that of mouse[18]. However, we have demonstrated here that the mouse S180 AT/3000 enzyme is different from the human KB/MTX enzyme in its isoelectric point, turnover number, and K_i for MTX. Although it is generally assumed that all mammalian enzymes will have similar properties, it seems this may not be the case at least for the dihydrofolate reductase. Thus, extrapolation of enzyme data from other mammalian sources to human enzymes is not warranted.

The kinetic properties of this human KB/MTX dihydrofolate reductase appear to be different from those reported by Coward et al.[5] for the human enzyme from AML and ALL cells and by Jackson and Niethammer[3] for the cultured WI-L2 lymphoblastic cells and their MTX resistant sublines. This difference in observations from various laboratories could be due to different properties of dihydrofolate reductases from different human sources. In addition, since our enzyme source was an MTX resistant subline, some of the properties may be due to the acquired resistance. Therefore, we are currently investigating other sources of human enzyme and preliminary observations indicate that the purified enzyme obtained from the lymphocytes of one patient with AML has a Km for $H_2PteGlu$ in the same range (Cheng and Domin, unpublished results) as reported herein.

Since the K_i for $PteGlu_5$ is the same when either $H_2PteGlu$ or $H_2PteGlu_5$ is the substrate and since the Km's for $H_2PteGlu$ and $H_2PteGlu_5$ are similar, it seems likely that this human dihydrofolate reductase cannot distinguish between the monoglutamate or polyglutamate folyl forms.

REFERENCES

1. Blakley, R.L. (1969) The Biochemistry of Folic Acid and Related Pteridines, pp. 139-187, North-Holland Publishing Company, Amsterdam.

2. Jackson, R.C., Hart, L.I. and Harrap, K.R. (1976) Cancer Res. 36, 1991-1997.

3. Jackson, R.C. and Niethammer, D. (1977) Europ. J. Cancer 13, 567-575.

4. Jackson, R.C., Niethammer, D., and Hart, L.I. (1977) Arch. Biochem. Biophys. 182, 646-656.

5. Coward, J.K., Parameswaren, K.N., Cashmore, A.R., and Bertino, J.R. (1974) Biochemistry 13, 19, 3899-3903.

6. Blakley, R.L. (1960) Nature 188, 231-232.

7. Godwin, H.A., Rosenberg, I.H., Ferenz, C.R., Jacobs, P.M. and Meinhoffer, J. (1972) J. Biol. Chem. 247, 2266-2271.

8. Meinhoffer, J., Jacobs, R.M., Godwin, H.A. and Rosenberg, I.H. (1970) J. Org. Chem. 35, 4137-4140.

9. Zakrzewski, S.F. and Sansone, A.M. (1971) Methods Enzymol. 18, 728-731.

10. Zakrzewski, S.F., Hakala, M.T., and Nichol, C.A. (1966) Mol. Pharmacol. 2, 423-431.

11. Haglund, H. (1967) Science Tools 14, 2, 17-23.

12. Hakala, M.T., Zakrzewski, S.F. and Nichol, C.A. (1961) J. Biol. Chem. 236, 952-958.

13. Hakala, M.T. and Ishihara, T. (1962) Cancer Res. 22, 987-992.

14. Ackermann, W.W. and Potter, V.R. (1949) Proc. Soc. Exp. Biol. Med. 72, 1-9.

15. Cha, S.(1975) Biochem. Pharmacol. 24, 2177-2185.

16. Cha, S., Agarwal, R.R. and Parks, R.E., Jr. (1975) Biochem. Pharmacol. 24, 2187-2197.

17. Cheng, Y.C., Domin, B.A., Piper, J.R., Temple, C. Jr., Elliott, R.D.,Rose, J.D., Montgomery, J.A., Rosowsky, A., Yu, C-S., and Modest, E.J., unpublished results.

18. Hakala, M.T. (1969) Feder. Eur. Biochem. Soc. 15, 31-47.

INHIBITION OF ESCHERICHIA COLI DIHYDROFOLATE REDUCTASE
BY SOME NEWER PYRIMIDINE ANALOGUES

C.M. DWIVEDI[a] AND C.R. KRISHNA MURTI[b]
Division of Biochemistry, Central Drug Research Institute, Lucknow, INDIA

ABSTRACT

As part of a model system for screening of newer antimetabolites, effect of newer pyrimidine analogues was studied on purified E. coli dihydrofolate reductase. Diaminopyrimidines and substitution at position-5 appeared to play an important role in determining the nature of enzyme inhibition.

INTRODUCTION

Inhibitors of dihydrofolate reductase [E.C.1.5.1.3] have acquired a unique position in the chemotherapy of cancer. Poor intake within the tissues and severe toxicity of potent antifolates (methotrexate and aminopterin, etc.) necessitated need for the search of other inhibitors of this enzyme[1-5]. Successful appearance of pyrimethamine a pyrimidine analogue as powerful antifolate led extensive investigations on small molecular inhibitors of DHFR[4,5]. As a result derivatives of pyrimidines, pteridines and triazines were studied in detail of which 2,4-diaminopyrimidines appeared to be the most effective inhibitors of this enzyme[4-6]. Substitution with alkyl and aralkyl side chains at position-1,5 and 6 further potentiated inhibitory properties of 2,4-diaminopyrimidines and 2,4-diamino-S-triazines[7-10].

Fairly large number of newer pyrimidine analogues substituted at 4,5 and 6 positions were synthesized in this laboratory. Our preliminary observations on growth inhibitory activities of these analogues against germinating Cicer arietinum seeds (unpublished data) were quite encouraging and led us to investigate their effect on purified E. coli DHFR. A close similarity between inhibition of seed germination and microbial DHFR was observed during these studies. In this communication, we report our findings on the inhibition of DHFR and kinetics of inhibition by newer pyrimidines and discuss a tentative structure activity relationship.

MATERIALS AND METHODS

An E. coli strain 113-3 MCIM Poona wild type was used during these investigations. Chemicals were obtained as follows: NADPH, 2-ME, DTT, EDTA, Protamine sulphate and Tris from Sigma Chem. Co.; DEAE-Cellulose from Mann Res. Labs.; pCMB from Upjohn Co.; Sephadex G-75 from Pharmacia Fine Chem. Ltd. and Methotrexate from Lederle Labs.,

[a]Present address: Tufts University School of Medicine, Department of Biochemistry and Pharmacology, 136 Harrison Avenue, Boston, Mass., 02111.
[b]Present address: Industrial Toxicology Research Centre, Lucknow, INDIA.

Div. Am. Cyn. Co. All other chemicals used were of analytical reagent grade. Dihydrofolic acid was synthesized according to the method of Futterman as modified by
Blakley[11].

E. coli cells were grown in a nutrient broth containing 1% peptone, 0.5% NaCl and
0.3% yeast extract pH 7.2. The 18 hr. old cells were suspended in 0.1 M tris-HCl
buffer pH 7.4 containing 5 mM 2-ME. The cells were then sonicated at 20 Kc/Sec. for
15 min at 4°C and centrifuged at 15000 g for 20 min at 0°C. This supernatant served
as crude enzyme preparation. DHFR was purified from this crude extract employing
conventional purification procedures including protamine sulphate treatment.
$(NH_4)_2SO_4$ fractionation (35-85%), gel filtration on Sephadex G-75 and DEAE-cellulose
chromatography. The enzyme was assayed spectrophotometrically by measuring the formation of N^5-N^{10}-methenyltetrahydrofolic acid (m-THF) at 350 nm according to the
method of Rosenthal et al.[12]. The protein was estimated according to the method of
Lowry et al.[13]. The nature of inhibition and K_m values were determined according to
the method of Lineweaver and Burk[14]. K_i values were determined according to the
method of Dixon[15]. I_{50} values were measured from the plots of inhibitor conc. versus
% inhibition.

RESULTS AND DISCUSSION

DHFR purified 185-fold with an overall recovery of 27% appeared to be quite similar in all its biochemical properties to the one studied by Burchall and Chan[16].
(Table 1 and 2). On the basis of our preliminary observations, 28 newer pyrimidine
analogues which blocked 80-100% germination (1 mM) of C. arietinum seeds were subjected to secondary screening on E. coli DHFR. It was of interest to find that these
agents also inhibited microbial DHFR. It was observed that 2,4-diaminopyrimidines
were better inhibitors of DHFR than 2-aminopyrimidines. However, substitution at
position-5 in both the cases enhanced inhibitory potencies of these analogues. The
results indicate that substitution with unsaturated groups like vinyl or propenyl and
saturated groups like ethyl, propyl, thioalkyl, thioaryl, chlorophenyl and bromo
groups at position-5 resulted in increased inhibition, whereas alteration at position
-6 with various groups did not show any effect. It was also noticed that compounds
substituted with thioalkyl groups at position-5 showed increased inhibition than
5-sulphonyl substituted compounds. Comparison of the I_{50} and K_i values of newer
pyrimidine analogues (Table 3) indicated that monoaminopyrimidines having vinyl
(7b and 8b) or thioalkyl (8f) group at position-5 and diaminopyrimidines having
chlorophenyl group at the same position (4c and 4d) had lower values than other
analogues and hence seem to be better inhibitors of DHFR. Methotrexate, a well-known
anti-leukemic agent, had even lower values.

In general substitution at 5 and 6 positions of the pyrimidine nucleus was found
to play an important role in establishing inhibitory potency of the compounds. 2,4-
Diaminopyrimidines having aryl, aralkyl or halogen substituted aryl groups at

TABLE 1
PROPERTIES OF E. COLI DHFR

Purification	185-fold
Homogeneity	Single band on polyacrylamide gels
Mol. Wt. (by gel fitration)	20.5×10^3 daltons
pH Optimum	7.2
Temp. Optimum	37-45°C
K_m DHFA	12.5 µM
K_m NADPH	20.0 µM

TABLE 2
ACTIVATION AND INHIBITION OF E. COLI DHFR

Agent	Conc.	% Org. Activity	Agent	Conc.	% Org. Activity
None	----	100.0	$FeSO_4$	1 mM	14.2
2-ME	100 mM	168.00	$PbNO_3$	1 mM	35.7
DTT	2.5 mM	143.00	$COCl_2$	1 mM	28.5
EDTA	1 mM	60.7	$MnCl_2$	1 mM	42.8
pCMB	1 mM	35.7	$CdCl_2$	1 mM	67.8
$MgCl_2$	1 mM	132.2	KCN	1 mM	85.7
$HgCl_2$	1 mM	25.0	MTX	10 nM	53.5

The reaction mixture contained in 0.4 ml: 80 mM tris-HCl buffer pH 7.4, 0.4 mM DHFA
and 0.3 mM NADPH. The enzyme was incubated with the agents for 5 min at r.t. and
then reaction was initiated by the addition of NADPH.

position-5 and heavier side chains at position-6 (alkoxy and phenoxy groups), however
appeared to be ideal inhibitors. Kinetic studies on nature of enzyme inhibition
(Table 3) further strengthened above observations. It was found that analogues substituted with unsaturated groups like vinyl (7b and 8b) at position-5 showed non-
competitive inhibition, while those substituted with saturated groups like chlorophenyl (4c and 4d), n-propyl (7f) and ethyl (8c) exhibited competitive inhibition.
Compound 5a having no substitution at position-5 also showed competitive inhibition.
However, analogues with propenyl (8d) and α-methylthioethyl (8f) groups at position-
5 showed mixed inhibition. Methotrexate exhibited non-competitive inhibition.
Our findings appear to be in agreement with the earlier observations[3,5,7-10].
The mechanism of non-competitive inhibition by 2-aminopyrimidines having unsaturated groups at position-5 may be via protonation of the antagonist and subsequent
tight binding with the enzyme. Probably after protonation these antagonists bind in
the same fashion as MTX. The mechanism of competitive and mixed inhibition by 2-
aminopyrimidines and 2,4-diaminopyrimidines having alkyl thioalkyl and aryl side

TABLE 3

KINETIC DATA ON THE INHIBITION OF E. COLI DHFR BY METHOTREXATE AND SOME NEWER PYRIMI-
DINE ANALOGUES.

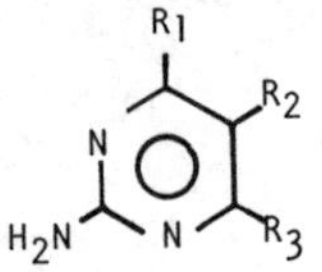

Comp. No.	Substituents R_1	R_2	R_3	I_{50}^{a}	K_i^{a}	Nature of[b] Inhibition
7b	H	$CH=CH_2$	C_6H_5	37 µM	13 µM	Non-competitive
8b	H	$CH=CH_2$	$C_6H_4OCH_3$ (p)	38 µM	8 µM	Non-competitive
8c	H	C_2H_5	$C_6H_4OCH_3$ (p)	130 µM	60 µM	Competitive
8d	H	$CH=CH-CH_3$	$C_6H_4OCH_3$ (p)	68 µM	35 µM	Mixed
7f	H	C_3H_7	C_6H_5	81 µM	81 µM	Competitive
8f	H	$CH(CH_3)SCH_3$	$C_6H_4OCH_3$ (p)	40 µM	10 µM	Mixed
5a	CH_3	H	C_6H_5	100 µM	60 µM	Competitive
4c	NH_2	C_6H_4Cl (p)	OC_2H_5	43 µM	25 µM	Competitive
4d	NH_2	C_6H_4Cl (p)	OC_3H_7	44 µM	30 µM	Competitive
	Methotrexate			10.5 nM	1 nM	Non-competitive

[a] The reaction mixture contained in 0.4 ml: 80 mM tris-HCl buffer pH 7.4, 0.1 mM DHFA
and 0.3 mM NADPH. The enzyme was incubated with respective analogues for 5 min at
r.t. and then reaction was initiated by the addition of NADPH.

[b] The reaction mixture contained in 0.4 ml: 80 mM tris-HCl buffer pH 7.4, 0.3 mM
NADPH, different concentrations of DHFA and inhibitor. The reaction was started
as described above.

chains at position-5 may be by forming hydrogen and ionic bonds with pyrimidine
moiety of the inhibitors to the DHFR[17-21].

ACKNOWLEDGEMENTS

We are thankful to Dr. H. Junjappa, ex-Scientist of this Institute, (presently at
North Hill University, Shillong, India) for providing analogues and to Indian Council
of Medical Research, New Delhi for financial support to one of us (CMD). We are also
thankful to Prof. Roy L. Kisliuk for valuable suggestions and critical assessment
of the present study.

REFERENCES

1. Hitchings, G.H. and Burchall, J.J. (1965) Advan. Enzymol., 27, 417.

2. Heidelberger, C. (1967) Ann. Rev. Pharmacol., 7, 101.

3. Baker, B.R. (1967) Design of Active Site Directed Irreversible Enzyme Inhibitors, John Wiley and Sons, New York

4. Blakley, R.L. (1969) The Biochemistry of Folic Acid and Related Pteridines, North Holland Press, Amsterdam, Netherlands

5. Baker, B.R. (1971) Ann. N. Y. Acad. Sci., 186, 214.

6. Townsend, L.B. and Cheng, C.C. (1974) Antineoplastic and Immunopressive Agents, Vol. I, Sartorelli, A.C. and Johns, D.G. eds., Springer Verlag, Berlin, Heidelberg, New York, pp. 112.

7. Baker, B.R., Ho, B.T. and Santi, D.V. (1965) J. Pharm. Sci., 54, 1415.

8. Baker, B.R. and Ho., B.T. (1965) J. Heterocyclic. Chem., 2, 162.

9. Baker, B.R. and Ho, B.T. (1965) J. Pharm. Sci., 55, 470.

10. Baker, B.R. (1970) Ann. Rev. Pharmacol., 10, 35.

11. Blakley, R.L. (1960) Nature, 188, 231.

12. Rosenthal, S., Smith, L.C. and Buchanan, J.M., (1965) J. Biol. Chem., 240, 836.

13. Lowry, O.H., Rosenbrough, N.J., Farr, A.L. and Randall, R.J. (1951) J. Biol. Chem., 193, 265.

14. Lineweaver, H. and Burk, D. (1934) J. Am. Chem. Soc., 56, 658.

15. Dixon, M. (1953) Biochem. J., 55, 170.

16. Burchall, J.J. and Chan, M. (1969) Fed. Proc. Fed. Am. Soc. Exptl. Biol., 28, 352.

17. Huennekens, F.M. (1968) Biological Oxidations, Singer, T.P. ed., Interscience Publishers, New York, pp. 439-513.

18. Blakley, R.L., Schronk, M., Sommer, K. and Nixon, P.F. (1971) Ann. N.Y. Acad. Sci., 186, 119.

19. McCullough, J.L., Nixon, P.F. and Bertino, J.R. (1971) Ann. N.Y. Acad. Sci., 186, 131.

20. Baker, B.R. and Jordan, J.H. (1965) J. Heterocyclic. Chem., 2, 162.

21. Baker, B.R. and Shapiro, H.S. (1966) J. Pharm., Sci., 55, 308.

REGULATION OF FOLATE ENZYMES IN CULTURED HUMAN CELLS

RICHARD W. ERBE

Genetics Unit, Massachusetts General Hospital, Boston, MA   02114

ABSTRACT

Folate enzyme activities can be measured in extracts of cultured human skin
fibroblasts, lymphoblastoid lines and amniotic fluid cells. The cellular levels of
methionine synthetase are related to the cobalamin concentrations in culture media.
Diploid fibroblasts show a coordinate, reciprocal pattern of changes in folate
enzyme activities during the growth cycle. One of the inborn errors of folate
metabolism, methylenetetrahydrofolate (methyleneTHF) reductase deficiency, has been
studied in cells cultured from patients. The inability of SV40 virus transformed
human cells to grow in medium in which homocysteine replaced methionine despite
high levels of endogenous methionine synthetase activity has been used study altered
growth control.

INTRODUCTION

The folate pathway enzymes offer many potential advantages for biochemical-genetic
studies of regulation in cultured human and other mammalian cells. The number of
folate enzymes in the pathway is relatively large and extensive information regarding
many of these has been gained from studies in bacteria, animal tissues and whole
animals. Most of the metabolic reactions involved are essential to cell survival and
growth. Moreover, most of the reactions appear to be unique, with no alternative
means of generating the product, so that mutational deficiencies should be expressed
and might provide a means for selecting mutant cell lines. In addition, patients
with putative inborn errors of folate metabolism could provide cells for study in
culture. Despite these potential advantages we found only a single published
report[1] involving measurement of a folate enzyme activity in cultured human cells
when we initiated our studies.

MATERIALS AND METHODS

Skin fibroblasts, derived from punch biopsy specimens, and amniotic fluid cells,
obtained by amniocentesis, were grown on the surface of petri dishes or in roller
bottles of 690 cm^2 surface area containing 100 ml of medium consisting of 85-90%
Eagle's minimum essential medium (MEM) plus nonessential amino acids and 10-15% un-
dialyzed or dialyzed fetal calf serum, modified where indicated. Lymphoblasts,
initiated from peripheral blood and containing Epstein-Barr virus, were grown in
suspension in MEM or RPMI 1640 medium with 10% fetal calf serum. Crude extracts
consisted of the supernatants (100,000 X g for 1 hr) from cell pellets that had been

sonicated in an isotonic sucrose solution. Folate enzyme activities were measured as described previously[2-4].

RESULTS AND DISCUSSION

Crude extracts of human skin fibroblasts, lymphoblasts and amniotic fluid cells grown in standard culture media contain measurable quantities of at least nine of the 15 major enzyme activities that interconvert or utilize folates[5]. Of the remainder, two activities (viz., glutamate formiminotransferase and formiminoTHF cyclodeaminase) are apparently not expressed in these cells while the assays for the others appear unsuitable for use with crude extracts (e.g., GAR transformylase and AICAR transformylase).

In order to test the effects on the folate enzyme activities of various metabolically relevant substances, cells were grown in test media altered in one or more components. We observed early, however, that changes in growth rate alone, e.g., with serum deprivation, could greatly influence enzyme activity. Thus constancy of growth rate was taken as a criterion for selecting the range of concentrations tested. Variations over several logs in the concentrations of L-serine, glycine, L-methionine and choline as well as the addition of L-homocysteine, thymidine and hypoxanthine produced no substantial (i.e., less than two-fold) change in the folate enzyme levels. Increasing the concentration of folic acid from the 2.3 μM present in MEM to 100 μM likewise was without effect. For fibroblasts in medium in which homocysteine replaced methionine and which contained dialyzed fetal calf serum 2.3 μM folic acid was barely sufficient for growth, whereas the restoration of methionine allowed growth at even lower folic acid levels [6]. The addition of 1.5 μM hydroxocobalamin to the growth medium resulted in an over two-fold increase in methionine synthetase activity[4], although we found no derepression upon substitution of homocysteine for methionine of the magnitude we had observed in aneuploid baby hamster kidney cells[2]. Rigorous interpretation of the change or lack thereof in these folate enzyme activities would require knowing more about the intracellular concentrations of the test substances under these conditions. Although substrate- and cofactor-induced stabilization could be produced by increasing their concentrations, enzyme derepression might be seen only when the relevant metabolite was growth limiting.

In diploid fibroblasts, extensive changes in folate enzyme activities were observed during the lag, log and confluent phases of the growth cycle. Cells passaged at a 1:10 dilution entered logarithmic growth and doubled about every 24 hr until forming a confluent monolayer by day six or seven. The activities of four folate enzymes involved in nucleic acid biosynthesis (namely, dihydrofolate reductase, serine hydroxymethyltransferase, thymidylate synthetase and 10-formylTHF synthetase) increased two to twenty times during the log phase of growth. Figure 1 shows the activity of dihydrofolate reductase. The specific activity (which is

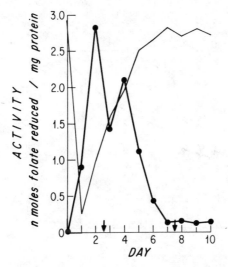

Fig. 1. Dihydrofolate reductase activity in crude extract of cultured human fibroblasts. The thin solid line indicates the relative cell number while the arrows
indicate refeeding. Modified from ref. 3 with permission.

identical to the activity per cell under the conditions used) increased rapidly to
a maximum that was 20-fold higher than the activity in the subsequent stationary
phase. The transient changes may relate to refeeding or to partial cell synchrony
or both. The magnitude of the increases in the three other log-phase enzymes was
less but the pattern was similar.

In contrast, the activities of two folate enzyme activities involved in regulating the levels of 5-methylTHF showed a reciprocal pattern during the culture
cycle (Figure 2). MethyleneTHF reductase activity decreased about three fold during
the log phase of growth, increasing rapidly between days six and eight. Methionine
synthetase (5-methylTHF: homocysteine methyltransferase) activity decreased and
remained low throughout the log phase but increased more slowly thereafter and did
not return to maximal activity until the cells had been confluent for nearly three
weeks. The low levels of both activities during log growth and the delayed increase
in methionine synthetase activity could, if the synthetase is rate limiting in early
confluency, result in accumulation of 5-methylTHF at the expense of the folates
needed for nucleic acid synthesis. For diagnostic purposes it is important to be
aware that these normal changes in activities during the culture cycle could cause
normal activity to be mistaken for heterozygous or even homozygous deficiency in the
absence of appropriate controls. Although fluctuations related to cell density and
growth rate have been observed in lymphoblasts and various aneuploid cells, the
interpretation of these changes is complicated by the fact that such cells lack a
quiescent stationary phase.

410

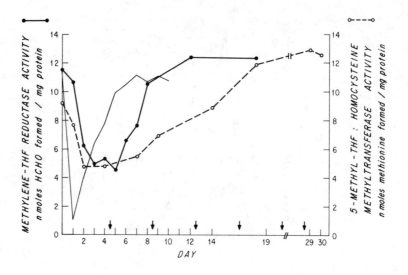

Fig. 2. MethyleneTHF reductase and methionine synthetase (5-methylTHF: homocysteine methyltransferase) activities in crude extracts of cultured human fibroblasts. The thin solid lines and arrows are as in Fig. 1. Modified from ref. 3 with permission.

Since 1961, five and possibly six new disorders have been attributed to primary congenital defects in the uptake or utilization of folic acid[5]. These disorders and the number of patients identified are shown in Table 1.

Of these disorders specific defects in cultured cells from patients have been demonstrated only in methyleneTHF reductase (MTHFR) deficiency[7-11]. All patients have shown some degree of neurological abnormality, often severe, and low serum

TABLE 1.   INBORN ERRORS OF FOLATE METABOLISM

Defect	No. of Cases Reported
Defective folate absorption:	
Congenital malabsorption of folate	4
Defective folate interconversion:	
Dihydrofolate reductase deficiency	3*
MethenylTHF cyclohydrolase deficiency	3*
MethyleneTHF reductase deficiency	12
Defective folate utilization:	
Methionine synthetase deficiency	1*
Glutamate formiminotransferase deficiency	9

*Evidence for the existence of the disorder in these patients is equivocal.

folate levels before treatment. Homocystinuria of moderate degree and homocys-
tinemia but with low or normal plasma methionine levels have been characteristic.
Residual MTHFR activity in cultured skin fibroblasts has ranged from about 20% of
normal[7,11] to undectable[10]. Evidence of allelic differences was found in studies
of thermal stability of the residual MTHFR activity in crude extracts of cells from
four patients, two of whom were sibs. Figure 3 shows that, when incubated at 55°
in the absence and presence of added FAD cofactor, the MTHFR activity of the sisters,
B.M. and L.M., was inactivated in a normal pattern, while that from patient C.P.
showed marked thermolability and that from patient W.Ma. was intermediate. The data
suggest that in C.P. and W.Ma. there is structural mutation altering cofactor binding
and provide strong evidence that the reductase deficiency in these three families is
due to different alleles.

Like the patients, the fibroblasts manifest a defect in homocysteine metabolism.
As first noted by Mudd et al.[7], MTHFR deficient cells are unable to grow in folic
acid- and cobalamin-supplemented medium containing dialyzed fetal calf serum and in
which methionine is replaced by homocysteine, its immediate metabolic precursor.
This methionine dependency presumably results from deficiency of methionine synthetase activity secondary to deficient cellular levels of 5-methylTHF both as substrate
and perhaps for stabilization. Indeed, deficiency of 5-methylTHF has been noted in
such cells by Cooper and Rosenblatt[12]. As yet unexplained, however, is the observation that MTHFR deficient fibroblasts also do not grow in methionine-deficient,
homocysteine-containing medium even when supplied with exogenous 5-methylTHF, the
product of the deficient enzyme[13]. Understanding this defect in the utilization of
5-methylTHF would contribute not only to knowledge of these pathways but also

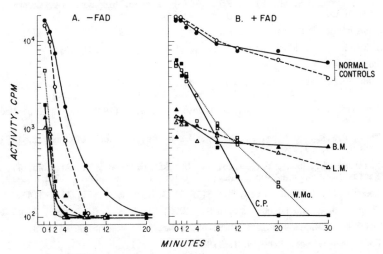

Fig. 3. Thermal stability of methyleneTHF reductase activity in extracts of fibroblasts from normal controls and four reductase-deficient patients. Reprinted from
ref. 11 with permission.

probably to therapy. Deficiency of de novo synthesis of labile methyl groups may
well contribute to the neurological abnormalities found in MTHFR deficient patients.

Finally, SV40 transformed human fibroblasts also require exogenous methionine[14].
This methionine dependence seems paradoxical in that endogenous methionine synthesis
in these growth-altered cells occurs in at least normal amounts and the dependency
is not related to cell density, making simple leakage of methionine unlikely. The
inability of transformed cells to grow in homocysteine-containing, methionine-
deficient medium has been used to select sublines that have spontaneous regained
methionine independence[16]. Studies of four such sublines indicate that increased
methionine biosynthesis is not a prerequisite for reversion to methionine independence and are consistent with our hypothesis that the original defect in the transformed cells is not in methionine biosynthesis.

Thus cultured human cells provide a useful system for studying many aspects of
the regulation of folate pathway enzymes.

ACKNOWLEDGEMENTS

This work was supported by USPHS Research Grant No. HD06356 from the National
Institute of Child Health and Human Development.

REFERENCES

1. Mudd, S.H., Uhlendorf, B.W., Hinds, K.R. and Levy, H.L. (1970) Biochem. Med.,
   4, 215-239.

2. Kamely, D., Littlefield, J.W. and Erbe, R.W. (1973) Proc. Natl. Acad. Sci. USA,
   70, 2585-2589.

3. Rosenblatt, D.S. and Erbe, R.W. (1973) Biochem. Biophys. Res. Commun., 54,
   1627-1633.

4. Rosenblatt, D.S. and Erbe, R.W. (1977) Pediat. Res., 11, 1137-1141.

5. Erbe, R.W. (1975) N. Engl. J. Med., 293, 753-758 and 807-811.

6. Hoffman, R.M. and Erbe, R.W. Unpublished data.

7. Mudd, S.H., Uhlendorf, B.W., Freeman, J.M., Finkelstein, J.D. and Shih, V.E.
   (1972) Biochem. Biophys. Res. Commun., 46, 905-912.

8. Freeman, J.M., Finkelstein, J.D. and Mudd, S.H. (1975) N. Engl. J. Med., 292,
   491-496.

9. Wong, P.W.K., Justice, P., Hruby, M., Weiss, E.B. and Diamond, E. (1977)
   Pediatrics, 59, 749-756.

10. Narisawa, K., Wada, Y., Saito, T., Suzuki, H., Kudo, M., Arakawa, T.,
    Katsushima, N. and Tsuboi, R. (1977) Tohoku J. Exp. Med., 121, 185-194.

11. Rosenblatt, D.S. and Erbe, R.W. (1977) Pediat. Res., 11, 1141-1143.

12. Cooper, B.A. and Rosenblatt, D.S. (1976) Biochem. Soc. Trans., 4, 1921-1922.

13. Hoffman, R.M., Rosenblatt, D.S. and Erbe, R.W. Unpublished data.

14. Hoffman, R.M. and Erbe, R.W. (1976) Proc. Natl. Acad. Sci. USA, 73, 1523-1527.

15. Hoffman, R.M., Jacobsen, S.J. and Erbe, R.W. (1978) Biochem. Biophys. Res.
    Commun., 82, 228-234.

BINDING OF 1-ANILINONAPHTHALENE-8-SULFONATE AND 2-p-TOLUIDINONAPHTHALENE-6-SULFONATE TO DIHYDROFOLATE REDUCTASE FROM METHOTREXATE-RESISTANT L1210/R6 CELLS

CHINAN C. FAN

Department of Biochemistry, Scripps Clinic & Research Foundation, La Jolla, CA 92037

ABSTRACT

The fluorescent probes, 1-anilinonaphthalene-8-sulfonate (ANS) and 2-p-toluidino-naphthalene-6-sulfonate (TNS), bind at neutral pH to dihydrofolate reductase from L1210 cells. Binding causes large enhancements of fluorescence and blue shifts in the emission maxima (524 → 475 nm for ANS and 495 → 450 nm for TNS). Fluorescence titrations show that the enzyme binds an equimolar amount of either probe; dissociation constants for the enzyme-ANS and enzyme-TNS complexes are 23.8 and 4.5 μM, respectively. ANS competes with dihydrofolate (K_i = 54 μM) and NADPH (K_i = 79 μM), while TNS competes only with dihydrofolate (K_i = 73 μM). In the presence of NADPH or NADP$^+$, the fluorescence emission of the enzyme-TNS complex undergoes a red shift. Methotrexate displaces the probes from the complexes; concentrations of the drug for half-maximum effect are 0.34 and 0.44 μM for the ANS and TNS complexes, respectively. These results provide further evidence for the existence of a hydrophobic domain at the dihydrofolate/Methotrexate binding site and for the ability of the enzyme to assume conformational forms varying in affinity for the drug.

INTRODUCTION

Previous studies from several laboratories[1-3] have suggested that dihydrofolate reductases (E.C. 1.4.1.6) are characterized by hydrophobic domains, particularly at the dihydrofolate binding site. Since the fluorescent probes 1-anilinonaph-thalene-8-sulfonate (ANS) and 2-p-toluidinonaphthalene-6-sulfonate (TNS) are extremely useful for examining the hydrophobicity of proteins[4], it was of interest to

1-Anilinonaphthalene-8-Sulfonate
(ANS)

2-$\underline{p}$-Toluidinonaphthalene-6-Sulfonate
(TNS)

investigate their interaction with the L1210 dihydrofolate reductase. Quantitative data have been obtained for the number and nature of the hydrophobic binding sites on the enzyme, dissociation constants for the enzyme-ANS and enzyme-TNS complexes, and effects of dihydrofolate, NADPH and Methotrexate upon these complexes.

MATERIALS AND METHODS

ANS and TNS were obtained from Eastman and Sigma, respectively. Sources of other materials and the preparation of homogeneous dihydrofolate reductase from L1210/R6 cells will be given elsewhere[5].

Enzyme activity was measured in a standard assay system[6]. Inhibition by ANS and TNS was determined by analysis of the data via Cleland's computer programs[7].

Fluorescence measurements, obtained with an Aminco-Bowman instrument using the general procedures described previously[8], were performed at 25° and in 50 mM potassium phosphate, pH 7.1. Enzyme concentrations ranged from 0.6 to 1.5 μM. The quantum yield (ϕ_1) of a probe under given conditions was calculated by the equation $\phi_1/\phi_2 = F_1/F_2$ where F_1 is the fluorescence under those conditions, F_2 is the fluorescence of the probe (at the same concentration) in n-butanol, and ϕ_2 is the known quantum yield of the n-butanol (0.56 for ANS and 0.57 for TNS)[8-10]. Dissociation constants (K_D) and number of binding sites (n) for enzyme-probe interactions were obtained from titration data[8]; molecular weight for the enzyme is 20,000.

RESULTS AND DISCUSSION

Fluorescence of free and enzyme-bound ANS and TNS. At neutral pH, fluorescence emission maxima of free ANS and TNS were located at 524 and 495 nm, respectively (excitation at 374 and 323 nm). In the presence of excess dihydrofolate reductase, the emission maxima of the bound probes shifted to 475 and 450 nm, and there was considerable enhancement of the fluorescence intensities (Fig. 1). Quantum yields

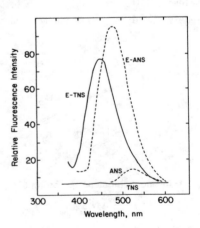

Fig. 1. Fluorescence emission spectra of ANS (10 μM), ANS (10 μM) plus enzyme (E)(6.64 μM), TNS (0.83 μM), and TNS (0.83 μM) plus enzyme (5.81 μM). Buffer, 50 mM potassium phosphate, pH 7.1. Temperature, 25° Excitation wavelengths, 374 nm for ANS and 323 nm for TNS.

TABLE I

FLUORESCENCE EMISSION MAXIMA AND QUANTUM YIELDS OF FREE AND ENZYME-BOUND ANS AND TNS

Medium	ANS[a]		TNS[a]	
	λ_{max}	ϕ	λ_{max}	ϕ
	nm		*nm*	
50 mM Potassium phosphate, pH 7.1	524	0.0017	495	0.0006
Dihydrofolate reductase	475	0.084	450	0.42
n-Propanol	475	0.48	435	0.53
n-Butanol	470	0.56	425	0.57

[a] Excitation at 374 and 323 nm for ANS and TNS, respectively. Emission maxima (λ_{max}) and quantum yields (ϕ) at indicated wavelengths.

TABLE II

DISSOCIATION CONSTANTS (K_D) AND NUMBER OF BINDING SITES (n)
FOR INTERACTION OF ANS AND TNS WITH ENZYME

Probe	n	K_D
		μM
ANS	1.10	23.8
TNS	1.06	4.5

TABLE III

INHIBITION OF ENZYME BY ANS AND TNS[a]

Inhibitor	Variable Substrate			
	Dihydrofolate		NADPH	
	Type[b]	K_i	Type[b]	K_i
		μM		μM
ANS	C	54	C	79
TNS	C	73	NC	220

[a] Standard assay system[6] in which concentrations of fixed substrates were 56 μM for dihydrofolate and 150 μM for NADPH.

[b] C, competitive; NC, non-competitive.

of the fluorescence of ANS and TNS under these conditions, as well as in the free state in n-propanol and n-butanol, are summarized in Table I. The quantum yield of enzyme-bound TNS was nearly identical to that of the compound in propanol, but the emission maximum occurred at a slightly shorter wavelength in the latter medium. In contrast, enzyme-bound ANS had a reduced quantum yield relative to that of the free compound in propanol, but the emission maxima were the same.

Analysis of the data for interaction of the probes with the enzyme yielded values of 23.8 μM for the dissociation constant of the enzyme-ANS complex and a stoichiometry of 1.10 moles of ligand bound per mole of protein, while corresponding values for the enzyme-TNS complex were 4.5 μM and 1.06 (Table II). These results suggested that the probes were interacting on an equimolar basis with a specific hydrophobic domain of the enzyme, the apolar characteristics of which were similar to those of n-propanol. In addition, however, ANS appeared to have some contact with an adjacent hydrophilic domain.

Inhibition of enzyme activity by ANS and TNS. Both of these compounds inhibited the activity of the L1210 dihydrofolate reductase. Analysis of the inhibition data (Table III) revealed that TNS was a competitive inhibitor (K_i = 73 μM) with respect to dihydrofolate and non-competitive (K_i = 220 μM) with respect to NADPH. ANS, alternatively, was competitive (K_i = 54 μM and 79 μM, respectively) with both dihydrofolate and NADPH. These results further support the hypothesis that ANS and TNS interact in a similar, but not identical, manner with the enzyme. Binding of either probe compromises the dihydrofolate site, while ANS has an additional effect upon the NADPH site.

Effect of substrates upon enzyme-TNS interaction. As anticipated from the above data, dihydrofolate competitively inhibited formation of the enzyme-TNS complex. The complex had identical fluorescence characteristics in the presence or absence of dihydrofolate, but the apparent dissociation constant increased from 4.5 to 18 μM when the substrate was present (Table IV).

TABLE IV

EFFECTS OF SUBSTRATES ON FLUORESCENCE PARAMETERS OF ENZYME-TNS INTERACTION

Addition	Emission Maximum	K_D	n	ϕ
	nm	μM		
None	450	4.5	1.06	0.42
Dihydrofolate (75 μM)	450	18	1.01	0.42
NADPH (64 μM)	464	9.6	1.00	0.28
NADP$^+$ (64 μM)	467	5.8	1.01	0.13

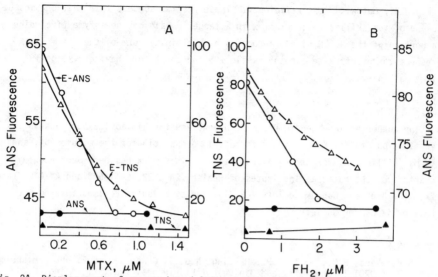

Fig. 2A. Displacement of enzyme-bound ANS and TNS by Methotrexate (MTX).
o, enzyme (0.65 μM) plus ANS (85 μM); Δ, enzyme (0.65 μM) plus TNS (42 μM);
●, ANS (85 μM); ▲ TNS (42 μM). MTX added as indicated. Other conditions
as in Fig. 1. 2B. Ditto, displacement by added dihydrofolate (FH$_2$ at
indicated concentrations.

A different set of results was obtained when NADPH or NADP$^+$ was present during
interaction of TNS with the enzyme (Table IV). With the former nucleotide, the
fluorescence maximum of the bound probe occurred at 464 nm and the quantum yield
was 0.28. An equimolar amount of TNS was bound, and the dissociation constant was
9.6 μM. With NADP$^+$, the corresponding values were 467 nm, 0.13 and 5.8 μM. One
interpretation of these results is that binding of the pyridine nucleotide induces
a conformational change in the enzyme which, in turn, renders the dihydrofolate/TNS
site more polar. The latter is indicated by the red shift and reduced quantum
yield when the fluorescence characteristics of the ternary complex are compared to
those of the enzyme-TNS complex.

Displacement of enzyme-bound probes by Methotrexate. Addition of Methotrexate
to the enzyme-ANS or enzyme-TNS complexes markedly reduced the fluorescence of
the latter due to displacement of the probes (Fig. 2A). This experiment is similar
to ejection of enzyme-bound dihydrofolate by Methotrexate, which can also be followed by the difference in fluorescence between the free and bound ligand[1]. Titration data for the enzyme-ANS complex gave a linear plot, and the concentration
of Methotrexate required to achieve half-maximum displacement of ANS was 0.34 μM.
For the enzyme-TNS complex, the plot was hyperbolic and the corresponding value
for Methotrexate was 0.44 μM. Dihydrofolate can also displace these probes

418

(Fig. 2B), but with less efficiency. These results suggest that ANS, perhaps because of its ability to interact with a larger domain on the enzyme (including
a portion of the NADPH site), induces a high-affinity form of the enzyme with
respect to Methotrexate binding, while TNS induces a form having a slightly
lower affinity.

ACKNOWLEDGMENTS

The author is indebted to Dr. F.M. Huennekens for his advice during this investigation, to Ms. Karin Vitols for aid in preparation of the manuscript, and
to Ms. Linlin Ding for technical assistance. This work has been supported by
grants from the National Institutes of Health (CA 6522, CA 16600 and AM 07097) and
from the American Cancer Society (CH 31), and by a Junior Fellowship from the
California Cancer Society.

REFERENCES

1. Huennekens, F.M., Mell, G.P., Harding, N.G.L., Gundersen, L.E. and Freisheim,
    J.H. (1970) in Chemistry and Biology of Pteridines, Iwai, K., Akino, M.,
    Goto, M., and Iwanami, Y., eds., International Academic Printing Co., Tokyo,
    pp. 329-350.

2. Matthews, D.A., Alden, R.A., Bolin, G.T., Freer, S.T., Hamlin, R., Xuong, Y.,
    Kraut, J., Poe, M., Williams, M. and Hoogsteen, K. (1977) Science, 197, 452-455.

3. Blakley, R.L., Schrock, M., Sommer, K. and Nixon, P. (1971) Ann. N.Y. Acad.
    Sci., 186, 119-130.

4. Brand, L. and Gohlke, J.R. (1972) Ann. Rev. Biochem., 41, 843-868.

5. Fan, C.C. and Huennekens, F.M., in preparation.

6. Huennekens, F.M. and Fan, C.C. (1978) Proc. Am. Assoc. Cancer Res., 19, 33.

7. Cleland, W.W. (1963) Nature, 198, 463-465.

8. Fan, C.C., Tomcho, L.A. and Plaut, G.W.E. (1974) J. Biol. Chem., 249, 5607-5613.

9. McClure, W.D. and Edelman, G.M. (1966) Biochemistry, 5, 1908-1919.

10. Weber, G. and Young, L.B. (1964) J. Biol. Chem., 239, 1415-1431.

STRUCTURE-FUNCTION RELATIONSHIPS OF DIHYDROFOLATE REDUCTASES: SEQUENCE
HOMOLOGY CONSIDERATIONS AND ACTIVE CENTER RESIDUES

JAMES H. FREISHEIM, A. ASHOK KUMAR, and DALE T. BLANKENSHIP
Department of Biological Chemistry (522), University of Cincinnati
College of Medicine, Cincinnati, Ohio 45267 *and* BERNARD T. KAUFMAN,
NIAMD, National Institutes of Health, Bethesda, Maryland 20014

ABSTRACT

The amino acid sequence of chicken liver dihydrofolate reductase is
described. This enzyme is highly homologous in structure to those from
L1210 lymphoma cells and from bovine liver. In addition, certain regions, particularly the N-terminal region of the chicken liver reductase, are homologous to certain bacterial enzymes. Activation of the
chicken liver and bovine liver enzymes with organic mercurials appear
to involve cysteine residues within the first 11 amino acid residues of
each enzyme. Known binding residues for Methotrexate and NADPH in bacterial enzymes appear to be largely conserved in animal reductases,
based on sequence homology alignments.

MATERIALS AND METHODS

Purification of Chicken Liver and Bovine Liver Dihydrofolate Reductases. These enzymes were purified as described by Kaufman and
Kemerer[1,2].

Amino Acid Sequence Analyses. Automated sequenator analyses were
performed as previously described[3,4]. Both bovine liver and chicken
liver enzymes were carboxymethylated (CM) using [14C]-iodoacetic acid.
Cleavage of the CM-chicken liver reductase at Met residues was done
with cyanogen bromide (CNBr) and at Arg residues with trypsin, following maleylation of the lysines with maleic anhydride. Subdigests of
these fragments were also carried out.

RESULTS AND DISCUSSION

The amino acid sequence of chicken liver dihydrofolate reductase
(DHFR) has been determined primarily by automated sequenator analyses
of the intact enzyme and certain cleavage fragments derived therefrom,
as described in *Materials and Methods*. The complete primary structure
of the reductase is indicated in Fig. 1.

The chicken liver enzyme contains 3 Trp, 5 Met, 8 Arg, and a single
CySH.

```
      5         10        15        20        25        30        35
V-R-D-L-N-S-I-V-A-V-C-Q-N-M-G-I-G-K-D-G-N-L-P-W-P-P-L-R-N-E-Y-K-Y-F-Q-
      40        45        50        55        60        65        70
-R-M-T-S-T-S-H-V-E-G-K-Q-N-A-V-I-M-G-K-K-T-W-F-S-I-P-E-K-N-R-P-L-K-D-R-
      75        80        85        90        95       100       105
-I-N-I-V-L-S-R-E-L-K-E-A-P-K-G-A-H-Y-L-S-K-S-L-D-D-A-L-A-L-L-D-S-P-E-L-
     110       115       120       125       130       135       140
-K-S-K-V-D-M-V-W-I-V-G-G-T-A-V-Y-K-A-A-M-E-K-P-I-N-H-R-L-F-V-T-R-I-L-H-
     145       150       155       160       165       170       175
-E-F-E-S-D-T-F-F-P-E-I-D-Y-D-K-F-K-L-L-T-E-Y-P-G-V-P-A-D-I-Q-E-E-D-G-I-
     180       185
-Q-Y-K-F-E-V-Y-E-K-K-N
```

Fig. 1. Amino acid sequence of chicken liver dihydrofolate reductase.

Carboxymethylation of the chicken liver DHFR with [^{14}C]-iodoacetate and subsequent sequenator analysis of the CM-protein revealed that 96% of the label was released as [^{14}C]-CM-cysteine at position 11. This result proves that the chicken liver enzyme contains only a *single* CySH, in agreement with previous results of amino acid analysis and titration with p-hydroxymercuribenzoate (pHMB)[1]. A similar treatment of the *bovine* liver reductase with [^{14}C]-iodoacetate showed the presence of a single CySH residue at position 6, based on sequenator analyses (Fig.2). The L1210 lymphoma enzyme also contains a CySH located at position 6 in the sequence[5].

The amino acid sequence of the chicken liver DHFR is highly homologous to that of the L1210 enzyme and to the first 34 residues of the bovine liver reductase (cf. Fig.2). The first 25 residues of the sarcoma-180 enzyme are identical to that found for the reductase from L1210 cells[6].

The chicken liver enzyme (0.023 µmoles/ml) is activated 12-to-13 fold by a stoichiometric amount of methylmercuric hydroxide (MeHgOH) within 5 min at 0°C and a 2-fold molar excess of pHMB results in an 8-fold maximum stimulation of enzyme activity. By contrast, bovine liver DHFR (0.022 µmoles/ml) is inhibited 20% by a 3-fold molar excess of MeHgOH after 35 hr at 0°C. Preincubation of the bovine enzyme with 5.7-fold molar excess of NADPH, however, followed by reaction with MeHgOH does result in a 1.5-fold enzyme activation after 24 hr at 0°C. In the absence of NADPH, pHMB *stimulates* the bovine enzyme *ca.* 1.8-fold after incubation for 20 hr at 0°C (Fig.3). This activation phase is followed by inhibition. A 4.5-fold molar excess of NADPH to enzyme delays the onset of maximum activation by pHMB (2.5-fold after *ca.* 50 hr), but does not prevent the reaction with the mercurial (Fig.3). The binding of NADPH to the bovine enzyme appears to stabilize the tertiary structure of the protein while not interfering with the reaction with

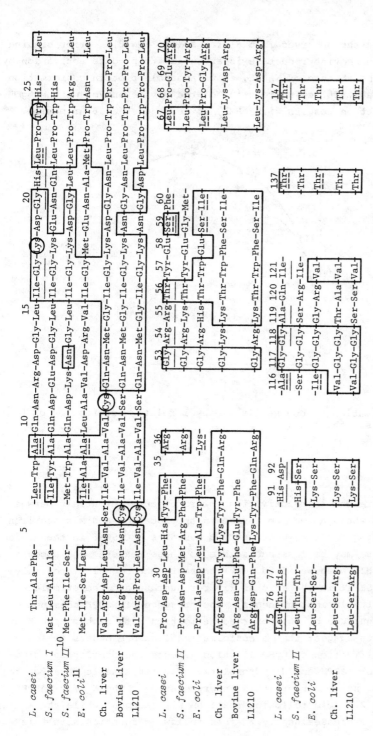

Fig. 2. Comparison of the amino acid sequences of dihydrofolate reductases in selected regions. Position numbers are based on the chicken liver sequence and identical residues from other species are enclosed. Gaps are introduced to achieve maximum homology. Circled residues indicate those which have been chemically modified. Residues implicated in MTX (---) or NADPH (——) binding are indicated.

422

pHMB, based on the observed initial rates (cf. Fig.3). Prior binding
of NADPH to the bovine reductase is essential to produce activation by
MeHgOH. In the absence of NADPH, an unfavorable protein conformation
appears to result following reaction of the bovine enzyme with MeHgOH,
whereas activation results with pHMB, at least over a 20 hr period.

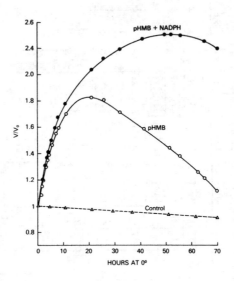

Fig. 3. Activation of bovine liver dihydrofolate reductase by pHMB.
For details, see the text.

Such differences in reactivities toward organic mercurials between
these enzymes would appear to reside in the location and microenvironment surrounding their respective CySH residues. CySH-6 in the bovine
liver reductase may be less accessible to these reagents and appears to
be more unstable when modified. By contrast, the organic mercurials
react with CySH-11 in the chicken liver reductase and the stimulation
at 0°C is virtually instantaneous. The presence of NADPH does not
affect the magnitude of the observed activation with either MeHgOH or
pHMB. The data suggest that a conformational change occurs following
mercurial modification of CySH-11 which affects the overlapping binding regions for NADPH and dihydrofolate. Certain kinetic data for the
chicken liver enzyme support this interpretation. The K_M for NADPH
increases *ca*. 2.5-fold following reaction with MeHgOH, while the K_M for
dihydrofolate increases nearly *50-fold* following reaction with this

organic mercurial. The V_{max} values for both NADPH and dihydrofolate increase dramatically following the modification.

By contrast, bacterial reductases which contain one or more CySH residues are inhibited by mercurials. The *Streptococcus faecium* reductase (isozyme I) contains a single CySH which is not located in the N-terminal 25 amino acid residues (Fig.2). Nearly stoichiometric amounts of pHMB lead to complete inactivation of this enzyme[7]. Thus, it is tentatively concluded that, for animal reductases stable to such treatment, activation by mercurials is directly related to the presence of a CySH residue in the amino-terminal region of their amino acid sequence.

Recent primary structural studies of bacterial DHFRs have shown them to contain from 159 to 167 amino acid residues, depending on the source. The reductase from *Lactobacillus casei* consists of 162 residues, including 2 Met and 4 Trp, but lacks CySH[3,4]. Chemical modification studies have implicated Trp-24 in the function of the *L. casei* reductase[8]. The position of this Trp is conserved in enzymes from at least seven different species (Fig.2). Dansyl chloride modification of 1 of 9 Lys residues of the *L. casei* reductase results in complete enzyme inactivation[9]. The location of the modified Lys has been established, using [3][H]-dansyl chloride at position 18 (Fig.2). The sequence, -Ile-Gly-Lys-, is conserved in 6 of the 7 species indicated in Fig. 2.

As discussed by Dr. Matthews, there are a number of binding residues for Methotrexate (MTX) in both *E. coli*[12] and *L. casei* enzymes which are conserved in their respective amino acid sequences. Many of these MTX (and NADPH) binding residues are also conserved in the chicken liver and L1210 reductases, based on homology alignments (cf. Fig.2). The Ala-9 is identical in all bacterial and animal reductases and is involved in both MTX and NADPH binding in the *L. casei* enzyme. The Trp-24 is conserved in all species and appears to interact with the nicotinamide portion of NADPH. The Asp-30, implicated by Matthews *et al.*[12] in MTX binding in the *L. casei* and *E. coli* enzymes, is Glu in the chicken liver and bovine liver enzymes, but is Gln in the L1210 reductase based on our alignments (Fig.2). The Arg-54 and Arg-55 residues implicated in binding of the phosphoryl moieties of NADPH in the *L. casei* enzyme are also conserved in other species. The Arg-70, involved in the binding of the γ-carboxyl group of MTX, is identical in all species.

Subsequent x-ray analyses of the chicken liver or of other animal reductases should aid in clarifying the exact interactions involved in MTX and NADPH binding in animal vs bacterial dihydrofolate reductases.

ACKNOWLEDGEMENTS

This work was supported by grant CA 11666, NIH, DHEW, and grant CH 80B from the American Cancer Society.

REFERENCES

1. Kaufman, B.T. and Kemerer, V.F. (1977) Arch. Biochem. Biophys., 179, 420-431.

2. Kaufman, B.T. and Kemerer, V.F. (1976) Arch. Biochem. Biophys., 172, 289-300.

3. Bitar, K.G., Blankenship, D.T., Walsh, K.A., Dunlap, R.B., Reddy, A.V. and Freisheim, J.H. (1977) FEBS Lett., 80, 119-122.

4. Freisheim, J.H., Bitar, K.G., Reddy, A.V. and Blankenship, D.T. (1978) J. Biol. Chem. (in press).

5. Stone, D. and Phillips, A.W. (1977) FEBS Lett., 74, 85-87.

6. Rodkey, J.A. and Bennett, C.D. (1976) Biochem. Biophys. Res. Commun., 72, 1407-1413.

7. Warwick, P.E. and Freisheim, J.H. (1975) Biochemistry, 14, 664-668.

8. Freisheim, J.H., Ericsson, L.H., Bitar, K.G., Dunlap, R.B. and Reddy, A.V. (1977) Arch. Biochem. Biophys., 180, 310-317.

9. Vehar, G.A., Reddy, A.V. and Freisheim, J.H. (1976) Biochemistry, 15, 2512-2518.

10. Gleisner, J.M., Peterson, D.L. and Blakley, R.L. (1974) Proc. Natl. Acad. Sci. USA, 71, 3001-3005.

11. Stone, D., Phillips, A.W. and Burchall, J.J. (1977) Eur. J. Biochem., 72, 613-624.

12. Matthews, D.A., Alden, R.A., Bolin, J.T., Freer, S.T., Hamlin, R., Xuong, N., Kraut, J., Poe, M., Williams, M. and Hoogsteen, K. (1977) Science, 197, 452-455.

QSAR OF COMPARATIVE INHIBITION OF MAMMALIAN AND BACTERIAL
DIHYDROFOLATE REDUCTASE BY TRIAZINES

CORWIN HANSCH, STEPHEN DIETRICH, AND R. NELSON SMITH
Department of Chemistry, Pomona College, Claremont, California 91711

ABSTRACT

Quantitative structure-activity relationships (QSAR) for triazines
inhibiting mammalian and bacterial dihydrofolate reductase (DHFR) have
been formulated. These equations are compared with QSAR for the inhibition of bacteria by triazines. The results show that there definitely is a hydrophobic pocket in which substituents bind which is different for bacterial enzyme.

INTRODUCTION

We have been concerned with developing QSAR for the inhibition of
DHFR by various nonclassical heterocyclic inhibitors, especially triazines of type I. We have formulated[1] eq 1 from an analysis of an ex-

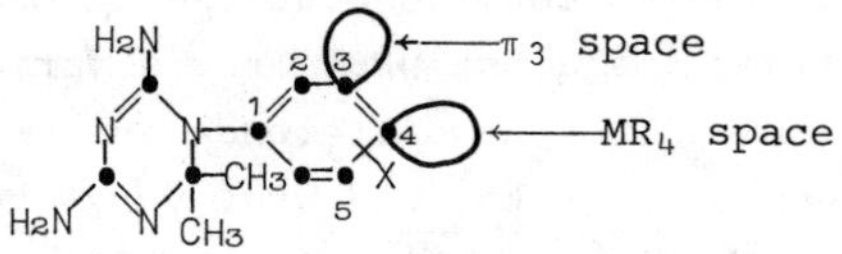

I

tensive study by B. R. Baker and his students of the inhibition by
triazines of type I of DHFR from Walker 256 tumor and L-1210 leukemia
tumor. C in eq 1 is the molar concentration of inhibitor producing

$$\log 1/C = 0.68\pi_3 - 0.12\pi_3^2 + 0.23MR_4 - 0.024MR_4^2 + 0.24I_1 - 2.53I_2$$
$$- 1.99I_3 + 0.88I_4 + 0.69I_5 + 0.70I_6 + 6.49 \tag{1}$$

$n = 244$; $r = 0.923$; $s = 0.377$; optimum $\pi_3 = 2.9$; optimum $MR_4 = 4.7$

50% inhibition, π_3 is the hydrophobic substituent constant for substituents in position 3 of the N-phenyl moiety, MR_4 is the molar refractivity (scaled by 0.1) of substituents in the 4-position of the
phenyl group, n is the number of data points, r is the correlation coefficient, and s is the standard deviation. The indicator variables
I_1-I_6 take the value of 1 or 0 for features which cannot be parameterized by the continuous variables π and MR. I_1 is assigned the value
of 1 for enzyme from Walker tumor and the value of 0 for enzyme from

L-1210 leukemia. I_2 is given the value of 1 for groups in the 2-position. As its large negative coefficient shows, such groups depress activity by a factor of 300, other features being constant. Rigid substituents (such as C_6H_5) attached directly to either the 3- or 4-position reduce activity; I_3 is given the value of 1 for such groups. I_4 takes the value of 1 for groups of the type $-SO_2OC_6H_4-X$ attached to position 4; the highly inhibitory effect (large coefficient with I_4) of these groups may result from alkylation of the enzyme. Flexible side chains in position 4 are parameterized by I_5 and I_6, which are given the value of 1 for certain amide bridges between two phenyl groups.

A subsequent analysis of the work of Hynes on the inhibition of rat liver DHFR yielded a QSAR[2] which was parallel to that of eq 1 in a number of ways. In addition, this QSAR gave numerical definition to the loss of inhibitory power which resulted by replacing the 2- and 4-NH_2 groups with either OH or SH. Another analysis of Hynes' studies of the inhibition of bacterial (*S. faecium*) DHFR by quinazolines yielded a QSAR which is quite different from that obtained for mammalian enzyme.[3]

These initial studies convinced us that a more careful study of the action of triazines I against DHFR from a variety of sources would be helpful in understanding the difference in structure between mammalian and bacterial enzymes. Baker had used very crude enzyme preparations and many of the substituents he selected for study are difficult to parameterize for QSAR. Finally, his studies were mostly limited to mammalian enzyme. We have studied only derivatives of I substituted in position 3 in our initial research.[4] From this work we have formulated eq 2-4 for the inhibition of DHFR from bovine liver, rat liver, and *L. casei*, with C defined as for eq 1.

Bovine DHFR

$$\log 1/C = 1.05\pi_3 - 1.21 \log(\beta \cdot 10^{\pi_3}+1) + 6.64 \tag{2}$$
$n = 28; \quad r = 0.955; \quad s = 0.210; \quad \pi_0 = 1.6; \quad \log \beta = -0.733$

Rat DHFR

$$\log 1/C = 1.12\pi_3 - 1.34 \log(\beta \cdot 10^{\pi_3}+1) + 6.29 \tag{3}$$
$n = 18; \quad r = 0.963; \quad s = 0.210; \quad \pi_0 = 1.7; \quad \log \beta = -0.978$

L. casei DHFR

$$\log 1/C = 0.53\pi_3 - 0.67 \log(\beta \cdot 10^{\pi_3}+1) + 0.79MR + 3.13 \tag{4}$$
$n = 28; \quad r = 0.949; \quad s = 0.302; \quad \pi_0 = 4.03; \quad \log \beta = -3.46$

These equations differ from eq 1 in that we have found much better

correlations using Kubinyi's bilinear model[5] than the parabolic model
used for eq 1. The bilinear model fits the data to two straight lines
with rounding of the curve in the region of intersection. This model
has a great advantage over the symmetrical parabola used for eq 1 in
that the positive and negative (slopes) portions of the curve may take
any slope. The slopes of the negative portions of eq 2-4 are: bovine
= 1.05 - 1.21 = -0.16; rat = 1.12 - 1.34 = -0.22; *L. casei* = 0.52 - 0.67
= -0.15. Equations 2-4 show that activity rises rapidly, especially
for mammalian DHFR, as the hydrophobicity of the 3-substituent is increased until π_0 is reached. There is a rather sharp break in the
curve at this point and activity begins to decrease very slowly as hydrophobicity is increased. While there is a large difference in the
initial increase in activity with hydrophobicity of substituents, after the point of π_0, the fall off in activity is the same (within experimental error) for all three enzymes. We interpret this to mean
that for large, lengthy substituents a point is reached with each enzyme where the substituent begins to protrude beyond the hydrophobic
pocket. The size of this pocket is set by π_0 which is relatively
small for the two mammalian enzymes (1.6 and 1.7) and larger (4)
for *L. casei*

The use of the bilinear model with the data used to formulate eq 1
does not give an improved correlation; this may be due to the fact
that the data upon which eq 1 is based contain more experimental
noise. Why π_0 is so much higher for eq 1 than for eq 2 and 3 is
also not clear but it may be due to the presence of other enzymes
in the crude preparation used by Baker.

There are other significant differences between mammalian and bacterial enzyme which are brought out by three special substituents:
$3-CH_2NHC_6H_4-4'-SO_2NH_2$, $3-CH_2OC_6H_4-3'-NHCONH_2$, and $3-CH_2NHC_6H_3-3',5'-$
$(CONH_2)_2$. The polar groups (SO_2NH_2, $NHCONH_2$, $CONH_2$) on these lengthy
groups require special parameterization for eq 2-4. In the case of
bovine and rat DHFR, π for the polar groups is set at 0; that is, π
for these substituents is taken as π for $CH_2NHC_6H_5$ or $CH_2OC_6H_5$. It
is presumed that these polar groups fall into the aqueous phase outside of the enzymic hydrophobic pocket off of position 3 of the tri-
azine and hence make no contribution to $\log 1/C$. In the case of *L.
casei*, these polar substituents actually increase $\log 1/C$ and we have
found that assigning a value of MR (molar refractivity) to them so
that a term in MR can be introduced into eq 4 allows us to account
reasonably well for their increased activity. We believe that this
striking difference in activity for these three congeners acting on

L. casei DHFR indicates that a special polar interaction takes place with the enzyme. Such an interaction is not possible with the two mammalian enzymes. This special effect must be studied with a better selection of derivatives

Another striking difference in mammalian and bacterial DHFR can be seen in the intercepts of eq 2-4. The mammalian intercepts are similar and close to those of eq 1. The intercept of the *L. casei* equation is over 3 units lower, showing that the parent compounds and compounds which do not differ much from it hydrophobically are about 1000 times less effective against this enzyme.

There is considerable difference in the slope of the π_3 term for the mammalian and bacterial equations. The slope of about 1 for the mammalian equations brings out the close relationship between partitioning in octanol/water and partitioning between enzyme/water. The lower slope in the *L. casei* equation suggests less effective desolvation of the substrate or possibly a less flexible hydrophobic pocket. In the case of *L. casei* DHFR, we can increase inhibition at the rate of $0.53 \cdot \pi$ up to 4 (π_0); that is, we can obtain about 200 (0.53×4) units increase in log $1/C$. With the mammalian enzyme, we can achieve 1.7×1 or 1.7 units increase in log $1/C$. Viewed in this way, the pockets in the two types of enzymes are similar (*L. casei* is a little larger); however, the mammalian enzyme behaves more like the octanol/water model of hydrophobicity.

The QSAR with *L. casei* can be compared with the QSAR obtained for the inhibitor of growth of *S. aureus* and *E. coli* by triazines I. We have formulated eq 5 and 6 from the data by Walsh et al.[6] In correlating their

S. aureus

$$\log 1/C = 0.59 \pi_3 - 1.52 \log(\beta \cdot 10^{\pi_3} + 1) + 2.83 \tag{5}$$
$$n = 23; \quad r = 0.986; \quad s = 0.218; \quad \pi_0 = 5.79; \quad \log \beta = -5.99$$

E. coli

$$\log 1/C = 0.51 \pi_3 - 1.09 \log(\beta \cdot 10^{\pi_3} + 1) + 2.57 \tag{6}$$
$$n = 22; \quad r = 0.960; \quad s = 0.307; \quad \pi_0 = 5.06; \quad \log \beta = -5.12$$

work Walsh et al. used the parabolic model for optimization of activity vs π. We have found a better correlation using the bilinear model. C in eq 5 and 6 is the minimum inhibitory concentration. It is interesting that the coefficients with π_3 in eq 4-6 are essentially identical and that the intercepts are close to each other. In these respects, inhibiting purified DHFR is very similar to inhibiting growth in the bacteria; however, π_0 is larger, especially for *S. aureus*, than for DHFR from *L. casei*. One can contribute 3.4 units to log $1/C$ for *S. aureus* (0.59×5.79) by increasing hydrophobicity before reaching π_0. The reasons behind this will be most interesting to uncover. An intriguing possibility is that DHFR is so situated in the bacterium that large groups in position 3 of I extend beyond the hydrophobic pocket of the enzyme but reach hydrophobic material adjacent to this hydrophobic region.

Another difference between QSAR for *L. casei* DHFR and the inhibition of *E. coli* and *S. aureus* is the slope of the negative part of the curve: -0.93 for *S. aureus* and -0.58 for *E. coli*. Once the optimum hydrophobicity with the intact bacteria has been reached, further increases in hydrophobicity cause rapid decrease in inhibitory power of these supraoptimal lipophilic congeners. This is no doubt connected with the penetration of the bacterial membrane by these very lipophilic drugs.[7]

REFERENCES

1. Silipo, C. and Hansch, C. (1975) J. Am. Chem. Soc., 97, 6849-6861.

2. Fukunaga, J. Y., Hansch, C., and Steller, E. E. (1976) J. Med. Chem. 19, 605-611.

3. Hansch, C., Fukunaga, J. Y., Jow, P. Y. C., and Hynes, J. B. (1977) J. Med. Chem. 20, 96-102.

4. Unpublished results, Dietrich, S., Smith, R. N., Fukunaga, J. Y., Olney, M., Brendler, S., and Hansch, C.

5. Kubinyi, H. (1977) J. Med. Chem. 20, 625-629.

6. Walsh, R. J. A., Wooldridge, K. R. H., Jackson, D., and Gilmour, J. (1977) Eur. J. Med. Chem. 12, 495-500.

7. Hansch, C. and Clayton, J. M. (1973) J. Pharm. Sci. 62, 1-21.

431

INHIBITION OF THYMIDYLATE SYNTHETASE BY POLY-γ-GLUTAMYL DERIVATIVES OF FOLATE AND METHOTREXATE

ROY L. KISLIUK AND YVETTE GAUMONT

Department of Biochemistry and Pharmacology, Tufts University School of Medicine, Boston, Massachusetts 02111

CHARLES M. BAUGH

Department of Biochemistry, University of South Alabama College of Medicine, Mobile, Alabama 36688

JOHN H. GALIVAN, GLADYS F. MALEY AND FRANK MALEY

Division of Laboratories and Research, New York State Department of Health, Albany, New York 12201

ABSTRACT

Pteroyl-γ-glutamates containing one through seven glutamate residues were tested as inhibitors of thymidylate synthetases derived from Lactobacillus casei, Escherichia coli and Coliphage T2. The three enzymes can be distinguished by differing patterns of inhibitory response to the pteroylpolyglutamates. The L. casei enzyme was the most sensitive being inhibited 50% by 8×10^{-7} M pteroyltriglutamate. This inhibition was noncompetitive with respect to (l)-tetrahydropteroylmonoglutamate but competitive with respect to (l)-tetrahydropteroyltriglutamate.

Poly-γ-glutamyl derivatives of methotrexate were found to be potent inhibitors of thymidylate synthetase. For example, 2,4-diamino-10-methylpteroyltriglutamate inhibited the L. casei enzyme 50% at 2×10^{-7} M. This inhibition was greatly diminished in the presence of 0.5 M NaCl.

INTRODUCTION

In view of the formation of poly-γ-glutamyl derivatives of folate[1,2] and methotrexate[3,4] in tissues and their possible role in chemotherapy we undertook a study of these compounds as inhibitors of thymidylate synthetases from Lactobacillus casei, Escherichia coli and Coliphage T2. We investigated the effect of increasing the number of γ-glutamyl residues on inhibitory potency, the type of inhibition involved and reversal of inhibition of NaCl.

MATERIALS AND METHODS

The γ-glutamyl derivatives of folate were synthesized by the solid phase method and purified by DEAE-cellulose chromatography. They were analysed quantitatively for their glutamate and folate content[6]. Pteroylpentaglutamate was also analysed by high performance liquid chromatography by Dr. M. Archer[7] and found to be 94% pure. The γ-glutamyl derivatives of methotrexate were synthesized by an analogous procedure[8].

Thymidylate synthetase was assayed spectrophotometrically in a mixture consisting of 3×10^{-4} M (dl)-tetrahydropteroylglutamate, 1.2×10^{-2} M formaldehyde, 2.1×10^{-2} M MgCl$_2$, 4×10^{-5} M dUMP, 0.11 M 2-mercaptoethanol, 0.05 M Tris-HCl and 8×10^{-4} M ethylenediaminetetraacetic acid. The final pH was 7.4 and the reaction incubated at 30°. (dl)-Tetrahydropteroylglutamate was replaced with the appropriate (l) derivative[6] where indicated (Fig. 1). The symbols (l) and (d) are used to denote, respectively, the natural and unnatural configurations of tetrahydropteroylglutamate at carbon 6 and do not denote optical activity or absolute configuration. In all cases glutamyl residues have the L configuration.

The specific activities of the thymidylate synthetases expressed as μmoles/hr/mg protein were L. casei 90, E. coli 15 and Coliphage T2 900. For the L. casei and E. coli enzymes protein was determined by absorption at 280 nm[10]. For the T2 enzyme[11] the method of Lowry[12] was employed.

RESULTS

The sensitivity of three thymidylate synthetases to inhibition by pteroyl-γ-glutamates is shown in Table 1. The most pronounced effect is seen with the L. casei enzyme, the inhibition by pteroyltetraglutamate being 375 fold that achieved with the monoglutamate. The increased inhibitory potency with increasing γ-glutamate chain length was 5, 37.5, and 2 fold on adding glutamates 2, 3 and 4 respectively. Further increasing the number of glutamate residues to 7 did not alter inhibitory potency appreciably. With the E. coli enzyme the inhibition by pteroyltriglutamate is 36 times greater than with the monoglutamate. The largest increase in inhibitory potency, 16.4 fold, occurred on adding glutamate 2, in contrast with the L. casei enzyme where the largest increase in inhibitory potency occurred on adding glutamate 3. The T2 enzyme shows only one increase in inhibitory potency, 8.7 fold, which occurred on adding glutamate 2.

TABLE 1

INHIBITION OF THYMIDYLATE SYNTHETASE BY PTEROYLGLUTAMATES

Glutamate residues	Concentration for 50% inhibition, M $\times 10^6$		
	L. casei	E. coli	T2
1	150	180	70
2	30	11	8
3	0.8	5	8
4	0.4	4	8
5	0.4	4	8
6	0.6	5	9
7	0.7	4	10

with <u>L</u>. <u>casei</u> thymidylate synthetase is therefore postulated to be similar to that observed with abortive complexes of NAD linked dehydrogenases in which inhibition can be noncompetitive or competitive depending on the rate of dissociation of the abortive complex[16].

The sensitivity of three thymidylate synthetases to inhibition by methotrexate and poly-γ-glutamyl derivatives thereof is shown in Table 2. In every instance metho-trexate derivatives are more inhibitory than the corresponding folates. In addition the increase in inhibitory potency on adding γ-glutamyl residues is more pronounced with methotrexate derivatives than with the corresponding folates. With the <u>E</u>. <u>coli</u> enzyme for example pteroyltriglutamate is 36 times as inhibitory as folate whereas 2,4-diamino-10-methylpteroyltriglutamate is 100 times as inhibitory as methotrexate. As was observed with the corresponding folates, the γ-heptaglutamate of 2,4-diamino-10-methylpteroate is no more inhibitory than the γ-triglutamate.

TABLE 2

INHIBITION OF THYMIDYLATE SYNTHETASE BY 2,4-DIAMINO-10-METHYL PTEROYLGLUTAMATES

Glutamate Residues	Concentration for 50% inhibition, $M \times 10^6$		
	L. casei	E. coli	T2
1	44	100	20
3	0.2	1	1.5
7	0.2	1	2

We observed earlier[6] that the inhibition of <u>L</u>. <u>casei</u> thymidylate synthetase by pteroylhexaglutamate was completely abolished by addition of 0.4 M NaCl. A similar effect is seen with 2,4-diamino-10-methylpteroyl tri and hepta glutamates, however the inhibition is not completely abolished even at 0.5 M NaCl (Table 3).

TABLE 3

EFFECT OF NaCl ON THE INHIBITION OF <u>L</u>. <u>casei</u> THYMIDYLATE SYNTHETASE BY METHOTREXATE AND ITS POLY-γ-GLUTAMYL DERIVATIVES

NaCl Conc. M	Control rate ΔOD/min	% Inhibition of control rate		
		Glu_1	Glu_3	Glu_7
0	0.021	54	65	82
0.1	0.020	-	55	67
0.2	0.019	-	40	60
0.3	0.019	47	29	36
0.4	0.018	-	23	28
0.5	0.016	40	14	19

Glu_1- 6.4×10^{-5} M, Glu_3- 6.9×10^{-7} M, Glu_7- 1.2×10^{-6} M

The inhibition of <u>L</u>. <u>casei</u> thymidylate synthetase by pteroylmono or triglutamate is noncompetitive when (l)-tetrahydropteroylmonoglutamate is the variable substrate and competitive when (l)-tetrahydropteroyltriglutamate is the variable substrate (Fig. 1). We interpret these results to indicate that a dUMP-inhibitor-enzyme complex is formed which is dissociated more readily in the presence of (l)-tetrahydropteroyltriglutamate than in the presence of (l)-tetrahydropteroylmonoglutamate.

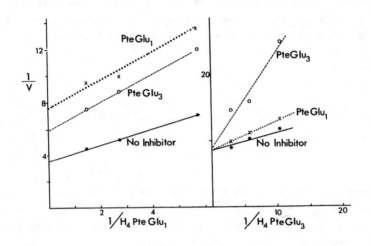

Fig. 1. Inhibition kinetics of <u>L</u>. <u>casei</u> thymidylate synthetase using pteroylmonoglutamate (PteGlu₁) and pteroyltriglutamate (PteGlu₃) as inhibitors and (l)-tetrahydropteroylmonoglutamate (H₄PteGlu₁) and (l)-tetrahydropteroyltriglutamate (H₄PteGlu₃) as substrates.

Two lines of evidence consistent with this view are: 1) a ternary complex containing pteroylmonoglutamate, dUMP and thymidylate synthetase is known to be formed[13] and 2) the binding of (l)-tetrahydropteroylmonoglutamate to thymidylate synthetase is much weaker than that of (l)-tetrahydropteroyltetraglutamate. No binding of (l)-tetrahydromonoglutamate was observed in equilibrium dialysis studies under conditions where (l)-tetrahydropteroyltetraglutamate had a dissociation constant of 2×10^{-5} M[14]. Furthermore the Km for (l)-tetrahydropteroylmonoglutamate is 1.5×10^{-5} M whereas that for (l)-tetrahydropteroyltriglutamate is 2.2×10^{-6} M[15]. The situation

ACKNOWLEDGEMENTS

Supported by grants CA10914 from the National Cancer Institute, USPHS (RLK), Cl-86-O from the American Cancer Society (CMB), and GM 20371 from the National Institute of General Medical Sciences, USPHS (FM).

REFERENCES

1. Corrocher, R. and Hoffbrand, A.V. (1972) Clinical Science, 43, 815-822.

2. Leslie, G.I. and Baugh, C.M. (1974) Biochemistry, 13, 4957-4961.

3. Baugh, C.M., Krumdieck, C.L. and Nair, M.G. (1973) Biochem. Biophys. Res. Commun., 52, 27-34.

4. Whitehead, M.V. (1977) Cancer Res., 37, 408-412.

5. Krumdieck, C.L. and Baugh, C.M. (1969) Biochemistry, 8, 1568-1572.

6. Kisliuk, R.L., Gaumont, Y. and Baugh, C.M. (1974) J. Biol. Chem., 249, 4100-4103.

7. Reed, L.S. and Archer, M.C. (1976) J. Chromatog. 121, 100-103.

8. Nair, M.G. and Baugh, C.M. (1973) Biochemistry, 12, 3923-3927.

9. Wahba, A.J. and Friedkin, M. (1962) J. Biol. Chem., 237, 3794-3801.

10. Layne, E. (1967) in Methods in Enzymol. vol. III, Colowick, S.P. and Kaplan, N.O. eds., Academic Press, N.Y., pp. 447-454.

11. Galivan, J., Maley, G.F. and Maley, F. (1974) Biochemistry, 13, 2282-2289.

12. Lowry, O.H., Rosebrough, N.J., Farr, A.L. and Randall, R. (1951) J. Biol. Chem.. 196, 265-275.

13. Galivan, J.H., Maley, G.F., and Maley, F. (1976) Biochemistry, 15, 356-362.

14. Galivan, J.H., Maley, F., and Baugh, C.M. (1976) Biochem. Biophys. Res. Commun., 71, 527-534.

15. Kisliuk, R.L., Gaumont, Y., Baugh, C.M., Galivan, J.H., Maley, F., and Maley, G.F. (1978) Fed. Proc., 37, 1427.

16. Dalziel, K. (1975) in The Enzymes, vol. XI, Part A, 3rd Edition, Boyer, P.D., ed., Academic Press, New York, pp. 2-59.

PRIMARY SEQUENCE OF BOVINE LIVER DIHYDROFOLATE REDUCTASE[*]

POR-HSIUNG LAI, YU-CHIN PAN, JOHN M. GLEISNER, DARRELL L. PETERSON, AND RAYMOND L. BLAKLEY

Dept. of Biochemistry, College of Medicine, Univ. of Iowa, Iowa City, IA   52242

ABSTRACT

Determination of the sequence of dihydrofolate reductase from bovine liver is described. Bovine and mouse L1210 reductases have considerable homology (85% identical and a mean of 0.16 minimum base changes/codon). Many residues of bacterial reductases previously shown to participate in ligand binding are identical in the bovine sequence; almost all changes in these residues are conservative.

INTRODUCTION

Dihydrofolate reductase (DHFR), the target of a group of antimicrobial and anti-cancer drugs, has been intensively studied for two decades. Certain 2,4-diaminopyrimidines exhibit differential inhibition of bacterial DHFR as compared with mammalian DHFR, and methotrexate (MTX) binds much more strongly to both than the substrate.[1] Structural studies offer the prospect of explaining such selective affinity in molecular terms and in addition of elucidating the catalytic mechanism.

Sequences of DHFR from *Streptococcus faecium*[2], *Escherichia coli*[3,4] and *Lactobacillus casei*[5], have been published, but the only complete sequence of a mammalian DHFR previously published is that of DHFR of mouse L1210 cells[6]. We now report the primary strucutre of DHFR from bovine liver.

MATERIALS AND METHODS

Bovine liver DHFR was prepared and carboxymethylated as previously described[7]. CNBr cleavage, citraconylation at Lys, followed by tryptic digestion, and separation of peptide mixtures by phosphocellulose chromatography and gel filtration were performed as previously[2]. Some tryptic peptides were further purified by preparative paper electrophoresis in pyridine/acetic acid/water (100/4/900) and eluted from the paper with 20% acetic acid.

Edman degradations were performed with a JEOL JAS47-K automatic sequence analyzer. Manual Edman degradation according to Tarr[8] was employed to analyze sequences of peptides obtained in small amounts. Treatment with carboxypeptidase A and B was according to Guidotti[9] except that protein was boiled for 5 min before digestion.

RESULTS AND DISCUSSION

The sequence of DHFR from bovine liver is shown in Fig. 1 where the peptides

---

[*]Work supported by US PHS Research Grant CA 13840 from the Natl. Cancer Institute.

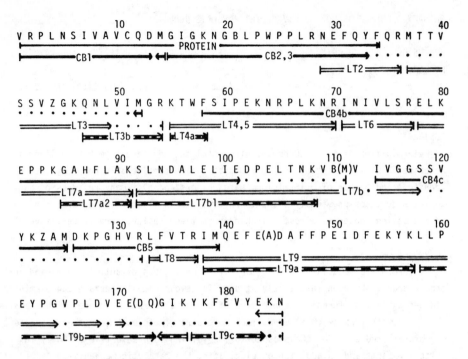

Figure 1. Sequence of bovine DHFR and of the peptides used in its determination. → signifies residues identified by Edman degradation. ← signifies residues identified by carboxypeptidase A + B digestion. • were not identified in that particular sequence study. ( ) indicates residues whose identity must be confirmed.

obtained from the various fragmentation procedures are also indicated. It may be seen that most of the sequence was obtained from data on the CNBr and tryptic peptides. CNBr treatment apparently did not cleave the Met-37-Thr-38 bond since the homoserine peptides corresponding to residues 15-37 and 38-52 were not detected, and in CB2,3 the bond was still intact. Similar results occurred in sequencing L1210 DHFR[6]. CNBr apparently cleaved at two Trp residues of bovine DHFR since the N-termini of two homoserine peptides, CB4b and CB4c, appear to follow Trp-57 and Trp-113, respectively.

Limited tryptic digestion was complicated by some cleavage at Lys residues (due either to incomplete citraconylation or to hydrolysis of some of the blocking groups) and by chymotryptic-like cleavage of the enzyme during prolonged digestion with trypsin. Autolytic development of chymotryptic activity has been reported previously[10].

The sequences of bovine and L1210 enzymes are very similar (Fig. 2). The mean minimum base change per codon to interconvert these two sequences is 0.16, and 85% of the residues are identical, including all aromatic residues. All the amino

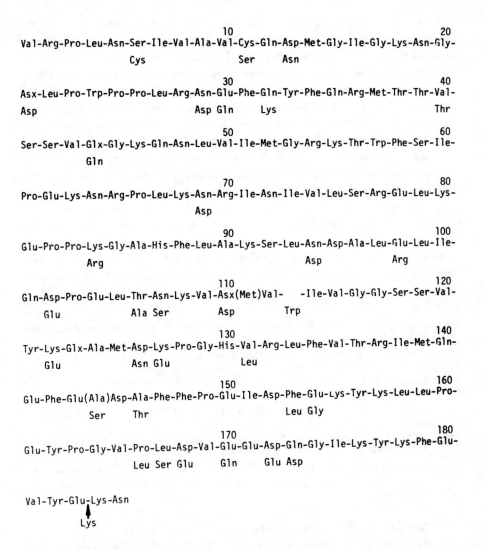

Figure 2. Comparison of sequences of dihydrofolate reductases from bovine liver and mouse L1210. The sequences are identical except in those positions where the different residue of the L1210 sequence is shown below the bovine liver sequence.

acid replacements in converting one of these sequences to the other can be produced by a single base change except at residues 40 (Val/Thr), 98 (Glu/Arg), and 173 (Glu/Asp) which require two base changes. The bovine sequence appears to be shorter than the L1210 by one Lys near the C-terminus.

Recently Matthews et al. reported X-ray diffraction studies on the structure

of the binary MTX complex with *E. coli* DHFR[11] and on the ternary MTX-NADPH complex
with *L. casei* DHFR[12,13]. This has provided information on the interaction of MTX
and NADPH with sidechains of DHFR. Of 12 sidechains of *L. casei* DHFR involved
in interactions with MTX, 7 are identical in bovine DHFR and substitutions are
conservative with two exceptions, Asp-26 in the bacterial sequences (*L. casei*
numbering) corresponds to Asn-28 in bovine DHFR, and His-28 to Gln-35. However,
the mammalian enzyme has Glu and Arg residues at positions 29 and 36 respectively,
and the latter may assume the functions of the replaced Asp and His.

Twenty residues of *L. casei* DHFR have sidechains interacting with NADPH. Corresponding residues in bovine DHFR are identical in 11 of the positions and 5 of the
replacements are conservative. In these interactions, 7 of the *L. casei* residues
have sidechain interactions with the ribosyl nicotinamide fragment of NADPH. At
six of the corresponding positions in the bovine sequence the residues are identical to those in *L. casei* and the single replacement in this series is conservative.
Consequently it may be concluded that the binding sites for MTX and NADPH, and
particularly for the ribosyl nicotinamide moiety, have been highly conserved.

REFERENCES

1. Blakley, R.L. (1969) The Biochemistry of Folic Acid and Related Pteridines
   (North-Holdland, Amsterdam).

2. Gleisner, J.M. Peterson, D.L., and Blakley, R.L. (1974) Proc. Natl. Acad.
   Sci. U.S.A., 71, 3001-3005.

3. Bennett, C.D., Rodkey, J.A., Sondey, J.M., and Hirschmann, R. (1978) Biochemistry, 17, 1328-1337.

4. Stone D., Phillips, A.W., and Burchall, J.J. (1977) Eur. J. Biochem., 72, 613-
   624.

5. Bitar, K.G., Blankenship, D.T., Walsh, K.A., Dunlap, R.B., Reddy, A.V.,
   and Freisheim, J.H. (1977) FEBS Lett., 80, 119-122.

6. Stone, D., and Phillips, A.W. (1977) FEBS Lett., 74, 85-87.

7. Peterson, D.L., Gleisner, J.M., and Blakley, R.L. (1975) Biochemistry, 14,
   5261-5267.

8. Tarr, G.E. (1977) Methods in Enzymol., 47, part E, 335-357.

9. Guidotti, G. (1960) Biochim. Biophys. Acta, 42, 177-179.

10. Keil-Dlouhá, V., Zylber, N., Imhoff, J.-M., Tong, N.-T., and Keil, B. (1971)
    FEBS Lett., 16, 291-295.

11. Matthews, D.A., Alden, R.A., Bolin, J.T., Freer, S.T., Hamlin, R., Xuong, N.,
    Kraut, J., Poe, M., Williams, M., Hoogsteen, K. (1977) Science, 197, 452-455.

12. Matthews, D.A., Alden, R.A., Bolin, J.T., Filman, D.J., Freer, S.T.,Hamlin,
    R., Hoe, W.G.T., Kisliuk, R.L. Pastore, E.J., Plante, T., Xuong, N-h., and
    Kraut, J. (1978) J. Biol. Chem., in press.

13. Matthews, D.A., Alden, R.A., Freer, S.T., Xuong, N-h., and Kraut, J., in press.

SUBSTRATE SPECIFICITY OF 10-FORMYLTETRAHYDROFOLATE SYNTHETASE

GARRY P. LEWIS, MAGGIE E. SALEM AND PETER B. ROWE
Department of Child Health, University of Sydney, N.S.W. AUSTRALIA 2006

INTRODUCTION

In mammals formate is derived from two major sources, the oxidation
of methionine and other methylated compounds and the catabolism of
tryptophan. Formate is salvaged primarily by the enzyme formyltetrahydrofolate synthetase for use in the folate-mediated one-carbon donor
reactions of purine biosynthesis. This enzyme has been found in
virtually all tissues and species studied, and has been reported as
existing in the form of a multifunctional protein with two other folate
pathway enzymes in mammalian liver. Since folates exist in the
mammalian cell primarily as polyglutamates, and the polyglutamate forms
are preferentially utilized by several folate dependent enzymes, we
have studied the utilization of polyglutamates by mammalian formyltetrahydrofolate synthetase. The only previously reported studies of
polyglutamate specificity of this enzyme used enzyme from a purine
fermenting bacterium and were concerned with the reverse (formate-
releasing) activity[1].

METHODS

Polyglutamate derivatives of folic acid were synthesized using solid
phase techniques. Polyglutamate chain length was analyzed by high performance anion-exchange liquid chromatography using Partisil 10 SAX
columns. Reduction of folic acid polyglutamates to the tetrahydro
derivatives was achieved by both chemical and electrochemical methods.
Enzyme used was an ammonium sulphate fraction from bovine or rat liver,
stabilized in solution with 1M ammonium sulphate.

RESULTS

Using $H_4PteGlu_1$ as folate substrate, the reaction had absolute
requirements for formate and ATP, and the optimal temperature was 30°.
Bovine enzyme Km values were 0.1mM for $H_4PteGlu_1$ and 7mM for formate.
Rat liver Km values were 0.4mM for $H_4PteGlu_1$ and 5mM for formate.

Using $H_4PteGlu_5$ as folate substrate, the reaction had an absolute
requirement for ATP but an only partial requirement for added formate
and the optimal temperature was 41°. The degree of formate independence was decreased using electrochemically reduced instead of chemically reduced $H_4PteGlu_5$. Bovine liver had Km values of 10μM for

442

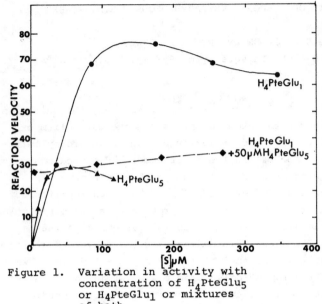

Figure 1. Variation in activity with
concentration of $H_4PteGlu_5$
or $H_4PteGlu_1$ or mixtures
of both.

$H_4PteGlu_5$ and 0.1mM
for formate, while rat
enzyme Km values were
6μM for $H_4PteGlu_5$ and
0.8mM for formate.
The maximum velocity,
as well as the folate
Km, was lower using H_4
$PteGlu_5$ (Fig.1). When
a mixture of $H_4PteGlu_5$
and $H_4PteGlu_1$ was used
a fivefold excess of
$H_4PteGlu_1$ over H_4Pte
Glu_5 caused negligible
increase of activity
over that due solely
to $H_4PteGlu_5$, illust-
rating the preferen-
tial utilization of
the polyglutamate.

DISCUSSION

As has been reported for several other folate dependent enzymes,
formyltetrahydrofolate synthetase exhibits a lower Km for a polyglutamate substrate than for a monoglutamate. Most reported $H_4PteGlu_1$
Km values have been 1 or 2mM but ranging from 0.1 to 10mM, while
formate Km has been reported from 1 to 25mM. Since the tissue concentrations of these substrates are likely to be orders of magnitude below
these Km values, the significance of the enzyme has remained question-
able. Our results indicating a Km for $H_4PteGlu_5$ of 6-10μM, a figure
much closer to the reported total folate concentration in liver of 10-
20μM, are therefore of use in ascribing a possible role for the enzyme
in cellular folate metabolism and purine biosynthesis. Although
cellular formate concentration is unknown, the lower formate Km values
obtained using $H_4PteGlu_5$ are probably of similar significance.

The nature of the formate independent activity observed with H_4Pte
Glu_5 is currently under investigation, but its existence invalidates
the use of formate omission as a suitable blank for assays using
polyglutamate substrates.

REFERENCES

1. Curthoys, N.P. and Rabinowitz, J.C. (1972) J. Biol.Chem.,
    247, 1965-1971.

FORMIMINOTRANSFERASE-CYCLODEAMINASE, A BIFUNCTIONAL PROTEIN FROM PIG LIVER

ROBERT E. MACKENZIE

Department of Biochemistry, McGill University, Montreal Canada H3G 1Y6

ABSTRACT

Proteolysis of native transferase-deaminase with low levels of chymotrypsin destroys the deaminase activity and is greatly accelerated by the presence of the inhibitor folic acid; this effect can be reversed by the inclusion of 10 mM KCl in the digestion medium. Purification of the digest demonstrated that the native octomeric structure was destroyed and that a 39,000 dalton fragment of the 64,000 dalton uncleaved subunit retains the transferase activity. From measurements of the time course of appearance of products it is concluded that the bifunctional enzyme is designed to utilize tetrahydropteroylpentaglutamate in order to channel the product of the transferase through the deaminase site and avoid accumulation of the formiminotetrahydrofolate intermediate.

INTRODUCTION

Formiminoglutamate: tetrahydrofolate formiminotransferase (EC 2.1.2.5.)-formiminotetrahydrofolate cyclodeaminase (EC 4.3.1.4.) activities were first co-purified from acetone powders of pig liver[1,2]. A crystalline, homogeneous protein prepared from frozen liver[3] was used to demonstrate that the protein is an octomer of identical polypeptides of 64,000 daltons arranged in a circular structure[3,4]. This protein belongs to the general class of multifunctional proteins where a single polypeptide is responsible for two different functions[5]. The transferase and deaminase sites are distinct since chymotryptic digestion[1] and sulfhydryl reagents[6] inactivate the deaminase while high pH less specifically inactivates the transferase[1]. In this paper we report isolation of a chymotryptic fragment containing transferase activity, and demonstrate a unique advantage of poly-glutamate substrates with this bifunctional protein.

MATERIALS AND METHOD

Transferase-deaminase was purified as described previously[3]; chymotrypsin, phenylmethylsulfonyl fluoride (PMSF) and formiminoglutamate were from Sigma. Pteroylpolyglutamates were provided by Dr. Charles Baugh, University of South Alabama and dihydrofolate reductase by Dr. Roy Kisliuk, Tufts University.

Chymotryptic digestion. Purified octomeric enzyme (500 μg/ml) was treated with 10 μg chymotrypsin in 0.1 M triethanolamine.HCl pH 7.3 at room temperature for 15 to 45 minutes, and the proteolysis was halted with PMSF. The digest was applied to a column of Ultragel AcA 34 (LKB), and the fractions assayed for transferase activity. Samples were subjected to dodecyl sulfate electrophoresis[7].

Preparation of tetrahydropteroylpolyglutamates. ℓ-Tetrahydropteroyl (glutamate)$_n$
(n = 1, 3 and 5) were prepared by reduction of 5 μmoles of the folate to the dihydro-
derivative with sodium dithionite in ascorbic acid at pH 6.0[8] followed by conversion
to the tetrahydrocompounds using dihydrofolate reductase. The tetrahydrofolates
were purified by chromatography on DEAE-cellulose and assayed enzymatically.

RESULTS

Proteolysis of the transferase-deaminase by chymotropsin is shown in Figure 1 and
requires the inhibitor folic acid at these low chymotrypsin concentrations.
Digestion could not be obtained in phosphate buffer, and even the addition of 10 mM
KCl to the mix prevented proteolysis. Purification of the products of digestion by
gel chromatography showed that the native octomeric structure was destroyed and the
bulk of the transferase activity eluted after the position of the native enzyme
(Figure 2). Dodecyl sulfate gel electrophoresis indicated that this transferase
activity was due to a polypeptide chain of 39,000 daltons Figures 3 and 4).

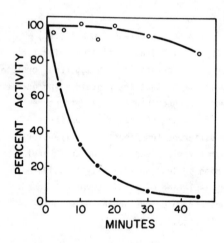

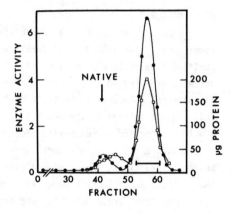

Fig. 1. Digestion of transferase-
deaminase by chymotrypsin as described
in methods; no folic acid (o) and 2 mM
folic acid (●).

Fig. 2. Purification of chymotryptic
digest on a column of Ultrogel AcA 34 in
0.1 M potassium phosphate pH 7.3.

Because the transferase and deaminase are sequential activities in the pathway of
formiminoglutamate metabolism, a possible kinetic advantage for this bifunctional
enzyme was sought. The time course of appearance of the products of the transferase
and of the deaminase were followed using formiminoglutamate and ℓ-tetrahydropteroyl-
glutamate as substrates. A significant lag was observed in the appearance of the

final product methenyltetrahydropteroylglutamate, indicating that the intermediate formiminotetrahydrofolate is released into the medium. However, the lag was reduced with the triglutamate substrate and disappeared with the pentaglutamate (Figure 5). The polyglutamates showed the same values of Vmax but the values of Km were 48, 31 and 3.5 μM for 1, 3 and 5 glutamates respectively.

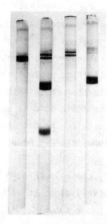

Fig. 3. Dodecyl sulfate gel electro-phoresis of formiminotransferase cyclodeaminase. From left to right the gels contain: control; enzyme after digestion with chymotrypsin; aliquot from the first transferase peak (native size); purified fragment.

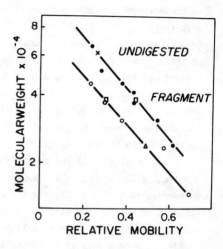

Fig. 4. Molecular weight of fragment on 10 and 12 percent polyacrylamide gels determined with standard proteins.

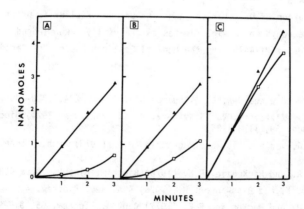

Fig. 5. Time course of appearance of products with 5 mM formiminoglutamate and 25 μM A. Tetrahydropteroyl glutamate B. Tetrahydropteroyl (glutamate)$_3$ and C. Tetrahydropteroyl (glutamate)$_5$.

SUMMARY

Formiminotransferase-cyclodeaminase is a very large protein composed of eight identical polypeptides of about 64,000 daltons[3,4] and is a bifunctional protein[5]. The number of active sites have not been determined directly, although eight sulfhydryl groups are responsible for deaminase activity[6] thereby suggesting eight deaminase sites. The interactions between the two active sites and their location in the polypeptide chain must be clarified in order to better understand the advantages of the bifunctionality of the protein. The isolation of a fragment having transferase activity suggests that the two sites are contained in different domains of the polypeptide. The deaminase domain becomes susceptible to proteolysis in the presence of folic acid, although it is interesting to note that this inhibitor protects the enzyme from modification with DTNB[6]. Because folic acid is an inhibitor of both activities it is not clear whether binding to the deaminase or transferase or both is required to effect the conformational changes necessary for susceptibility to proteolysis.

The observation that the pentaglutamate preferentially channels through the deaminase site suggests that the two sites must be relatively close to each other. However it is not clear whether the two sites are on the same subunit, different subunits or whether one site is formed by interaction between subunits. Nevertheless it is clear that the bifunctionality of the protein and the pentaglutamate substrate combine to make a very efficient system to utilize the one carbon fragment of formiminoglutamate, both from a kinetic stand point as well as in avoiding the accumulation of a labile folate intermediate.

ACKNOWLEDGEMENTS

The cooperation of Dr. Charles Baugh and Dr. Roy Kisliuk in providing the means to obtain ℓ-tetrahydropteroylglutamates is gratefully acknowledged. This work was supported by grant MT-4479 from the Medical Research Council of Canada.

REFERENCES

1. Tabor, H. and Wyngarden, L. (1959) J. Biol. Chem. 234, 1830-1846.
2. Slavik, K., Zizkovsky, V., Slavikova, V. and Fort, P. (1974) Biochem. Biophys. Res. Commun. 59, 1173-1184.
3. Drury, E.J., Bazar, L.S. and MacKenzie, R.E. (1975) Arch. Biochem. Biophys. 169, 662-668.
4. Beaudet, R. and MacKenzie, R.E. (1976) Biochim. Biophys. Acta 453, 151-161.
5. Kirschner, K. and Bisswanger, H. (1976) Ann. Rev. Biochem. 45, 143-166.
6. Drury, E.J. and MacKenzie, R.E. (1977) Can. J. Biochem. 55, 919-923.
7. Weber, K. and Osborn, M. (1969) J. Biol. Chem. 244, 4406-4412.
8. Blakley, R.L. (1960) Nature 188, 231-232.

STUDIES ON IDENTIFYING THE SUBSTRATE BINDING SITES OF <u>LACTOBACILLUS</u> <u>CASEI</u>
THYMIDYLATE SYNTHETASE

GLADYS F. MALEY, RONALD L. BELLISARIO, DON U. GUARINO AND FRANK MALEY
Division of Laboratories and Research, New York State Department of Health
Albany, New York 12201

ABSTRACT

Procedures for obtaining the complete amino acid sequence of <u>Lactobacillus</u> <u>casei</u>
thymidylate synthetase are described in part. The enzyme consists of two identical
subunits, each composed of 316 amino acids which yield a molecular weight for the
holoenzyme of 73,176. The nucleophile involved in ternary complex formation and
reactive with sulfhydryl reagents in the native enzyme has been identified as
Cysteine-198. A second apparently unreactive cysteine was located at Residue 244.
Preliminary experiments are described in attempting to fix the position of the folate
binding site.

INTRODUCTION

The elucidation of the primary sequence of thymidylate synthetase (EC 2.1.1.45)
would provide an opportunity to clearly identify functional groups involved in substrate binding and would also possibly clarify their role in the unique reductive
methylation reaction catalyzed by this enzyme. Much of what is known about this
reaction is based on model systems[1] and the stable ternary complex resulting from the
interaction of the enzyme with FdUMP and $5,10\text{-}CH_2H_4PteGlu_1$[2,3]. However, this complex
while representing a plausible transition-state intermediate may in reality be a
dead-end complex which has been side-tracked from the main reaction pathway. If this
is the case, it could explain why the enzyme binds two moles each of FdUMP and 5,10-
$CH_2H_4PteGlu_1$, while apparently only binding one of dUMP[4]. As shown previously by us
through kinetic studies with chick embryo thymidylate synthetase[5] and equilibrium
dialysis studies with <u>Lactobacillus</u> <u>casei</u> thymidylate synthetase[4], the reaction is an
ordered one with dUMP (or deoxynucleotide analogue) adding first, which in turn pro-
motes the binding of $5,10\text{-}CH_2H_4PteGlu_1$. This order of addition is supported by

recent kinetic studies with the human blast cell[6] and L. casei synthetases[7].

There is little doubt now that the reaction is initiated by the nucleophilic addition of an enzyme cysteinyl residue to the 6-position of the pyrimidine ring of dUMP to saturate the 5,6-position. By sequencing the L. casei synthetase we have been able to locate the residues involved, which is the major focus of this report. In addition, we will report on our initial attempts to identify the sites involved in folate binding.

MATERIALS AND METHODS

L. casei thymidylate synthetase was obtained from the New England Enzyme Center, Boston, Massachusetts, as a dialyzed ammonium sulfate fraction and purified to homogeneity[8]. The guanidine-HCl denatured enzyme was reduced and S-carboxymethylated with [1-^{14}C]iodoacetate[9] and after dialysis was converted by enzymatic and chemical cleavages to the peptides necessary for these studies. For studies with the ternary complex, [2-^{14}C]FdUMP was used[9]. The methodology employed for sequencing either form of the synthetase is to be described[10]. Folylpolyglutamates were generously provided by Dr. Charles Baugh of the Department of Biochemistry, University of South Alabama, Mobile, Alabama. These compounds were coupled to the synthetase with a water soluble carbodiimide as described by Chu and Whitely[11].

RESULTS AND DISCUSSION

Sequence Methodology. The critical peptides necessary for initiating the sequence analysis were derived by the unique extraction procedure described in Fig. 1. The demonstration of only five CNBr peptides on SDS-acrylamide gel electrophoresis or by the isolation procedures indicated in Fig. 1 suggested the presence of four methionines in each of the enzyme's apparently identical subunits. However, the finding of six methionines in each subunit raised a serious complication, which was fortunately resolved by the demonstration of a methionyl residue on the NH$_2$-terminal end and the presence of a methionine resistant to cleavage in CNBr 2 (Met-101, Fig. 2).

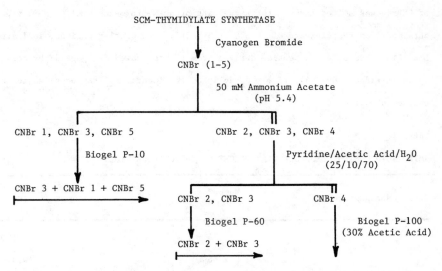

SCM—THYMIDYLATE SYNTHETASE

Cyanogen Bromide

CNBr (1-5)

50 mM Ammonium Acetate
(pH 5.4)

CNBr 1, CNBr 3, CNBr 5   CNBr 2, CNBr 3, CNBr 4

Biogel P-10   Pyridine/Acetic Acid/H$_2$O
                                (25/10/70)

CNBr 3 + CNBr 1 + CNBr 5   CNBr 2, CNBr 3   CNBr 4

                            Biogel P-60   Biogel P-100
                                                  (30% Acetic Acid)

                            CNBr 2 + CNBr 3

Fig. 1. Isolation of peptides from SCM-thymidylate synthetase hydrolyzed with cyanogen bromide. Horizontal arrows indicate order of elution of peptides from the Biogel columns.

As indicated in Fig. 1, the extracted CNBr peptides were easily separated in pure form by Biogel chromatography, with the largest peptide, CNBr 4, solubilized in 30% acetic acid and purified on Biogel P-100. This peptide was shown previously (designated at that time as CN2[9]) to encompass the site containing the inhibitory FdUMP-ternary complex, which is presumably the same as the active site of the enzyme. Residue analysis of each peptide (Table 1) provided a true measure of their size, which in turn confirmed that Biogel chromatographic elution was more accurate than SDS-gel electrophoresis for establishing the size of the CNBr peptides.

Table 1 reveals that each peptide subunit contains 316 amino acid residues with the resultant molecular weight of the holoenzyme being 73,176 on summing the amino acid residues comprising the enzyme. To locate the CNBr peptides relative to one another in the linear array of an enzyme subunit, the presence of an NH$_2$-terminal methionine established CNBr 1 at the NH$_2$-end of each subunit, while the presence of valine at the COOH-terminus of CNBr 5 clearly fixed this peptide on the COOH-terminal end of a subunit. Limited tryptic (LT) and BNPS-skatole peptides were used primarily to place CNBr 2, 3, and 4. The amino acid residues at which cleavage was effected to yield the desired peptides is shown in Fig. 2. The difficult COOH-terminal sequence of CNBr 4 was solved through the sequencing of an N-bromosuccinimide (NBS) peptide obtained from the cleavage of BNPS 8 at Tyr-261. The overlap regions, indicated by LT2, LT6, BNPS 8, and a peptide derived from the indicated NBS peptide by acid hydrolysis (Residues 289-304), firmly established the location of the peptides in the enzyme subunit.

TABLE 1

AMINO ACID CONTENT AND MOLECULAR WEIGHT OF THE CNBr PEPTIDES

CNBr peptide	Number of residues	MW
1	36	4,100
2	86	10,300
3	71	8,100
4	103	11,800
5	20	2,200
Total	316	36,500

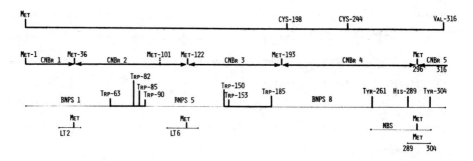

Fig. 2. Peptides used to establish the sequence of thymidylate synthetase.

The Active Site Peptide. Sequencing of S-carboxymethylated synthetase or the FdUMP containing ternary complex revealed in both cases that labeled products were associated with CNBr 4. In the case of [1-^{14}C]iodoacetate inactivated enzyme the radioactivity was associated with only one of the enzyme's four sulfhydryls, the same residue as that involved in ternary complex formation, Cys-198. In the latter case, however, Cys-198 in each subunit had reacted. The reason for this perplexing result is not apparent, but has been repeated numerous times and with other thiol reagents[12]. As indicated in Fig. 2, the second thiol resides at Cys-244.

Folylpolyglutamate Binding. While most kinetic studies have employed $5,10$-CH_2H_4-$PteGlu_1$ as a substrate, the corresponding naturally occurring folates exist in the polyglutamate state. As revealed previously[13], there is a clear dichotomy in the binding of the two substrates, with nucleotide binding being prevented by sulfhydryl inhibitors and folate binding by carboxypeptidase treatment of the synthetase. Although $5,10$-$CH_2H_4PteGlu_1$ or $PteGlu_1$ do not bind in the absence of FdUMP[4,13], $PteGlu_4$ and $PteGlu_7$ bind effectively in the absence of dUMP or FdUMP, the extent of which is greatly impaired with carboxypeptidase treated enzyme, particularly in the case of $PteGlu_4$[14]. Since binding of the folylpolyglutamates is so effective, we attempted to determine if $PteGlu_7$ can be fixed to the protein in a site specific manner, a possibility suggested from kinetic studies which revealed that unreduced folylpolygluta-mates are competitive inhibitors of $5,10$-$CH_2H_4PteGlu_1$[15,16]. Through the use of water soluble carbodiimide, the fixation of $Pte[^{14}C]GluGlu_6$ was measured and found to occur as shown in Table 2.

TABLE 2

EFFECT OF TIME ON THE BINDING OF PTEROYLGLUTAMATE TO THYMIDYLATE SYNTHETASE

Time	$[^{14}C]PteGlu_7$ bound	Ratio
(min)	(nmoles)	$PteGlu_7$/enzyme
30	4.24	0.61
60	6.49	0.93
120	8.88	1.27
180	9.57	1.38

The reaction mixture contained L. casei thymidylate synthetase (7 nmoles), dUMP (0.1 µmole), $Pte[^{14}C]GluGlu_6$ (0.13 µmole) (1 µC per µmole) and 1-ethyl-3-(dimethyl-aminopropyl)-carbodiimide hydrochloride (0.15 µmole) in 0.05 M $NaHCO_3$, pH 7.0, at 25°. Aliquots were removed at the indicated times and bound radioactivity determined by a filter assay[2].

Less fixation occurred in the presence of dUMP (data not presented) suggesting that the specificity of the reaction is promoted by the nucleotide. The labeled protein has been digested with trypsin and a peptide isolated containing the folate is being purified in preparation for sequencing. With the aid of the complete linear sequence of the synthetase, which is now available, it should not be difficult to locate the site to which the folate is bound.

REFERENCES

1. Pogolotti, A. L., Jr. and Santi, D. V. (1977) Bioorganic Chem., 1, 277-311.

2. Santi, D. V. and McHenry, C. S. (1972) Proc. Natl. Acad. Sci. U.S.A., 69, 1855-1857.

3. Langenbach, R. J., Dannenberg, D. V. and Heidelberger, C. (1972) Biochem. Biophys. Res. Commun., 48, 1565-1571.

4. Galivan, J. H., Maley, G. F. and Maley, F. (1976) Biochemistry, 15, 356-362.

5. Lorenson, M. Y., Maley, G. F. and Maley, F. (1967) J. Biol. Chem., 242, 3332-3344.

6. Dolnick, B. J. and Cheng, Y.-C. (1977) J. Biol. Chem., 252, 7697-7703.

7. Daron, H. H. and Aull, J. L. (1978) J. Biol. Chem., 253, 940-945.

8. Galivan, J. H., Maley, G. F. and Maley, F. (1975) Biochemistry, 14, 3338-3343.

9. Bellisario, R. L., Maley, G. F., Galivan, J. H. and Maley, F. (1976) Proc. Natl. Acad. Sci. U.S.A., 73, 1848-1852.

10. Maley, G. F., Bellisario, R. L., Guarino, D. U. and Maley, F. (1978) J. Biol. Chem., in press.

11. Chu, B. C. F. and Whitely, J. M. (1977) Mol. Pharm., 13, 80-88.

12. Galivan, J., Noonan, J. and Maley, F. (1977) Arch. Biochem. Biophys., 184, 336-345.

13. Galivan, J. H., Maley, F. and Baugh, C. M. (1976) Biochem. Biophys. Res. Commun., 71, 527-534.

14. Galivan, J., Maley, F. and Baugh, C. M. (1977) Arch. Biochem. Biophys., 184, 346-354.

15. Kisliuk, R. L., Gaumont, Y. and Baugh, C. M. (1974) J. Biol. Chem., 249, 4100-4103.

16. Dolnick, B. J. and Cheng, Y.-C. (1978) J. Biol. Chem., 253, 3563-3567.

THE EVALUATION OF FOLATE ANALOGUES AS INHIBITORS OF FOLATE ENZYMES

JOHN H. MANGUM, SANDRA L. BLACK, MICHAEL J. BLACK, C. DENIS PETERSON,
SANHA PANICHAJAKUL, AND JEFFREY BRAMAN
Brigham Young University Cancer Research Center, Provo, Utah 84602
(U.S.A.)

ABSTRACT

An enzyme screen for antifolates has been established that currently
includes dihydrofolate reductase, serine transhydroxymethylase, 5,10-
methylene tetrahydrofolate reductase, methionine synthetase, 5,10-
methylenetetrahydrofolate dehydrogenase, glycinamide ribotide transformylase, aminoimidazole carboxamide ribotide transformylase, cyclohydrolase, 10-formyltetrahydrofolate synthetase, and thymidylate synthetase. The availability of these enzymes coupled with the fact
that assays for each of these enzymes have been standardized has
enabled us to evaluate the inhibitory properties of approximately 100
potential antifolates.

INTRODUCTION

The antifolate drug, methotrexate, has been shown to interact primarily with dihydrofolate reductase. The inhibition of this enzyme results in an accumulation of dihydrofolate and leads to the eventual
lowering of the cellular levels of free tetrahydrofolate as well as the
coenzyme forms of tetrahydrofolate. The primary consequence of these
events appears to be a diminished rate of synthesis of deoxythymidylate
which then in turn limits DNA synthesis.

It has been suggested that it might be necessary to look beyond
dihydrofolate reductase in order to obtain a more complete understanding of the mechanism of action of methotrexate since the possibility
exits that the administration of this agent might also inhibit other
essential folate enzymes. In order to carefully examine this possibility, four years ago we initiated a research effort with the following
objectives: (1) to isolate a series of folate-dependent enzymes from
both normal and tumor animal tissues; (2) to determine the extent to
which methotrexate as well as certain other folate analogues inhibited
these enzymes; and (3) to use these determinations as a screen for
potential antifolates. This manuscript summarizes the progress we
have made in this endeavor.

RESULTS AND DISCUSSION

In Table 1 we have listed the ten enzymes that are employed in our screen for antifolates. Each of these enzymes have been purified to the extent and from the source indicated. In those situations where we have relied primarily on a published purification scheme we have referenced this in the Table. The absence of a reference implies that we have worked out the purification procedure and currently the details have not been published. Similarily, we have also indicated the type of assay employed for each enzyme and have also provided a reference when the assay used was based primarily on a previously published method.

TABLE 1

ENZYMES CURRENTLY INCLUDED IN THE SCREEN

Enzyme	Source	Fold Purification	Type of Assay
Dihydrofolate Reductase	Beef Liver	$11,400^1$	Spectrophotometric[1]
Serine Transhydroxy-methylase	Beef Liver	400^2	Formation of $[^{14}C]$-HCHO[3]
5,10-Methylenetetrahy-drofolate Reductase	Pig Kidney	300^4	Formation of $[^{14}C]$-HCHO[4] Spectrophotometric[5]
Methionine Synthetase	Pig Kidney	$1,800^6$	Formation of $[^{14}C]$-Met[7]
5,10-Methylenetetrahy-drofolate Dehydrogenase	Pig Liver	$100^{8,9}$	Spectrophotometric[8]
Glycinamide Ribotide Transformylase	Pigeon Liver	32	Spectrophotometric[10]
Aminoimidazole Carbox-amide Ribotide Trans-formylase	Pigeon Liver	392	Spectrophotometric[11]
Cyclohydrolase	Pig Liver	$100^{8,9}$	Spectrophotometric[8]
Formate Activating Enzyme	Pig Liver	$100^{8,9}$	Spectrophotometric[8]
Thymidylate Synthetase	Calf Thymus	100^{12}	Formation of $[^3H]$-H_2O

To date we have used this enzyme screen to evaluate approximately 100 potential antifolates. Those compounds which we have examined have been supplied primarily by the Division of Cancer Treatment, National Cancer Institute, who have provided the financial support for the development of this screen. We have received and evaluated thirty aminopterin-methotrexate analogues, homofolate and 5-methyl tetrahydrohomofolate, sixteen pteroylglutamic acid analogues, twenty substituted diamino triazines (Baker antifols), two quinoliniums, two quinazolines, ten pteridine derivatives, and 20 other agents that cannot be conveniently placed into any particular category.

Table 2 contains representative data for two of the inhibitors we have evaluated. Methotrexate appears to be quite specific for dihydrofolate reductase since it failed to inhibit any of the other enzymes to any appreciable extent. This would strongly suggest that methotrexate _in vivo_ would not directly interfere with purine ring biosynthesis.

TABLE 2

INHIBITION OF FOLATE ENZYMES BY FOLATE ANALOGUES

Enzyme	Inhibition (%)	
	Methotrexate	5-MethylH_4homofolate
Dihydrofolate Reductase	$63(10^{-8})$ [a]	$30(10^{-4})$
Serine Transhydroxymethylase	$8(10^{-4})$	$3(10^{-4})$
5,10-Methylenetetrahydrofolate Reductase	$43(10^{-4})$	$25(10^{-4})$
Methionine Synthetase	$0(10^{-4})$	$25(10^{-4})$
5,10-Methylenetetrahydrofolate Dehydrogenase	$20(10^{-4})$	$7(10^{-4})$
Glycinamide Ribotide Transformylase	$0(10^{-4})$	$17(10^{-4})$
Aminoimidazole Carboxamide Ribotide Transformylase	$0(10^{-5})$	$21(10^{-4})$

[a] This number indicates the molar inhibitor concentration which resulted in the indicated % inhibition.

5-Methyltetrahydrohomofolic acid has been shown to possess anti-tumor activity in methotrexate insensitive tumors.[13] However, the inhibition data we have accumulated on this compound failed to provide a molecular rational for this activity (Table 2).

We have examined several Baker Anifols (substituted diamino triazines) containing a reactive sulfonyl fluoride group and have found that a few of them inhibit serine transhydroxymethylase and methionine synthetase. Furthermore, the inhibition is greatly increased by preincubating the enzyme and the inhibitor. This time dependent enhancement is compatable with there being a subsequent covalent attachment of the inhibitor to the enzyme.

A specific inhibitor of methionine synthetase would result in the buildup of 5-methyltetrahydrofolate with the concomitant diminishing of the cellular levels of tetrahydrofolate and its other coenzyme forms. This represents potentially as lethal a metabolic block as the inhibition of dihydrofolate reductase.

The inhibition of serine transhydroxymethylase would adversely affect cellular 5,10-methylene tetrahydrofolate formation which in turn would dramatically interfere with thymidylate and DNA biosynthesis. This represents an alternate basis for chemotherapy involving folate analogues, namely, depleting the cell of an essential one-carbon source rather than tetrahydrofolate stores.

SUMMARY

We have established a folate-dependent enzyme screen for antifolates that currently includes the following enzymes:

      (1)   dihydrofolate reductase

      (2)   serine transhydroxymethylase

      (3)   5,10-methylenetetrahydrofolate reductase

      (4)   methionine synthetase

      (5)   5,10-methylenetetrahydrofolate dehydrogenase

      (6)   glycinamide ribotide transformylase

      (7)   aminoimidazole carboxamide ribotide transformylase

      (8)   cyclohydrolase

      (9)   formate activating enzyme

    (10)   thymidylate synthetase

Over the last four years we have used these enzymes to screen a large number of antifolates. The majority of the compounds we tested were designed to inhibit dihydrofolate reductase. Obviously, many of the compounds we examined were analogues of methotrexate; we also looked at several diaminotriazines containing the reactive sulfonyl fluoride group. The homofolates were examined as well as a number of other compounds. From these studies it was readily apparent that those heterocyclic rings (pteridines, triazines, quinazolines) which contained the basic diamino structure of methotrexate were the most effective inhibitors of dihydrofolate reductase.

The majority of those compounds which inhibited dihydrofolate reductase failed to inhibit the other nine folate enzymes employed in our screen.

One of the primary objectives of the research described in this presentation is to identify the essential structural features that are required in order to design antifolates that will inhibit folate-dependent enzymes other than dihydrofolate reductase. We would like to provide an alternate way of placing one-carbon metabolism under stress where one might realize a beneficial chemotherapeutic effect equivalent to that of the classical antifolate, methotrexate.

ACKNOWLEDGMENTS

This work was supported by Contract No. NO1-CM-43790 from the Division of Cancer Treatment, National Cancer Institute, NIH, DHEW.

REFERENCES

1. Kaufman, B. and Kemerer, V. (1976) Arch. Biochem. Biophys., 172, 289-300.

2. Jones, C. and Priest, D. (1976) Arch. Biochem. Biophys., 174, 305-311.

3. Taylor, R. amd Weissbach, H. (1965) Anal. Biochem., 13, 80-84.

4. Kutzbach, C. and Stokstad, E. (1971) Biochim. Biophys. Acta, 250, 459-477.

5. Donaldson, K. and Keresztesy, J. (1962) J. Biol. Chem., 237, 1298-1304.

6. Mangum, J. and North, J. (1971) Biochem., 10, 3765-3769.

7. Weissbach, H., Peterkofsky, A., Redfied, B. and Dickerman, H. (1963) J. Biol. Chem., 238, 3318-3324.

8. MacKenzie, R. (1973) Biochem. Biophys. Res. Commun., 53, 1088-1095.

9. Tan, L., Drury, E. and MacKenzie, R. (1977) J. Biol. Chem., 252, 1117-1122.

10. Flaks, J. and Lukens, L. (1963) in Methods in Enzymology, VI, Colowick, S. and Kaplan, N. eds., Academic Press, New York, pp. 65-99.

11. Black, S., Black, M. and Mangum, J. (1978) Anal. Biochem., 89, in press.

12. Dolnick, B. and Cheng, Y. (1977) J. Biol. Chem., 252, 7697-7703.
13. Mishra, L. C. and Mead, J. A. R. (1972) Proc. Am. Assoc. Cancer Res. 13, 76.

INHIBITION OF PIG LIVER METHYLENETETRAHYDROFOLATE REDUCTASE BY DIHYDROFOLATE

ROWENA G. MATTHEWS AND BOBBIE J. HAYWOOD

Department of Biological Chemistry, University of Michigan and Veterans Administration
Hospital, Ann Arbor, Michigan (U.S.A.)

ABSTRACT

Pig liver methylenetetrahydrofolate reductase (E.C. 1.1.1.68) has been purified
3800 fold by a new method. The kinetics of the NADPH-methylene-FH_4 reductase
reaction catalyzed by this enzyme are consistent with a ping-pong bi bi mechanism
in which the enzyme reacts alternately with NADPH and methylene-FH_4. The K_m for
methylene-FH_4 is about 5 μM, and that for NADPH is 16 μM. Dihydrofolate inhibits
the NADPH-methylene-FH_4 reductase reaction. It is linearly competitive with respect
to methylene-FH_4 and has a K_i of 5 μM. The K_i for dihydrofolate inhibition of the
NADPH-methylene-FH_4 reductase reaction is 5-10X lower than the K_i values associated
with inhibition due to methyl-FH_4, folic acid, FH_4 or methenyl-FH_4.

INTRODUCTION

Methylenetetrahydrofolate reductase (E.C. 1.1.1.68) is one of five enzymes which
are known to utilize methylene-FH_4 as substrate. The enzyme catalyzes the reaction:

$$NADPH + H^+ + methylene\text{-}FH_4 \longrightarrow NADP^+ + methyl\text{-}FH_4$$

This reaction, which is effectively irreversible in vivo[1], commits one carbon units
to the pathways of S-adenosylmethionine dependent methylation in mammalian systems.
The mammalian enzyme was first identified by Donaldson and Keresztesy[2] who showed
that FAD was required for maximal activity. It was purified about 400-fold by
Kutzbach and Stokstad[3], who demonstrated that the enzyme was inhibited by S-adenosylmethionine. However, regulation of the enzyme by metabolites in competing pathways
had not been demonstrated. Since methylenetetrahydrofolate is also required for
biosynthesis of thymidylate, purines, serine and glycine, mechanisms for assuring an
equitable distribution of substrate might be expected.

MATERIALS AND METHODS

NADPH-methylene-FH_4 reductase activity was measured at 25° under nitrogen in 50
mM phosphate buffer pH 6.7, 0.3 mM in EDTA, 2.5 μM in FAD, and 12.5 mM in β-mercaptoethanol. Methylene-FH_4 was prepared each day by dissolving FH_4 annerobically in
carbonate buffer, pH 9.2, 50 mM in formaldehyde. Preincubation of the enzyme in a
solution containing 2 μM FAD and 100 μM NADPH was necessary in order to obtain
maximal activity in assays.

For the inhibition studies, dihydrofolate was prepared by the method of Futterman[4] and fresh stock solutions were prepared daily and stored under nitrogen. Methyl-FH_4 was obtained from Sigma; methenyl-FH_4 was prepared by the method of Tatum et al[5], and diluted into the assay mixtures at the start of the assay from a stock in 0.1 N HCl-0.1 β-mercaptoethanol. The FH_4 used in inhibition studies was purified by chromatography on DEAE-cellulose and stored under nitrogen. For the experiments in which FH_4 was used as an inhibitor, a solution of methylene-FH_4 prepared from a 1:1 mixture of FH_4 and formaldehyde was used as the substrate.

RESULTS

The procedure used for the purification of methylenetetrahydrofolate reductase is summarized in the table which follows. The data shown are for 1 kg of pig liver homogenate.

Purification of methylenetetrahydrofolate reductase from pig liver

Step	Activity units*	Specific activity (units/mg)	Relative purification	Yield
Crude homogenate	90,000	0.3	1x	100%
pH 5.8 supernatant	61,200	1.2	4x	68%
Eluate from DEAE-52 adsorption	55,060	23.9	80x	61%
Eluate from Affi-Gel Blue column	41,850	1141	3800x	46%

*nmoles methyl-FH_4 oxidized per minute at 37° determined as described by Kutzbach and Stokstad[3] with menadione as the electron acceptor.

The absorption spectrum of the enzyme after purification as outlined above shows elements characteristic of flavin absorption, and addition of NADPH leads to spectral changes characteristic of the bleaching of a flavoprotein. However, there is still significant contamination of the spectrum with colored impurities, and the protein is heterogeneous on disc gel electrophoresis.

Figure 1 (below)shows the kinetics of the NADPH-methylene-FH_4 reductase reaction catalyzed by the enzyme. The ratio of V_{max} in the NADPH-methylene-FH_4 reductase reaction to V_{max} in the NADPH-menadione reductase reaction is 0.28 which is substantially higher than the ratio previously reported.[3] The kinetics are consistent with a ping-pong bi bi mechanism in which the enzyme is alternately reduced by NADPH and reoxidized by methylene-FH_4. The K_m for methylene-FH_4 varies between 2 and 10 µM with different enzyme preparations. The K_m for NADPH is 16 µM.

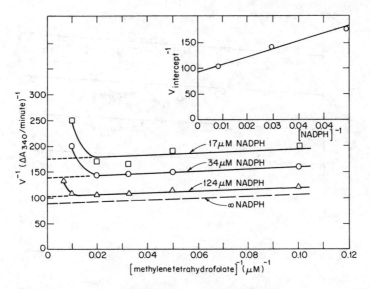

Figure 1. Kinetics of the NADPH–methylene-FH$_4$ reductase reaction. 10 µL of an enzyme solution which was approximately 0.07 µM in enzyme bound FAD was used for each assay (2 ml total volume).

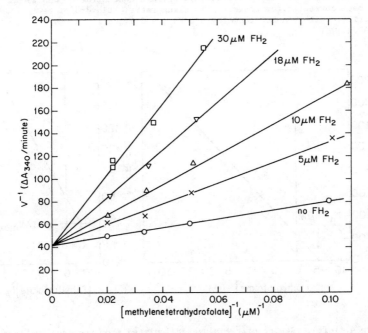

Figure 2. Effect of dihydrofolate on the methylene-FH$_4$ reductase reaction. 25 µL of an enzyme solution which was approximately 0.07 µM in enzyme bound FAD was used for each assay. The NADPH concentration was 124 µM. The data have been corrected for nonenzymatic blank rates.

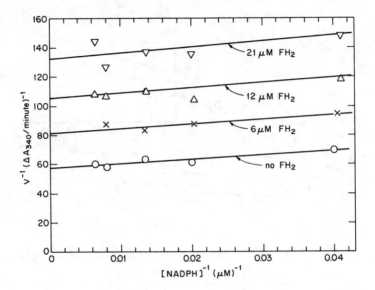

Figure 3. Effect of dihydrofolate on methylene-FH$_4$ reductase reaction. Conditions as in figure 2. The methylenetetrahydrofolate concentration was 29 μM. The data have been corrected for nonenzymatic blank rates. Dihydrofolate is linearly competitive with respect to methylene-FH$_4$, and linearly uncompetitive with respect to NADPH.

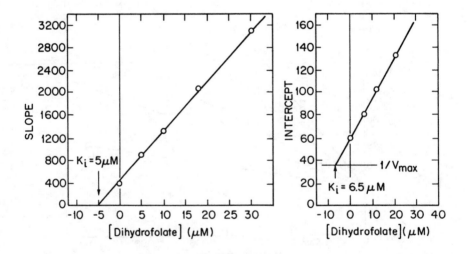

Figure 4.(left). Replot of the slopes calculated from the data in Figure 2 versus the concentration of dihydrofolate.
Figure 5. (right). Replot of the intercepts in Figure 3 as a function of the dihydrofolate concentration.

The data presented in Figures 2-5 are consistent with a simple competition of dihydrofolate for the methylene-FH$_4$ binding site on reduced enzyme. Although the inhibition caused by S-adenosylmethionine occurs slowly, requiring almost 5 minutes after addition of this inhibitor to exert its maximal effect[3], the inhibition exerted by dihydrofolate is effected immediately on addition of this compound, and preincubation with dihydrofolate does not increase the level of inhibition seen. When the effect of dihydrofolate on the methyltetrahydrofolate-menadione reductase reaction catalyzed by methylene-FH$_4$ reductase was examined, it was found that dihydrofolate was competitive with respect to methyl-FH$_4$ and uncompetitive with respect to menadione.

Figure 6 compares the inhibition exerted by dihydrofolate with the effects of other folate derivatives on the NADPH-methylene-FH$_4$ reductase reaction.

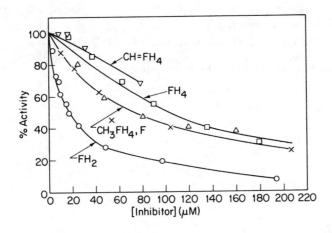

Figure 6. Inhibition exerted by folate derivatives on the NADPH-methylene-FH$_4$ reductase reaction. Each assay contained 25 µL of an enzyme solution which was approximately 0.07 µM in enzyme bound FAD, 124 µM NADPH, and 29 µM methylene-FH$_4$. The data shown have been corrected for blank rates measured in the absence of enzyme. Data points are for inhibition by dihydrofolate (o), methyl-FH$_4$ (x), folic acid (Δ), FH$_4$ (□) and methenyl-FH$_4$ (∇).

The observed order of effectiveness of inhibition is dihydrofolate, methyl-FH$_4$, folic acid, FH$_4$, and methenyl-FH$_4$, in decreasing order. There is a 5-fold difference between the concentration of dihydrofolate required for 50% inhibition, and the concentration of methyltetrahydrofolate required.

SUMMARY

Dihydrofolate has been shown to be a competitive inhibitor with respect to methylene-FH$_4$ in the NADPH-methylene-FH4 reductase reaction. This inhibition is characterized by a K_i which is 5-6 μM, in the same concentration range as the K_m for methylene-FH_4. While these results have been obtained <u>in vitro</u>, it is possible that dihydrofolate also inhibits the enzyme <u>in vivo</u>, serving to spare methylene-FH_4 under conditions where the rate of thymidylate biosynthesis is elevated.

ACKNOWLEDGEMENTS

This work has been supported by the Medical Research Service of the Veterans Administration and in part by Grant GM 24908 from the National Institute of General Medical Sciences, National Institutes of Health, Public Health Service and Michigan Memorial Phoenix Project 534. This work was done during the tenure of an Established Investigatorship of the American Heart Association (R.G.M.).

REFERENCES

1. Katzen, H.M., and Buchanan, J.M. (1965) J. Biol. Chem., 240, 825-835.

2. Donaldson, K.O., And Keresztesy, J.C. (1959) J. Biol. Chem., 234, 3235-3240.

3. Kutzbach, C., and Stokstad, E.L.R. (1971) Biochem. Biophy. Acta, 250, 459-477.

4. Futterman, S. (1957) J. Biol. Chem., 228, 1031-1038.

5. Tatum, C.M., Jr., Benkovic, P.A., Benkovic, S.J., Potts, R., Schleicher, E., and Floss, H.G. (1977) Biochemistry, 16, 1093-1102.

X-RAY STRUCTURAL STUDIES OF DIHYDROFOLATE REDUCTASE

D. A. MATTHEWS, R. A. ALDEN, J. T. BOLIN, D. J. FILMAN, S. T. FREER,
N. XUONG AND J. KRAUT
Department of Chemistry, University of California, San Diego,
La Jolla, California 92093 (USA)

Introduction

Dihydrofolate reductase (DHFR) catalyzes the NADPH linked reduction of dihydrofolate to tetrahydrofolate. Tetrahydrofolate is
in turn an essential cofactor in the synthesis of important metabolites, including thymidylate. Clinically useful dihydrofolate
reductase inhibitors such as methotrexate (MTX) and trimethoprim
operate by blocking the synthesis of these metabolites. In order to
better understand the structure, function, evolution and ligand
binding properties of this important enzyme we are studying the
x-ray structure of several DHFRs and of their complexes with certain
inhibitors.

We have recently determined the structure of bacterial DHFRs from
E. coli[1] and L. casei[2,3] and are currently working on a third DHFR
from chicken liver. Both of the bacterial enzymes were crystallized
in the presence of MTX and crystals of L. casei DHFR contain bound
NADPH in addition. These two structures were determined from electron
density maps at 2.5 Å resolution. High resolution refinement of
both initial models is now in progress.

General Structural Features

The overall folding of the backbone chain is dominated by a large
eight-stranded beta sheet which starts at the amino terminus and
ends with a single antiparallel strand at the carboxy terminus
(Fig. 1). Thirty percent of the backbone chain is involved in this
piece of secondary structure. The individual beta strands are connected by four helices and by a number of loops. Taken together
the helices incorporate about 23% of the backbone chain.

MTX binds near the top of a 15 Å deep cavity that cuts across one
whole face of the enzyme. The lower portion of this cavity also
binds the nicotinamide portion of NADPH. The remainder of the
coenzyme occupies a shallow groove that winds back across the carboxyl
ends of beta strands B-E. Unlike other pyridine nucleotide linked
reductases that have been characterized crystallographically, DHFR

does not contain separate domains for binding substrate and coenzyme. In fact, binding of MTX and NADPH is carried out by overlapping portions of the primary amino acid sequence.

When 142 out of the 159 α-carbon coordinates in *E. coli* DHFR are matched by least squares to structurally equivalent α-carbon coordinates for the *L. casei* enzyme, the rms deviation is 1.7 Å. Thus, despite the rather low sequence homology for these two bacterial reductases (27%) and despite the fact that NADPH is bound to the *L. casei* enzyme complex but not the *E. coli* enzyme complex, the backbone geometries of the two are very similar. There are, however, several definite differences in backbone conformation between the *L. casei* DHFR ternary complex and the *E. coli* DHFR binary complex. Some of these differences are evidently due to coenzyme binding and are discussed below.

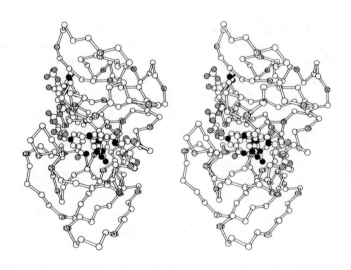

Fig. 1. Stereo drawing of the 162 α-carbon atoms in *L. casei* DHFR. Also shown are bound molecules of NADPH and MTX. Nitrogen and oxygen atoms are indicated by blackening and shading respectively.

Binding of Methotrexate

Methotrexate binds to DHFR in an extended conformation with its pteridine ring nearly perpendicular to the aromatic ring of its p-aminobenzoyl group. Every residue interacting with MTX in the *L. casei* complex (with the exception of Leu-19) has its counterpart in the *E. coli* complex. Indeed in only four out of thirteen cases are the interacting side chains merely analogous rather than identical. The inhibitor is draped over alpha helix αB with the pyrimidine end deeply buried in a primarily hydrophobic pocket formed by side chains from helix αB and from the amino terminal strand βA.

The aromatic ring of the p-aminobenzoyl portion of MTX resides in a second hydrophobic pocket formed, in *E. coli* DHFR, by the side chains of Leu-28, Ile-50 and Leu-54. These two leucines are also present in the *L. casei* enzyme where they perform the same binding function. However, the residue structurally corresponding to Ile-50 in *E. coli* DHFR is Phe-49 in the *L. casei* enzyme. This substitution could account for a 10-20° difference between the dihedral angle $C_{(9)}-N_{(10)}-C_{(3')}-C_{(4')}$ that is observed when the conformation of MTX is compared in the *E. coli* binary and the *L. casei* ternary complex.

The glutamate portion of the inhibitor is bound at the enzyme surface with the side chain of Arg-57 hydrogen bonded to the α-carboxyl group. Identically the same interaction occurs in both bacterial reductases. However, because the γ-carboxyl group interacts with non-conserved residues it is held in different conformations in these two enzymes.

The affinity of MTX for most DHFRs is 10^3 to 10^4 greater than that of folate, even though the only difference between methotrexate and folate that can significantly affect binding is substitution of a 4-oxo group in folate by a 4-amino group in the inhibitor. It was first suggested by Baker[4] that enhanced binding of MTX results from increased basicity at $N_{(1)}$. In both bacterial enzymes we find that the side chain carboxyl of an invariant aspartate (Asp-26 and Asp-27 in *L. casei* and *E. coli* DHFRs respectively) closely approaches $N_{(1)}$ and the 2-amino group of bound MTX. Such an interaction is consistent with donation of an aspartate proton to $N_{(1)}$ of MTX and supports Baker's initial hypothesis. The possible significance of this interaction for the mechanism of DHFR is further discussed below.

NADPH Binding to *L. casei* Dihydrofolate Reductase

a) Conformation of bound NADPH. Both NADH and NADPH in solution, as well as their oxidized counterparts, are thought to exist predominantly in a folded conformation with their two bases stacked parallel to one another. In contrast, the NADPH molecule binds to

DHFR in an extended conformation, as does NAD^+ bound to lactate dehydrogenase (LDH), glyceraldehyde 3-phosphate dehydrogenase (GAPDH) and malate dehydrogenase (MDH).[5] Somewhat surprisingly, however, these bound conformations for NADPH on the one hand and NAD^+ on the other are quite different. This difference is most readily quantified by comparing the distance between the two bases ($C6_a$-$C2_n$) and by comparing the dihedral angle α relating the relative rotations of the two bases about the P_a-P_n direction. The nucleotide bases in bound NADPH are 17 $\overset{o}{A}$ apart ($C6_a$-$C2_n$), to be compared with a distance of 14 $\overset{o}{A}$ in the NAD^+-dehydrogenase complexes.[5] Viewed down the P-P axis, the six oxygen atoms (excluding the pyrophosphate bridge oxygen) are arranged hexagonally in a staggered conformation, with the ester oxygens *trans* to one another. In contrast, bound NAD^+ assumes a less extended conformation, with a twist at the pyrophosphate group resulting in *gauche-gauche* positioning of the ester oxygens.[5] This difference in pyrophosphate conformation also accounts for most of the 120° difference between α in pyridine dinucleotides bound to dihydrofolate reductase on the one hand and to the dehydrogenases on the other.

b) Interaction with the enzyme. In general terms, the interaction between DHFR and NADPH can be briefly described by noting that the ribose phosphate portions of the coenzyme are involved in numerous specific hydrogen-bonded interactions, that the adenine ring resides in an apparently nonspecific hydrophobic cleft and that the nicotinamide ring is bound in an intricately constructed cavity, a portion of which includes the pyrazine ring of bound MTX.

The 2'-phosphate of NADPH apparently serves as an important anchor for the adenine ribose. All three available 2'-phosphate oxygens are involved in charge-charge or hydrogen bonded interactions with the enzyme: the positively charged guanidinium group of Arg-43 is close to the negatively charged $O_{(1)}$; a hydrogen bond to $O_{(2)}$ is donated by the side chain of Thr-63; and $O_{(3)}$ accepts a hydrogen bond from Nδ1 of His-64. Taken together these interactions between the enzyme and the 2'-phosphate group must account for much of the hundred-fold greater K_m value for NADH relative to NADPH bound to *L. casei* DHFR.[6]

c) Possible changes in enzyme structure induced by NADPH binding. Preliminary comparisons of the α-carbon backbones in *E. coli* and *L. casei* DHFR show that there are three regions where corresponding parts of the structures differ by 2 $\overset{o}{A}$ or more. In the following discussion we assume that only when they occur in backbone regions directly interacting with NADPH are these differences attributable

to coenzyme binding. Thus a structural variation between the backbone chain segment connecting βG and βH is assumed to be due to
species specific sequence differences and crystal packing effects.
On the other hand, the remaining two regions of significant structural
difference between the *E. coli* and *L. casei* enzymes in their respective
binary and ternary complexes are assumed to result from NADPH binding
to the latter.

The structure of the *E. coli* DHFR:MTX complex revealed that two
rather extended loops (residues 10-24 and 117-135) connect βA to
αB and βF to βG respectively. Because these regions are represented
by relatively weak electron density in the original 2.5 Å map, it
is likely that they are rather flexible. In contrast, the main chain
and side chain electron density for these two loops is strong and
well defined in the *L. casei* ternary complex. Moreover, both of
these polypeptide chain segments in the *L. casei* DHFR complex appear
to move slightly relative to the corresponding segments in the *E.coli*
dihydrofolate reductase complex. The largest movements of up to 3 Å
involve residues 12-21 and 125-128 in the *L. casei* enzyme. Within
these loops residues 13-14, 17-19, 21 and 126 directly interact with
bound NADPH.[3] Strict conservation of four of these residues in all
known DHFR primary sequences confirms their functional importance
and supports the assumption that these observed conformation differences between the *E. coli* and *L. casei* DHFR complexes are caused
by coenzyme binding.

Relevance to Enzyme Mechanism

Enzyme catalyzed reduction of dihydrofolate occurs across the
$N_{(5)}$-$C_{(6)}$ bond of the dihydropteridine ring. Hydride transfer from
nicotinamide to $C_{(6)}$ of dihydrofolate is known to proceed with A
side specificity and with incorporation of a proton at $N_{(5)}$. As
shown in Fig. 1, in the *L. casei* DHFR:MTX:NADPH structure the
pteridine ring of MTX and the nicotinamide ring of NADPH are close
together in the active site of the enzyme with the $C_{(4)}$ carbon of
the nicotinamide ring close to the $N_{(5)}$-$C_{(6)}$ bond of the inhibitor.
Examination of Fig. 1 confirms that the transferable hydride ion at
$C_{(4)}$ must come from the A side of the nicotinamide ring; the B side
points down and away from the pyrazine ring.

We noted above that an invariant aspartate interacts closely with
$N_{(1)}$ of MTX in the two bacterial reductases. In addition, the
hydrophobic crevice in which Asp-26 (in *L. casei* DHFR) resides is,
in the ternary complex, completely blocked off from access to

surrounding solvent by the nicotinamide ring of NADPH and the pteridine ring of MTX. Consequently the pK of this side chain in the complex must be considerably higher than that of a solvent-exposed aspartic acid. It seems likely therefore that Asp-26 is the required proton source in the enzyme reaction. But herein lies a slight apparent complication, which has led us to suggest that the pteridine ring in MTX may possibly be turned over relative to the "productive" orientation of the substrates pteridine ring.[2] Although a proton is ultimately delivered to $N_{(5)}$ in the enzymic reduction, the carboxylate group of the Asp-26 side chain in our structure interacts most closely with $N_{(1)}$. However, if the pteridine ring in the substrate were to be turned over, the carboxylate group of Asp-26 would instead be close to $N_{(5)}$. In fact there may be no need to consider such a possibility, for it is not unreasonable to invoke a proton jump within the pteridine ring, or a proton rearrangement mediated by water, either during the enzymic reaction or after release of products.[7] Thus at present we can only say that during productive binding of substrate the pteridine ring *may* be turned over from the orientation of the pteridine ring observed in bound MTX, but the evidence does not *require* it.

References

1. Matthews, D. A, Alden, R. A., Bolin, J. T., Freer, S. T., Hamlin, R., Xuong, N., Kraut, J., Poe, M, Williams, M. and Hoogsteen, K. (1977) Science, 197, 452-455.

2. Matthews, D. A., Alden, R. A., Bolin, J. T., Filman, D. J., Freer, S. T., Hamlin, R., Hol, W. G. J., Kisliuk, R. L., Pastore, E. J., Plante, L. T., Xuong, N., and Kraut, J. (1978) J. Biol. Chem. in press.

3. Matthews, D. A., Alden, R. A., Freer, S. T., Xuong, N. and Kraut, J., submitted for publication.

4. Baker, B. R. (1959) Cancer Chemotherapy Rept 4, 1-10.

5. Rossman, M. G., Liljas, A., Bründén, C. I. and Banaszak, L. J. (1975) in The Enzymes, Boyer, P. D. ed., Academic Press, New York, ed. 3, 61-102.

6. Feeney, J., Birdsall, B., Roberts, G. C. K. and Burgen, A. S. V. (1975) Nature (London) 257, 564-566.

7. Dreyfus, M., Dodin, C., Bensaude, O. and Dubois, J. E. (1976) J. Am. Chem. Soc. 97, 2369-2376.

CHARACTERIZATION OF MAMMALIAN FOLYLPOLYGLUTAMATE SYNTHETASES

JOHN J. McGUIRE, YASUNORI KITAMOTO, PEARL HSIEH, JAMES K. COWARD AND JOSEPH R.BERTINO
Dept. of Pharmacology, Yale University School of Medicine, New Haven, Conn. 06510

INTRODUCTION

Folates extracted from natural sources are nearly always poly-γ-glutamyl conjugates of the more familiar reduced and 1-carbon substituted pteroylmonoglutamate (folate) derivatives. Within any single source there is generally a characteristic distribution of the lengths of these polyglutamate chains. The function of these polygluta- mates in folate metabolism is still unclear although their universal presence, even in organisms lacking the ability to biosynthesize folic acid, suggests they are physi- ologically important. A substantial body of indirect evidence suggests that polyglu- tamylation "traps" folate monoglutamates that are transported into cells[1] and also that the polyglutamates serve as the actual cofactors for folate mediated reactions in vivo.[2]

Despite the accumulation of data suggesting the physiological importance of the folylpolyglutamates, relatively little information has been obtained in vitro about their biosynthesis. Griffin and Brown[3] first demonstrated the presence of a folyl- polyglutamate synthetase (FPGS) in E. coli which catalyzed the following reaction:

$$H_4PteGlu + ATP + Glutamate \xrightarrow{Mg^{++}} H_4PteGlu\text{-}\gamma\text{-}Glu_x + ADP + P_i$$

Both di- and triglutamate derivatives were detected when the reaction mixture was analyzed by electrophoresis and bioautography. Since this initial observation, how- ever, little progress has been made in understanding this reaction chiefly because no simple assay has been available. In order to fill this gap in our knowledge of folate metabolism we have developed an in vitro assay for the folylpolyglutamate synthetase and begun an investigation of this enzyme from rat liver and several cultured cell lines.

ASSAY

A reproducible, sensitive chromatographic assay using DEAE-cellulose was developed to monitor the incorporation of ^{3}H-glutamate into folylpolyglutamates catalyzed by folylpolyglutamate synthetase. By a combination of chemical and enzymatic syntheses a variety of reduced and/or substituted standards were prepared from chemically syn- thesized pteroyldiglutamate (PteGlu$_2$). Chromatographic conditions were established which allowed the separation of ^{3}H-glutamate and the standard folyldiglutamates (as well as longer polyglutamates) with a simple buffer wash. Standard assay mixtures (0.25 ml; pH 8.3 at 37°) which contain Tris-Cl (0.1M), ATP (5 mM), MgCl$_2$ (10 mM),KCl (20 mM), 100 mM 2-mercaptoethanol (2-ME), 35 μM dl-tetrahydrofolate, 4 mM ^{3}H-glutamate (7x10^6 cpm/μmole), and enzyme are incubated at 37°C. The reaction is terminated by the addition of 1 ml ice cold 25 mM 2-ME. The entire reaction mixture is rapidly transferred to a DEAE-cellulose column (0.4x6 cm). Unreacted ^{3}H-glutamate is eluted with 10 mM Tris-Cl, pH 7.5; 110 mM NaCl; 25 mM 2-ME while all polyglutamyl forms of tetrahydrofolate are retained. The polyglutamates are eluted with HCl and quantitated by liquid scintillation counting as a measure of total ^{3}H-glutamate incorporation. For product analysis by high pressure liquid chromatography (HPLC)[4], the polyglutamates are eluted with phosphoric acid. An independently developed assay based on the same principle has been recently described.[5]

RESULTS AND DISCUSSION

This assay has been employed in an investigation of the organ distribution of FPGS activity in the rat. The subcellular localization of the enzyme in rat liver has also been determined and a partial purification of the cytoplasmic activity has been obtained. Further purification and characterization of this enzyme is underway.

Organ Distribution. Organs were obtained from four male Sprague-Dawley rats (150-240g) and rapidly cooled. Cold 0.9% saline was used to perfuse the livers and flush the heart, stomach, and small intestine. Organs were minced, homogenized, and centrifuged at 105,000 x g for 60 min. The supernatants were assayed. The results (Table 1) show that liver is the richest source of this enzyme. This is not unexpected because liver contains the highest amounts of folate, and folate occurs in that organ predominantly as pteroylpentaglutamates.

TABLE 1

ACTIVITIES OF FOLYLPOLYGLUTAMATE SYNTHETASE IN SOLUBLE FRACTIONS FROM DIFFERENT RAT ORGANS[a]

Organ	Specific Activity pmoles/h/mg
Heart	N.D.[b]
Spleen	38 $\pm$ 14
Stomach	33 $\pm$ 4
Lung	19 $\pm$ 8
Small Intestine	50 $\pm$ 21
Brain	23 $\pm$ 0
Kidney	N.D.[b]
Liver	100 $\pm$ 10

[a]Values from 2 experiments were pooled
[b]Not detectable

Subcellular Distribution. Fresh livers were perfused with 0.9% saline and homogenized in 9 volumes of 250 mM sucrose; 10 mM Tris-Cl,pH 8.4. Nuclear, mitochondrial/
lysosomal, and microsomal fractions were obtained by differential centrifugation at
600 x g for 10 min., 10,000 x g for 10 min., and 105,000 x g for 60 min., respectively. The final supernatant was designated as the soluble fraction. The mitochondrial
fraction was prepared separately.[6] Marker enzymes (succinate cytochrome c reductase
for mitochondria and NADPH cytochrome c reductase for microsomes) indicated the fractionation procedure was effective. Each fraction was assayed for FPGS activity
(Table 2) and the soluble fraction was found to have both the highest specific activity and the largest per cent of total activity. Gawthorne and Smith[7] reported that
sheep liver FPGS was also predominantly cytoplasmic.

TABLE 2

SUBCELLULAR DISTRIBUTION OF RAT LIVER FOLYLPOLYGLUTAMATE SYNTHETASE[a]

Fraction	Specific Activity pmoles/h/mg	Total Activity as % of Activity in Homogenate
Whole Homogenate	61 + 45	100
Nuclear	34 + 21	20
Mitochondrial/Lysosomal	33 + 12	13
Mitochondrial	33	
Microsomal	42 + 24	9
Soluble	139 + 12	75

[a]Values for 3 experiments were pooled

Purification. Our earlier studies[8] of this enzyme in crude extracts of rat liver
were performed at pH 8.0 (37°), 100 mM KCl, with 35 μM dl-tetrahydrofolate (H_4PteGlu)
as substrate. HPLC analysis of the products from the H_4PteGlu dependent reaction
showed the major peak of radioactivity chromatographed at the same position as chemically synthesized H_4Pte Glu$_2$. Although there was substantial incorporation in the
absence of dl-H_4PteGlu, HPLC analysis of the products showed no radioactivity eluted
at the position of H_4PteGlu$_2$ or any longer polyglutamate. When the total incorporation was corrected for this endogenous incorporation, a net of 110 pmoles ^{3}H-gluta-
mate/h/mg were incorporated into polyglutamates. Further experimentation has revealed that optimal incorporation requires pH 8.3 (37°C) and 20 mM KCl. Using this refined assay the rat liver FPGS has been purified 75 fold (Table 3).

TABLE 3

PURIFICATION OF RAT LIVER FOLYLPOLYGLUTAMATE SYNTHETASE

Fraction	Total Protein (mg)	Total Units[a]	Specific Activity (units/mg)	Yield (%)
Crude Extract	6900	1.8×10^6	270	100
0-35% Am SO$_4$ Pellet	1670	1×10^6	600	56
Phosphocellulose	275	0.6×10^6	2250	33
Sephadex G-150	34	0.7×10^6	20600	39

[a]One unit of enzyme is defined as the amount that allows the conversion at 37° of 1 pmole/h of ^{3}H-glutamic acid to a product which elutes in the HCl wash of the assay column.

Characterization of Reaction Conditions. Partially purified FPGS displays absolute dependence on the addition of ATP and an exogenous folate cofactor. Incorporation of ^{3}H-glutamate is maximal with 4 mM ^{3}H-glutamate, 5 mM ATP, and 10 mM MgCl$_2$. Lower Mg/ATP ratios give decreased incorporation. The pH optimum is 8.3 (37^oC). High levels (100 mM) of KCl are slightly inhibitory and maximum incorporation is achieved at 20 mM. The last result differs from data obtained with sheep liver FPGS,[7] where 100 mM KCl is optimal, and with the E. coli FPGS[9] where 200 mM KCl gave maximum stimulation.

Specificity for L-glutamate. A number of compounds were tested for their ability to inhibit the incorporation of L-^{3}H-glutamate (at 3 mM, a subsaturating level) into polyglutamates. Unlabeled L-glutamate at 3 mM reduced incorporation by 45%. D-glutamate, L-glutamine, L-aspartate, glycine, and p-aminobenzoic acid at 3 mM did not inhibit. L-methionine-DL-sulfoximine at 1.2 mM also was not inhibitory. Thus the enzyme displays rigorous specificity for L-glutamate. Extension of the polyglutamate chain one residue at a time is suggested because 3 mM γ-L-glutamyl-L-glutamate also did not inhibit.

Folate Specificity. The specificity of FPGS for different folates and folate analogs is crucial for understanding how the intracellular polyglutamate pool is generated. The specificity of the partially purified enzyme has been investigated, at 5 and 35 μM levels, using purified samples of various oxidized, reduced, and one carbon substituted pteroylmonoglutamates (Table 4).

TABLE 4

FOLATE SPECIFICITY OF RAT LIVER FOLYLPOLYGLUTAMATE SYNTHETASE

Substrate	5 μM		35 μM	
	pmoles ^{3}H-Glu[#] incorp./3h	% Activity Relative to THF	pmoles ^{3}H-Glu[#] incorp./3h	% Activity Relative to THF
None	0	0	0	0
Folic Acid[*]	270	16	1200	47
Dihydrofolic Acid[*]	960	56	2150	84
dl-Tetrahydrofolate (THF)	1700	100	2550	100
dl-5,10-methylene-tetrahydrofolate	1150	68	1640	64
dl-5-CH$_3$-THF	330	19	1225	48
l-5-CH$_3$-THF[**]	170 (2.5μM)	10	1075 (17.5μM)	42
dl-5-CH$_3$-H$_4$homo-folate[##]	70	4	380	15
dl-10-formyl THF[***]	1500	88	1380	54

[#]Value is mean of duplicates.

[*]1 μM JB-11 (quinazoline inhibitor of dihydrofolate reductase[10])present

[**]Solution of l-5-CH$_3$-THF enzymically synthesized according to Horne, D.W., Briggs, W.T., & Wagner, C. (1977) Anal. Biochem., 83, 615-621. Generously supplied by Dr. C. Wagner.

[##]Supplied by NCI.

[***]
With dl-10-formyl-THF as substrate the DE-52 columns are washed with only 80 mM NaCl in the buffer. Incorporation is corrected for an appropriate blank lacking 10-formyl-THF.

All the naturally occurring folates tested can be utilized as substrates although with different efficiencies. Although dl-tetrahydrofolate is the best substrate at both levels the determination of an absolute order of specificity requires complete concentration dependence studies with all these folates. Of significance, 5-CH$_3$-tetrahydrofolate, the main serum folate, serves as a substrate. Its relatively low activity may explain why conflicting reports regarding its activity have appeared. In addition, the l-isomer is active which rules out the possibility that the activity with the dl-mixture is the result of slow metabolism of the unnatural d-isomer[11] only. Assays with folate and dihydrofolate contained a potent quinazoline inhibitor of dihydrofolate reductase to eliminate their possible conversion to tetrahydrofolate. This quinazoline is not a substrate for FPGS and it does not inhibit FPGS activity with dl-tetrahydrofolate as a substrate.

HPLC analysis of the reaction products with dl-tetrahydrofolate (THF) as sub-strate yield a striking result. At 5μM THF the di-and triglutamate products are synthesized in approximately equal amounts. However, at 35μM THF the diglutamate is the predominant product with only a small amount of triglutamate detectable. Thus low substrate concentrations favor formation of longer polyglutamates while high substrate concentrations favor formation of shorter polyglutamates. This ob-servation has also been made with the Chinese Hamster Ovary cell enzyme[5]. The potent chemotherapeutic agent methotrexate is also a substrate. This result corre-lates with findings that polyglutamates of methotrexate are formed in vivo. Chemi-cally synthesized $H_4Pteglu_2$ is also a substrate and HPLC analysis shows that besides the predominant product, $H_4Pteglu_3$, there are some higher polyglutamates formed.

Enzyme Activity in Cell Culture. FPGS activity has also been detected in ex-tracts from a number of cell culture lines. Extracts of the murine leukemia L1210S and a methotrexate resistant sub-line have specific activities 3-4 times that of crude rat liver. Extracts of a second murine leukemia, L5178Y, catalyze the reac-tion at 460 pmoles/h/mg. Detection of this enzyme in cultured cells will allow studies of the regulation of the enzyme activity.

REFERENCES

1. McBurney, M.W. and Whitmore, G.F. (1974) Cell, 2, 173-182.
2. Coward, J.K., Parameswaran, K.N., Cashmore, A.R. and Bertino, J.R. (1977) Biochemistry, 13, 3899-3904.
3. Griffin, M.J. and Brown, G.M. (1964) J. Biol. Chem., 239, 310-316.
4. Cashmore, A.R., Dreyer, R.N., Horvath, C., Coward, J.K., Knipe, J.O. and Bertino, J.R., Methods in Enzymology. In press.
5. Taylor, R.T. and Hanna, L.M. (1977) Arch. Biochem. Biophysics, 181, 331-344.
6. Simpson, M.V., Fournier, M.J., and Skinner, D.M. (1967) Methods in Enzymology, 10, 755-762.
7. Gawthorne, J.M. and Smith, R.M. (1973) Biochem. J., 136, 295-301.
8. McGuire, J.J., Coward, J.K., Hsieh, P., Bertino, J.R. (1978) Fed. Proc., 37, 1347.
9. Masurekar, M. and Brown, G.M. (1975) Biochemistry, 14, 2424-2430.
10. Bertino, J.R. and Sawicki, W.L. (1977) Proc. Am. Assoc. Cancer Res., 18, 168.
11. Shane, B. and Stokstad, E.L.R. (1977) J. Gen. Microbiol., 103, 249-259.

THE INTERACTION OF [13]C(BENZOYLCARBONYL)-FOLATE AND [13]C(BENZOYL-
CARBONYL)-AMINOPTERIN WITH DIHYDROFOLATE REDUCTASE

E.J. PASTORE, L.T. PLANTE*, J.M. WRIGHT, R.L. KISLIUK*, and N.O. KAPLAN
Dept. of Chemistry, University of California (San Diego), La Jolla, CA
92093, and *Dept. of Biochemistry and Pharmacology, Tufts University
Medical School, Boston, MA 02111

ABSTRACT

The chemical shift of the benzoylcarbonyl carbon of folate bound to
Lactobacillus casei dihydrofolate reductase appears 2.5 ppm upfield
from its position in free solution, while the corresponding position
in bound aminopterin appears 2.8 ppm upfield. Inspection of the crystal structure of this enzyme suggests that such strong shielding is
attributable to proximity of this carbonyl to ring currents of PHE-49.

INTRODUCTION

Our earlier studies of binding interactions between dihydrofolate
reductase (DHFR) and its ligands by ^{1}H-NMR spectroscopy demonstrated
changes in protein conformation but did not permit direct observation
of the ligands because of marked line broadening[1,2]. Using CMR spectroscopy and ligands specifically enriched with carbon-13, we have
been able to obtain excellent resolution of individual carbon atoms of
bound folate and aminopterin. This method provides a means of observing positions throughout the substrate and inhibitor molecules and is
potentially more informative than ^{1}H-NMR spectroscopy since the
pteridine ring contains six carbon atoms compared to only one proton
(Fig. 1).

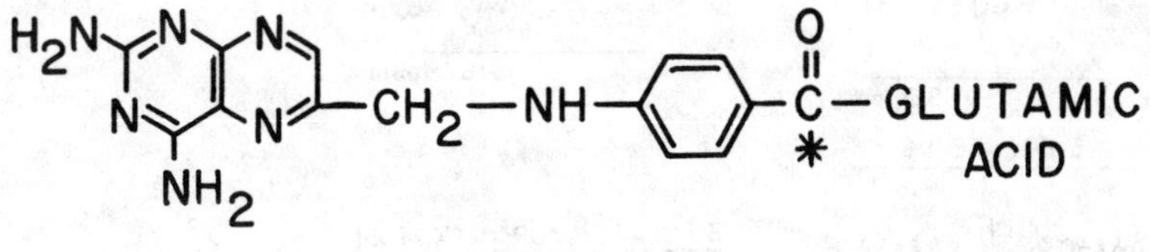

Fig. 1. Aminopterin: an asterisk (*) indicates the benzoylcarbonyl.

MATERIALS AND METHODS

Folate and aminopterin labeled with ^{13}C in the benzoylcarbonyl carbon

(Fig. 1) were synthesized according to the procedures of Plante et al.[3,4] DHFR was purified from extracts of L. casei by affinity chromatography on pteroyllysine sepharose[5]. ^{13}C-NMR spectra were obtained at 25.03 MHz with a JEOL PFT-100 NMR spectrometer equipped with a Nicolet 1085 computer using conditions described previously[6]. Chemical shifts were measured relative to 0.02 M internal dioxane and referred to tetramethylsilane (TMS) by adding 67.4 ppm.

RESULTS

Figure 2 shows the ^{13}C(benzoylcarbonyl)-folate chemical shift changes ($\Delta\delta$) observed in the presence of L. casei DHFR. Spectrum A shows a 1:1 binary complex of enzyme and ^{13}C-folate. There is a single peak at 168.0 ppm which represents a $\Delta\delta$ of -2.5 ppm relative to the δ of 170.5 ppm for free folate. Spectrum B is the 1:2 binary complex of DHFR and ^{13}C-folate. Marked broadening of both peaks in this complex does not permit accurate measurement of the chemical shift difference. Spectrum C is the ternary complex DHFR:NADP$^+$:^{13}C-folate, 1:2:2. The sharp peaks centered at 170.4 and 167.9 ppm represent free and bound folate, respectively, and the $\Delta\delta$ is again -2.5 ppm which is the same value obtained for the binary complex. Addition of methotrexate (MTX) to C gives the spectrum shown in D which consists of a single peak representing only free ^{13}C-folate since the bound form has been displaced from the enzyme by the unlabeled MTX.

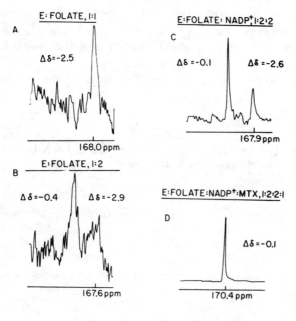

Figure 2. ^{13}C-NMR spectra at 25.03 MHz. ^{13}C(benzoylcarbonyl)-folate chemical shift changes ($\Delta\delta$) observed in the presence of L. casei DHFR.

Figure 3 shows the ^{13}C(benzoylcarbonyl)-aminopterin δ's and $\Delta\delta$'s observed in the presence of DHFR. Spectrum A shows the δ of free ^{13}C-aminopterin. A single sharp peak at 167.5 ppm in B represents bound aminopterin with a $\Delta\delta$ = -3.0 ppm.

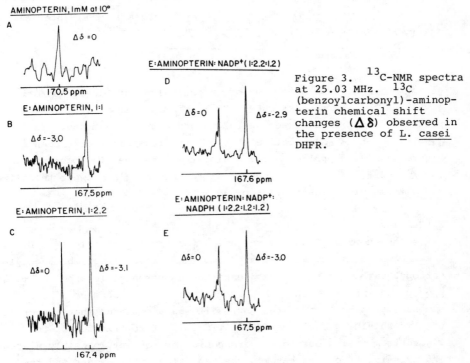

AMINOPTERIN, ImM at 10°

A

$\Delta\delta$ =0

170.5 ppm

E: AMINOPTERIN, 1:1

B

$\Delta\delta$ =-3.0

167.5 ppm

E: AMINOPTERIN, 1:2.2

C

$\Delta\delta$ =0 $\Delta\delta$ =-3.1

167.4 ppm

E:AMINOPTERIN: NADP⁺(1:2.2:1.2)

D

$\Delta\delta$=0 $\Delta\delta$=-2.9

167.6 ppm

E: AMINOPTERIN: NADP⁺:
NADPH (1:2.2:1.2:1.2)

E

$\Delta\delta$=0 $\Delta\delta$=-3.0

167.5 ppm

Figure 3. ^{13}C-NMR spectra at 25.03 MHz. ^{13}C (benzoylcarbonyl)-aminopterin chemical shift changes ($\Delta\delta$) observed in the presence of L. casei DHFR.

The spectrum for the 1:2.2 binary complex of DHFR and ^{13}C-aminopterin is shown in Spectrum C. Two peaks representing free (δ=170.5) and bound (δ=167.4) aminopterin are seen and the $\Delta\delta$ between the two forms is -3.1 ppm. Spectrum D is the ternary complex of DHFR:^{13}C-aminopterin: NADP⁺, 1:2.2:1.2, and it shows free and bound peaks at 170.5 and 167.6 ppm, respectively. Finally Spectrum E shows the ternary complex of DHFR:^{13}C-aminopterin: NADPH, 1:2.2:1.2, consisting of two peaks, free (170.5 ppm) and bound (167.5 ppm) with a $\Delta\delta$ of -3.0.

Figure 4 shows the results of a separate experiment in which both ^{13}C(benzoylcarbonyl)-folate and ^{13}C(benzoylcarbonyl)-aminopterin have been added sequentially to the same enzyme sample. Spectrum A is the ternary complex of DHFR:^{13}C-folate:NADP⁺, 1:4:2. Two peaks representing free and bound ^{13}C-folate are seen at 170.5 and 168.0 ppm, respectively,

480

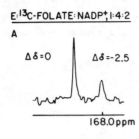

E:¹³C-FOLATE:NADP⁺, 1:4:2

A

Δδ=0   Δδ=-2.5

168.0ppm

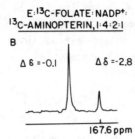

E:¹³C-FOLATE:NADP⁺:
¹³C-AMINOPTERIN, 1:4:2:1

B

Δδ=-0.1   Δδ=-2.8

167.6ppm

Figure 4. ^{13}C-NMR spectra at 25.03 MHz. Comparative binding of ^{13}C (benzoylcarbonyl)-folate and -aminopterin to L. casei DHFR: Internal Control.

giving a $\Delta\delta$ of -2.5. Addition of an equivalent of ^{13}C-aminopterin gives the ternary complex DHFR:NADP^{+}:^{13}C-aminopterin, 1:2:1. Two peaks again represent free ^{13}C-folate and bound ^{13}C-aminopterin (δ =167.6) and a $\Delta\delta$ relative to the δ for free aminopterin seen in Figure 2A (170.5 ppm) of -2.9. Using the δ observed in Spectrum B, the $\Delta\delta$ =-2.8. The results show a difference in δ's between these two bound forms of at least 0.3 ppm.

DISCUSSION

Results shown in Figure 2 reviewing the binding of folate to L. casei DHFR in binary and ternary complexes[6] reveal that the benzoyl-carbonyl carbon of this ligand experiences strong shielding (2.5+0.1 ppm) during interaction with this enzyme. In the absence of a 3-dimensional structure of the enzyme it was speculated that the origin of this shielding could be attributed in part to transfer of the ligand from an aqueous to a hydrophobic environment, possibly disrupting existing H-bonding between the benzoylcarbonyl oxygen and the aqueous solvent, and an aromatic amino acid side chain residue close to this position of the ligand. Each of these events could contribute to increased shielding observed upon interaction with the active site.

Recently, in a collaborative effort with this laboratory, Kraut's group[7] has succeeded in obtaining a 3-dimensional structure for the enzyme-NADPH-methotrexate ternary complex by X-ray crystallography. Inspection of this structure reveals that PHE-49 of the enzyme lies close to the benzoylcarbonyl of the methotrexate. Exact distances are not yet available to us at the present time since the model is still being refined, but the present model indicates that the diamagnetic anisotropy of the aromatic ring of PHE could account for a large part of the observed shielding.

Since there is some question about the similarity in enzyme interaction of folate compared to diamino pteridines such as aminopterin

TABLE 1

COMPARISON OF LIGAND BINDING TO L. casei DHFR: ^{13}C(BENZOYLCARBONYL) CHEMICAL SHIFTS OF FOLATE AND AMINOPTERIN

Enzyme Complex	Exp. 1 ^{13}C-Folate	Exp. 2 ^{13}C-Aminopterin	Difference[a]
(1) Binary	167.96	167.46	-0.50
(2) Ternary with NADP$^+$	167.92	167.60	-0.32
(3) Ternary with NADPH	--	167.51	--

[a]Chemical shift difference between bound folate and bound aminopterin

and methotrexate, it was of considerable interest to obtain binding data for a diamine containing ^{13}C in the benzoylcarbonyl carbon. Data presented in Figure 3 reveal that this position in aminopterin is also strongly shielded upon binding to L. casei DHFR. The chemical shift difference between free and bound ^{13}C(benzoylcarbonyl)-aminopterin is 2.9 ppm (Figure 3D) for the enzyme:^{13}C-aminopterin:NADP$^+$ complex. Comparative results for ^{13}C-folate and ^{13}C-aminopterin binding to L. casei DHFR are summarized in Table 1. As shown in Row 2, the difference in shielding between bound folate and bound aminopterin is -0.32 ppm, with aminopterin being more shielded than folate.

The results shown in Table 1 were obtained from separate experiments carried out at different times with different enzyme preparations. Since we are planning to study other ^{13}C-labeled ligands, we were interested to see if these relatively small chemical shift differences, e.g., less than 0.5 ppm, were reproducible. Therefore, we carried out another experiment, shown in Figure 4, in which we added both ^{13}C-folate and ^{13}C-aminopterin sequentially to the same enzyme sample. The labeled ligands are in each case present in ternary complexes with the enzyme and NADP$^+$. The results summarized in Table 2 again show chemical shift differences ($\Delta\delta$) between free and bound folate of -2.42 and free and bound aminopterin of -2.75. The difference between bound folate and bound aminopterin in column 4 is -0.33 ppm, which reproduces the result obtained in separate experiments and confirms the reliability of our methodology in measuring even relatively small differences in local shielding of specific positions within a ligand.

Our results show that as far as the benzoylcarbonyl position is concerned, folate and aminopterin are bound similarly. The 0.3 ppm increased shielding for aminopterin probably reflects small changes in the geometrical orientation of this position to the aromatic ring of

TABLE 2

COMPARISON OF ^{13}C(BENZOYLCARBONYL) FOLATE and AMINOPTERIN[a] DURING
BINDING TO L. casei DHFR: INTERNAL CONTROL

	E:NADP^{+}:^{13}C-Folate	E:NADP^{+}:^{13}C-Aminopterin	Difference
Free	170.46	170.37	--
Bound	168.04	167.62	--
Δδ	-2.42	-2.75	-0.33[b]

[a]Ligands contain ca. 90 percent ^{13}C enrichment of the benzoylcarbonyl carbon.
[b]Chemical shift difference between bound folate and bound aminopterin.

PHE-49. These conclusions may be tested by comparing binding of the
two ligands to DHFR's which lack an aromatic amino acid at the corresponding position of their primary structure, e.g., S. faecium or
E. coli. Such experiments are in progress in this laboratory.

ADDENDUM

Recent results in this laboratory with S. faecium DHFR from R.L.
Blakley show that the benzoylcarbonyls of bound folate and aminopterin are not strongly shielded by this enzyme, thereby affirming our
prediction.

ACKNOWLEDGMENTS

We are indebted to Y. Gaumont for early stages of enzyme purification and to M.E. Fisher for his outstanding contributions in all
phases of this work. This work was supported by CA 19094, CA 10914,
CA 20539, NSF PCM77-20858, NIH RR-00708, Amer. Ca. Soc. ACrS BC60S
and personal funds of EJP.

REFERENCES

1. Pastore, E.J., R.L. Kisliuk, L.T. Plante, J.M. Wright and N.O.
   Kaplan, Proc. Nat. Acad. Sci. U.S.A. 71, 3849 (1974).

2. Pastore, E.J., R.L. Kisliuk, L.T. Plante, J.M. Wright, N.O. Kaplan
   and M. Friedkin, Fed. Proc. 34, 1700 Abs (1975).

3. Plante, L.T., E.J. Pastore and K.L. Williamson, Methods in Enzymol,
   (in press).

4. Plante, L.T., Methods in Enzymol, (in press).

5. Pastore, E.J., L.T. Plante, R.L. Kisliuk, Methods in
   Enzymol., Jakoby, W.B. and M. Wilchek, editors, Acadmic Press
   34B, 281 (1974).

6. Pastore, E.J., L.T. Plante, J.M. Wright, R.L. Kisliuk and N.O.
   Kaplan, Biochem. Biophys. Res. Comm. 68, 471 (1976).

7. Matthews, D.A., R.A. Alden, J.T. Bolin, D.J. Filman, S.T. Freer,
   R. Hamlin, W.G. Hol, R.L. Kisliuk, E.J. Pastore, L.T. Plante,
   N. Xuong and J. Kraut, J.Biol. Chem. 253, 6946 (1978).

PMR STUDIES ON *E. COLI* MB 3746 DIHYDROFOLATE REDUCTASE

MARTIN POE, JOSEPH K. WU, CHARLES SHORT, jr., JAMES FLORANCE AND
KARST HOOGSTEEN
Department of Biophysics, Merck Institute for Therapeutic Research,
Rahway, New Jersey 07065

Nuclear magnetic resonance studies on dihydrofolate reductase (DHFR)
by Roberts and coworkers (see 1, refs. therein), by Blakley and
coworkers (2 and refs. therein) and by Pastore and collaborators (3
and references therein) have provided insight into the role of
various residues of the protein and of the functional groups on
ligands in the binding of substrates and inhibitors. We have done
nmr studies on *E. coli* DHFR (4 and refs. therein) and seek to cor-
relate this data to the crystal structure of the binary methotrexate
(MTX) complex of the enzyme which was solved by Matthews *et al*[5].

One important aspect of our nmr studies has been the study of
specifically-deuterated forms of *E. coli* DHFR, for which we have used
the DHFR isolated and purified from the DHFR-megaoverproducing,
trimethoprim-resistant strain MB 3746 of *E. coli* K12[6]. This enzyme
appears to be almost identical to DHFR from *E. coli* MB 1428[7] and
RT-500[8]. This strain will incorporate exogenous deuterated aromatic
amino acids into its proteins in good yield, when the deuterated
aromatic amino acids are made according to Matthews *et al*[9] or
Griffiths *et al*[10].

The five histidine residues of *E. coli* MB 3746 DHFR exhibit values
of pK' and $\delta(HA^+)$, the chemical shift of the protonated form of the
histidine, which are equal within experimental error (±0.2 for pK',
±10 Hz for $\delta(HA^+)$) to the values for corresponding histidines of
E. coli MB 1428 DHFR, when the histidines are numbered in pK' order.
See Table I. The pK' and $\delta(HA^+)$ values given in Table I were measured
for binary MTX complexes at 25° in buffer A, 0.10 M NaCl, 0.02 M
borate, 0.02 M bis Tris, 0.01 M $CaCl_2$ in D_2O, from the visual fitting
of standard histidine titration curves to experimental plots of
chemical shift versus pH*, the direct reading of a pH meter in D_2O
solution. The similarity in pK' and $\delta(HA^+)$ values for corresponding
histidines in the 1428 and 3746 enzymes suggests that they correspond
to the same residue in both proteins and further suggests that the local
environment of charged groups, polar groups and aromatic rings is
similar for each of the five histidines in the binary MTX complex of

the two proteins. This supports our proposition that the MB 1428 and
MB 3746 reductases have similar tertiary and quaternary structure, in
consonance with their similarity in amino acid composition and molecular weight[6] and in amino terminal sequence (Bennett *et al*, this
volume).

TABLE I

COMPARISON OF HISTIDINE pK' VALUES AND $\delta(HA^+)$ FOR BINARY MTX COMPLEXES
OF DHFR FROM *E. COLI* MB 1428 AND MB 3746

	Histidine				
	1	2	3	4	5
Assignment	124	141	149	114	45
pK'					
MB 1428	8.0	7.2	6.6	6.2	5.7
MB 3746	8.1	7.5	6.9	6.4	5.9
$\delta(HA^+)$, Hz					
MB 1428	2605	2664	2637	2608	2646
MB 3746	2603	2648	2626	2600	2642

Replotted for Figure 1 are the aromatic regions of the 300 MHz pmr
spectra of the binary MTX complex of five different preparations of
E. coli MB 3746 DHFR. These spectra were obtained at 25° in buffer A,
at the pH* and concentration noted in the legend. For these preparations, *E. coli* MB 3746 were grown in the complex synthetic medium
described by Matthews *et al*[9] but with certain of the aromatic amino
acids, His Phe Trp and Tyr, replaced by 20-fold higher levels of the
corresponding deuterated aromatic amino acid. The large excess of
deuterated aromatic amino acid was used to attempt to dilute the endogenous pool of protonated aromatic amino acids, which this *E. coli*
strain can readily biosynthesize. In the bottom spectrum, the
bacteria were grown on fully protonated medium components. For the
spectrum second from the bottom in Fig. 1, the DHFR was isolated from
bacteria grown on protonated media with D,L-[α,3,5]-D3-Tyr in place
of Tyr. For the spectrum third from the top in Fig. 1, the DHFR was
isolated from bacteria grown on protonated media with D,L-[α,2,4]-D3-
His, D,L-[α,2,4,5,6,7]-D6-Trp and D,L-[α,2,3,5,6]-D5-Tyr replacing
His, Trp and Tyr, respectively. In the top two spectra, the deuterated aromatic amino acids used are indicated on the figure; D6-PHE
is D,L-[α,2,3,4,5,6]-D6-Phe.

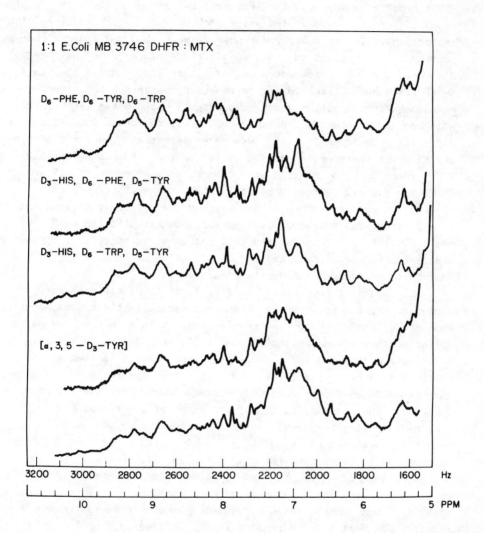

Fig. 1. Aromatic regions of 300 MHz pmr spectra of binary MTX complex of *E. coli* MB 3746 DHFR. The DHFRs contained deuterated aromatic amino acids, as indicated at the upper left of each spectrum. The spectra from bottom to top were run on samples at the following concentrations and pH* values, respectively: 1.34 mM, 7.78; 0.29 mM, 7.4; 1.81 mM, 7.4; 1.30 mM, 7.42; 1.25 mM, 7.2.

The broad resonances to the left or low-field of 2500 Hz in Fig. 1 probably correspond to buried amide protons that do not exchange with the solvent. The narrower resonances between 1800 and 2500 Hz correspond mostly to protons on the aromatic rings of the side chains of His, Phe, Trp and Tyr residues of the enzyme and of MTX. The His C-2-H resonances discussed in the preceding paragraph are narrow resonances in the bottom spectrum of Fig. 1 just to the left of the main body of resonances. Because the pH* of the spectra in Fig. 1 are different (see legend), these resonances appear at somewhat different positions in the upper spectra. It is apparent that there are His C-2-H resonances in DHFR isolated from *E. coli* grown on [α,2,4]-D3-His. The His C-2 deuterium possibly back-exchanges for protons of the medium, or the protonated His may have been freshly biosynthesized from protonated precursors. In general, the substitution of His by deuterated His was least successful, and substitution of Tyr by deuterated Tyr most successful, and the substitution of Phe and Trp by their deuterated counterparts moderately successful.

By comparison of the spectra in Fig. 1, it is possible to make a number of partial assignments of the resonances in the bottom spectrum. Upon comparison of the bottom two spectra, it is seen that resonances corresponding to two protons at 1942, 1998 and 2080 Hz are missing in the spectrum labelled [α,3,5]-D3-Tyr; these resonances thus are assigned as 3,5-protons (O- to OH) of the four Tyr residues. The two unassigned C-3,5-Tyr protons may be single proton resonances. See Table II. The standardization of the areas of the resonances is done by comparing the areas to the total area under the narrow aromatic resonances between 1800 and 2500 Hz, assuming that this area corresponds to 86 protons (5 on MTX, and 25, 30, 16 and 10 on the aromatic rings of the 5, 6, 4 and 5 residues of Trp, Phe, Tyr and His, respectively) and also to the areas of the methyl resonances to highfield of 0 ppm. Both methods of standardization give equivalent results. In regions of extensive resonance overlap, it is not possible to reliably calculate how much area corresponds to each separate maximum, so data for several resonances are aggregated.

Comparison of the middle spectrum with the bottom spectrum and the two top spectra in Fig. 1 suggests that the two protons of the 3-proton resonances centered at 2282 Hz, two protons in the four-proton resonances at 2239 and 2256 Hz, two protons in the six-proton resonances at 1998 Hz, and one proton in the two-proton resonances at 1871 and 1900 Hz correspond to 7 of the 30 ring protons of the six Phe residues. The other 23 presumably correspond to resonances

TABLE II

PARTIAL ASSIGNMENT OF RESONANCES IN THE AROMATIC REGION OF 300 MHz
PMR SPECTRUM OF BINARY MTX COMPLEX OF *E. COLI* MB 3746 DHFR

δ	N	Assignment
1748 Hz	1	Not assigned
1812 } 1824	2.5	0.5 proton, C-3',5'-2H of MTX
1871 } 1900	2	1 Phe
1942	2	2 C-3,5-2H-Tyr
1998	6	2 C-3,5-2H-Tyr, 2 Phe, 2 Trp
2054	9	1 C-3',5'-2H of MTX
2080 to 2184	46	2 C-3,5-2H Tyr
2206	5	
2239 } 2256	4	2 Phe, 2 Trp
2282	3	2 Phe, 1 Trp
2397	2	1 Trp
2468 } 2489	1	C-7-H of MTX

in the 2054 to 2206 Hz region. Analogous arguments were used to make
Trp assignments in Table II. More complete assignments will be made
when more extensively deuterated enzyme is obtained.

Also given in Table II are the assignments for the protons on C-7,
C-3' and C-5' of MTX[11]. MTX has been proposed[11] to bind to *E. coli*
DHFR in two forms in slow conformational equilibrium; one form was
proposed to be identical to the conformation in the crystalline
complex with MTX.

REFERENCES

1. Feeney, J., Roberts, G.C.K., Birdsall, B., Griffiths, D.V.,
    King, R.W., Scudder, P. and Burgen A. (1977) Proc. Roy. Soc.
    Lond. B., 196, 267-290.

2. Cocco, L., Blakley, R.L., Walker, T.E., London, R.E. and
    Matwiyoff, N. (1977) Biochem. Biophys. Res. Commun., 76,
    183-188.

3. Pastore, E.J., Plante, L.T., Wright, J.M., Kisliuk, R.L. and Kaplan, N.O. (1976) Biochem. Biophys. Res. Commun., 68, 471-475.

4. Poe, M., Williams, M.N., Greenfield, N.J. and Hoogsteen, K. (1975) Biochem. Biophys. Res. Commun., 67, 240-247.

5. Matthews, D.A., Alden, R.A., Bolin, J.T., Freer, S.A., Hamlin, R., Xuong, N., Kraut, J., Poe, M., Williams, M.N. and Hoogsteen, K. (1977) Science, 197, 452-455.

6. Poe, M., Breeze, A.R., Wu, J.K., Short, C.R. and Hoogsteen, K. (1978) J. Biol. Chem., in press.

7. Bennett, C.D., Rodkey, J.A., Sondey, J.M. and Hirschmann, R.F. (1977) Biochemistry, 17, 1328-1337.

8. Stone, D., Phillips, A.W. and Burchall, J.J. (1977) Europ. J. Biochem., 72, 613-624.

9. Matthews, H.R., Matthews, K.S. and Opella, S.J. (1977) Biochim. Biophys. Acta, 497, 1-13.

10. Griffiths, D.V., Feeney, J., Roberts, G.C.K. and Burgen, A.S.V. (1976) Biochim. Biophys. Acta, 446, 479-485.

11. Poe, M., Hoogsteen, K. and Matthews, D.A. (1978) J. Biol. Chem., in preparation.

THYMIDYLATE SYNTHETASE (EC 2.1.1.45) FROM L1210 MOUSE LEUKEMIA CELLS - CELL CYCLE
PATTERN AND AFFINITY CHROMATOGRAPHY PURIFICATION

WOJCIECH RODE[§], KEVIN J. SCANLON AND JOSEPH R. BERTINO[θ]
Departments of Pharmacology and Medicine, Yale University School of Medicine, New
Haven, Connecticut 06510 (USA)

INTRODUCTION

In order to understand the regulation and properties of mammalian tumor thymidylate synthetase (TS), a target enzyme in cancer chemotherapy, the enzyme in L1210
cells has been studied. Since both the phase of the cell cycle[1] and availability of
a proper methylenetetrahydropteroyloligoglutamate[2] have been reported to influence TS
activity, L1210 cells have been synchronized and changes of the enzyme activity
followed throughout the cell cycle both in cell extracts and in the intact cells (in
situ).

A new method of TS purification based on affinity chromatography has been developed. The method and electrophoretic properties of the purified L1210 enzyme are
presented.

MATERIALS AND METHODS

L1210 cells were maintained in Fischer's medium containing 10% horse serum and
antibiotics (penicillin and streptomycin).

Cell synchronization was achieved by isoleucine deprivation (18 hrs) followed by
treatment with 1mM hydroxyurea (10 hrs).[3]

Enzyme assays. TS activity in cell extracts and purified preparations was assayed
by a modification of Roberts' procedure.[4] The in situ assay[5] was carried out by incubating cell suspensions (up to $2x10^6$ cells/ml) with 10μM 5-^{3}H-deoxyuridine and
estimating tritium not absorbable on charcoal.

Biospecific adsorbent. N[10]-formyl-5,8-deazafolate, a potent inhibitor of TS
($I_{50}=1.5x10^{-7}$M for the L1210 enzyme), was coupled to aminoethyl-Sepharose in a 1-
ethyl-3(3-dimethyl-aminopropyl)-carbodiimide-promoted reaction.

Affinity chromatography. All buffers contained 0.1% Triton X-100 and 0.01M 2-
mercaptoethanol. The 30-70% ammonium sulphate fraction prepared from crude extract
was dissolved in 0.01M phosphate buffer pH 7.5 containing 20μM dUMP, dialyzed against
the same buffer and passed through a 7x2 cm affinity column. The column was then
extensively washed with 0.2M phosphate pH 7.5 containing 0.5M KCl and 20μM dUMP.
After subsequent equilibration of the column with 0.01M phosphate pH 7.5 containing
20μM dUMP, TS was eluted with 1L of the same buffer without dUMP. The enzyme was
concentrated by absorbing the eluate on a 1.5x5 cm DEAE-cellulose column, and eluting

§ Leukemia Society of America Fellow;   θ American Cancer Society Professor

490

with 0.2M phosphate buffer pH 7.5 containing 20% sucrose.

RESULTS AND DISCUSSION

Cell cycle pattern. Synchronization of the cells was evaluated on the basis of
cell count (per cent phasing over 60%) and rate of DNA synthesis changes (Fig. 1).
Due to the method used[3], the cells were arrested in late G1 and entered S phase after
removal of hydroxyurea.

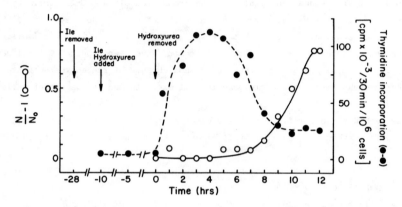

Fig. 1. Cell count and DNA synthesis patterns of synchronized L1210 cells.

TS activity assayed in extracts did not show significant changes during the cell
cycle (Fig. 2). However, TS activity assayed in situ showed considerable changes
(Fig. 2), parallel to the changes of the rate of DNA synthesis (Fig. 1). The latter
TS pattern remained the same with or without 20μM leucovorin (Fig. 2), suggesting
that availability of tetrahydrofolate was not rate-limiting. On the other hand,
availability of a specific methylenetetrahydropteroyloligoglutamate (which would
increase the V_{max} of the reaction[2]) is a possible explanation of the much higher TS
activity assayed in situ than that assayed in extracts during S phase (Fig. 2).

Results of the in situ assay may also depend on deoxyuridine transport properties
and thymidine kinase activity of cells. Both factors have been found to change in
synchronized mouse cells[6-9], but patterns of these changes show that neither of the
factors could be responsible for the changes of TS activity in situ. Thus the
pattern of TS activity observed in the intact cells may be due to the presence of a
regulatory system(s) for this enzyme in the cell.

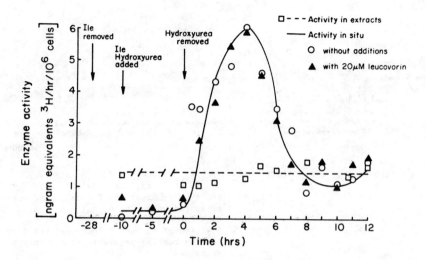

Fig. 2. Cell cycle pattern of changes of TS activity assayed in extracts and _in situ_ in L1210 cells.

Purification of TS takes advantage of the fact that the enzyme binds to the affinity adsorbent (Fig. 3) in the presence of dUMP, while other proteins are eluted from the column with a high ionic strength buffer. Elimination of dUMP from the buffer then results in elution of the enzyme. The affinity chromatography system presented here differs from that described earlier[10] in that a stable affinity adsorbent is used and Triton X-100 is included in all buffers. Neutral detergents (Triton X-100, Nonidet P40) appear to cause release of L1210 TS bound to high molecular weight complexes and to stabilize the enzyme.

Polyacrylamide gel electrophoresis of a preparation obtained as a result of affinity chromatography showed that TS was the main constituent but other proteins were present (Fig. 4). Electrophoresis of the preparation treated with an excess of 5-fluorodeoxyuridylate (FdUMP) and 5,10-methylenetetrahydrofolate (5,10-CH_2H_4PteGlu) showed the presence of two forms of TS-FdUMP-5,10-CH_2H_4PteGlu complex (Fig. 4). This result is similar to that obtained with bacterial TS[12], indicating that there are two binding sites of FdUMP present on the enzyme. Molecular weight of the L1210 TS subunit was found to be 38,500 (Fig. 5).

Repeating the affinity chromatography step resulted in an electrophoretically homogeneous enzyme (Fig. 6). A summary of the purification is presented in Table 1.

492

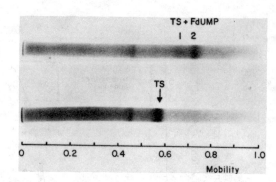

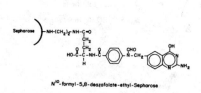

N^{10}-formyl-5,8-deazafolate-ethyl-Sepharose

Fig. 3. Structure of the affinity adsorbent.

Fig. 4. Polyacrylamide gel electrophoresis (7.5% gel, 0.1% Triton X-100) of TS (affinity chromatography I step). The sample separated on the upper gel was treated with 20µM FdUMP and 100µM 5,10-CH_2H_4PteGlu. The position of TS on the lower gel was identified by testing parallel gel for enzyme activity[11].

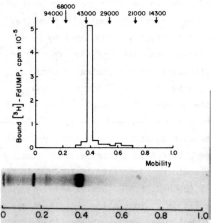

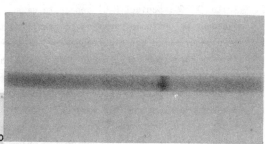

Fig. 5. SDS polyacrylamide gel electrophoresis (10% gel) of TS (affinity chromatography I step) treated with 20µM [^{3}H]-FdUMP and 100µM 5,10-CH_2H_4PteGlu.

Fig. 6. Polyacrylamide gel electrophoresis (7.5% gel, 0.1% Triton X-100) of TS after affinity chromatography II.

TABLE 1

PURIFICATION OF THYMIDYLATE SYNTHETASE FROM L1210 CELLS

Purification stage	Volume (ml)	Total activity (units[a])	Specific activity (units/mg protein)	Purification	Yield (%)
Crude extract	79	11,845	11.7	1.0	100
30-70% $(NH_4)_2SO_4$ fraction	38	9,480	16.5	1.4	80
Pooled fractions after affinity chromatography I	103	8,215	16,400	1,402	70
Pooled fractions after affinity chromatography II	110 (17)[c]	8,250 (4,600)	>33,500[b]	>2,863[b]	70 (39)

[a] TS activity unit = 1 mg equivalent of ^3H released per hour at 37°.
[b] Protein concentration under limit of sensitivity (8μg/ml) of protein assay used.
[c] Most active fractions

SUMMARY

Thymidylate synthetase activity was measured both in cell extracts and in intact L1210 cells (in situ) throughout the cell cycle. The per cell activity assayed in extracts did not change significantly during the cell cycle whereas that assayed in situ changed markedly following the pattern of DNA biosynthesis. In S phase much higher activity in situ than in cell extracts was observed.

L1210 TS was purified as a result of an affinity chromatography procedure based on reversible deoxyuridylate-dependent binding of the enzyme to a stable biospecific adsorbent, N^{10}-formyl-5,8-deazafolate, immobilized on aminoethyl-Sepharose. The presence of Triton X-100 stabilized TS during purification.

ACKNOWLEDGEMENTS

The authors would like to thank Ms. Barbara A. Moroson for skillful technical assistance and Dr. John Hynes for generously supplying N^{10}-formyl-5,8-deazafolate. This work was supported by grant CA08010.

REFERENCES

1. Conrad, A. H. (1971) J. Biol. Chem., 246, 1318-1323.
2. Dolnick, B. J., and Cheng, Y. (1978) J. Biol. Chem., 253, 3563-3567.
3. Tobey, R. A. and Crissman, H. A. (1972) Exptl. Cell Res. 75, 460-464.
4. Roberts, D. W. (1966) Biochemistry, 5, 3546-3548.
5. Kalman, T. J. and Yalowich, J. (1977) 177th ACS Meeting Abstract 127.
6. Sander, G. and Pardee, A. B. (1972) J. Cell Physiol., 80, 267-272.
7. Cunningham, D. D. and Remo, R. A. (1973) J. Biol. Chem. 248, 6282-6288.

8. Stubblefield, E. and Murphree, S. (1967) Exptl. Cell Res., 48, 652-656.

9. Mittermayer, C., Bosselmann, R. and Bremerskov, V. (1968) Eur. J. Biochem., 4, 487-489.

10. Slavik, K., Rode, W. and Slavikova, V. (1976) Biochemistry, 15, 4222-4227.

11. Dolnick, B. J. and Cheng, Y. (1977) J. Biol. Chem., 252, 7697-7703.

12. Donato, H., Jr., Aull, J. L., Lyon, J. A., Reinsch, J. W. and Dunlap, R. B. (1976) J. Biol. Chem., 251, 1303-1310.

PROPERTIES OF THE MULTIFUNCTIONAL ENZYME FORMYL-METHENYL-METHYLENETETRAHYDROFOLATE SYNTHETASE (COMBINED) FROM RABBIT LIVER

LaVerne Schirch, Elizabeth D. Mooz, and Darrell Peterson
Department of Biochemistry, Medical College of Virginia, Richmond, Virginia 23298

ABSTRACT

Titration of sulfhydryl groups of formyl-methenyl-methylenetetrahydrofolate synthetase with DTNB led to a concommitant loss of activity of dehydrogenase and cyclohydrolase activities. 10-Formyltetrahydrofolate synthetase activity disappeared more rapidly than the other two activities.

The multifunctional enzyme in combination with an equivalent amount of the enzyme serine transhydroxymethylase converts formate to the third carbon of serine. Tetrahydrofolate functions in this system in catalytic amounts. High concentrations of tetrahydrofolate, 0.1 mM, inhibit the conversion of formate to serine.

Sucrose density centrifugation and affinity column chromatography of mixtures of serine transhydroxymethylase and the multifunctional enzymes from rabbit liver suggest that they do not form a stable complex in solution.

INTRODUCTION

The conversion of the third carbon of serine to formate involves 4 reactions (reactions 1 through 4). Reaction 1 is catalyzed by serine transhydroxymethylase (STHM)* while reactions 2, 3, and 4 are catalyzed by a single multifunctional protein[1-3]. The activity of $5,10$-CH_2-H_4-folate dehydrogenase (MTFD)* (reaction 2) and $5,10$-CH^+-H_4-folate cyclohydrolase* (reaction 3) appear to be catalyzed at the same active site[3] or at least to closely linked sites[4,5]. The activity for 10-CHO-H_4-folate synthetase (reaction 4) appears to be catalyzed at a site different from the site catalyzing reactions 2 and 3.

$$\text{L-serine} + H_4\text{-folate*} \rightleftharpoons \text{glycine} + 5,10\text{-}CH_2\text{-}H_4\text{-folate} \qquad (1)$$

$$5,10\text{-}CH_2\text{-}H_4\text{-folate} + NADP^+ \rightleftharpoons 5,10\text{-}CH^+\text{-}H_4\text{-folate} + NADPH + H^+ \qquad (2)$$

$$5,10\text{-}CH^+\text{-}H_4\text{-folate} + H_2O \rightleftharpoons 10\text{-}CHO\text{-}H_4\text{-folate} + H^+ \qquad (3)$$

$$10\text{-}CHO\text{-}H_4\text{-folate} + ADP + Pi \rightleftharpoons H_4\text{-folate} + ATP + HCO_2^- \qquad (4)$$

Reactions 1 through 4 are an important series of reactions since they generate

---

*Abbreviations: STHM, serine transhydroxymethylase; MTFD, 5,10-methylene tetrahydrofolate dehydrogenase; BES, N,N-bis(2-hydroxyethyl)-2-amino-ethane sulfonic acid; DTNB, 5,5'-dithiobis-(2-nitrobenzoic acid); H_4-folate, tetrahydrofolate; 5-CH_3-H_4-folate, 5-methyl tetrahydrofolate; 5-CHO-H_4-folate, 5-formyl tetrahydrofolate.

many of the intermediates required in the biosynthetic pathways using one-carbon compounds. We have initiated a study to probe the properties of each of the 4 reactions and to also study the properties of the 4 reactions when they are acting in concert. With all four reactions combined H_4-folate needs to be present in only catalytic amounts, which more closely resembles its true physiological situation. This paper is a brief account of some of our recent observations.

MATERIALS AND METHODS

All materials were prepared and purchased as previously described[3].

The titration of the sulfhydryl groups of the multifunctional enzyme were performed as follows. To 0.4 ml of a 50 mM potassium phosphate - 50 mM ascorbate buffer, pH 7.3, was added 356 μgrams of the multifunctional enzyme. DTNB, 1 mM, was added to this solution in μL aliquotes. After each addition of DTNB the enzyme solution was incubated for 20 min at 30⁰ to allow the DTNB to react. At the end of each incubation period 2 μL aliquotes were removed to assay for dehydrogenase and cyclohydrolase activities[3]. Ten μL aliquotes were removed to determine the synthetase activity[3].

The determination of the rate of conversion of formate to serine was done as follows. In 1 ml of 50 mM potassium BES* buffer, pH 6.6, the following reagents were added: sodium formate, 4 μmoles; adenosine triphosphate, 1 μmole; magnesium sulfate, 2 μmoles; glycine, 2 μmoles; NADPH, 1 μmole; 2-mercaptoethanol, 10 μmoles; STHM*, 60 μg; multifunctional enzyme, 56 μg; and H_4-folate in concentrations up to 0.26 μmoles. The solution was incubated at 30⁰. At several time intervals 0.1 ml aliquotes were removed and added to 0.3 ml of 0.2 M sodium citrate, pH 2. Forty μL of this solution was analyzed for serine on a Durrum Model MBF amino acid analyzer.

Sucrose density gradient centrifugation of a mixture of STHM and the multifunctional enzyme were performed as follows. The multifunctional enzyme, 40 μg, and STHM, 200 μg, were layered on top of 5 ml of a 5% to 20% sucrose gradient in 50 mM potassium phosphate - 5 mM 2-mercaptoethanol, pH 7.3. The solutions were run at 4⁰ for 16.5 hours at 30,000 rpm in a Beckman SW 50.1 rotor. At the end of the run small holes were punctured in the bottom of each tube and the drops collected in several small test tubes. The activities for MTFD and STHM were determined for the solutions in each of the tubes.

Affinity chromatographic columns were prepared in Pasteur pipetts. Solutions of STHM and the multifunctional enzyme were added to the column in 10% sucrose - 10 mM potassium phosphate buffer, pH 6.8. The columns were washed with the 10 mM phosphate buffer until no enzyme activity was being eluted. One mM solutions of the appropriate substrate in 10 mM potassium phosphate was then added to the column to elute the enzymes. One ml sample volumes were collected and assayed for STHM and MTFD activities.

Fig. 1. Inhibition patterns for the
three reactions catalyzed by the multifunctional enzyme with increasing concentrations of DTNB.

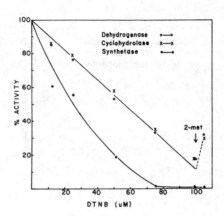

RESULTS AND DISCUSSION

Titration with DTNB: Even though a single enzyme catalyzes the three reactions
in converting 5,10-CH$_2$-H$_4$-folate to formate and H$_4$-folate it has not been clear
whether each reaction is catalyzed at a different site on this multifunctional
enzyme. It has been suggested that the first two reactions, the dehydrogenase and
cyclohydrolase activities, are catalyzed by a single active site[3]. This was
supported by similarities in dissociation constants for substrates and inhibitors
for these two reactions and by spectral changes observed in the conversion of
5,10-CH$_2$-H$_4$-folate to 10-CHO-H$_4$-folate[3]. That a single site may catalyze these
two reactions is also supported by the experiments of MacKenzie et al. who have
isolated a tryptic fragment from the multifunctional enzyme containing only the
dehydrogenase and cyclohydrolase activities[4]. To further investigate this point,
experiments have been undertaken to test the sensitivity of the three enzymatic
activities to sulfhydryl reagents. As shown in Fig. 1, addition of the reagent
DTNB to a solution of the multifunctional enzyme leads to identical inhibition
patterns for the dehydrogenase and cyclohydrolase activities. However, 10-CHO-
H$_4$-folate synthetase activity is more sensitive to inhibition by DTNB. After
incubation of the DTNB inhibited enzyme with 2-mercaptoethanol about 20 per cent
of the dehydrogenase and cyclohydrolase activities were recovered. Similar inhibition patterns were found when iodoacetamide was used as the sulfhydryl
reagent.

The identical sensitivity of the dehydrogenase and cyclohydrolase activities to
sulfhydryl reagents lends further support to these reactions being catalyzed by a
single active site.

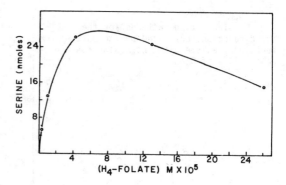

Fig. 2. Rate of formation of serine from formate as a function of H_4-folate concentration.

Conversion of Formate Serine: The metabolic coupling of the multifunctional enzyme to STHM permits the interconversion of formate and serine with catalytic amounts of H_4-folate. To our knowledge the conversion of formate to serine has not been demonstrated by a purified enzyme system. To investigate this reaction, we incubated STHM and the multifunctional enzyme with formate, glycine and the necessary cofactors and measured the amount of serine formed. We found that serine was formed in several-fold excess to the amount of H_4-folate present. Since H_4-folate is a competitive inhibitor for the other 1-carbon-H_4-folate intermediates in this system, you would predict that increasing concentrations would be inhibitory by competing for the active sites of the intermediate steps. The data in Fig. 2 show that this is indeed the case.

We have also tested the inhibitory effect of 5-CH_3-H_4-folate and 5-CHO-H_4-folate on this system. These two compounds inhibited the formation of serine about 50% when their concentration was in a 3 to 1 excess over H_4-folate.

STHM and Multifunctional Enzyme Complex Formation: Recently we have observed that adding the multifunctional enzyme to a solution of STHM, which has been tagged with a fluorescent probe, increased the fluoresence polarization of the enzyme. This increase in polarization could be explained by the formation of a complex between STHM and the multifunctional enzyme. Such a complex is also suggested by our previous observation that STHM and the multifunctional enzyme copurify through 5 of 6 purification steps[3]. Recently others have observed that a number of H_4-folate enzymes stick together on affinity columns[6]. This suggests that perhaps H_4-folate enzymes form some type of large multiple enzyme complex in

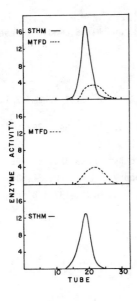

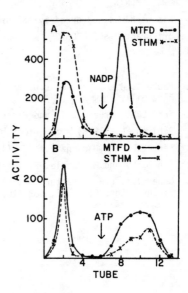

Fig. 3. Sucrose density centrifugation patterns for
serine transhydroxymethylase
(STHM) and 5,10-CH₂-H₄-folate
dehydrogenase (MTFD).

Fig. 4. Affinity chromatography
elution patterns for serine trans-
hydroxymethylase (STHM) and 5,10-
CH₂-H₄-folate dehydrogenase
(MTFD). A. NADP-agarose column.
B. ATP-agarose column.

the cell. We have done two experiments to test this hypothesis. First, we performed a sucrose density gradient centrifugation with a mixture of STHM and the
multifunctional enzyme. The results, as shown in Fig. 3, do not indicate the
formation of any complex under these conditions. The second experiment involved
the affinity of mixtures of STHM and the multifunctional enzyme for columns of
NADP-agarose and ATP-agarose both of which bind the multifunctional enzyme[5]. The
data are shown in Fig. 4. STHM shows no affinity for the NADP column. However,
STHM does stick to ATP-agarose and is eluted by ATP which is a substrate for the
multifunctional enzyme. However, in an experiment where STHM alone was tested
with the ATP-agarose column an essentially identical elution pattern was observed to that shown in Fig. 4B. We conclude from this that complex formation
between STHM and the multifunctional enzyme is not necessary to explain the
affinity of STHM for the ATP-agarose column. However, these experiments do not
rule out the formation of a transient complex between STHM and the multifunctional enzyme.

ACKNOWLEDGMENTS

This work was supported by NSF grant PCM 77-25748, and NIH Biomedical research support grant 5-S07-RR05725.

REFERENCES

1. Paukert, J.L., Srauss, L.D. and Rabinowitz, J. (1976) J. Biol. Chem. 251, 5104-5111.

2. Tan, L.L., Drury, E.J. and MacKenzie, R.E. (1977) J. Biol. Chem. 252, 1117-1122.

3. Schirch, L. (1978) Arch. Biochem. Biophys. 189, 283-290.

4. Tan, L.L. and MacKenzie, R.E. (1977) Biochim. Biophys. Acta 485, 52-59.

5. Cohen, L. and MacKenzie, R.E. (1978) Biochim. Biophys. Acta 522, 311-317.

6. Caperelli, C.A., Chettur, G., Lin, L.Y. and Benkovic, S.J. (1978) Biochem. Biophys. Res. Comm. 82, 403-410.

STUDIES ON METHYLENETETRAHYDROFOLATE REDUCTASE FROM OX BRAIN

ANTHONY J. TURNER, ANDREW G.M. PEARSON AND ROBERT J. MASON

Department of Biochemistry, University of Leeds, 9 Hyde Terrace, Leeds LS2 9LS, England

ABSTRACT

5,10-Methylenetetrahydrofolate reductase (EC 1.1.1.68) has been partially purified from ox brain and was found to be inseparable from the enzyme responsible for the synthesis of tetrahydro-β-carboline from methyltetrahydrofolate (CH_3FH_4) and tryptamine. Serine hydroxymethyltransferase could also mediate in β-carboline synthesis, supporting the role of methylene-FH_4 in this process. Methylene-FH_4 reductase could be substantially purified by chromatography on Procion Red HE3B-Sepharose. This resin could also be used for the purifications of certain pteridine-enzymes.

INTRODUCTION

Incubation of a brain cytosol fraction with CH_3FH_4 and tryptamine has been shown to generate the alicyclic alkaloid, 1,2,3,4-tetrahydro-β-carboline[1-3]. It has been suggested that the mechanism of this reaction involves the formation of methylene-FH_4 from CH_3FH_4 catalysed by methylene-FH_4 reductase[4-7]. Methylene-FH_4 can dissociate to FH_4 and formaldehyde, and the latter compound can then condense non-enzymically with tryptamine to form tetrahydro-β-carboline. We report here a purification of methylene-FH_4 reductase from ox brain. The final product retained tetrahydro-β-carboline synthetase activity. The purification procedure included chromatography on the novel affinity resin Procion Red HE3B-Sepharose. We have previously shown the general value of this resin for the purification of nucleotide-dependent enzymes[8], and demonstrate here that it can be used for the purifications of dihydropteridine reductase and dihydrofolate reductase.

A number of properties of purified methylene-FH_4 reductase are reported, including sensitivity to anti-folate drugs. Furthermore the ability of serine hydroxymethyltransferase to mediate in the formation of tetrahydro-β-carboline alkaloids is reported.

MATERIALS AND METHODS

Reagents   1,2,3,4-Tetrahydro-β-carboline was synthesized by the method of Vejdelek et al.[9], and the melting point, i.r. and mass spectra of the product were in agreement with previously published data[3,9]. Procion Red HE3B was a gift from ICI Organics Division, Blackley, Manchester, U.K. and the dye was immobilized to Sepharose by the method of Dudman and Bishop[10]. NADP-Sepharose was prepared

by the method of Larsson and Mosbach[11] and 2'5'ADP-Sepharose was purchased from
Sigma Chemical Co. 5-[^{14}C]Methyl FH$_4$ (57-61 mC$_i$/mmol) and L-[3-^{14}C]serine
(60 mC$_i$/mmol) were from the Radiochemical Centre, Amersham, U.K. Folate analogues
were provided by Dr. D. Mercer, Department of Biophysics, University of Leeds.
All other chemicals were purchased from British Drug Houses Ltd. or from Sigma
Chemical Co.

__Enzyme assays__ Methylene-FH$_4$ reductase was assayed either spectrophotometrically
or radiometrically as described by Kutzbach and Stokstad[12]. Serine hydroxymethyltransferase was measured by the method of Jones and Priest[13]. Dihydropteridine
reductase and dihydrofolate reductase were assayed as described by Craine et al.[14],
and Kaufman and Kemerer[15] respectively.

__Purification of methylene-FH$_4$ reductase__ Ox brain (650 g) was homogenised in
5 vol. distilled water and the high-speed supernatant fraction submitted to
(NH$_4$)$_2$SO$_4$ fractionation. The fraction precipitating between 35 and 55% saturation
was re-suspended in 10 mM KH$_2$PO$_4$/KOH, pH 7 (buffer A) and was dialysed exhaustively.
The enzyme preparation was then applied to a column of DEAE-cellulose (14.5 x 7 cm)
equilibrated in buffer A. The column was washed with 1 l. buffer A followed by
a linear gradient of KCl (0 - 0.5 M), pH 7. Fractions containing methylene-FH$_4$
reductase activity were pooled and applied to a column (15 x 4 cm) of Procion Red
HE3B-Sepharose equilibrated with 50 mM KH$_2$PO$_4$/KOH, pH 7.2. Enzyme activity was
eluted with a linear gradient of KCl (0 - 3 M), pH 7.2. The reductase was
concentrated by ultrafiltration and applied to a column (144 x 2 cm) of Sepharose
4B equilibrated with 50 mM KH$_2$PO$_4$/KOH, pH 7.5. Active fractions were pooled,
concentrated and stored at -20° C in 35% (v/v) glycerol.

__Purification of serine hydroxymethyltransferase__ Serine hydroxymethyltransferase
was purified from ox liver by the method of Jones and Priest[12]. The purified
enzyme contained no detectable methylene-FH$_4$ reductase activity.

RESULTS

The purification procedure for methylene-FH$_4$ reductase resulted in an overall
enrichment of approx. 360-fold from the cytosol fraction. The reductase retained
tetrahydro-β-carboline synthetase activity which co-purified throughout the
procedure. Chromatography of proteins on Procion Red HE3B-Sepharose has previously
been applied to the purifications of certain dehydrogenases[8]. Methylene-FH$_4$
reductase was adsorbed to the dye-resin and activity could subsequently be eluted
by an increase in ionic strength. This procedure resulted in 50-fold purification
(fig.1). Although the reductase uses NADPH as cofactor, neither NADP-Sepharose
nor 2'5'ADP-Sepharose were successful in adsorbing enzyme activity. The use of
Red HE3B-Sepharose was then extended to the purifications of pteridine and folate
reductases. Rat liver was homogenised in 5 vol. buffer A and 1 ml of the cytosol
fraction (13 mg) applied to a column (1.2 x 10 cm) of Red HE3B-Sepharose equilibrated

with buffer A. Both activities were adsorbed to the resin and could be selectively eluted with their respective coenzymes resulting in substantial purification (fig.2). The recovery of both enzymes was greater than 70%.

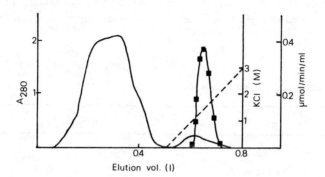

Fig.1   Purification of methylene-FH$_4$ reductase by chromatography on Procion Red HE3B-Sepharose. Methylene-FH$_4$ reductase activity (■-■) was eluted by a linear gradient of KCl (0 - 3 M). See text for details.

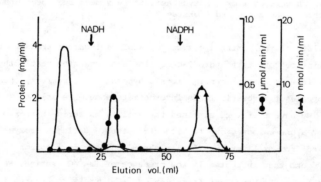

Fig.2   Purification of dihydropteridine and dihydrofolate reductases by chromatography on Procion Red HE3B-Sepharose. Dihydropteridine reductase (●-●) was eluted by including 1 mM NADH in the eluant buffer and dihydrofolate reductase (▲-▲) by the inclusion of 1 mM NADPH.

A number of properties of the purified methylene-FH_4 reductase were investigated. The molecular weight was estimated by gel filtration to be 180 000 ± 20 000. The reductase was reversibly inhibited by trimethoprim (K_i = 8 μM) and a number of other anti-folate drugs were also effective as inhibitors (table 1). The enzyme was also inhibited by dicoumarol which is consistent with its ability to reduce menadione[12]. Similar behaviour has been observed with the pig liver enzyme[12].

TABLE 1

EFFECT OF ADDITIVES ON METHYLENE-FH_4 REDUCTASE ACTIVITY

Additive	% Activity
Folic acid	90
Aminopterin	70
Methotrexate	60
Dichloromethotrexate	55
Dicoumarol	60
S-Adenosyl methionine (Ado-Met)	29
Ado-Met + Ado-Homocysteine	51
Procion Red HE3B	<1

All inhibitors were at a concentration of 0.1 mM except Ado-Met and Ado-Homo-cysteine which were at 1 mM. Enzyme activity was measured spectrophotometrically by the method of Kutzbach and Stokstad[12]

The ability of the purified enzyme to catalyse 1-carbon transfer from CH_3FH_4 to tryptamine to form tetrahydro-β-carboline has suggested that methylene-FH_4 is an intermediate in this process. If this hypothesis is correct, then other enzymes capable of generating this intermediate should be able to mediate in this reaction. We have therefore examined the ability of serine hydroxymethyltransferase to transfer a one-carbon group to biogenic amines. Serine hydroxymethyltransferase was purified from ox liver by affinity chromatography on a column of folate-Sepharose[13] and then incubated in the presence of [3-^{14}C]-serine, FH_4 and tryptamine. The FH_4-dependent formation of ^{14}C-tetrahydro-β-carboline could be demonstrated (table 2). The mechanism of this reaction is presumed to be:

$$\text{Serine} + FH_4 \rightleftharpoons \text{glycine} + \text{methylene-}FH_4$$

$$\text{Methylene-}FH_4 + \text{tryptamine} \longrightarrow \text{tetrahydro-β-carboline} + FH_4 \quad \text{(non-enzymic)}$$

TABLE 2

THE TRANSFER OF A ONE-CARBON GROUP FROM $[3-^{14}C]$-SERINE TO TRYPTAMINE *IN VITRO*

	Incubation conditions	Radioactivity recovered from product zone (d.p.m.)	
		THBC	NMT
1.	SHMT	1500	360
2.	SHMT (boiled)	200	20
3.	SHMT ($-FH_4$)	130	–

SHMT: Serine hydroxymethyltransferase; THBC: Tetrahydro-β-carboline;
NMT: N-Methyltryptamine.

SHMT (0.05 unit) was incubated in a total vol. of 0.5 ml at 30° C with 30 μmol KH_2PO_4/KOH, pH 7.4, 0.1 μmol pyridoxal phosphate, 0.1 μmol (0.5 μCi) L-$[3-^{14}C]$-serine, 0.8 μmol FH_4, 4 μmol mercaptoethanol and 10 μmol tryptamine HCl. Blank incubations were performed with boiled enzyme and in the absence of FH_4. The products were extracted into toluene, evaporated to dryness and taken up into acetone. Samples were applied to a silica gel t.l.c. plate and developed in butan-1-ol/acetic acid/H_2O (60 : 30 : 10).

DISCUSSION

Methylene-FH_4 reductase has previously been partially purified from mammalian liver[12]. The brain enzyme reported here exhibited many properties similar to the liver enzyme but differed in degree of sensitivity to the feedback regulator Ado-Met. Whether Ado-Met functions as a physiological regulator of brain reductase requires further investigation. The ability of both methylene-FH_4 reductase and serine hydroxymethyltransferase to participate in alicyclic alkaloid formation *in vitro* raises the possibility that such alkaloids may be formed *in vivo*. Tetrahydro-β-carboline and tetrahydroisoquinoline alkaloids both possess pharmacological activity[16-18].

Chromatography on Procion Red HE3B-Sepharose provided 50-fold purification of methylene-FH_4 reductase and the free dye was a potent inhibitor of reductase activity. The dye-resin also proved useful in purifying folate and pteridine reductases and in the latter cases, elution could be effected with coenzyme. Procion Red HE3B-Sepharose provides a cheap, re-usable affinity resin that does not require the use of cyanogen bromide in its preparation. It may therefore have wide applications to enzyme purification.

ACKNOWLEDGEMENTS

This work was supported by a MRC project grant to AJT. We should like to thank John Hryszko for excellent technical assistance.

REFERENCES

1. Mandel, L.R., Rosegay, A., Walker, R.W. and Vandenheuvel, W.J.A. (1974) Science, 186, 741-743.

2. Meller, E., Rosengarten, H., Friedhoff, A.J., Stebbins, R.A. and Silber, R. (1975) Science, 187, 171-173.

3. Wyatt, R.J., Erdelyi, E., DoAmaral, J.R., Elliott, G.R., Renson, J. and Barchas, J.D. (1975) Science, 187, 853-855.

4. Pearson, A.G.M. and Turner, A.J. (1975) Nature, 258, 173-174.

5. Ordonez, L.A. and Caraballo, F. (1975) Psychopharmacol. Commun., 1, 253-260.

6. Stebbins, R.D., Meller, E., Rosengarten, H., Friedhoff, A. and Silber, R. (1976) Archs. Biochem. Biophys., 173, 673-679.

7. Taylor, R.T. and Hannah, M.L. (1975) Life Sci., 17, 111-120.

8. Stockton, J., Pearson, A.G.M., West, L.J. and Turner, A.J. (1978) Biochem. Soc. Trans., 6, 200-203.

9. Vejdelek, Z.J., Trcka, V. and Protiva, M. (1961) J. Med. Pharm. Chem., 3, 427-440.

10. Dudman, W.F. and Bishop, C.T. (1968) Can. J. Chem., 46, 3079-3084.

11. Larsson, P.-O. and Mosbach, K. (1971) Biotechnol. Bioeng., 13, 393-398.

12. Kutzbach, D. and Stokstad, E.L.R. (1971) Biochim. Biophys. Acta, 250, 459-477.

13. Jones, C.W. and Priest, D.G. (1976) Archs. Biochem. Biophys., 174, 305-311.

14. Craine, J.E., Hall, E.S. and Kaufman, S. (1972) J. Biol. Chem., 247, 6082-6091.

15. Kaufman, B.T. and Kemerer, V.F. (1976) Archs. Biochem. Biophys., 172, 289-300.

16. Meller, E., Friedman, E., Schweitzer, J.W. and Friedhoff, A.J. (1977) J. Neurochem., 28, 995-1000.

17. Buckholtz, N.S. and Boggan, W.D. (1976) Biochem. Pharmacol., 25, 2319-2321.

18. Rommelspacher, H., Strauss, S.M. and Rehse, K. (1978) J. Neurochem., 30, 1573-1578.

D-FLUOROALANINE: A SUICIDE SUBSTRATE FOR SERINE TRANSHYDROXYMETHYLASE

ELIZABETH WANG, ROLAND KALLEN AND CHRISTOPHER WALSH
Departments of Chemistry and Biology, Massachusetts Institute of
Technology, and Biochemistry and Biophysics, University of Pennsylvania
Medical School

INTRODUCTION

Serine transhydoxymethylase (SHM) (E.C. 2.1.2.1.) is a pyridoxal-
phosphate (PLP) dependent enzyme that catalyzes the following reversible physiological reaction[1-3]:

$$\text{L-serine} + \text{tetrahydrofolate} \rightleftharpoons \text{glycine} + N^{5,10}\text{-methylene tetrahydrofolate} \tag{1}$$

The enzyme also carries out transformations (2) through (6)[4-8].

$$\text{L-allothreonine} \rightleftharpoons \text{glycine} + \text{acetaldehyde} \tag{2}$$
$$\text{L-phenylserine} \rightleftharpoons \text{glycine} + \text{benzaldehyde} \tag{3}$$
$$\text{aminomalonate} \rightleftharpoons \text{glycine} + CO_2 \tag{4}$$
$$\alpha\text{-methylserine} + \text{THF} \rightleftharpoons N^{5,10}\text{-methylene-THF} + \text{D-alanine} \tag{5}$$
$$\text{D-alanine} + \text{E-PLP} \rightleftharpoons \text{pyruvate} + \text{E-PMP} \tag{6}$$

Tetrahydrofolate (THF) is required as a cosubstrate for reactions (1)
and (5). The enzyme forms a glycyl-α-carbanion intermediate in the
synthesis of serine (1)[4]. We expected that such enzyme-mediated α-
carbanion formation with a serine analogue such as β-fluoroalanine
could lead to net α,β-elimination of HF[9-11]. In this paper we have
tested the interaction of SHM with this and other β-substituted serine
analogues and find that D-fluoroalanine (DFA) is processed as a suicide
substrate, partitioning between formation of pyruvate, NH_4^+, F^-, and
enzyme inactivation. Examination of this and other β-elimination reactions catalyzed by SHM and the degree of dependence on tetrahydrofolate
indicates the nature of that cofactor requirement.

RESULTS AND DISCUSSION

Turnover of D-fluoroalanine leads to enzyme inactivation. SHM, homogeneous from lamb liver or rabbit liver, catalyzes a very slow elimination of fluoride ion from D- or L-fluoroalanine to produce pyruvate,
F^-, and ammonia. As catalysis progresses with D-fluoroalanine, there
is a concomitant time-dependent loss of enzyme activity (Figure 1). The
rate of α,β-elimination from D-fluoroalanine at 20 mM is stimulated
about 200-fold with lamb enzyme by 0.5 mM THF (d,l mixture) and the

508

inactivation rate is increased proportionately with a pseudo first
order rate constant of 0.12 min^{-1}.

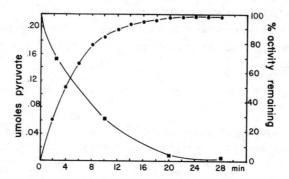

Fig. 1.   Turnover and Inactivation of SHM by DFA. 50 µg of lamb SHM
was incubated in 20 mM DFA, 0.5 mM THF, 50 mM Hepes, pH 7.5, 25 mM
Na$_2$SO$_4$, 1 mM EDTA, in a final volume of 0.5 ml. Pyruvate production
was followed by its reduction to lactate by NADH and lactate dehydrogenase. Aliquots were removed from a similar incubation at indicated
times and assayed for activity by allothreonine cleavage.

At complete inactivation there are 60 equivalents of pyruvate and F$^-$
generated per mole of lamb enzyme subunit (the enzyme is tetrameric).
This partition ratio of 60/1 reflects the frequency of harmless hydrolytic release of PLP-bound aminoacrylate versus the rare alkylative
capture by an enzyme nucleophile prior to release[9].

Covalent labeling by [^{14}C]-D-fluoroalanine. The UV-visible spectrum
of cytoplasmic lamb SHM was recorded during inactivation with 1,2-[^{14}C]-
D-fluoroalanine[9] in the presence of THF as shown in Figure 2: a time
dependent loss of A$_{425}$ occurs with a first order rate constant equal to

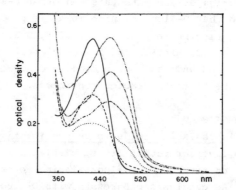

Fig. 2.   Spectral Changes Upon Inactivation by D-fluoroalanine. 3.4 mg
of lamb SHM, 18 µmoles 1,2-[^{14}C]-2-[^{2}H]-D-fluoroalanine, 0.3 µmole
THF incubated at 10°. —— =0, ----=12, ······=22,—·—=40,—---=65,—····=146 min.

that for inactivation measured simultaneously (k = 0.07)[10]. An increase in A_{460} occurs with a slower rate constant, k = 0.03. Separation on G-25 column produced enzyme with 0.83 labels per subunit, no absorbance at 460 nm, and less than 1% of the original 425 nm absorbance and activity. (The nature of the 460 nm absorbing species is as yet unknown.) Prolonged dialysis in the presence of dithiothreitol and PLP yielded 19% recovery of initial activity. This partial reactivation could reflect a 20% transamination of SHM during DFA processing, in competition with β-elimination, in which case labeling stoichiometry adjusted for transamination would yield 1.1 labels per subunit, or could reflect partial decomposition of a somewhat labile covalent enzyme adduct which will be examined further.

Role of THF. To examine the nature of the specific acceleration of the elimination/inactivation sequence with DFA, several folate oxidation states and analogues were tested at 20 mM DFA. While THF gives 200-fold rate increases, 7,8-dihydrofolate and folate are inactive as is 5-methyl-THF, in some parallel to their activity to labilize the pro S hydrogen of glycine[12].

Results of examination of other β-substituted alanine or aminobutyrates are summarized in Table I.

Table I
SUBSTRATES FOR ELIMINATION

Substrate	Elimination rate (min⁻¹)		Acceleration (20 mM)	t 1/2 for inactivation (min)	
	+THF	-THF		+THF	-THF
L-fluoroalanine[a]	0.65	0.01	50	>380	nd (20 mM)
D-fluoroalanine[a]	8.8	0.04	220	5.7	340 (20 mM)
L-chloroalanine	1.0	0.05	20	nd	nd
D-chloroalanine	1.2	0.25	5	57	nd (20 mM)
L-difluoroalanine[a]	0.65	0.07	9	nd	nd
D-difluoroalanine[a]	1.0	0.015	60	>150	nd (15 mM)
L-erythro-fluoro-aminobutyrate[a]	0.08	0.01	8	not detectable (20 mM)	
D-erythro-fluoro-aminobutyrate[a]	0.01	0.01	none	nd	nd
L-fluoroalanine	1.0[b]	1.0	none	nd	nd
D-fluoroalanine	95.0[b]	0.8	120	4.4	1500 (10 mM)

[a] provided by Dr. J. Kollonitsch and colleagues, Merck, Inc.
[b] rabbit liver enzyme

The V_{max} for serine synthesis in rabbit SHM is 80 min^{-1} in the presence of THF and 0.5 min^{-1} in its absence.

Several points can be noted about these data. First, the lamb liver enzyme will accelerate the α,β-HF elimination with both D- and L-fluoroalanine in the presence of THF by ca. 200-fold and 60-fold respectively. With rabbit liver enzyme the DFA reaction is selectively accelerated, expressing the expected specificity for its removal at the α-carbon. The broader lamb liver specificity is consistent with the observation[5] that this enzyme will generate a PLP-quinoid adduct (λ_{max} = 503 nm) with L-phenylalanine while the rabbit enzyme will not. Second, there is no detectable inactivation of rabbit serine hydroxymethylase and only slow inactivation of lamb enzyme with L-fluoroalanine in sharp contrast to the 60/1 turnover to inactivation ratio from the DFA. The respective bound aminoacrylate-PLP intermediates may be oriented in different directions at the active site and only the DFA eneamino-PLP is close to an active site nucleophile.

Third, although the eliminations rates at 20 mM for DFA and D-chloroalanine are only 7-fold different (8.8 vs. 1.2 min^{-1}), THF stimulates the basal rate only 5-fold with D-chloroalanine. The ratios for t 1/2 in the presence of THF for inactivation are 10-fold different, suggesting at this preliminary stage a similar partition ratio for catalytic turnover/inactivation event with these β-substituted D-alanines.

With the difluoroalanines, THF selectively stimulates D-isomer-HF elimination. The monofluoro-aminoacrylate-PLP product inactivates SHM at a much lower frequency than the aminoacrylate-PLP from D-monofluoroalanine based on the estimated partition number of 1400 for D-difluoroalanine.

Substrate kinetic isotope effect. V_{max} rates for β-elimination were determined with 2-[^{1}H]- and 2-[^{2}H]-D-fluoroalanine[10] with and without THF present. In the absence of THF there is a 2.2 fold deuterium kinetic isotope effect on V_{max} (V_H/V_D = 2.2) but no effect on the K_m (20 mM), indicating that α-proton abstraction from DFA is rate-limiting. At 0.5 mM THF the isotope effect on the elementary C-H cleavage step is no longer expressed on V_{max} (V_H/V_D = 1) and the maximal rate of pyruvate formation is enhanced 800-fold so that the intrinsic deuterium isotope effect is not expressed on V_{max}. This corresponds to an increase of $\sim$3 pKa units in the kinetic acidity of the α-hydrogen at the active site when THF is added.

D-cycloserine inhibits SHM solely by transamination. D-cycloserine is inhibitory to SHM activity in crude tissue preparations[13,14]. We noted that both DFA and D-cycloserine are suicide substrates for the alanine racemase of *E. coli* [9].D-cycloserine inactivates homogeneous SHM in a time dependent manner which is accelerated 7-fold by addition of THF (t 1/2 = 38 min - THF, t 1/2 = 5 min + THF). However, addition of exogenous PLP completely reverses this inactivation. The formation of pyridoxamine-P after D-cycloserine incubation implies that transamination, rather than covalent modification of the enzyme, is the molecular inactivation mechanism with the cyclic oxazolidinone. The L-isomer of cycloserine inactivates at 14 mM with a t 1/2 of about 20 min. and shows no rate enhancement on THF addition.

CONCLUSION

The pterin THF has previously been ascribed two roles in SHM catalysis[1-4]. It carries formaldehyde away from the active site in serine cleavage and serves as a source of unhydrated formaldehyde in serine synthesis. The second role is seen in serine synthesis where THF may aid in enzymic removal of the pro S hydrogen of the PLP-bound glycine[8] for the glycyl carbanion requisite for C-C bond formation.

The present studies with suicide substrates illuminates this second α-proton labilization role. The large variation in THF dependence on the nature of the leaving group and the substrate chain length attests to the sensitivity of the active site to tertiary complex interactions, and clear explanation may require an X-ray map at high resolution. The requirement for the tetrahydro oxidation state of folate could mean a specific role for N^5 as the active site base and/or the puckered conformation that the tetrahydropyrazine ring will assume[15].

With a partition ratio of 60/1 at saturating THF and a reasonable turnover number (6-8 min^{-1}) for D-fluoroalanine, rapid inactivation of both cytoplasmic and mitochondrial isozymes is obtained *in vitro*. However, the relatively high K_m (15-20 mM) and the low likelihood of obtaining such intracellular concentrations (even if D-fluoroalanine were being used for antibiotic purposes[9,16]) strongly decrease the probability that rapid inactivation of SHM will occur *in vivo* or in tissue culture. These results at least beckon one to develop more efficient SHM suicide substrates and evaluate physiological responses obtained by blocking cellular folate metabolism at this key point.

REFERENCES

1. Benkovic, S. and Bullard, W. (1973) Progress in Bioorganic Chemistry, 2, 133.
2. Blakeley, R.L. (1969) The Biochemistry of Folic Acid and Related Pteridines, North-Holland , Amsterdam, pp. 267-291.
3. Benkovic, S.J. (1978) Accts. Chem. Res., 11, 314-320.

512

4. Schirch, L. and Jenkins, W.T. (1964) J. of Biol. Chem., 239, 3797-3800.

5. Ulevitch, R.J. and Kallen, R.G. (1977) Biochem., 16, 5342-5350.

6. Palekar, A.G., Tate, S.S. and Meister, A. (1973) J. of Biol. Chem., 248, 1158-1167.

7. Schirch, L.G. and Mason, M. (1963) J. of Biol. Chem., 238, 1032-1037.

8. Schirch, L. and Jenkins, W.T. (1964) J. of Biol. Chem., 239, 3801-3807.

9. Wang, E. and Walsh, C. (1978) Biochem., 17, 1313-1321.

10. Walsh, C.T. (1977) in Horizons in Biochemistry and Biophysics, Quagliariello, E., Palmieri, F. and Singer, T.P. eds., Addison-Wesley, Reading, MA, pp. 36-81.

11. Walsh, C. (1978) Ann. Rev. Biochem, 47, 881-931.

12. Jones, C.W., Hynes, J.B. and Priest, D.G. (1978) Biochim. Biophys. Acta, 524, 55-59.

13. Draudin-Krylenko, V.A. (1976) Khim.-Farm. Zh., 10, 3-7.

14. Bukin, Y.V. and Sergeev, A.V. (1968) Biochim., 33, 1092-1101.

15. Poe, M. and Hoogsten, K. (1978) J. of Biol. Chem., 253, 543-546.

16. Kahan, F.M., Kropp, H., Woodruff, H.B., Kollonitsch, J., Borash, L., Jenson, N.P., Marburg, S., Perkins, L., Miller, S.M., Shen, T.Y., Onishi, H.R. and Jacobus, D.P. (1975) Interscience Conference on Antimicrobial Agents and Chemotherapy, Abstracts 101-103, Washington, D.C.

513

FOLIC ACID AND THE ACID MICROCLIMATE

JOHN A. BLAIR, MICHAEL L. LUCAS & SARA K. SWANSTON
Chemistry Department, the University of Aston in Birmingham, Gosta Green,
Birmingham B4 7ET, Great Britain

The effects of compounds implicated in folate malabsorption were tested both on folic acid transport and on surface pH in rat proximal jejunum in vitro. Transport studies (Blair, Johnson, and Matty, 1975) involved 3 cm everted sacs (serosal volume 0.2 mls) incubated for one hour in Krebs-Phosphate containing $1\mu M$ folic acid with C^{14} isotope (sp.act.58.2mCi:/mol) as a tracer. Surface pH studies were done as described elsewhere (Lucas & Blair, 1978).

In a wide variety of circumstances (Table 1) water movement paralleled folate transfer, except when high oral doses 10mg/kg methotrexate (MTX) were given; here water transported increased yet folate uptake fell, showing that solvent drag is not the mechanism for transfer. Low sodium buffer, oral MTX and in vitro 3% ethanol reduced both surface pH and transfer. There was a better correlation between transfer and surface pH alterations ($p < 0.02$) than with water movement (NS).

Concentration changes in the mucosal, tissue and serosal compartments of the everted sac preparation resembled diffusion through a three-compartment catenary system: this was as good a model as the Michaelis-Menten kinetics of a "pump-and leak" system. Where appropriate, relative apparent first order kinetic constants could be derived for two permeability barriers in series (Table 2). The values for the first barrier encountered (k_1) were smaller than the second set of 'downstream' constants (k_2) indicating that the first barrier was rate limiting. Where surface pH was elevated, corresponding k_1 values were depressed significantly, often with increases in the k_2 values.

In summary, both experimental results and kinetic analyses are consistent with an acid microclimate controlling a diffusion mechanism for folic acid transfer.

TABLE I

Treatment	Folic acid uptake (pmol/h per mg)	Change in surface pH (ΔpH)	Mucosal fluid uptake (mg/h per mg)
20% Ethanol ad lib.	$23.5 \pm 1.9(6)$**	$+0.09(8)$	$7.9 \pm 0.8(6)$**
Phenytoin	$20.6 \pm 0.9(6)$	$+0.06 \pm 0.20(8)$	$6.3 \pm 0.4(6)$**
Control	$17.0 \pm 0.8(12)$	0.0	$4.9 \pm 0.3(12)$
1μM- Methotrexate	$14.5 \pm 1.4(6)$	$-0.03 \pm 0.09(6)$	$4.5 \pm 0.8(6)$
3% Ethanol in vitro	$13.9 \pm 1.5(6)$	$-0.33 \pm 0.10(6)$*	$4.2 \pm 0.3(6)$
30mM-Na$^+$	$13.0 \pm 1.0(6)$**	$-0.42 \pm 0.10 (12)$***	$3.9 \pm 0.2(6)$**
Methotrexate (10mg/kg orally)	$10.0 \pm 2.1(6)$***	$-0.39 \pm 0.11(4)$*	$9.2 \pm 1.2(6)$***

Differences from control *$P<0.05$; **$P<0.02$; ***$P<0.01$

Regressions folic acid versus water transport $r = 0.1360$

P is not significant

folic acid versus change in surface pH $r = 0.8564$

$P < 0.02$.

TABLE 2

Relative Apparent First Order
Kinetic Constants (min^{-1} x 10^3)

	k_1	k_2
Control	5.3 ± 0.6	20 ± 3
20% Ethanol ad lib	4.8 ± 0.6	18 ± 1
Oral Methotrexate	2.9 ± 0.2*	169 ± 53**
3% Ethanol in vitro	2.3 ± 0.2*	48 ± 7
30mM Na+	2.8 ± 0.1*	25 ± 5

Differences from control   *$P<0.05$;   **$P<0.02$

Blair, J.A., Johnson, I.T. & Matty, A.J. (1975) J.Physiol. 236
653-661
Lucas, M.L. & Blair,J.A. (1978) Proc.Roy.Soc. B 200 27-41.

SEPARATION OF ρ-AMINOBENZOYL(GLUTAMATE) BINDING FROM FOLATE BINDERS

J. Douglas Caston and Barton A. Kamen

ABSTRACT

Binding of ρ-aminobenzoyl(glutamate) (ρABG) has been identified in porcine plasma and kidney, human umbilical cord serum, and bovine milk and β-lactoglobulin. ρABG binding can be separated from folate binding by affinity chromatography. Binding was proportional to binder concentration and ligand concentration but was not saturable at any ρABG concentration up to 10 mM. Similar binding of other simple ring compounds was also demonstrated and appears to be due to low affinity binding sites.

INTRODUCTION

Many attempts to quantify high affinity binders of folate during their preparation and to ascertain their physical and chemical characteristics yield confusing results. Often recoveries of more than 400% of the initial binding activity are noted during the early steps of purification whereas the final yield might appear to be only 1-5%. Moreover, it is not uncommon to record unstable alterations in binding affinity and specificity for different folate derivatives as the purification proceeds.

The identification and purification of high affinity binders of folate rely heavily on radioactive folic acid for the detection and quantification of binding activity. Most of the difficulties encountered in studies on folate binders seem to arise from impurities that form spontaneously in commercial preparations of high specific radioactivity folic acid. As illustrated by data presented herein, of the several radioactive compounds that are generated from the decomposition of ^{3}H-folic acid, ^{3}H-ρABG derivatives are most noteworthy. Crude and partially purified preparations of folate binder from all sources studied to date contain sizable quantities of binding sites for these compounds.

MATERIALS AND METHODS

DEAE-cellulose or DEAE-Sephadex column chromatography was used to purify ^{3}H-ρABG, ^{3}H-ρABA (ρ-aminobenzoic acid), ^{3}H-ptCHO (pterin-6-carbox aldehyde) and several unidentified labelled compounds from preparations of ^{3}H-folic acid that had been allowed to undergo spontaneous decomposition. Two different batches were obtained from Amersham/Searle Corporation, Batch 50 (26 Ci/mmole) and Batch 63 (47 Ci/mmole). From data furnished by the vendor, specific activities of 23 and 27 Ci/mmole for ρABG (and ρABA) and 2.9 and 19.7 Ci/mmole for ptCHO generated from Batches 50 and 63, respectively, were calculated.

The tritiated compounds ATP (24 Ci/mmole), cAMP (30 Ci/mmole), CTP (21 Ci per mmole), GTP (10 Ci/mmole), TTP (50 Ci/mmole), UTP (45 Ci/mmole), tyrosine (38 Ci per mmole), phenylalanine (48 Ci/mmole) and tryptophan (21 Ci/mmole) were purchased from Amersham/Searle. Folic acid (ICN Life Sciences), ρABG, ρABA (ICN), ptCHO and pterin-6-carboxylic acid (Sigma) were purified by column chromatography and quantified by published spectral absorption tables.[1]

Porcine kidney[2], porcine plasma[3], umbilical cord serum[4], bovine milk[5] and bovine β-lactoglobulin[5] were prepared for folate binder as described elsewhere. To assay binding activity, an aliquot of material was incubated with radioactive ligand as indicated in a final volume of 1.0 ml of 0.05 M phosphate buffer, usually pH 7.6, at 4°C in the dark for 20 minutes which was optimal for maximal binding. Reactions were terminated by addition of 1.0 ml of charcoal-Dextran solution and processed for liquid scintillation counting as detailed elsewhere[2].

RESULTS AND DISCUSSION

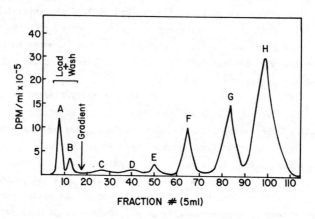

Figure 1. Separation of Labelled Decomposition Products of ^{3}H-Folic Acid.

As seen in figure 1, several radioactive compounds can be isolated from preparations of ^{3}H-folic acid that have been stored at -40°C for several months. Refractionation of purified folic acid (Fraction H) after 4 hours in the dark at 4°C showed that about 5% of the ^{3}H initially purified as folic acid was now in ρABG and ρABA which appeared as a minor component in the leading boundry of ρABG (Fraction G) and another 1-2% was in water (Fraction A), thus indicating the instability of ^{3}H-folic acid preparations under these conditions.

Each fraction was diluted about 100-fold with 0.05 M phosphate buffer and tested immediately for its ability to bind to either crude preparation of binder or affinity chromatography (AFC) purified folate binder. Results are given in table 1 and show that Fractions B (aniline?), C and D (unidentified), G (ρABG) and H (folic acid) all bound to crude binder preparation with ρABG and folic acid showing the highest level of binding. Of these fractions, only folic acid bound to AFC folate binder. Fraction F (ptCHO) was not bound by either binder preparation.

Table 1. Binding of Radioactive Fractions Separated on DEAE-Sephadex Columns by Crude and AFC Purified Preparations of Folate Binder.

| | | NET DPM BOUND (% of Imput DPM) | |
	FRACTION	CRUDE BINDER PREPARATION	AFC FOLATE BINDER
A	WATER	- -	- -
B	ANILINE (?)	4,800 (12%)	<200
C	UNKNOWN	4,400 (11%)	<200
D	UNKNOWN	4,700 (12%)	<200
F	PTERIN-6-CARBOXALDEHYDE	<200	<200
G	p-AMINOBENZOYL(GLUTAMATE)	18,100 (35%)	<200
H	FOLIC ACID	34,200 (70%)	48,100 (100%)

Results presented in table 1 also show that at some step during purification of folate binder from crude porcine kidney preparations, ρABG binding and folate binding activities become separated. This separation is better illustrated by figure 2 which outlines the purification scheme and summarized the estimated ρABG and folate binding activities as total pmoles of each ligand bound at each step. About half of the ρABG binding activity precipitated in solutions of 50% ethanol; the remainder and all of the folate binding activity precipitated in solutions of 75% ethanol. Folate and ρABG binding activities were completely separated from each other by passing the 75% ethanol precipitate, dissolved in 0.05 M phosphate buffer, pH 7.6, through an affinity column of methotrexate-Sepharose. The folate binder adhered to the matrix whereas the ρABG binding activity ran through. Addition of ethanol to the "run through" to a concentration of 75% yielded a white flocculus and a red precipitate each of which contained ρABG binding sites.

Figure 2. Scheme for Separation of pABG Binding from Folate Binder of Porcine Kidney.

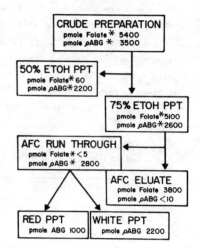

At a constant pABG concentration, binding was proportional, but not strictly linear, to binder concentration until about 75% of the ligand had been bound (figure 3). This deviation from linear binding is no doubt responsible for much of the error encountered in estimation of total pABG binding activity (figure 2). This parameter of pABG binding contrasts sharply with high affinity folate binder of porcine kidney which shows strict linearity until virtually 100% of the available folic acid has been bound[4].

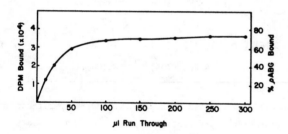

Figure 3. Binding of pABG by AFC Run Through. Amounts of binder indicated were incubated with 1.0 pmole of ^{3}H-pABG as detailed in the text.

It was not possible to saturate pABG binding sites. Binding by a given amount of "run through" was strictly linear with respect to pABG concentration with about 30% of the available ligand being bound at each concentration (figure 4). In a separate series of experiments, non-radioactive pABG at concentrations up to 10 mM were used to compete with 2 pmoles of ^{3}H-pABG; again, about 30% of the radioactivity was bound at each concentration. Care was taken to ensure that the charcoal adsorptive system was adequate to separate free and bound ligand over the entire concentration range of ligand used. Although indaequate to use in calculation of a precise binding constant, these results illustrate the low affinity of pABG binding.

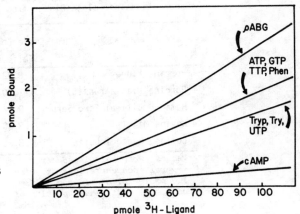

Figure 4. Binding of pABG and Other Compounds by AFC Run Through

Binding was not restricted to pABG. Several other simple ring compounds were also bound by AFC "run through" (figure 4). Because saturation of binding sites was not possible, competitive and displacement experiments could not be conducted. Thus, we cannot ascertain whether these compounds were all bound by the same sites.

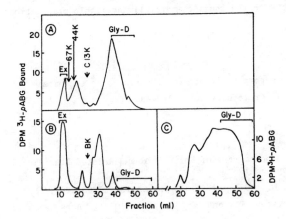

Figure 5. Sephadex Filtration of pABG Binding Sites. DPMx10[3].

pABG binding activity separated into several molecular weight fractions on Sephadex G-100 (figure 5A) and G-25 (figure 5B), with the major activity fraction having an apparent molecular weight of about 6-8,000. Filtration of pABG-binder complexes on Sephadex G-25 (figure 5C) yielded a broad fraction of ^{3}H-pABG in the lower molecular weight region and probably indicates the instability of the complexes which also reflects the low affinity of the binding.

Table 2. Binding of Folic Acid and pABG by Crude
Preparations of Folate Binder from Several Sources.

	pmole Bound per mg Protein*	
	Folic Acid	pABG
Porcine Kidney	0.42	0.18
Porcine Plasma (unsat)	1.30	1.61
Human Umbilical Cord Serum	0.07	0.20
Bovine Milk	3.80	0.11
Bovine β-Lactoglobulin	8.20	0.02

*Values were calculated from results obtained from
several concentrations of binder preparation with
1.0 pmole folic acid and 2.0 pmole pABG/ml reaction
using the most linear portion of the binding curves.

pABG binding activity has also been identified in other sources of folate binder. Table 2 summarizes and compares folate binding activity with pABG binding activity for porcine kidney, native unsaturated activity in porcine plasma, umbilical cord serum, bovine milk and bovine β-lactoglobulin. Hence, it appears that pABG binding activity, though perhaps non-specific and of low affinity, may be widely distributed in biological materials. Certainly, it must be controlled for when studying folate binder with the usual commercially available preparations of radioactive folic acid.

ACKNOWLEDGEMENTS

This work was supported in part by grants for the NIH. The technical assistance of Mrs. Radka Vatev is gratefully acknowledged.

REFERENCES

1. Blakley, R. L. (1969) The Biochemistry of Folic Acid and Related Pteridines, North-Holland, Amsterdam, pp. 58-105.

2. Kamen, B. A. and Caston, J. D. (1975) J. Biol. Chem., 250, 2203-2205.

3. Mantzos, J. D., Terzaki-Alevizou, V., and Gyftaki, E. (1974). Acta Haemat., 51, 204-210.

4. Kamen, B. A. and Caston, J. D. (1975) Proc. Nat. Acad. Sci., 72, 4261-4264.

5. Ford, J. E., Salter, N. and Scott, K. J. (1969) J. Dairy Res., 36, 435-446.

FOLATE ANALOG TRANSPORT BY ISOLATED MURINE INTESTINAL EPITHELIAL CELLS

P. L. CHELLO, F. M. SIROTNAK, D. M. DORICK AND J. GURA

Memorial Sloan-Kettering Cancer Center, New York, NY 10021

ABSTRACT

Epithelial cells were removed from both the villi and the crypts of mouse small intestine by treatment with hyaluronidase. Suspensions of these cells transported methotrexate. Influx of drug was temperature-dependent, exhibited Michaelis-Menton saturation kinetics, and was inhibited in a competitive manner by natural folates. Efflux of drug showed first-order kinetics. The transport system exhibited structural specificity for substituents at the 10 position of the folate molecule: affinity during influx was in the order aminopterin >> 10-methylamino-pterin (methotrexate) $\simeq$ 10-ethylaminopterin. The values for the V_{max} for influx and the rate constant for efflux were similar for each ana-log. These data support the notion of carrier-mediated transport of methotrexate and other folate analogs.

INTRODUCTION

In murine tumor models, the epithelial lining of the small intestine is the host tissue most sensitive to folate analog toxicity[1]. Although the transport of natural folates and folate analogs has been studied with a variety of murine tumor cells in vitro[2], similar studies are lacking for these normal proliferative cells of the mouse. We now de-scribe a procedure for the isolation of epithelial cells from the mu-cosa of the small intestine, and present evidence which suggests that methotrexate and other folate analogs accumulate in these cells as in tumor cells by a carrier-mediated process.

MATERIALS AND METHODS

Epithelial cells were isolated by incubating intestinal mucosa with hyaluronidase, a procedure originally developed by Kimmich[3]. Small intestines from BD_2F_1 mice were everted on applicator sticks and incubated at 37° in a Tris-salts isolation medium (see Kimmich[3]), pH 6.9, containing 0.1% BSA and 0.1% hyaluronidase. After 20 min, epithelial cells were separated from the lamina propria by gentle agitation, filtered through nylon hose, washed twice with isolation medium less hyaluronidase, pH 7.4, and resuspended in transport medium[4], pH 7.4. The cell suspension was composed predominantly of two cell species[4], present in approximately equal amounts. The first species was the columnar-shaped adsorptive epithelia from villi; the second, considered to be proliferative cells released from the crypts, was smaller, more spherical, and less dense under phase contrast microscopy. Procedures for the measurement of folate analog influx and efflux by these cell suspensions have been described[4].

RESULTS AND DISCUSSION

The uptake of methotrexate by isolated epithelial cells was characterized by a rapid, temperature-independent component assumed to represent drug nonspecifically adsorbed to the cell surface, and a temperature-dependent influx which was linear for approximately 20 min, after which there was an exponential approach to steady-state. The concentration dependence of methotrexate influx (uptake corrected for nonspecific cell surface adsorption) at 0° and at 37° is shown in Figure 1. Influx at 0° was linear with concentration. At the lower concentrations, methotrexate influx at 37° exhibited saturation kinetics, while at the higher concentrations, influx was more proportional to concentration. A double reciprocal plot of the 37° influx is shown in the insert. Both a saturable (K_m: 83.3 µM; V_{max}: 2.0 nmoles/min/g dry wt) and a nonsaturable component of influx are delineated. The Q_{10}

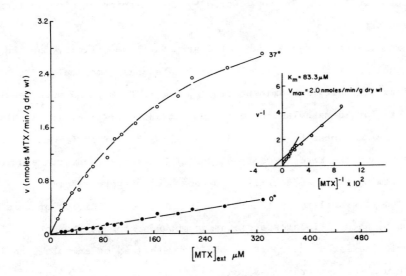

Fig. 1. Concentration dependence of methotrexate influx.

ratio for influx at 37° versus influx at 27° was 3.5. Influx at 37° but not at 0° was competitively inhibited by dl-L-5-formyltetrahydrofolate (K_i: 357.6±61.8 μM), dl-L-5-methyltetrahydrofolate (K_i: 371.5± 61.5 μM) and folic acid (K_i: 1745.2±78.2 μM).

Intracellular methotrexate was distributed as an exchangeable and a nonexchangeable fraction. Drug effluxed from preloaded cells to a constant level of 0.56 nmoles/g dry wt of cells. The efflux of drug showed first-order kinetics and a $t_{1/2}$ of 9.0 min. The fraction of methotrexate which did not efflux from the cells is assumed to represent drug bound to dihydrofolate reductase.

The initial 37° influx of methotrexate (at 22 μM) was moderately inhibited by 5.0 mM ouabain (44%), 10 mM sodium azide (25%) and 0.25 mM

524

p-chloromercuribenzoate (65%). Neither reagent affected methotrexate influx at 0°. The steady state for methotrexate but not the initial rate of influx at 37° was lowered by the omission of glucose from the transport medium.

The transport system exhibited structural specificity for the substituent at the 10-position of the folate analog molecule. It had the highest affinity for aminopterin (K_m: 7.2±3.6 µM), and much less affinity for 10-methylaminopterin (methotrexate) (K_m: 87.1±6.3 µM) and 10-ethylaminopterin (K_m: 123.8±17.9 µM). The values for the V_{max} for influx and the kinetic constant for efflux for aminopterin and 10-ethylaminopterin were similar to those for methotrexate.

The saturability of the 37° influx and the inhibition of this influx by natural folates and other compounds support the notion of carrier-mediated transport of methotrexate (and other folate analogs). Although the temperature-dependence of influx and the effect of metabolic poisons and glucose deprivation is suggestive of an energy-requiring process, demonstration of drug accumulation against an electrochemical gradient will be required before it can be concluded that "active" transport is actually involved.

ACKNOWLEDGEMENTS

Supported in part by NCI grants CA-08748, CA-18856, CA-22764 and ACS grant CH-26.

REFERENCES

1. Philips, F.S., Thiersch, J.B. and Ferguson, F.C., Jr. (1950) Ann. N.Y. Acad. Sci., 52, 1349-1359.

2. Sirotnak, F.M. and Donsbach, R.C. (1976) Cancer Res., 36, 1151-1158.

3. Kimmich, G.A. (1970) Biochemistry, 9, 3659-3668.

4. Chello, P.L., Sirotnak, F.M., Dorick, D.M. and Donsbach, R.C. (1977) Cancer Res., 37, 4297-4303.

KINETIC AND CHROMATOGRAPHIC EVIDENCE FOR HETEROGENEITY OF THE HIGH
AFFINITY FOLATE BINDING PROTEINS IN SERUM

NEVILLE COLMAN AND VICTOR HERBERT
Veterans Administration Hospital and SUNY-Downstate Medical Center,
Bronx, New York 10468

INTRODUCTION

Serum contains at least two binding systems for folate[1]. The low
affinity, high capacity binders became apparent in early studies using
equilibrium dialysis, gel filtration and ultrafiltration. Only the
first of these appears a valid technique, since binding is overestim-
ated using ultrafiltration due to adsorption of free folate onto filter
membranes[2] and using gel filtration due to an artifact of the dilute
buffer system[3]. This binding is often called "non-specific" because it
was not saturable over a wide range of concentration[4], was easily dissociated by electrophoresis[5] or coated charcoal adsorption[6], and has
not been shown to require a specific conformational structure[7]. The
low affinity binders comprise a variety of serum proteins[8] which are
profoundly affected by aspirin acetylation[9,10] and bind PGA with an
association constant less than 10^4 1/mol[1,7]. Folate bound in this
system is apparently not available for glomerular filtration[11] but is
accessible to the active, carrier-mediated cell transport systems[12].

The high affinity, low capacity folate binders were first identified
in milk[6,13]. In serum, they were first identified in 3 patients with
chronic granulocytic leukemia[14] and were subsequently observed in serum
of women who were pregnant or taking oral contraceptives[15], folate
deficient[16], cirrhotic and uremic patients[17,18]. By developing a technique which strips endogenous folate from the high affinity binder, we
have demonstrated the presence of folate binder in all sera[19]. This
technique has been used to prepare the folate binder for studies of
binding kinetics and possible functional and structural heterogeneity.

TOTAL FOLATE BINDING CAPACITY (TFBC)

Our studies in this area developed from an investigation of the
effect of pH on the folate binding capacity of serum. It was observed
that binding at pH 4.2 was less than 5% of optimal binding[19], and that
neutralisation of the acidified material restored the original binding
capacity, indicating that acidification had dissociated rather than
denatured the binder. By adding coated charcoal at the low pH, dissociated endogenous folate was removed from the system. The newly

available folate binding sites were then measured using ^{3}H-PGA. Using
this technique, the TFBC was measureable and substantially greater than
unsaturated folate binding capacity (UFBC) in all plasma and serum
samples, irrespective of whether they contained large amounts of unsaturated binder. The increase of TFBC over UFBC was evaluated by gel
filtration on Sephadex G-200 of TFBC and UFBC supernatants (see Fig 1).
Both peaks eluted at an identical rate, corresponding to an apparent
molecular weight of 42,000[19], with the entire increase in binding
eluted in the major bound peak. The minor peak is non-folate tritium.

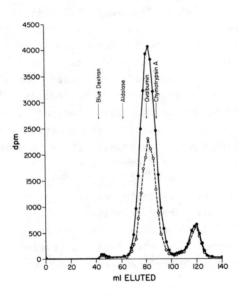

Fig. 1. Sephadex G-200 gel filtration of unsaturated (o----o) and
total (o——o) serum folate binder (from Colman and Herbert[19]).

The normal mean UFBC (61 ± 11 pg/ml) increased to TFBC = 171 ± 6 pg/ml,
and the L. casei assay confirmed that this technique removed more than
enough bound folate to explain the elevation in serum binding capacity.
Sequential repetition of the acid-charcoal technique in the same
aliquot of serum yielded similar results, indicating that there was
denaturation of the binder when using this technique.

KINETIC DATA

The apparent association constant of the serum binder for ^{3}H-PGA has been studied by addition of increasing amounts of the ligand, previously purified on DEAE cellulose, to constant amounts of the same normal serum prepared and buffered by the TFBC method. The Scatchard plot after removal of endogenous folate followed a linear function (r=.9921) indicating a single class of binding sites with apparent k_a=2.8 X 10^{10} 1/mol. Binding of nonradioactive folate analogues to these sites was studied by estimating ^{3}H-PGA binding inhibition[20] in hepatitis serum.

Pteroic acid was as potent an inhibitor as PGA whereas pterin, p-aminobenzoic acid, glutamate and p-aminobenzoylglutamate had no effect on binding; compounds with N-5 substituents showed apparent steric inhibition proportional to the size of the side-chain[21]. Alerted to this possibility by another[22], we observed that folate triglutamate and heptaglutamate displaced more ^{3}H-PGA than equimolar monoglutamate.

There was heterogeneity in affinity of the serum folate binder for different folate analogues. In contrast to binder of probable hepatic origin, used above, binder of probable granulocytic origin appearing in 15-20% of sera after incubation of whole blood for a few hours[18] had only half as much inhibition of ^{3}H-PGA binding by methyltetrahydrofolate compared with PGA. Other evidence for functional heterogeneity was obtained in studies of pH optima for binding, in which the former serum bound optimally at pH 6.3 whereas the latter did this at pH 5.4.

CHROMATOGRAPHIC HETEROGENEITY

Two prior reports indicated that serum folate binders eluted from ion exchange columns essentially as one low-molarity peak[24,25]. We confirmed the first report which used a dual buffer elution method designed for separation of transcobalamins[26], and obtained similar results with a batchwise method[27]. However, clearcut separation into two binder peaks was achieved by eluting in other buffers from DEAE Sephadex A-50 and assaying the fractions by a modification of the TFBC technique in which more dilute acid is used to allow for decreased buffering capacity of the samples. Elution of the binders from a linear gradient yielded a peak at 75-90mM and another at 115-125mM phosphate-buffered saline, with separation only being achieved when the gradient was sensitive enough to resolve eluents at these 2 molarities[28-30]. This sensitivity requirement may explain the failure of prior workers to detect the two different peaks in gradient elution[25].

The use of appropriate stepwise gradients resulted in elution of the binders in two sharply defined peaks, as shown in Fig. 2. Peak 1 had identical UFBC and TFBC, and thus contained only unsaturated binder. In peak 2, UFBC was only 60% of TFBC.

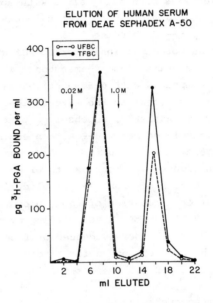

ELUTION OF HUMAN SERUM
FROM DEAE SEPHADEX A-50

Fig. 2. Elution of human serum folate binders from DEAE Sephadex A-50, with comparison of UFBC (o----o) and TFBC (o———o).

The state of saturation of the binder thus appeared to affect its elution from the column, consistent with the observation that the binding site was mainly at the pterin moiety whereas the glutamate carboxyl groups are chiefly responsible for the compound's retention on a DEAE column. Addition of PGA to peak 1 or removal of endogenous folate from peak 2 resulted in some shift to the opposite peak but some binder still eluted in the original position, indicating that saturation differences did not account for all the elution differences. This data suggests that there are inherent differences between these binders.

Further evidence supporting the presence of heterogenous serum folate binders appeared in hydrophobic interaction chromatography[28] and ammonium sulphate precipitation, which suggested at least two binders. When combined with data obtained using ion exchange, this data may explain paradoxical results of prior studies of the function of folate binders. This suggests that future studies of their function should distinguish and separate the effects of different folate binders.

SUMMARY

Serum folate binders were studied after removal of endogenous folate by charcoal exposure at acid pH. Although Scatchard plot analysis suggested a single class of folate binding sites, considerable evidence for heterogeneity emerged. Competitive inhibition of ^{3}H-PGA binding by methyltetrahydrofolate was twice as great using serum from a subject with liver disease than in "granulocyte-derived" binder present in normal serum, with optimal pH for binding differing greatly in the two sera. Serum folate binders eluted from DEAE Sephadex A-50 in two distinct peaks at 75-90mM and 115-125mM phosphate-buffered saline, with the low molarity peak containing unsaturated binder only. The evidence for heterogeneity gathered in these studies suggests that the different serum folate binders should be studied separately to determine possible distinct functions of each. The preference of folate binders for polyglutamate suggests a possible source of error in folate radioassays.

REFERENCES

1. Colman, N. and Herbert, V. (1977) in Topics in Hematology, S. Seno, F. Takaku and S. Irino, eds., Excerpta Medica, Amsterdam, p. 720.

2. Lavoie, A. and Cooper, B.A. (1974) Clin. Sci. Mol. Med. 46, 729.

3. Colman, N. and Herbert, V. (1976) Clin. Res. 24, 305A.

4. Johns, D.G., Sperti S. and Burgen, A.S.V. (1961) J. Clin. Invest. 40, 1684.

5. Condit, P.T. and Grob, D. (1958) Cancer 2, 525.

6. Metz, J., Zalusky, R. and Herbert, V. (1968) Amer. J. Clin. Nutr. 22, 289.

7. Rothenberg, S.P., da Costa, M. and Fischer, C. (1977) in Folic Acid Biochemistry and Physiology in Relation to the Human Nutrition Requirement, Food and Nutrition Board, National Research Council, Washington, D.C., p. 82.

8. Markannen, T. and Peltola, O. (1971) Acta Haemat. (Basel) 45, 106.

9. Alter, H.J., Zvaifler, N.J. and Rath, C.E. (1971) Blood 38, 405.

10. Colman, N. and Herbert, V. (1976) Abstracts, 16th Int. Congr. Hemat., Kyoto, Japan, 1976, p. 64.

11. Goresky, C.A., Watanabe, H. and Johns, D.G. (1963) J. Clin. Invest. 42, 1841.

12. Goldman, I.D. (1971) Ann. N.Y. Acad. Sci. 186, 400.

13. Ghitis, J. (1967) Amer. J. Clin. Nutr. 20, 1.

14. Rothenberg, S.P. and da Costa, M. (1971) J. Clin. Invest. 50, 719.

15. da Costa, M. and Rothenberg, S.P. (1974) J. Lab. Clin. Med. 83, 207.

530

16. Waxman, S. and Schreiber, C. (1973) Blood 42, 281.

17. Hines, J.D., Kamen, B. and Caston, D. (1973) Progr., 16th Ann. Mtg., Amer. Soc. Hematol., p. 57.

18. Colman, N. and Herbert, V. (1974) Progr., 17th Ann. Mtg., Amer. Soc. Hematol., p. 155.

19. Colman, N. and Herbert, V. (1976) Blood 48, 911.

20. Edsall, J.Y. and Wyman, J. (1958) Biophysical Chemistry, Academic Press, New York, p. 651.

21. Longo, D.L., Colman, N. and Herbert, V. (1975) Fed. Proc. 34, 904.

22. Gutcho, S. (1977) Personal Communication.

23. Colman, N. and Herbert, V. (1975) Clin. Res. 23, 270.

24. Waxman, S. and Schreiber, C. (1973) Blood 42, 291.

25. Retief, F.P., Gottlieb, C.W., Kochwa, S., Pratt, P.W. and Herbert, V. (1967) Blood 29, 501.

26. Silverstein, E. and Herbert, V. (1968) Blood 31, 518.

27. Zettner, A. and Duly, P.E. (1976) Clin. Chem. 22, 1047.

28. Colman, N., Pfeffer, R.D. and Herbert, V. (1977) Blood 50, (Suppl. 1), 91.

29. Colman, N. and Herbert, V. (1978) Fed. Proc. 37, 493.

30. Colman, N. and Herbert, V. (1978) Abstr., 17th Int. Congr. Hematol., 1, 49.

These investigations were supported by the Medical Research Service of the Veterans Administration and by NIH Grant AM-20526.

THE METABOLISM OF 10 FORMYLFOLATE IN THE NORMAL RAT AND THE RAT BEARING THE WALKER 256 CARCINOMA

MICHAEL J. CONNOR AND JOHN A. BLAIR

Dept of Chemistry, University of Aston in Birmingham, Birmingham, U.K.

INTRODUCTION

10 Formylfolate (10CHOFA) is an oxidation product of 10CHOTHF found in food.   An earlier study using $[2^{14}C]$ 10CHOFA suggested that it was only slowly metabolised by the rat and was thus unavailable to the folate pool[1].   We have reinvestigated 10CHOFA metabolism in the normal rat and in the rat bearing the Walker 256 carcinoma (W256) using a dual label.

MATERIALS AND METHODS

Dual labelled $[2^{14}C]$ $[3',5',9(n)-^{3}H]$ 10CHOFA synthesised from folic acid by modification of the method of Blakley[2], was dosed orally to normal Wistar rats (200g) at 10.5, 52.35 or 104.7µg per kg.   They were then housed in sealed metabolism cages and urine and air sampled over 48 hr.   The rats were then killed and the radioactivity of the faeces and tissues examined.   Metabolites in urine and tissues were characterised using paper, Sephadex G15 and DE52 ion exchange column chromatography.   Rats bearing implanted W256 received an oral dose of 52.35µg per kg and were treated in a similar manner.

RESULTS

Normal Rats.   The ratio of isotopes in the tissues (liver, kidney, gut, spleen, sternum, heart, brain, testis, lung) was the same as the dose at all dose levels;   the faeces contained more ^{14}C than ^{3}H and this was reversed in the urine; $^{14}CO_2$ (c.3%) and $^{3}H_2O$ (c.5%) were detected in the expired air.   Tissue retention decreased as the dose increased (e.g. liver 9.6% ^{14}C at 10.5µg to 6.3% ^{14}C at 104.7µg) and the retained folate was largely 10CHOTHF polyglutamates.

Analysis of urine revealed at least nine metabolites;   intact folates included 10CHOFA, 10CHOTHF, 5MeTHF and an unidentified folate (A), microbiologically active for L.casei and S.faecalis but not P.cerevisiae;   catabolites included p-acetamidobenzoic acid (p AcBA), $^{3}H_2O$, an unidentified minor ^{3}H metabolite (B) (possibly p-acetamido-

benzoyl-L-glutamate), an unidentified reduced pterin (C) and a
^{14}C derivative which may be urea.   The % of the dose excreted as
C and urea was constant; pAcBA, ^3H_2O and B excretion decreased
with dose.

W256 Rats.   These metabolised lOCHOFA in a similar manner to the
controls with the following differences (i) the presence of an extra
urinary metabolite (W) in the first 24 hr, possibly a reduced pterin
(but not pterin 6 CHO)[3] or an intact folate which has lost some
^3H during metabolism (ii) hot extracts of tumours and host livers
showed that these both contained mainly lOCHOTHF polyglutamates
whereas autolysis of cold extracts produced intact folates in liver
but chemical degradation products such as pterin and p-aminobenzoyl-
L-glutamate polyglutamates in the tumour (iii) increased hepatic
uptake (12.6%^{14}C in W256 rats, 7.6%^{14}C in controls) (iv) urinary
5MeTHF excretion was 63% controls.

DISCUSSION

Although lOCHOFA is reported to be a poor substrate for dihydrofolate reductase[4], it does enter the folate pool in the rat where its
metabolism is similar to that of folic acid.   Once metabolised into
the pool catabolism can evidently occur,possibly by gut microflora
or gut enzymes.   Evidence for the former is suggested by (i) absence
of tissue imbalance of isotopes but imbalance in the faeces
(ii) pAcBA in the urine suggesting carboxypeptidase Gl activity, this
being a microbial enzyme[5] (p-NH$_2$benzoic acid produced in the mammal
would be excreted as the glycine conjugate, p-NH$_2$ hippuric acid)
(iii) urinary ^3H metabolites increase relatively with time suggesting requisite prior metabolism.   Evidence for biliary excretion of
only intact folates is presented in the next paper.

The increased hepatic uptake by W256 rats, probably due to diminished
biliary excretion since faecal radioactivity was reduced by a reciprocal
amount, and the depressed 5MeTHF excretion are indicative of tumour
induced folate deficiency observed by others[6].   The disruptive effect
of the tumour on the folate pool was sufficient to produce a novel
urinary metabolite (w) and thus the pool is a potential source of
tumour markers.

REFERENCES
1.Beavon, J.R.G. & Blair, J.A. (1975) Brit.J.Nutr. 33, 299-308.
2.Blakley, R.L. (1959) Biochem.J. 72, 707-715.
3.Halpern, R et.al. (1977) Proc.Nat.Acad.Sci. 74, 587-591.
4.Bertino, J.R. et.al. (1965) Biochem., 4, 839-846.
5.Valerino, D.M. et.al. (1972) Biochem.Pharmacol. 21, 821-831.
6.Poirier, L.A. (1973) Cancer Res. 33, 2109-2113.

THE DISTRIBUTION OF ^{3}H AND ^{14}C MIXED LABEL FOLATES IN RAT LIVER CELLS

ROBERT J. COOK* and JOHN A. BLAIR

Department of Chemistry, University of Aston in Birmingham, B4 7ET,UK

*Present address: Biochemistry Department, Vanderbilt University
                   School of Medicine, Nashville, Tennessee 37232

ABSTRACT

Subcellular fractionation of rat liver cells revealed that a mixture of ^{14}C and ^{3}H labelled folic acid was distributed approximately equally between the mitochondria and the cytosol from 2-72h. Subfractionation of liver mitochondria 48h after dosing with ^{14}C and ^{3}H folic acid showed the majority of the radioactivity to be associated with the inner membrane and the matrix. The nature of these folates is discussed.

INTRODUCTION

This paper describes the distribution of a mixture of $(2-^{14}$C) and $(3', 5', 9-^{3}$H) folic acid in rat liver cells and mitochondrial subfractions. The use of a mixture of labelled folic acid should reveal any scission of the folate molecule by showing a segregation of label in the recovered fractions.

MATERIALS AND METHODS

Male Wistar rats (200-300g) were orally dosed with a mixture of $(2-^{14}$C) and $(3', 5', 9-^{3}$H) folic acid in the ratio of 1μCi ^{14}C: 2.5μC ^{3}H/100g body weight. Animals were killed after 2, 24, 48 or 72h and the livers fractionated[1] to give: nuclei, mitochondria 1, mitochondria 2 + lysosomes, microsomes and cytosol. Liver mitochondrial subfractionations[2] were performed on rats dosed with ^{14}C/^{3}H folic acid 48h before killing. Radioactivity in subcellular and submitochondrial fractions and in fractions obtained from column chromatography was determined as described by Barford et al[3]. Column chromatography was performed as described by Barford et al[3] with the exception of G-150 Sephadex procedures which were described by Andrews[4].

RESULTS AND DISCUSSION

Subcellular fractionation of liver showed that ^{3}H and ^{14}C activities were almost exclusively associated with mitochondrial and cytosol fractions, in approximately equal amounts. A significant level of

^{14}C/^{3}H activity was associated with the microsomal fraction after
2h; this activity decreased with time. These results agree with
Shin et al[5] and Zamierowski and Wagner[6]. The recoveries of ^{3}H and
^{14}C were very similar indicating that there was no apparent scission of
the folate molecule in all the subcellular fractions up to 72h after
oral dosing.

Subfractionation of liver mitochondria from rats orally dosed with a
mixture of ^{14}C/^{3}H folic acid 48h prior to killing showed very little activity
(2%) associated with the outer mitochondrial membrane. The soluble
intermembrane proteins contained 18% of the recovered ^{3}H/^{14}C. The
majority of the label was associated with the mitoplast fraction; 28%
with the inner membrane and 52% with the matrix. In all the fractions
the percentage recoveries of ^{14}C and ^{3}H were very close indicating
intact folate molecules.

G-15 Sephadex chromatography of mitochondrial matrix showed a single
mixed label peak close to the void volume in which the percentage
recoveries of ^{14}C and ^{3}H were exactly matched. Chromatography of the
matrix on G-75 Sephadex showed a mixed label peak close to the void
volume which accounted for 40-45% of the recovered ^{14}C and ^{3}H. The
remainder of the radioactivity was recovered in two singly labelled
peaks which eluted in a similar region to folate monoglutamates. A
similar result was obtained if a sample of the mixed label peak from a
G-15 column was run on G-75. Chromatography of the pooled, singly
labelled peaks from the G-75 column on a G-15 column showed the ^{3}H peak
eluted in a similar position to p-aminobenzoylglutamate while the ^{14}C
peak eluted in the same region as pterin. Extraction of matrix with
boiling phosphate buffer (0.05M; pH 7.0) + ascorbate (2%) followed by
G-15 chromatography showed the great majority of the radioactivity
eluted as a mixed label peak close to the void volume indicating folate
polyglutamates.

Zamierowski and Wagner[6] reported that in a sonicated extract of
mitochondria folate was bound to a protein with an estimated molecular
weight of 90,000. G-150 Sephadex chromatography of the mitochondrial
matrix showed approximately 25% of recovered ^{14}C and ^{3}H eluted in a
position consistent with a molecular weight of 90,000. The remainder
of the radioactivity eluted as two separate ^{3}H and ^{14}C peaks in the
same region as folate monoglutamates. Chromatography of the pooled
^{3}H and ^{14}C peaks on G-15 showed two separate peaks which eluted in
similar positions to p-aminobenzoylglutamate and pterin respectively.
Treatment of the high molecular weight peak from the G-15 column with

with TCA (8% w/v) followed by G-15 chromatography of the neutralized supernatant showed two major peaks; one ^{3}H labelled which eluted close to p-aminobenzoylglutamate and the other ^{14}C labelled which eluted in the same region as pterin.   Also present was a minor mixed label peak which eluted close to 10-formylfolate.

The above results indicate that the mitochondrial matrix folates were predominantly polyglutamates some of which are bound to protein. The polyglutamates present were very unstable as evidenced by the scission of the molecule on G-75 and G-150 chromatography.   The scission products of the folates after acid treatment were consistent with the breakdown of tetrahydrofolates possibly 10-formyltetrahydrofolate polyglutamate[7].

The folates associated with the inner membrane gave similar results to those of the matrix with the exception that about 60% were still attached to the membrane after boiling or TCA precipitation suggesting covalent bonding to the inner membrane.   The exact role of mitochondrial folates is not known.

REFERENCES
1. Fleischer, S. and Kervina, M. (1974) Methods Enzymol. 31, 6-41.
2. Greenawalt, J.W. (1974).   Methods Enzymol. 31. 310-323.
3. Barford, P.A.,et al.(1977).   Biochem.J. 164, 601-605.
4. Andrews, P. (1966) Biochem.J. 96, 595-606.
5. Shin, Y.S. et al. (1976) B.B.A. 444, 794-801.
6. Zamierowski, M. and Wagner, C. (1977) J.Biol.Chem. 252, 933-938.
7. Connor, M.J., et al. Biochem.Soc.Trans. (1977), 5, 1319.

ACKNOWLEDGEMENTS
The authors of the above four papers are grateful to the Cancer Research Campaign, the Science Research Council and the Royal Society for financial support.

EFFECT OF COMMON DRUGS ON SERUM LEVEL AND BINDING OF FOLATE IN MAN

E.R. EICHNER, J.E. LOEWENSTEIN, C.R. McDONALD, and V.L. DICKSON
Departments of Medicine, University of Oklahoma Health Sciences Center
and Louisiana State University School of Medicine in Shreveport

INTRODUCTION

Common drugs have been associated with subnormal serum folate levels and, in some instances, tissue folate deficiency. We have shown that ethanol decreases the serum folate level and accelerates the onset of megaloblastic anemia[1,2]. The acute postoperative folate deficiency and pancytopenia caused by an intravenous solution of amino acids in ethanol can be prevented by intravenous folic acid[3]. Many patients taking aspirin for rheumatoid arthritis have subnormal serum folate levels[4]. Phenytoin and oral contraceptives may depress serum folate level and increase urinary folate excretion[5-8].

While such common drugs may alter folate metabolism through diverse mechanisms, one common denominator might be a decrease in serum binding of methyltetrahydrofolate (MTHF) caused by the drug or by one of its metabolic concomitants. We report here our research on the possibility that aspirin, phenytoin, and ethanol lower serum folate level by displacement of MTHF from serum protein.

MATERIALS AND METHODS

Serum and urine folate levels were assayed by our modification of Herbert's *L. casei* method[9]. Serum folate binding was assayed primarily by equilibrium dialysis and checked by ultrafiltration. For equilibrium dialysis, presoaked dialysis tubing was formed into bags for 1 ml of serum which was then dialyzed to equilibrium at 4° C against either 1 ml, 2 ml, or 10 ml of 0.1 M pH 7.4 sodium phosphate buffer. Aliquots of retentate and filtrate were assayed for MTHF by *L. casei* and percent binding of MTHF by the serum was calculated. We found an inverse relationship between percent serum binding and amount of buffer outside the bag, with the normal value for percent binding reaching a maximum of 50-60%. This value approximated that of 60-70% for normal serum we found by ultrafiltration. For the *in vitro* experiments, acetylsalicylic acid or phenytoin was dissolved in 95% ethanol and incubated 2-4 hours at room temperature in normal, fasting serum which was then dialyzed as above with appropriate ethanol and buffer controls. The avid serum binding of phenytoin was verified by enzyme-immunoassay. Ethanol at 100-1000 mg/dl and increments of acetate 20 mg/dl, lactate 4mM, urate 2 mg/dl and oleic acid 6mM in various combinations were added to normal, fasting serum and incubated with agitation for 1-2 hours at 4° before equilibrium dialysis as above. A normal man underwent a 6-day and 9-day aspirin protocol with a constant, normal diet and with serum folate assayed daily at 7:00 a.m. (fasting) and 6:00 p.m. (before dinner). Aspirin, 650 mg every 4 hours (omitting the 3:00 a.m. dose), was taken on days 3-4 of the 6-day proto-col and on days 4-6 of the 9-day protocol. A normal woman underwent a similar 11-day protocol with aspirin, 650 mg every 4 hours around the clock on days 4-7. Single doses of 650-1300 mg aspirin were given to 6 other subjects. A normal man drank 1 ounce of 95% ethanol in "7-Up" every 2 hours for 6 doses while fasting, as in protocols described ear-lier[1,10], and later while eating a standard, normal diet. Blood was drawn every 2 hours for assay of serum folate and blood ethanol.

RESULTS

Single doses of aspirin to 6 normals resulted in serum salicylate levels of 5-10 mg/dl but no fall in serum folate level after 45-120 minutes. However, there was an early, significant ($p<0.05$), reversible, 16-20% fall in serum folate level during both the 6-day and 9-day aspirin protocols, during which serum salicylate levels rose to a peak of 20 mg/dl. The more definitive 11-day aspirin protocol is shown in Figure 1. Aspirin, as it rose from a first-day serum level of 15 mg/dl to a third-day peak of 24 mg/dl, caused an acute but reversible 20-25% fall in serum binding of MTHF ($p<0.01$ by Student's t test) and a 30-40% fall in serum folate level ($p<0.001$), without increasing urinary folate excretion. Aspirin *in vitro* (30 mg/dl) on 2 occasions displaced 8% and 24% of serum MTHF ($p=0.10$ and 0.14); 40 mg/dl caused substantial ($45 \pm 12.4\%$), sig-nificant ($p<0.001$) displacement of MTHF from serum protein.

Two patients who received intravenous phenytoin (200-500 mg) had no significant change in serum folate level or in MTHF binding within one hour. Phenytoin *in vitro* had no effect on serum folate binding, which was $54 \pm 4.8\%$ at 0 µg/ml phenytoin, $52 \pm 4.0\%$ at 20 µg/ml, $52 \pm 4.4\%$ at 40 µg/ml, $56 \pm 1.9\%$ at 60 µg/ml, and $53 \pm 5.7\%$ at 80 µg/ml.

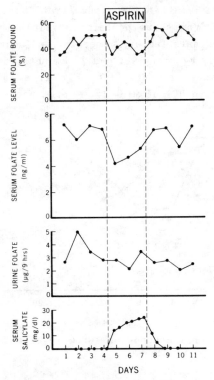

Fig. 1. Effect of aspirin on serum binding, serum concentration, and urinary excretion of folate in a normal woman.

The effect of ethanol in a fasting man is shown in Figure 2, where serum folate level and percent binding of MTHF both fall acutely by about 50% as the blood ethanol rose to a 10-hour peak of 80 mg/dl (the values for bound folate are lower here because the bag:buffer ratio was 1:10 rather than 1:1). Mixing experiments with normal serum suggested that the serum of this subject contained a folate-displacing agent in excess when his serum folate level was at its nadir. Although the serum folate level showed a brisk rebound to normal after ethanol was stopped, the percent of bound folate remained low. The important contribution of fasting was shown when the same man drank 95% ethanol as before, but ate a normal diet. As the blood ethanol rose to a 10-hour peak of 50 mg/dl, there was nonetheless a sharp rise in serum folate level after breakfast and dinner, and only a 15% general downward trend in serum folate level throughout the 16-hour study. Serum binding of MTHF was not assayed in

that study. Ethanol *in vitro* at concentrations up to 1,000 mg/dl did
not displace MTHF from serum protein; physiological concentrations of
the ethanol concomitants lactate, acetate, and urate in various combinations displaced only minor (<10%; p=0.1) amounts of MTHF. In contrast, a
similar physiological concentration of a free fatty acid (6 mM oleic
acid) displaced up to 90% of MTHF from serum protein.

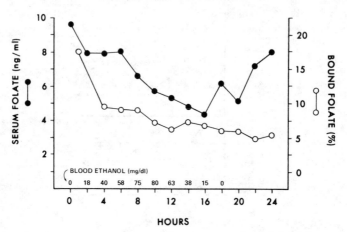

Fig. 2. Effect of oral ethanol on serum level and binding of folate.

DISCUSSION

   Our studies to date have shown that aspirin lowers serum folate level
by displacing MTHF from serum protein. Limited data suggest that phenytoin per se is not a displacing agent acutely, and that metabolic concomitants of ethanol oxidation may displace MTHF.

   Alter et al. showed that 71% of 51 patients with rheumatoid arthritis
had low serum folate levels but only one had a megaloblastic marrow;
in vitro work suggested that aspirin displaced radiolabeled pteroylglutamic acid from albumin. However, there is an undiscovered
correlation between serum albumin level and serum folate bound in their
data (p<0.05; Table 2), and they did not study binding of the principal
circulating folate, MTHF. Our data show that aspirin causes an acute,
reversible fall in serum MTHF level. Furthermore, the changes in binding of MTHF, which mirror the changes in serum folate level, largely
discount malabsorption of food folate as a contributor, and strongly
suggest that the principal or sole mechanism by which aspirin decreases
serum folate concentration is the displacement of MTHF from serum

protein. It is known that aspirin binds to, and acetylates, serum albumin[11]. The brisk rebound in total and bound folate concentration, along with the apparent lack of increased urinary excretion of folate, suggests that the displaced MTHF enters an extravascular compartment and returns to serum binding sites after aspirin is metabolized.

We do not yet know how aspirin affects cellular uptake of MTHF. The brisk rebound suggests that aspirin does not drive MTHF into cells. The aspirin-induced drop in serum MTHF level may impair cellular uptake. If a small portion of the displaced MTHF leaves the body via the urine or feces, daily aspirin could in time cause tissue folate deficiency. Finally, the displacing action of aspirin may explain the low serum ascorbic acid levels in rheumatoid arthritis[12] and may have implications for the transport of other water-soluble vitamins.

The chronic use of phenytoin can cause subnormal serum folate levels and occasionally megaloblastic anemia. Many causative mechanisms have been proposed, with recent studies excluding malabsorption of food folate[13] and indicating an increase in urinary excretion of folate[6]. Phenytoin, which binds avidly to albumin, could displace MTHF which could then be lost in part in the urine. Our data, however, indicate that bolus injections of phenytoin do not depress serum MTHF binding or serum folate level and that even high concentrations of phenytoin *in vitro* do not displace MTHF. Perhaps our *in vitro* conditions are not optimal; our aspirin experiments showed a greater displacing effect *in vivo* than *in vitro*, and an ever greater disparity has been seen with phenytoin's displacement of thyroxine from serum protein[14]. Then too, phenytoin does not acetylate albumin; perhaps displacement of MTHF is more specific than we have assumed. Finally, an *in vivo* metabolite of phenytoin may displace MTHF.

Ethanol may decrease serum folate level by diverse mechanisms such as malabsorption of dietary folate[15] and interference with enterohepatic cycling of folate[16]. Our work suggests a third mechanism, in certain fasting protocols at least, may be displacement of MTHF by a yet unidentified metabolite. We have shown that free fatty acids displace large amounts of MTHF *in vitro*. Free fatty acids rise[17], after an acute fall[18], in some protocols in which subjects drink ethanol while fasting. However, this is variable, and our earlier subjects who fasted without ethanol had no fall in serum folate level despite probable accumulation of free fatty acids because of caloric deprivation[10]. Perhaps the stress of our ethanol-fasting regimens outweighs the caloric contribution from ethanol to evoke a substantial net rise in serum free fatty acids with temporary displacement of MTHF from albumin. This possibility needs further research, as do other models in which serum free fatty acids are raised or lowered in the absence of ethanol.

Drug displacement of MTHF is a new mechanism for low serum folate levels which may have broad implications for the general population. Further research will determine if this phenomenon alters cellular uptake of folate or enhances loss of folate from the body.

ACKNOWLEDGEMENT: Supported by NIH Research Grant 5 R01 AM 21347-02

REFERENCES

1. Eichner, E.R. and Hillman, R.S. (1973) J Clin Invest, 52, 584.

2. Eichner, E.R., Pierce, H.I. and Hillman, R.S. (1971) New Engl J Med, 284, 933.

3. Wardrop, C.A.J., Lewis, M.H., Tennant, G.B., et al. (1977) Brit J Haemat, 37, 521.

4. Alter, H.J., Zvaifler, N.J. and Rath, C.E. (1971) Blood, 38, 405.

5. Richens, A. and Waters, A.H. (1971) Brit J Pharm, 41, 414p.

6. Krumdieck, C.L., Fukushima, K., Fukushima, T., et al. (1978) Am J Clin Nutr, 31, 88.

7. Shojania, A.M., Hornady, G.J. and Scaletta, D. (1975) J Lab Clin Med, 85, 185.

8. Paine, C.J., Grafton, W.D., Dickson, V.L. and Eichner, E.R. (1975) JAMA, 231, 731.

9. Eichner, E.R. and Dickson, V.L. (1974) Am J Clin Path, 62, 840.

10. Paine, C.J., Eichner, E.R. and Dickson V. (1973) Am J Med Sci, 266, 135.

11. Hawkins, D., Pinckard, R.N., Crawford, I.P. and Farr, R.S. (1969) J Clin Invest, 48, 536.

12. Sahud, M.A. and Cohen, R.J. (1971) Lancet, 1, 937.

13. Nelson, E.W., Cerda, J.J., Wilder, B.J. and Streiff, R.R. (1978) Am J Clin Nutr, 31, 82.

14. Larsen, P.R., Atkinson, A.J., Wellman, H.N. and Goldsmith, R.E. (1970) J Clin Invest, 49, 1266.

15. Halsted, C.H., Robles, E.A. and Mezey, E. (1973) Gastroenterology, 64, 525.

16. Hillman, R.S., McGuffin, R. and Campbell, C. (1977) Trans Assoc Am Phys, 90, 145.

17. Searle, G.L., Shames, D., Cavalieri, R.R., et al. (1974) Metabolism, 23, 1023.

18. Lieber, C.S., Leevy, C.M., Stein, S.W., et al. (1962) J Lab Clin M Med, 49, 8826.

TRANSPORT AND METABOLISM OF METHOTREXATE BY HEPATIC CELLS IN CULTURE

JOHN GALIVAN

Division of Laboratories and Research, New York State Department of Health,

Albany, New York 12201

ABSTRACT

Methotrexate (MTX) transport and metabolism have been measured in primary monolayer cultures of hepatocytes. After 24 h in culture the cells on Falcon dishes took several hours to reach steady state, and the intracellular concentration of MTX was several fold higher than the medium concentration. At 48 and 72 h in culture uptake was rapid, reaching steady state in 30 to 60 min, and over a 4 h period the intracellular concentration did not significantly exceed the media concentration. Cells in culture for 72 h converted 27% of the intracellular MTX to polyglutamates in 4 h, and this increased to 75% after 24 h (medium MTX = 10 μM).

Monolayer cultures of H35 hepatoma cells, in contrast, showed a prolonged (4 to 6 h) linear uptake which reached steady state at 12 to 16 h. When MTX was present in the media at 10 μM, the intracellular steady state concentration of all MTX species was between 60 and 80 μM. The percent of MTX occurring as polyglutamate derivatives at 1, 4, and 24 h was 84, 91, and 95% respectively. Evidence is presented to indicate that MTX polyglutamates are primarily responsible for inhibiting dihydrofolate reductase and thus contribute directly to the toxicity of MTX.

INTRODUCTION

The transport of MTX has been widely studied in a number of cell lines, but little is known about this process in hepatic tissue. Perfused liver preparations[1,2] and freshly isolated hepatocytes[3,4] have recently been used to investigate this problem. In this laboratory a monolayer culture system for hepatocytes[5] and an established hepatoma cell line (H35 cells[6]) have been used to further characterize the transport and metabolism of MTX in hepatic tissue.

544

MATERIALS AND METHODS

Cell isolation and culture procedures are described in Refs. 5 and 6. Collagen coated plates and the techniques for measuring uptake of radioactive compounds by cells in monolayer culture have been described[7]. The intracellular volume, which was measured with 3-O-methyl-D-glucose[8], was 2.15 µl/mg cell protein for hepatocytes and 3.1 µl/mg cell protein for H35 cells. Tyrosine aminotransferase (TAT) assays were conducted according to Diamondstone[9].

RESULTS

The capacity of hepatocytes to transport MTX was measured on collagen coated and uncoated plastic plates as a function of time in culture (Fig. 1, Table 1). On collagen, the steady state levels of intracellular MTX were close to or below the medium levels throughout three days of culture. On plastic, the cells are able to concentrate MTX from the media during the first 24 h in culture, but after that retain levels which are near or below media concentration. Horne et al.[3] and Gewirtz et al.[4] found that freshly isolated hepatocytes also have the ability to concentrate MTX several fold.

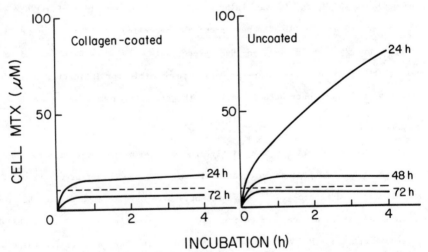

Fig. 1. Hepatocyte uptake of MTX as a function of time in culture. The cells were grown in Swims S-77 medium supplemented with insulin (10 mU/ml) and 4 mM glutamine. The time (h) adjacent to the curves indicates the length of time in culture before adding [³H]MTX. The dashed line indicates the medium concentration of MTX (10 µM).

TABLE 1

HEPATOCYTE MEMBRANE PROPERTIES AS A FUNCTION OF TIME IN CULTURE [a]

Hours in culture	[AIB] Int/Ext	TAT induction	[MTX] Int/Ext Plastic	[MTX] Int/Ext Collagen
24	4	3.5	5.6	1.1
48	12	5.4	1.0	
72	12	8.6	0.6	.62

[a] AIB and MTX are expressed as the ratio of intracellular to extracellular (medium) levels at steady state. Both were present in the medium at 10 μM. TAT induction is the increase in the level caused by exposure of the cells to 10 μM Dexamethasome for 16 h.

The loss of concentrative capacity does not appear to indicate general membrane dysfunction since the inducibility of TAT and the capacity to concentrate α-aminoisobutyric acid (AIB) from the media increased between 24 and 72 h in culture (Table 1). Two possible explanations for the change in MTX concentrative function are: (1) a loss in specific function, or (2) a change in transport due to the trauma of collagenase treatment and isolation, which is corrected with time. The latter explanation may apply to both AIB[7] and MTX[2] uptake, since the steady state concentrations observed with 72 h cultures are more representative of in vivo than those observed at 24 h.

The transport of MTX in H35 hepatoma cells was measured at medium MTX concentrations from 0.03 to 25 μM (Fig. 2). MTX uptake is linear for 4 to 6 h and reaches steady state between 12 and 16 h. Both the rate of uptake and the final intracellular concentration were saturable with a V_{max} of 1.1 nmol/g cell protein/min, and the Km for MTX uptake is 5.2 μM. The maximal intracellular concentration at steady state is 115 μM as measured by radioactivity or titration with dihydrofolate reductase.

The effect of analogs on MTX uptake was measured with both cell lines. In hepatocytes, a five fold excess of 5-methyltetrahydrofolate or folic acid did not inhibit MTX (10 μM in medium) uptake in hepatocytes over a 30 min period after 24 or 72 h in culture. In H35 cells, a five fold excess of 5-methyltetrahydrofolate completely blocked MTX uptake (2 μM in medium), but folic acid had no effect.

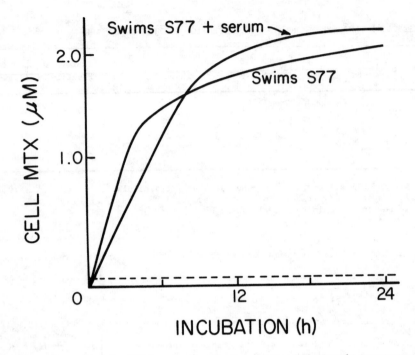

Fig. 2. Uptake of MTX by H35 hepatoma cells in culture. The uptake was measured on day five in culture in the presence or absence of serum, and the dashed line indicates the concentration of MTX in the medium (0.06 µM).

The metabolism of MTX was examined, and no breakdown products of MTX were observed in the media or within the cells. To examine the cell extracts for the presence of polyglutamate derivatives of MTX, Sephadex G-15 gel filtration[10] was used. Both hepatocytes and H35 cells catalyzed the conversion of MTX to its polyglutamate derivatives (Table 2). The H35 cells were particularly active with over 80% of intracellular MTX converted to polyglutamates throughout the incubation at a medium concentration of 10 µM. Conversion by the hepatocytes was much lower within the first 4 h, but by 24 h 75% of the MTX was converted to polyglutamates. The data in Fig. 1 indicated that steady state was reached by 30 min after 48 h in culture, but the intracellular MTX concentration (Table 2) indicated a slow incorporation must occur over a 24 h incubation, since the internal concentration of all MTX species reaches 40 µM.

TABLE 2

MTX CONVERSION TO POLYGLUTAMATES IN CULTURED HEPATOCYTES AND H35 HEPATOMA CELLS [a]

Time of Incubation (h)	$[MTX]_{Int}$ (µM)	$[Total\ MTX]_{Int}$ (µM)	Polyglutamates (%)
Hepatocytes (72 h culture) [b]			
2	6.5	7.5	13
4	7.3	10	27
24	10	40.7	75
H35 cells (120 h culture) [b]			
1	2.0	12.5	84
4	2.5	29	91
24	2.5	74	97

[a] [^{3}H]MTX (10 µM) was added, and at the indicated times boiled cell suspensions were chromatographed on Sephadex G-15[10,11] to determine the distribution of MTX and MTX polyglutamates. Total MTX is the sum of MTX and MTX polyglutamates.
[b] 0 time was at 72 h for hepatocytes and 120 h in culture (early stationary) for H35 cells.

In both cell types the polyglutamates corresponded to MTX(G_2) and MTX(G_3) standards, and treatment of these peaks with pancreatic conjugase resulted in the formation of MTX as indicated by Sephadex G-15 gel filtration and thin layer chromatography. A similar conversion has been observed in freshly isolated hepatocytes in suspension[4]. In other cells and tissues where MTX polyglutamate formation has been observed, MTX-(G_1) is more common, although MTX(G_2) has been observed in L1210 cells[10,11]. Both cell types examined here appear to have a relatively high capacity for polyglutamate formation. The unusually high conversion in the H35 cells appears responsible for the high intracellular levels and long period of linear uptake.

A role of MTX polyglutamates in the toxicity of MTX to the H35 cells is also suggested by these experiments. The minimal toxic dose of MTX, 0.03 µM, added at mid-log causes cell growth to decline over a period of 24 h after which the cells detach from the plate. At the end of the 24 h period, approximately 90% of the intracellular MTX is in the polyglutamate form and the molar ratio of all MTX species to dihydrofolate reductase is between 1.25 and 1.5 to 1. This finding strongly suggests that the polyglutamates are inhibiting dihydrofolate reductase and therefore are responsible for cell kill. A precedent for this possibility has been set by Jacobs et al.[12] and Whitehead[11], who found that MTX polyglutamates caused equal or greater inhibition of dihydrofolate reductase than did MTX. Similar studies in this laboratory have demonstrated that MTX(G_2) and MTX(G_3) are as effective as MTX in the inhibition of dihydrofolate reductase from <u>Lactobacillus</u> <u>casei</u> and extracts of H35 cells.

ACKNOWLEDGEMENTS

This work was supported in part by Grant NIA AG00207 from the National Institute on Aging. I gratefully acknowledge Joyce Becker and Dr. Van Potter of the McArdle Laboratories, University of Wisconsin, Madison, Wisconsin, for supplying H35 cells and Dr. Charles M. Baugh, Department of Biochemistry, University of South Alabama, Mobile, Alabama, for supplying MTX(G_3) and MTX(G_2) standards.

REFERENCES

1. Strum, W. B. and Liem, H. H. (1977) Biochem. Pharmacol., 26, 1235-1240.

2. Strum, W. B., Liem, H. H. and Müller-Eberhard, U. (1978) Clin. Res., 26, 113a.

3. Horne, D. W., Briggs, W. T. and Wagner, C. (1976) Biochem. Biophys. Res. Commun., 68, 70-76.

4. Gewirtz, D. A., White, J. C. and Goldman, I. D. (1978) Fed. Proc., 37, 1346.

5. Bonney, R. J. (1974) In Vitro, 10, 130-142.

6. Pitot, H., Periano, C., Morse, P. and Potter, V. R. (1964) Natl. Cancer Mono., 13, 229-245.

7. Kletzian, R. F., Pariza, M. W., Becker, J. E., Potter, V. R. and Butcher, F. R. (1976) J. Biol. Chem., 251, 3014-3020.

8. Kletzian, R. F., Pariza, M. W., Becker, J. E. and Potter, V. R. (1975) Anal. Biochem., 68, 537-544.

9. Diamondstone, T. I. (1966) Anal. Biochem., 16, 395-401.

10. Whitehead, V. M., Perrault, M. M. and Stelcner, S. (1975) Cancer Res., 35, 2985-2990.

11. Whitehead, V. M. (1977) Cancer Res., 37, 408-412.

12. Jacobs, S. A., Adamson, R. H., Chabner, B. A., Derr, C. J. and Johns, D. G. (1975) Biochem. Biophys. Res. Commun., 63, 692-698.

ENERGETICS OF METHOTREXATE TRANSPORT IN L1210 MOUSE LEUKEMIA CELLS

GARY B. HENDERSON AND EDWARD M. ZEVELY
Department of Biochemistry, Scripps Clinic & Research Foundation, La Jolla, CA 92037

ABSTRACT

Methotrexate (MTX) transport into L1210 mouse leukemia cells is inhibited by various components found in physiological buffers. Elimination of these inhibitors
from the medium leads to a considerable increase in the ability of these cells to
concentrate MTX. Two types of inhibitors have been identified: Compounds in one
group (bicarbonate and Ca^{++}) affect only the steady-state level for transported drug,
while those in the other group (phosphate and sulfate) decrease both the initial
rate and the steady-state phases of the transport process. Phosphate (K_i = 6.8 mM)
and sulfate (K_i = 10 mM) both act as *competitive* inhibitors of the MTX transport
rate. The MTX carrier protein thus appears to contain a substrate-binding site of
sufficient flexibility to accommodate both MTX and inorganic, divalent anions.
These results suggest that the energy source to drive MTX transport may be a phosphate ion gradient, although sulfate could presumably also function in the same capacity. A mechanism is proposed in which the MTX carrier protein can transport both
MTX and phosphate across the membrane in either direction. Thus, when the internal
phosphate concentration is high relative to that in the external medium, MTX can
enter the cell in exchange for phosphate. The latter is extruded into the medium
down a concentration gradient as the binding site on the carrier reorients to the
external membrane surface. The degree of phosphate asymmetry determines the ability
of the cells to achieve an MTX concentration gradient, the latter being about 10-fold
under optimum conditions. The fact that L1210 cells sustain MTX transport capabilities in the presence of azide can also be explained by the proposed mechanism.

INTRODUCTION

The transport of folate compounds by *Lactobacillus casei* has been extensively
studied in our laboratory[1-3] and elsewhere[4-6]. The uptake process is highly concentrative and energy-dependent, is regulated by the level of folate in the growth
medium, and occurs independently of folate metabolism. The binding component, which
mediates folate transport[3,7], has been solubilized from the cell membrane[7,8], and
purified to homogeneity[3,8]. The cellular location and physio-chemical properties
of this unusually hydrophobic protein suggest that it acts not only as the receptor but also as the carrier of folate across the cell membrane.

Considerably less is known about the mechanism and the components of the 5-methyl-
tetrahydrofolate-MTX transport system of L1210 cells. This transport process is
carrier-mediated and appears to be active[9-10], although sources of energy (such as

glucose) inhibit MTX transport. While previous investigators have suggested that this inhibition might result from energy-stimulated MTX efflux[12], our recent studies[13,14] suggest that glucose is inhibiting MTX transport by elevating the intracellular level of cyclic AMP (cAMP). A possible regulatory function for cAMP has been deduced from the observation that a variety of compounds which elevate cAMP levels produce a proportional inhibition of MTX transport[14].

The designation of MTX transport in L1210 cells as active and concentrative has been difficult to establish. Even though MTX enters these cells at a relatively rapid rate, free drug does not accumulate to high levels. Under the standard assay conditions, concentration gradients are generally in the range of only 1- to 2-fold, although higher values can be obtained by either the addition of metabolic inhibitors[11] or by measuring transport at low levels of substrate[9,10,15]. The modest capacity of L1210 cells to concentrate MTX could also be due, in part, to the fact that uptake is routinely measured in physiological salt solutions, which contain anions inhibitory to the transport process[12]. The effects of buffer constituents have also complicated earlier analyses of MTX transport kinetics and energetics and are of particular importance in light of the previous suggestions[12,16] that gradients of organic phosphate compounds across the membrane might provide the driving force for active transport of MTX. As part of our characterization of the MTX transport mechanism in L1210 cells, we have examined further the effects of anions on the uptake process. A critical step in these studies was the realization of a buffer whose inherent components had only minimal inhibitory effects on MTX transport.

RESULTS AND DISCUSSION

Figure 1 shows the time-dependence for MTX transport by L1210 cells in three buffer systems, 20 mM Hepes-140 mM KCl, a phosphate-buffered saline (PBS) employed previously in our laboratory[14], and the bicarbonate-buffered saline system (BC) used by Goldman and his associates[11]. The initial rates of MTX transport, although not affected to a large extent by the buffer composition, were about 2-fold higher in Hepes-KCl than in either the PBS or BC buffers. This difference increased further with time, resulting in a more pronounced effect on the steady-state levels for free intracellular drug. While a concentration ratio of two was achieved in both the PBS and BC buffers, the cells in the Hepes-KCl buffer concentrated MTX by nearly 10-fold. The exit rates for MTX were also affected by the buffer employed. Cells that were preloaded (20 min at 37°) with MTX (2 μM) in Hepes-KCl, washed and resuspended in either the PBS or Hepes-KCl buffers released the label at a faster rate in PBS ($t\frac{1}{2}$ = 6 min) than in Hepes-KCl ($t\frac{1}{2}$ = 9 min).

Inhibitory effects of several constituents of the PBS and BC buffers are shown in Figure 2. The latter depicts a time-course for MTX uptake in the presence of $CaCl_2$, $MgCl_2$, $KHCO_3$, K_2HPO_4, and K_2SO_4. Two classes of inhibitors are apparent from these data: Bicarbonate and Ca^{++} (and perhaps Mg^{++}) constitute one group in that they

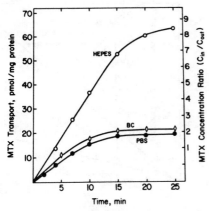

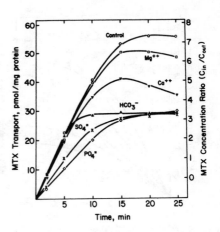

Fig. 1. Time-dependence for MTX transport in 20 mM Hepes-140 mM KCl (HEPES), a phosphate-buffered saline (PBS), and a bicarbonate-buffered saline (BC). Transport of 2 μM [3H]MTX was measured at 37° and pH 7.4 according to a previously described procedure[14]; protein concentrations were determined on cell suspensions by the Biuret method. MTX concentration ratios were calculated using a volume of 5 μl/10[7] cells[15] and a dihydrofolate reductase content of 7 pmoles/mg protein.

Fig. 2. Effect of salts on the time-dependent uptake of MTX in 20 mM Hepes-140 mM KCl. Indicated additions were as follows: Control, none; $MgCl_2$, 1 mM; $CaCl_2$, 1 mM; $KHCO_3$ (pH 7.4), 10 mM; K_2HPO_4 (pH 7.4), 10 mM; and K_2SO_4 (pH 7.4), 10 mM. [3H]MTX concentration, 2 μM. Other conditions as described in the legend to Fig. 1.

decreased only the steady-state for accumulated MTX; initial rates of uptake were unaffected by these compounds. The second type of inhibitor (exemplified by phosphate and sulfate) decreased both the initial rate and steady-state phases of MTX transport. Anions were generally better inhibitors than cations, although not all anions acted comparably as shown by the differing effects of bicarbonate and phosphate. Na^+ did not affect transport; uptake profiles for MTX were the same when measured in Hepes buffer containing either 140 mM NaCl or 140 mM KCl (data not shown). Transport rates in this buffer were also not affected by inclusion of 5 mM azide in the incubation mixture, although plateau values were slightly increased (ca. 10%) by this agent.

Since phosphate appeared to be the most pronounced inhibitor of MTX transport, the kinetics of phosphate inhibition were examined in more detail. Figure 3 shows the time-dependence for MTX transport at various levels of phosphate. Increasing concentrations of this anion produced proportional decreases in both the initial rate and steady-state level for MTX uptake. When the reciprocals of both the rates and steady-state levels of MTX transport were plotted against phosphate concentration (Dixon plot), linear relationships were observed (Fig. 4). From the

552

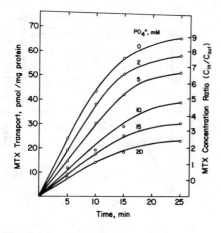

Fig. 3. Concentration-dependence for the inhibition of MTX transport by K_2HPO_4 (pH 7.4). Buffer, 20 mM Hepes-140 mM KCl. [^{3}H]MTX concentration, 2 μM.

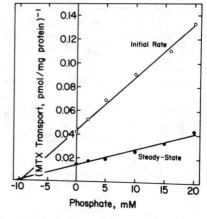

Fig. 4. Dixon plot of the data shown in Fig. 3 for the initial rates and steady-state levels for MTX transport achieved at various levels of K_2HPO_4.

x-intercepts, values of 9.5 mM and 10 mM were calculated for 50% inhibition of the initial rate and steady-state processes, respectively. Since essentially the same concentration of phosphate was required to reduce both transport parameters by 50%, it is tempting to speculate that phosphate may be inhibiting these processes via the same mechanism. The linearity of the replotted data also suggests that the inhibition of MTX transport would be increased further at higher levels of phosphate, and that 95% inhibition of both processes would occur at an inhibitor concentration of about 100 mM.

The double-reciprocal plots of MTX transport as a function of the MTX concentration in the absence and presence of 10 mM K_2HPO_4 are shown in Figure 5. The data are linear and yield a common y-intercept, indicating that phosphate is a competitive inhibitor of MTX transport. From this knowledge of the type of inhibition (competitive) and the experimentally determined K_t for MTX (5 μM), a K_i value of 6.8 mM could be calculated for phosphate from the data in Figure 3. In a separate experiment, MTX transport was measured in the presence of 10 mM K_2SO_4, and this compound was found to act (like phosphate) as a competitive inhibitor (K_i = 10 mM) of MTX transport.

Goldman[12,16] has suggested that co-transport of MTX and organic phosphates may account for the uphill transport of MTX into L1210 cells. It was postulated that compounds such as ATP, ADP, AMP, and glucose 6-phosphate are both bound and transported by the MTX carrier protein. The high intracellular concentration of the organic phosphate compounds could then serve as the energy source for the concentration of MTX within the cell. This hypothesis is attractive in that it provides a feasible explanation for the strong inhibition of MTX transport by adenine nucleotides and

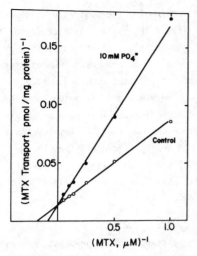

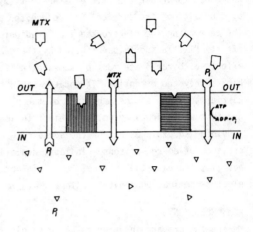

Fig. 5. Double-reciprocal plot of MTX
transport rate vs. MTX concentration
in the absence (o — o) and presence
(● — ●) of 10 mM K_2HPO_4 (pH 7.4).
Buffer, 20 mM Hepes-140 mM KCl;
time of incubation, 5 min.

Fig. 6. Model for phosphate-exchange mechanism
for energization of MTX transport in L1210
cells. Vertical bars, the MTX-phosphate exchange carrier; horizontal bars, a second
independent carrier specific for phosphate
and energized by ATP hydrolysis.

for the fact that the MTX transport system can sustain uphill transport in the presence of metabolic inhibitors. A disadvantage of the proposed mechanism is that the
cells would utilize high-energy compounds for a purpose typically fulfilled in other
systems by inorganic ions. Also implicit in this hypothesis is that a second transport system would be required to recover the organo-phosphates from the medium.
Carriers of the latter type, however, are not generally found in the plasma membrane.

An alternative hypothesis (Fig. 6) for energization of MTX transport by a gradient
of inorganic phosphate ions is suggested from the present data. The MTX carrier
protein (vertical bars, Fig. 6) is proposed to reside in the membrane and have a
common binding site for both inorganic phosphate (K_D = 6.8 mM) and MTX (K_D = 5 μM).
This commonality of binding sites is suggested by the competitive kinetics obtained
with these compounds (see Fig. 5). It is postulated that phosphate or MTX can be
facilitated across the membrane in either direction while bound to the carrier. Thus,
under the asymmetrical conditions depicted in Figure 6, in which phosphate is contained within the cells and MTX is present in the external medium, the antifol is
transported to the internal compartment and, during reorientation of the carrier,
phosphate exits. Recovery of the extruded phosphate would then occur via a second,
high-affinity transport system (horizontal bars, Fig. 6) dependent upon ATP. MTX
would be concentrated at the expense of, and to a level determined by, the phosphate
gradient. This MTX-phosphate exchange model is consistent with the effects illustrated in Figure 3; upon addition of phosphate to the external medium, the anion

would both decrease the rate of transport (by competing for the substrate at the binding site of the carrier) and reduce the ability of the system to concentrate MTX (by decreasing the electro-chemical gradient of phosphate). Sulfate apparently affects MTX transport (see Fig. 2) by the same mechanism as phosphate, whereas the effects of bicarbonate must be somewhat different. The latter compound, which inhibits only the extent of MTX uptake, could be acting via a general anion exchange carrier to diminish the magnitude of the phosphate gradient. Finally, a phosphate gradient would probably not be subject to immediate influence by ATP levels, thus providing an explanation for the sustaining of MTX transport capabilities in the presence of energy poisons. In fact, depletion of energy pools might, in itself, actually increase the internal level of inorganic phosphate ions thus elevating the electro-chemical phosphate gradient.

ACKNOWLEDGMENTS

The authors are indebted to Karin Vitols for assistance in the preparation of this manuscript, and to Drs. F.M. Huennekens and M.R. Suresh for discussions of the subject matter. This work was supported by Grants CA 6522 and CA 23970 from the National Cancer Institute, by Grant CH-31 from the American Cancer Society and by Grant PCM77-23414 from the National Science Foundation. G.B.H. is a recipient of a Senior Fellowship, California Division, American Cancer Society.

REFERENCES

1. Henderson G.B. and Huennekens, F.M. (1974) Arch. Biochem. Biophys., 164, 722-728.
2. Huennekens, F.M. and G.B. Henderson (1976) in Chemistry and Biology of Pteridines, Pfleiderer, W. ed., Walter de Gruyter, Berlin, pp. 179-196.
3. Henderson, G.B., Zevely, E.M. and Huennekens, F.M. (1977) J. Supramol. Struct., 6, 239-247.
4. Cooper, B.A. (1970) Biochim. Biophys. Acta, 208, 99-109.
5. Shane, B. and Stokstad, E.L.R. (1975) J. Biol. Chem., 250, 2243-2253.
6. Shane, B. and Stokstad, E.L.R. (1976) J. Biol. Chem. 251, 3405-3410.
7. Henderson, G.B., Zevely, E.M. and Huennekens, F.M. (1976) Biochem. Biophys. Res. Commun., 68, 712-717.
8. Henderson, G.B., Zevely, E.M., Huennekens, F.M. (1977) J. Biol.Chem.,252,3760-3765.
9. Kessel, D. and Hall, T.C. (1967) Cancer Res., 27, 1539-1543.
10. Goldman, I.D., Lichtenstein, N.S. and Oliverio, V.T. (1968) J. Biol. Chem., 243, 5007-5017.
11. Goldman, I.D. (1969) J. Biol. Chem., 244, 3779-3785.
12. Goldman, I.D. (1971) Ann. N.Y. Acad. Sci., 186, 400-422.
13. Henderson, G.B., Schrecker, A., Smith C., Gordon, M., Zevely, E.Z., Vitols, K.S. and Huennekens, F.M. (1977) Adv. Enzyme Regulation, 15, 141-151.
14. Henderson, G.B., Zevely, E.M. and Huennekens, F.M. (1978) Cancer Res., 38,859-861.
15. Dembo, M. and Sirotnak, F.M. (1976) Biochim. Biophys. Acta, 448, 505-516.
16. Goldman, I.D. (1977) Adv. Exp. Med. and Biol., 84, 85-111.

STUDIES ON THE TRANSPORT OF 5-METHYLTETRAHYDROFOLATE AND RELATED COMPOUNDS INTO
ISOLATED HEPATOCYTES

DONALD W. HORNE AND CONRAD WAGNER

VA Hospital Research Laboratory and Department of Biochemistry, Vanderbilt University
Nashville, Tennessee 37203 (U.S.A.)

ABSTRACT

Uptake of 5-Methyltetrahydrofolate (5-CH$_3$-H$_4$PteGlu) by isolated hepatocytes is a
complex process involving both a saturable (K_m=0.9 µM) system and a system which is
non-saturable up to 20 µM. Both systems were influenced by the presence of sodium.
The saturable component is an active process since 5-CH$_3$-H$_4$PteGlu was concentrated
against an electrochemical gradient and was inhibited by compounds affecting generation of energy. Efflux and influx of 5-CH$_3$-H$_4$PteGlu are controlled by different
processes since they responded differently to inhibitors such as azide.

Hepatocytes from vitamin B$_{12}$ and methionine deficient animals took up less
5-CH$_3$-H$_4$PteGlu than those from control animals. The Km and Vmax for influx of
5-CH$_3$-H$_4$PteGlu was no different in experimental and control animals suggesting that
efflux is more rapid in vitamin B$_{12}$ and methionine deficiency. Ethanol stimulated
uptake of 5-CH$_3$-H$_4$PteGlu when added in vitro. This was shown to be a result of a
decreased (more negative) redox potential brought about by the utilization of the
added ethanol.

INTRODUCTION

The transport of folic acid (PteGlu) and its naturally occurring derivative has
been studied in a wide variety of tissues including bacteria[1,2], tumor cells[3], the
choroid plexus[4], cells from the intestinal tract[5] and the hematologic system[6,7].
Because of the central role played by the liver in metabolism, we have developed a
system to study the transport of the major circulating form of folate, 5-CH$_3$-H$_4$PteGlu,
by isolated hepatocytes. Since studies of transport involve measurement of initial
rates of entry, they require very high specific radioactive 5-CH$_3$-H$_4$PteGlu. This was
accomplished by a novel enzymatic method[8] which was central to the establishment of
the use of isolated hepatocytes for measurement of 5-CH$_3$-H$_4$PteGlu transport[9]. This
system has enabled us to test various physiologic parameters which have been known
to affect the level of folic acid in vivo upon the transport process itself. Two
such parameters which have been investigated and are reported here are the effects
of vitamin B$_{12}$ deficiency and the effects of ethanol.

MATERIALS AND METHODS

Hepatocyte Isolation and Incubation Techniques. The procedures used for

556

isolation of hepatocytes and measurement of transport in these cells have been described previously[9]. Unless indicated otherwise, 170-300g male Sprague-Dawley rats were fed Wayne Lab-Blox <u>ad libitum</u> and used as a source of the hepatocytes. Radioactive (ℓ)-5-CH$_3$-H$_4$[G-^{3}H]PteGlu was prepared as described[8]. Radiochemical purity was greater than 96%. Other radioisotopes were obtained commercially and purified before use.

RESULTS

<u>Uptake kinetics</u>. The rate of uptake of 5-CH$_3$-H$_4$PteGlu by hepatocytes was linear for at least 10 min and then decreased to a steady state level. Fig. 1,a shows that sodium arsenate and 5-CHO-H$_4$PteGlu inhibited uptake, but that sodium azide stimulated it. Although the rates of uptake were decreased in medium where choline replaced sodium, the relative effects of these additions were the same (Fig. 1,b). When initial rates of uptake of 5-CH$_3$-H$_4$PteGlu was measured as a function of extracellular concentration, the data revealed that two components were involved. Fig. 2

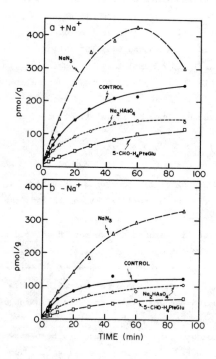

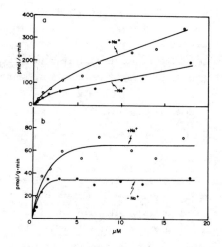

Fig. 2. Concentration dependence of 5-CH$_3$-H$_4$PteGlu uptake. Panel a is total uptake. Panel b is uptake after subtraction of non-saturable component in Na$^+$ (o) and choline ($\bullet$) containing medium.

Fig. 1. Time course of uptake of 0.25 μM 5-CH$_3$-H$_4$PteGlu by isolated hepatocytes. ($\bullet$—$\bullet$), control; ($\triangle$---$\triangle$), 10 mM sodium azide; (o----o), 10 mM sodium arsenate; ($\square$--$\square$), 0.1 mM folinic acid. Panel a is uptake in presence of Na$^+$; in panel b choline has replaced Na$^+$.

shows that there was a primary, saturable component which was evident at low concentrations and a secondary component which was linear up to concentrations of about 20 μM.

Analysis of the intracellular contents after incubation for 90 min revealed that about 88% of the $5\text{-CH}_3\text{-H}_4\text{PteGlu}$ taken up by the cells was non-metabolized and only about 20% was bound to macromolecules. When the distribution ratio of the tissue to medium concentration of $5\text{-CH}3\text{-H}_4\text{PteGlu}$ was measured after 60 min it showed that concentration had taken place against an electrochemical gradient in both the presence and absence of sodium, suggesting that transport was an active process.

Inhibitors. The effect of a number of inhibitors on uptake of 0.25 μM $5\text{-CH}_3\text{-H}_4$-PteGlu was measured. Table 1 shows that 2,4-dinitrophenol, cyanide and arsenate are inhibitory as would be expected if uptake is energy dependent. Sodium azide is paradoxical in that it stimulates uptake (see also Fig. 1). This action of azide was also noted by Goldman[3] in studies on methotrexate uptake by Ll210 cells. It was shown that net uptake of methotrexate was stimulated because efflux was inhibited by azide. Fig. 3 shows that addition of azide to hepatocytes preloaded with $5\text{-CH}_3\text{-H}_4$-PteGlu also resulted in inhibition of efflux.

Effect of vitamin B_{12} deficiency. One current theory to explain the observation that vitamin B_{12} deficiency often leads to a functional folate deficiency[10] is that vitamin B_{12} is required for membrane transport of folate into tissues[11]. We have tested this directly by measuring uptake of $5\text{-CH}_3\text{-H}_4\text{PteGlu}$ by hepatocytes from control rats and from rats deficient in vitamin B_{12} and limiting in methionine[12]. Fig. 4 shows that uptake by hepatocytes from the deficient animals was markedly decreased with the difference being significant as early as 10 min. When the kinetic parameters were measured in the two groups of animals, there was no significant difference (Table 2). These data suggest that the decreased uptake demonstrated

TABLE 1

INFLUENCE OF INHIBITORS ON $5\text{-CH}_3\text{-H}_4\text{PTEGLU}$ TRANSPORT

Uptake was measured for 5 min after 45 min preincubation with inhibitor. Each value is the mean of the number of measurements in parenthesis.

Addition	Concentration mM	% Control
2,4-DNP	1.0	9.5(7)
NaCN	10.0	59.6(8)
NaN_3	10.0	130 (8)
$Na_2H\ AsO_4$	10.0	53.4(8)
Ouabain	1.0	89.4(11)
Dithioerythritol	10.0	68.1(2)

558

TABLE 2

EFFECT OF B$_{12}$ AND METHIONINE ON KINETIC PARAMETERS OF 5-CH$_3$-H$_4$PTEGLU UPTAKE

Uptake was measured in hepatocytes isolated from rats fed a basal or B$_{12}$ deficient, limiting methionine diet. Measurements were made after 7.5 min of uptake and corrected for non-specific binding. Km and Vmax of the primary saturable component were calculated after subtracting the secondary, linear component; k is the first order rate constant of the latter.

Parameter	Basal Diet	Deficient Diet
Km (µM)	0.87 ± 0.37	0.71 ± 0.19
Vmax (pmol/g·min)	19.4 ± 1.3	18.4 ± 4.9
k (pmol/g·min·µM)	3.15 ± 0.34	5.10 ± 0.66

by the deficient hepatocytes is not due to a basic defect in the uptake mechanism but may be due to regulation of the transport mechanism. It should be noted that since there is very little metabolism of the 5-CH$_3$-H$_4$PteGlu taken up in a 90 min period (vida supra) it seems unlikely that the decreased uptake of the deficient cells seen as early as 10 min could be due to differences in metabolism of the transported substrate by control and deficient hepatocytes.

   Effect of ethanol. It is well established that alcohol can contribute to folate deficiency in malnourished individuals[13], and this may occur because alcohol may block release of folate from tissue stores to the plasma[14]. When ethanol is added to hepatocytes, the uptake of 5-CH$_3$-H$_4$PteGlu, but not PteGlu or methotrexate, is

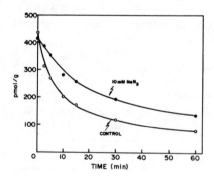

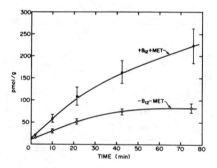

Fig. 3. Inhibition of 5-CH$_3$-H$_4$PteGlu efflux by 10 mM sodium azide. Cells were preloaded with 1.66 mM 5-CH$_3$-H$_4$-PteGlu in presence of 10 mM azide and efflux took place in presence (●) or absence (o) of azide.

Fig. 4. Effect of feeding diet deficient in vitamin B$_{12}$ and methionine on uptake of 0.25 µM 5-CH$_3$-H$_4$PteGlu by hepatocytes.

markedly stimulated (Table 3) confirming previous studies[9] that separate carriers are involved. This effect on $5-CH_3-H_4PteGlu$ uptake is similar to that seen by addition of sodium azide (Fig. 1) which was demonstrated to be due to an inhibition of efflux. Although we have not been able to consistently demonstrate an inhibition of $5-CH_3-H_4PteGlu$ efflux by ethanol, if it does prove to be the case, it would provide a cellular basis for the in vivo effects of ethanol on diminishing plasma levels of folate[15]. The stimulation of $5-CH_3-H_4PteGlu$ uptake by ethanol may be duplicated by other oxidizable alcohols and is inhibited by pyrazole. Uptake is also stimulated by decreased O_2 tension, suggesting that all these effects are mediated by a reduced redox potential.

TABLE 3

EFFECT OF ETHANOL ON UPTAKE OF FOLATE DERIVATIVES

Uptake was measured for 60 min and compared with that of control in absence of ethanol.

Substrate	Conc	% Control	p
$5-CH_3-H_4PteGlu$	0.34 μM	138.6 ± 4.2	<0.001
PteGlu	0.28 μM	93.9 ± 1.8	<0.05
Methotrexate	0.25 μM	75.6 ± 4.6	<0.01

SUMMARY

Data have been presented to show that isolated hepatocytes can be used as a convenient model to study transport of folate derivatives in liver. This model has been used to show that vitamin B_{12} and methionine deficiency results in reduced uptake of $5-CH_3-H_4PteGlu$ but that this is not due to an altered transport system. Ethanol and other treatments which produce a decreased redox potential stimulate uptake of $5-CH_3-H_4PteGlu$, which may be due to inhibition of efflux from the cell.

ACKNOWLEDGMENTS

This work was supported in part by funds from the Medical Research Service of the Veterans Administration and Grants No. 469 from the Nutrition Foundation and No. AM-15289 from the U. S. Public Health Service. We are pleased to acknowledge the excellent technical assistance of Mr. William T. Briggs.

REFERENCES

1. Henderson, G.B. and Huennekens, F.M. (1974) Arch. Biochem. Biophys. 164, 722-728.

2. Shane, B. and Stokstad, E.L.R. (1976) J. Biol. Chem. 251, 3405-3410.

3. Goldman, D. (1971) Ann. N. Y. Acad. Sci. 186, 400-422.

4. Chen, C.-P. and Wagner, C. (1975) Life Sci. 16, 1571-1582.

5. Momtazi, S. and Herbert, V. (1973) Am. J. Clin. Nutr. 26, 23-29.

6. Bobzien, W.F. and Goldman, D. (1972) J. Clin. Invest. 51, 1688-1696.

7. Corcino, J.J., Waxman, S. and Herbert, V. (1971) Br. J. Haematol. 20, 503.

8. Horne, D.W., Briggs, W.T. and Wagner, C. (1977) Anal. Biochem. 80, 615-621.

9. Horne, D.W., Briggs, W.T. and Wagner, C. (1978) J. Biol. Chem. 253, 3529-3535.

10. Stokstad, E.L.R. (1977) in Folic Acid: Biochemistry and Physiology in Relation to the Human Nutrition Requirement. National Academy of Sciences, Washington, D.C., pp. 122-135.

11. Gawthorne, J.M. and Smith, R.M. (1974) Biochem. J. 142, 119-126.

12. Thenen, S.W. and Stokstad, E.L.R. (1973) J. Nutr. 103, 363-370.

13. Sullivan, L.W. and Herbert, V. (1964) J. Clin. Invest. 43, 2048-2062.

14. Lane, F., Goff, P., McGuffin, R., Eichner, E.R. and Hillman, R.S. (1976) Brit. J. Haematol. 34, 489-500.

15. Eichner, E.R. and Hillman, R.S. (1973) J. Clin. Invest. 52, 584-591.

TRANSPORT OF FOLATE ANALOGS IN <u>STREPTOCOCCUS</u> <u>FAECIUM</u> AND <u>PEDIOCOCCUS</u> <u>CEREVISIAE</u>

FREDERIKA MANDELBAUM-SHAVIT and ROY L. KISLIUK

Department of Biochemistry and Pharmacology, Tufts University School of Medicine,
Boston, Massachusetts 02111

ABSTRACT

The transport of 5-methyltetrahydrofolate (5-CH_3H_4PteGlu) was studied in <u>Strepto-coccus</u> <u>faecium</u> and <u>Pediococcus</u> <u>cerevisiae</u>. Neither of these organisms metabolize this compound. Upon incubation for 1 min., <u>S</u>. <u>faecium</u> accumulated 5-CH_3H_4PteGlu to a 12 times higher intracellular concentration than that of the medium. The K_m for influx was 2.0 μM with a V_{max} of 0.1 nmol per min per mg of cells (dry weight). Folate homofolate and (dl)-tetrahydrohomofolate competitively inhibit the uptake of 5-CH_3H_4PteGlu with apparent K_i values of 1.8 μM, 1.4 μM and 2.0 μM respectively. The finding that both 5-CH_3H_4PteGlu and tetrahydrohomofolate compete with folate for transport, yet only the latter inhibits growth, indicates that the growth inhibition must be due to interaction with a target in addition to the transport system. With <u>P</u>. <u>cerevisiae</u> tetrahydrohomofolate and 5-methyltetrahydrohomofolate were taken up by the same carrier-mediated mechanism as CH_3H_4PteGlu (K_m 0.4 μM) with K_i values of 0.38 μM and 0.52 μM respectively. We conclude that an ability of a compound to inhibit folate transport in <u>S</u>. <u>faecium</u> and <u>P</u>. <u>cerevisiae</u> does not indicate that it will be able to inhibit growth.

INTRODUCTION

5-Methyltetrahydrofolate has been shown to be taken up by <u>P</u>. <u>cerevisiae</u>[1] and <u>S</u>. <u>faecium</u>[2] by a carrier-mediated mechanism, although neither of these microorganisms metabolize this compound. In the present study we use 5-CH_3H_4PteGlu as a model substrate for investigation of the transport of other folates with potential anti-tumor and antibacterial activities.

Tetrahydrohomofolate has been reported to be an effective antileukemic agent against a methotrexate-resistant subline of leukemia L1210 cells[3], an inhibitor of thymidylate synthetase from <u>Escherichia</u> <u>coli</u> and a growth inhibitor for <u>S</u>. <u>faecium</u> and <u>Lactobacillus</u> <u>casei</u>[4]. Another derivative, homofolate, is known to support growth of <u>S</u>. <u>faecium</u>, although less effectively than folate[5]. It was thus found of interest to examine whether the cell permeability is responsible for this phenomenon.

Since <u>P</u>. <u>cerevisiae</u> is not inhibited by relatively high concentrations of tetra-hydrohomofolate[4], we studied the route of uptake of this compound, as well as of a recently investigated antifol, 5-methyltetrahydrohomofolate[6].

MATERIALS AND METHODS

<u>Chemicals</u>. (dl)-5[^{14}C] Methyltetrahydrofolate, 57 mCi/nmol, was purchased from

Amersham Corp., Arlington Heights, Illinois 60005. Homofolate (NSC79249) and (dl)-5-methyltetrahydrohomofolate (NSC139490) were supplied by the Drug Synthesis and Chemistry Branch, Division of Cancer Treatment, National Cancer Institute, Bethesda, Maryland 20014. (dl)-Tetrahydrohomofolate (NSC89473) was prepared from homofolate by hydrogenation using platinum oxide as catalyst[7].

Growth of bacteria and transport assays. Streptococcus faecium (ATCC 8043) and Pediococcus cerevisiae (ATCC 8081) were grown in Folic Acid Assay Broth (Baltimore Biological Laboratories, Cockeysville, Maryland) supplemented with folic acid, 150 pg/ml for S. faecium and (dl)-5-formyltetrahydrofolate (folinate), 200 pg ml for P. cerevisiae. Logarithmic phase cells equivalent to 1 mg dry weight were incubated at 37° in potassium phosphate buffer, pH 6.0, 20 μmol, glucose 10 mg, and 5-[^{14}C]CH$_3$H$_4$PteGlu 0.1 nmol in a total volume of 1 ml. Uptake was terminated by rapid filtration and washing of the cells with cold saline.

RESULTS

Time course of 5-CH$_3$H$_4$PteGlu uptake in Streptococcus faecium. The data presented in Fig. 1 show that the uptake of 5-CH$_3$H$_4$PteGlu in S. faecium is linear for three minutes of incubation. At the steady state, the intracellular concentration is 37 times higher than that in the medium, assuming the intracellular water volume to be 4 μl/mg dry cells[8]. The accumulated radioactivity was identified as 5-CH$_3$H$_4$PteGlu (after extraction and paper chromatography)[1]. McElwee and Scott[2] also reported that S. faecium actively accumulates 5-CH$_3$H$_4$PteGlu, whereas no such accumulation against a concentration gradient was observed by Shane and Stokstad[9].

Effect of folate, homofolate and tetrahydrohomofolate on 5-CH$_3$H$_4$PteGlu transport in Streptococcus faecium. The initial rate of 5-CH$_3$H$_4$PteGlu uptake increased with increasing external concentration, exhibiting saturation kinetics. This process was linear up to 0.5 μM with saturation at 3.0 μM (data not shown). The K$_m$ for influx of 5-CH$_3$H$_4$PteGlu, as calculated from the Lineweaver-Burk plot in Fig. 2A, is 2.0 μM with a V$_{max}$ of 0.1 nmol/min/mg cells (dry weight). Folate, homofolate and (dl)-tetrahydrohomofolate competitively inhibited the uptake of 5-CH$_3$H$_4$PteGlu with K$_i$ values of 1.8 μM, 1.4 μM, and 2.0 μM respectively.

Effect of tetrahydrohomofolate and 5-methyltetrahydrohomofolate on 5-CH$_3$H$_4$PteGlu uptake by Pediococcus cerevisiae. The effect of (dl)-tetrahydrohomofolate and (dl)-5-methyltetrahydrohomofolate on 5-CH$_3$H$_4$PteGlu uptake by P. cerevisiae was also studied. The K$_m$ value for the uptake of 5-CH$_3$H$_4$PteGlu is 0.4 μM, as observed in earlier experiments[1]. As shown in Fig. 2B, tetrahydrohomofolate and 5-methyltetrahydrohomofolate competitively inhibited the uptake of 5-CH$_3$H$_4$PteGlu with respective K$_i$ values of 0.38 μM and 0.52 μM.

DISCUSSION

In the study described herein, we found that folate, homofolate, tetrahydrohomo-

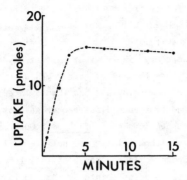

Fig. 1. Rate of 5-CH₃H₄PteGlu uptake by <u>S. faecium</u>.

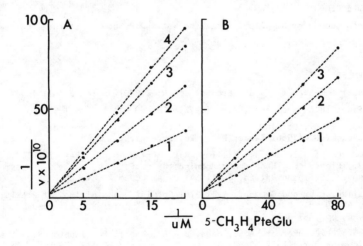

Fig. 2A. Reciprocal plot of 5-CH₃H₄PteGlu uptake by <u>S. faecium</u> (1) and the effect of (dl)-tetrahydrohomofolate 1 nmol (2), folate 2 nmol (3) and homofolate 2 nmol (4). V is the rate of uptake in mol/min/mg dry weight of cells. Incubation time 1 min.
Fig. 2B. Reciprocal plot of 5-CH₃H₄PteGlu uptake by <u>P. cerevisiae</u> (1) and the effect of (dl)-tetrahydrohomofolate 0.2 nmol (2) and (dl)-5-methyltetrahydrohomofolate 0.2 nmol (3).

564

folate and $5\text{-CH}_3\text{H}_4\text{PteGlu}$ enter S. faecium cells by a carrier-mediated process shared by the mentioned derivatives. The fact that $5\text{-CH}_3\text{H}_4\text{PteGlu}$ and tetrahydrohomofolate are equipotent as inhibitors of folate transport, yet only tetrahydrohomofolate inhibits growth indicates that growth inhibition must be due to interaction with a target in addition to the transport system.

Earlier studies from this laboratory[5] showed that (d)-tetrahydrohomofolate inhibits the growth of S. faecium whereas the (l) diastereomer supports growth and is active as a cofactor for serine hydroxymethylase and thymidylate synthetase. In subsequent unpublished work, we found that each diastereomer was equally potent in blocking folate uptake by cell suspensions of S. faecium. Our results also show that the low growth promoting activity of homofolate[5] was not due to its impaired uptake, since the K_i value for this compound is in the range of that for folate. We suggest that (d)-tetrahydrohomofolate after transport into S. faecium is metabolized to a growth inhibitor.

In P. cerevisiae tetrahydrohomofolate was taken up by the same carrier-mediated mechanism as $5\text{-CH}_3\text{H}_4\text{PteGlu}$ and folinate. However, the growth of this microorganism was not affected by tetrahydrohomofolate[4]. Therefore with P. cerevisiae as in S. faecium, the ability of a compound to compete with a folate for transport does not necessarily indicate that the compound will inhibit growth.

ACKNOWLEDGEMENT

Supported by grant CA10914 from the National Cancer Institute, United States Public Health Service.

REFERENCES

1. Mandelbaum-Shavit, F. and Grossowicz, N. (1970) J. Bacteriol. 104, 1-7.

2. McElwee, P.G. and Scott, J.M. (1972) Biochem. J. 127, 901-905.

3. Mead, J.A.R., Goldin, A., Kisliuk, R.L., Friedkin, M., Plante, L., Crawford, E.J. and Kwok, G. (1966) Cancer Res., 26, 2374-2379.

4. Goodman, L., DeGraw, J., Kisliuk, R.L., Friedkin, M., Pastore, E.J., Crawford, E.J., Plante, L., Nahas, A., Morningstar, J.F., Jr., Kwok, G., Wilson, L., Donovan, E.F. and Ratzan, J. (1964) J. Am. Chem. Soc., 86, 308-309.

5. Kisliuk, R.L. and Gaumont, Y. (1970) Chemistry and Biology of Pteridines, Iwai, K., Akino, M., Goto, M. and Iwanami, Y. eds. International Academic Printing Co., Toyko, pp. 357-364.

6. Mishra, L.C., Parmar, A.S., Mead, J.A.R., Knott, R., Taunton-Rigby, A., and Friedman, O.M. (1972) Proc. Am. Assoc. Cancer Res., 13, 76.

7. Kisliuk, R.L. (1971) in Methods in Enzymology, vol. XVIII, Vitamins and Coenzymes Part B, McCormick, D.B. and Wright, L.D. eds., Academic Press, New York, pp. 663-670.

8. Kepes, A. and Cohen, G.N. (1962) in The Bacteria, Gunsalus, I.C. and Stanier, R.Y. eds., vol. 4, Academic Press, New York, pp. 179-222.

9. Shane, B. and Stokstad, E.L.R. (1975) J. Biol. Chem., 250, 2243-2253.

PURIFICATION OF A METHOTREXATE BINDING PROTEIN FRACTION FROM L1210 LYMPHOCYTE PLASMA MEMBRANES

JOHN I. McCORMICK, SANDRA S. SUSTEN, JEANNE I. RADER, and JAMES H. FREISHEIM. Dept. of Biological Chemistry (522), University of Cincinnati College of Medicine, 231 Bethesda Ave., Cincinnati, OH 45267 USA

ABSTRACT

In characterizing plasma membrane-associated Methotrexate binding proteins in L1210 lymphoma cells, a protein species of molecular weight 56,000 has been identified using differential labeling with $[^{14}C]$-N-ethylmaleimide. A MTX binding protein fraction has also been isolated by MTX-affinity chromatography of solubilized plasma membrane proteins. This aggregate fraction consists of three major protein bands with molecular weights of 67,000, 63,000, and 56,000, based on SDS gel electrophoresis.

INTRODUCTION

Methotrexate (MTX), N^5-formyl-tetrahydrofolate (5-formyl-FAH_4) and N^5-methyl-tetrahydrofolate (5-methyl-FAH_4) are transported into L1210 lymphoma cells by an active carrier-mediated process involving protein components containing reactive sulfhydryl groups[1,2].

In the present study, attempts have been made to characterize the membrane components involved in the transport of MTX. The sensitivity of the transport system to N-ethylmaleimide (NEM) has been used to label MTX binding sites on the plasma membranes of L1210 lymphocytes. In addition, affinity chromatography has been used to isolate a MTX binding component from L1210 lymphocyte plasma membranes. The binding complex has been isolated from solubilized crude plasma membranes and also from a detergent extract of intact cells.

MATERIALS AND METHODS

Uptake Studies. $[^3H]$MTX uptake studies were performed with L1210 lymphocytes using methods already described[2].

Preparation of Crude Plasma Membranes. L1210 cells (10^9-10^{10} cells) were suspended in 40ml 10mM Tris/HCl, 150 mM NaCl, pH 7.4, and disrupted by passage through a French Press at 200 psi. The crude homogenate was subjected to differential centrifugation at 310 x g (15 min), 7,800 x g (30 min), and 20,000 x g (30 min). Each isolated pellet was assayed for membrane marker enzymes using standard methods[3].

Protection Studies. Washed L1210 cells were incubated for 5 min at
37°C with varying concentrations of MTX in phosphate buffered saline
(PBS), pH 6.8. Following incubation, NEM (100µM) was added and incubation continued for a further 10 min at which time β-mercaptoethanol
(10mM) was added and the cells were harvested by centrifugation and
washed in PBS buffer, pH 7.4. [^{3}H]MTX uptake in the cells was then
measured over a 10 min period[2].

Labeling with [^{14}C]-NEM. Two cell suspensions (5 x 10^6 cells/ml)
were prepared in PBS buffer, pH 6.8, and designated *protected* and *unprotected* fractions. The *protected* fraction was incubated for 5 min at
37°C with MTX (48µM). NEM (100µM) was then added, and following a 10
min incubation, β-mercaptoethanol (10mM) was added, and the incubation
continued for a further 5 min. The cells were harvested, washed, and
resuspended in PBS buffer, pH 6.8, to their original volume. [^{14}C]-NEM
(100µM) was added and the suspension incubated for 10 min at 37°C. The
cells were harvested and a crude plasma membrane pellet was prepared.

In the *unprotected* sample, pretreatment with MTX was omitted and
the cell suspension was incubated for 5 min prior to the addition of
NEM (100µM, 10 min) and β-mercaptoethanol (10mM, 5 min). The cells
were harvested, washed, and incubated with [^{14}C]-NEM as described above,
and a crude plasma membrane pellet prepared.

SDS Gel Electrophoresis. SDS gel electrophoresis was carried out on
protected and *unprotected* fractions on separate gels by a modified
Laemmli method[4,5]. Following electrophoresis, gels were sliced for
determination of radioactivity.

Extraction of Protein From Intact L1210 Lymphoma Cells. Washed L1210
cells were suspended (5 x 10^6 cells/ml) in PBS buffer, pH 7.4, containing 0.01% Triton X-100(w/v) and 0.014M β-mercaptoethanol, and incubated
at 37°C for 15 min. Following incubation, the cells were removed by
centrifugation and the supernatant stored at 4°C.

Affinity Chromatography. MTX-affinity resins were prepared by methods already described[6]. Before use, columns were extensively washed[6]
and finally equilibrated in 50mM KPO$_4$ buffer, pH 7.4, containing 0.01%
Triton X-100 and 0.014M β-mercaptoethanol. Proteins were extracted from
intact L1210 cells as described above and loaded onto an affinity column
(1.5cm x 8.0cm). Following loading and washing, proteins retained on
the column were eluted with solutions of 0.12mM 5-formyl-FAH$_4$ or MTX
in the equilibration buffer, and characterized on SDS gel electrophoresis.

Affinity chromatography was also carried out on a crude plasma membrane pellet following partial solubilization in PBS buffer, pH 7.4,
containing 0.01% Triton X-100 and 0.014M β-mercaptoethanol.

RESULTS AND DISCUSSION

MTX transport in L1210 lymphoma cells is sensitive to inhibition by NEM. This effect is substantially reduced when cells are pretreated with MTX (Table 1). Partial protection of transport is observed after pretreatment of cell suspensions with 4.8 or 9.3µM MTX, and complete protection occurred after treatment with 48µM MTX. These results formed the basis for the NEM labeling experiment.

TABLE 1

UPTAKE OF [^{3}H]-METHOTREXATE BY L1210 CELLS: EFFECT OF PRETREATMENT WITH METHOTREXATE ON INHIBITION BY N-ETHYLMALEIMIDE.

Pretreatment[a]		Uptake[b]	
MTX µM	NEM 100µM	pmoles/10^9 cells	Percent
None	−	773	100
	+	372	48
4.8	−	181	100
	+	129	72
9.3	−	154	100
	+	129	84
24.0	−	139	100
	+	126	91
48.0	−	149	100
	+	164	110

[a]Pretreatment: Methotrexate (MTX) 5 min; N-ethylmaleimide (NEM) 10 min.
[b]Uptake: 10 min; 1.7µM [^{3}H]-MTX.

For analysis of NEM labeled membrane proteins, crude plasma membranes were prepared from L1210 cells. The 20,000 x g pellet isolated by the methods described was enriched approximately 4- and 3-fold for 5'-Nucleotidase and Na$^+$-K$^+$-ATPase, respectively, and represents a crude plasma membrane preparation. The yield of membrane was approximately 20%.

The NEM labeling procedure resulted in the incorporation of 21% of the [^{14}C]-NEM into cells previously *protected* by exposure to MTX. Incorporation of approximately 16% of the label was observed in the *unprotected* fraction. Preincubation with MTX therefore results in a differential distribution of the label between *protected* and *unprotected* cells. SDS gel electrophoresis of the two fractions indicates that a number of proteins are labeled by the procedure described (Fig.1). However, the largest differential distribution of radioactivity consistently occurred in protein components with a minimum molecular weight of 56,000, indicating that this membrane component plays a role in the binding of MTX.

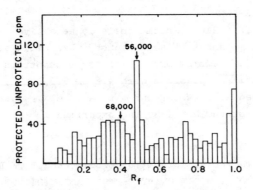

Fig. 1. Difference profile following SDS gel electrophoresis of *protected* and *unprotected* membrane fractions.

For the study of an active plasma membrane associated MTX binding complex, a novel procedure has been developed. The methodology for this procedure evolved from observations on the effect of Triton X-100 on MTX uptake in L1210 cells. This detergent inhibits MTX uptake, the maximum effect being at a concentration of 0.01% detergent (Fig. 2).

The cessation of MTX uptake observed is accompanied by a release of protein from the cell, a process which occurs in the absence of extensive cell destruction as determined by measurements of cell viability. Indications are that a substantial portion of the proteins released from the intact cell are plasma membrane derived. Thus, L1210 cell plasma membrane 5'-Nucleotidase is released, and in addition, SDS gels of the released or solubilized proteins are qualitatively similar to SDS gels of isolated crude plasma membranes. In contrast, the lack of succinic dehydrogenase activity in the intact cell solubilized material is indicative of some maintainance of cellular structure. Similar methods have been developed for the extraction of membrane proteins from other cell types[7].

When solubilization is carried out in the presence of [^{3}H]MTX, drug binding can be studied by application of an aliquot of the extracted material to a Sephadex G-25 column (Fig.3). Maximum binding is obtained only when extraction is carried out in the presence of [^{3}H]MTX.

Affinity chromatography of the intact cell solubilized material results in the purification of a protein fraction containing three major proteins of molecular weights 67,000, 63,000, and 56,000 (Fig. 4), based on SDS-PAGE. These same three proteins are also present as major components following affinity chromatography of a solubilized crude plasma membrane pellet.

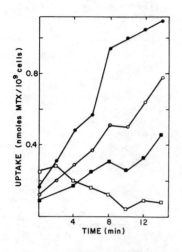

Fig. 2. The effect of Triton X-100 on [³H] MTX uptake in Ll210 cells. ●——●, normal uptake; O——O, uptake in the presence of 0.0025% (w/v) Triton X-100; ■——■ , uptake in the presence of 0.005% (w/v) Triton X-100; ▫——▫ , uptake in the presence of 0.01% (w/v) Triton X-100.

When the retained protein fraction is eluted from the affinity resin with [³H] MTX, binding activity can be demonstrated by use of Sephadex G-25 gel chromatography. On this basis, approximate estimations of binding give a figure of 10^{-12} moles for the concentration of binding protein molecule extractable from 10^9 cells, assuming one MTX molecule binds to one binding protein molecule.

Preliminary evidence indicates that the three proteins (Fig.4) represent sub-units of a high molecular weight complex. The component of molecular weight 56,000 is of particular interest since a protein of similar molecular weight has been identified using the NEM differential labeling technique (Fig.1). This indicates that a high molecular weight complex present in Ll210 lymphoma cell plasma membranes may play some role in the initial binding of MTX.

SUMMARY

The transport of MTX by Ll210 lymphoma cells is sensitive to inhibition by NEM. This effect is reduced when the cells are pretreated with MTX. [¹⁴C]-NEM has been used to label binding sites for MTX in the plasma membranes of cells previously *protected* from reaction with NEM by MTX. By this procedure, an MTX-binding protein of molecular weight 56,000 has been identified.

An active binding protein fraction has also been isolated by affinity chromatography of solubilized plasma membranes. This fraction consists of 3 major proteins with molecular weights of 67,000, 63,000, and 56,000, based on SDS-PAGE.

570

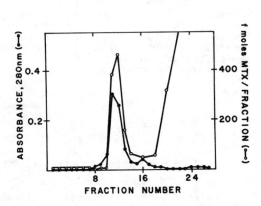

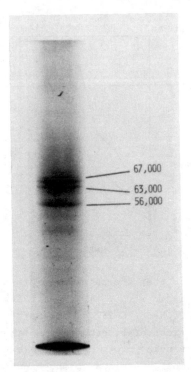

67,000

63,000
56,000

Fig. 3. Sephadex G-25 chromatography
of proteins extracted from the intact
cell in the presence of [^{3}H] MTX.

Fig. 4. SDS gel electro-
phoresis of the protein
fraction purified by affinity
chromatography.

ACKNOWLEDGEMENTS

This research was supported by grant CH 80B from the American
Cancer Society, and by grant CA 11666, NCI, NIH, DHEW.

REFERENCES

1. Goldman, I.D. (1971) Ann. N.Y. Acad. Sci., 186, 400-422.

2. Rader, J.I., Niethammer, D. and Huennekens, F.M. (1974)
   Biochem. Pharmacol., 23, 2057-2059.

3. Allan, D. and Crumpton, M.J. (1970) Biochem. J., 120, 133-143.

4. Laemmli, U.K. (1970) Nature, 227, 680-685.

5. LeSturgeon, W.M. and Rusch, H.P. (1973) Arch. Biochem. Biophys.,
   155, 144-158.

6. Kaufman, B.T. (1974) Methods in Enzymology, 34B, 272-281.

7. Pearlstein, E. and Seaver, J. (1976) Biochim. Biophys. Acta, 426,
   589-597.

571

STUDIES ON THE MECHANISM OF INTESTINAL FOLATE ABSORPTION

J.M. NORONHA AND V. KESAVAN

Biochemistry & Food Technology Division, Bhabha Atomic Research Centre, Trombay, Bombay 400 085 (INDIA)

ABSTRACT

Blair et al.[1,2,3] first suggested that dietary folates could be absorbed by passive diffusion of the neutral species in an acidic microenvironment generated at the intestinal site of absorption. Our experiments provide good supporting evidence for a Mg^{2+}-activated ATPase, located in the mucosal brush border, which has properties ideally suited for a role in generating the necessary acidic microenvironment for folate absorption.

A protein fraction has been identified from the mucosal brush border which instantly binds folate over a wide pH range (4 - 7). However, from the characteristics of its binding folate in vivo and in vitro it seems unlikely to be involved in folate transport across the mucosal cell. Other kinetic studies described suggest that the mechanism involves a non-carrier mediated, passive diffusion of the unionized folate species in an acid microenvironment. Respiratory energy is essentially utilized in order to sustain the required surface acidity.

INTRODUCTION

Our earlier experiments had indicated that 700 R whole-body x-irradiation had impaired folate absorption as judged by the the absence of the expected rise in blood folate levels after folate ingestion[4]. It was further shown that irradiation had adversely affected intestinal oxidative phosphorylation and ATP added in vitro could restore the defective transport[4]. Blair et al.[1,2,3] first suggested that folate transport could occur by a process of passive diffusion of the unionized form in which the vitamin would exist in the special acidic microenvironment generated at the intestinal glycocalyx. Our recent work[5] presents striking evidence for an acid microclimate-dependent mechanism for intestinal folate transport. Radiation, having depleted mucosal ATP reserves, had interfered with the acidification process which depended on the activity of a mucosal surface ATPase. Some properties of the ATP involved, as well as the possible role of a mucosal folate binding protein are now described, together with the overall mechanism of intestinal folate absorption that has emerged from these studies.

Abbreviations: 5-CH$_3$THFA, 5-methyl tetrahydrofolic acid; SDS, sodium dodecyl sulfate.

MATERIALS AND METHODS

Male Wistar rats weighing between 150 - 170 gm were used throughout the study. $2\text{-}^{14}C$ folic acid (specific activity 54.3 mCi/mmole) was obtained from Radiochemical Centre, Amersham. $5\text{-}CH_3THFA$ was obtained from Sigma Chemical Co., St. Louis.

ATPase activity. Rats were killed after a 20 hr fasting period, the jejunal small intestine (40 cm) removed and transferred to a beaker containing oxygenated isotonic saline at $0\text{-}4^{\circ}C$. The lumen was flushed out with cold isotonic saline and then washed with 0.25 M sucrose. The intestine was slit open lengthwise, the epithelial cells were gently scrapped off and a 10% homogenate prepared in 0.25 M sucrose. ATPase activity was determined as described earlier[5]. The effect of cations was studied as their chloride salts in the concentrations and combinations indicated.

Subcellular fraction of mucosal cells. The mucosal cells were fractionated by the method of Gitzelmann et al.[6] The brush border fraction of the mucosal cells were prepared by the method of Porteous[7].

Folate transport. The transport of $5\text{-}CH_3THFA$ at various concentrations across the everted intestinal segments was studied as described earlier[5].

Folate binding studies. Mucosal cells equivalent to 40 mg protein were suspended in 5 ml Krebs-Ringer phosphate medium pH 6.5 containing 5 mM folic acid and 0.2 μC of $2\text{-}^{14}C$ folic acid. Samples (0.1 ml) were removed at various time intervals after incubation at $37^{\circ}C$ washed thoroughly until the supernatant is free of radioactivity, dissolved in 0.5 ml hyamine hydroxide and the radioactivity determined. An aliquot corresponding to 6 mg protein of the brush border preparation that had been preincubated for 10 min with labelled folate was solubilized with 0.2% SDS for 2 hr at $4^{\circ}C$ and then fractionated on Sephadex G 150 (300 x 15 mm) columns with 25 mM Tris HCl buffer pH 7.5 containing 0.1% SDS as eluant.

The in vivo folate absorption and mucosal binding studies were carried out under conditions of saturated tissue stores as detailed earlier[4]. After oral administration of 40 μg $2\text{-}^{14}C$ folic acid/kg body weight (20 μCi), serum was sampled and jejunal mucosal cells isolated at various time intervals for radioactivity determinations. All radioactive measurements were made in a Beckmann liquid scintillation counter LS 100 using Bray's solution. Folate activity was determined by microbiological assay using Lactobacillus casei ATCC 7469.

Results presented are averages for at least three experiments.

RESULTS AND DISCUSSION

Mucosal surface ATPase activity. Recently published data indicate that maximal folate transport across everted rat intestinal sacs occurred at pH 4 and that at this pH its transport was insensitive to the irradiation induced lesion observed when transport was studied at the neutral pH (6.5) of the bulk intestinal chyme[5]. Under neutral conditions the radiolabile target was the build up of an acidic microclimate which in turn depended on a proton generating ATPase activity at the mucosal surface capable of hydrolyzing solution phase ATP[5].

In Table 1 it can be seen that mucosal cell homogenate ATPase is maximally stimulated by 4 mM Mg^{2+}. Ca^{2+} was only a third as stimulatory and in fact antagonised the effect of Mg^{2+} when these divalent cations were present together. Na^+ and K^+ separately or together were comparatively ineffective. In a previous paper[5] a mucosal surface ATPase of the intact intestinal everted segments which similar properties and which could hydrolyze solution phase ATP has been described.

TABLE 1

METAL ION REQUIREMENTS OF INTESTINAL MUCOSAL ATPase

Metal ion: mM	Mg^{2+}	Ca^{2+}	$Mg^{2+} + Ca^{2+}$	Na^+	K^+	$Na^+ + K^+$
			μg Pi released / mg protein / 30 min			
1	135	15	60	10	10	18
2	150	27	70	15	15	25
3	155	40	78	30	31	38
4	160	55	89	35	41	45
5	148	48	82	40	50	55
6	130	41	61	55	61	70
8	120	30	40	30	34	35

From the data in Table 2 it is seen that the ATPase activity is concentrated four fold in the purified brush border. The activity in the 1000xg fraction is due to the nuclei and brush border. To a lesser extent it is also associated with other particulate fractions but not with soluble cytoplasm. Its maximal concentration in the brush border and its well known role in the generation of hydrogen ions[8] suggest that its function is to sustain an acidic microclimate in the glycocalyx. Recently Lei et al. employing direct pH measurements have demonstrated that the proximal jejunum can maintain a low surface pH despite excessive luminal alkalinity[9].

A concentration of 4 mM ATP was also found to be optimal. Other properties described earlier[5] indicate that the enzyme is optimally active at the neutral pH (6.5) of the bulk intestinal chyme, and that the enzyme is essentially inactive below pH 5, although it could regain full activity (at pH 6.5) after as long as 30 min at pH 4. The activity is inhibited 85 - 90% by 50 mM sodium azide, in presence of which in vitro folate transport at neutral pH is similarly reduced. The ATPase inhibitor did not affect folate transport when studied under acidic conditions. The results taken together clearly point to a crucial role of the mucosal brush border ATPase in regulating the build up of an unstirred acidic microclimate 1 - 2 pH units below the pH of the bulk intestinal chyme which is essential for intestinal folate transport.

TABLE 2
SUBCELLULAR LOCALISATION OF INTESTINAL
MUCOSAL ATPase

Subcellular fractions	ATPase activity[a]
Homogenate	160
1000 g x 10 min	202
10300 g x 5 min	88
41000 g x 6 min	120
105000 g x 1 hr	72
Supernatant	Nil
Brush border	520

[a] μg Pi released/mg protein/30 min

TABLE 3
5-CH$_3$THFA TRANSPORT IN INTESTINAL
EVERTED SACS

Mucosal 5-CH$_3$THFA (M)	Serosal content[a]
10^{-7}	28.1
10^{-6}	32.8
10^{-5}	131.5
10^{-4}	423.0
10^{-3}	758.4

[a] mμg 5-CH$_3$THFA/5cm segment/hr

Mucosal folate-binding protein. Whole mucosal cells when incubated with labelled folate are found to instantly bind and retain folate at a saturation level of 1.0 μ mole/mg protein. This binding of folate to the mucosal surface is unaffected over a wide pH range (4 - 7). Isolated brush borders from such cells, after solubilization with 1% SDS could be fractionated on Sephadex G 150. As seen in Fig. 1 folate was found to be associated with a single protein fraction which elutes out as a symmetric peak.

We next attempted to ascertain whether the observed folate receptor has a role in folate transport across the mucosal cell. Simultaneous measurements of serum folate and mucosal receptor-bound folate were made at various time intervals after folate ingestion. It can be seen (Fig. 2) that there was no correlation between folate transport as indicated by rise in serum folate and the extent of folate bound to the mucosal cell receptor. Folate was transported maximally between 30 - 45 min after ingestion while the receptor-bound folate activity remained unaltered over the entire period of at least 5 hrs after folate ingestion.

In Table 3 it is observed that folate transport from the mucosal to the serosal compartment was dependent on the initial mucosal folate concentration over a range spanning four orders of magnitude. Had a protein carrier been involved in folate transport, saturation kinetics should have been observed. From similar data with different folate species Blair et al.[8] have concluded that the observed kinetics of folate transport can only be explained on the basis of the solubility of different folate derivatives, in a prevailing acidic microenvironment at the absorption site where the pH is below 4.5. Folates would then exist as the unionised species allowing a concentration dependent, passive folate uptake unhampered by the negatively charged

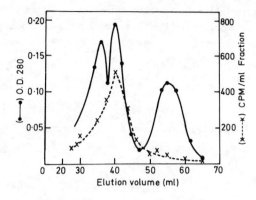

Fig. 1. Separation of the folate binding
Protein of the brush border.

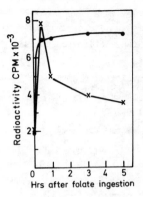

Fig. 2. Folate uptake in serum
(x—x) and mucosl cells (●—●)

phospholipid mucosal cell membrane. Further evidence that folate transport basically involved passive diffusion was the inability to measure differences between final serosal and final mucosal folate levels after 60 min.incubation in an initial zero concentration gradient[5]. The possibility that acidification had caused non-specific breakdown of the normal absorption barrier has also been eliminated[5]. It has also been established that the acidification did not interfere with some other active physiological process[5].

In 1971, after many conflicting mechanisms of folate transport had been proposed by various workers, Strum et al.[10] presented evidence which showed that mucosal folate transport occurred without metabolic transformation, by a non-carrier mediated, passive and nonsaturable system. Numerous experiments discussed above would confirm these observations and further explain them in terms of the observed requirement of an acidic microenvironment at the absorption site for successful folate transport. Our current work, begining with unravelling the nature of the radiation sensitivity of the system, has led us to conclude that a mucosal brush border, Mg^{2+}-dependent ATPase is involved in the acidification process. Direct mucosal surface pH measurements have indicated substantially lowered surface acidity in the intestines of the coeliac and Crohn's diseased[11]. The accompanying folate malabsorption in such diseases is often accompanied by a disruption of the normal continuity of the glycocalyx at the mucosal cell surface[12]. An understanding of the mechanisms involved should serve in formulating more rational approaches towards correcting folate malabsorption.

Although the present evidence would indicate that intestinal folate absorption per se occurs through passive diffusion, the requirement of an acidic microenvironment calls for the operation of a proton pump involving the hydrolysis of ATP at the mucosal cell surface. The sensitivity of the absorption process to an uncoupler of oxidative phosphorylation and to irradiation (which also decreased oxidative phosphorylation[4]) clearly points to the continual need of respiratory energy to maintain the surface acidity essential for folate absorption. External ATP could be utilized for this purpose in our in vitro experiments. However, the exact mechanism of proton translocation operative in vivo remains to be worked out.

ACKNOWLEDGEMENTS

We are grateful to the Symposium Organizing Committee and the Department of Atomic Energy, Government of India for financial assistance which has made this presentation possible.

REFERENCES

1. Blair, J.A., Johnson, I.T. and Matty, A.J. (1974) J. Physiol., 236, 653-661.
2. Blair, J.A., Matty, A.J. and Razzaque, A. (1975) J. Physiol., 250, 221-230.
3. Blair, J.A., Johnson, I.T. and Matty, A.J. (1976) J. Physiol., 256, 197-208.
4. Kesavan, V. and Noronha, J.M. (1971) Int. J. Radiat. Biol., 19, 205-214.
5. Kesavan, V. and Noronha, J.M. (1978) J. Physiol., in print.
6. Gitzelmann, R., Davidson, E.A. and Osinchak, J. (1964) Biochem. Biophys. Acta, 85, 69-81.
7. Porteous, J.W. (1972) in 'Subcellular components - Preparation and fractionation'. G.D. Birnie, ed. Butterworths, London. pp. 157-183.
8. Blair, J.A. and Matty, A.J., (1974) Clinics in Gastroenterol., 3, 183-197.
9. Lei, F.H., Lucas, M.L. and Blair, J.A. (1977) Biochem. Soc. Trans., 5, 149-152.
10. Strum, W., Nixon, P.F., Bertino, J.B. and Binder, H.J. (1971) J. Clin. Invest., 50, 1910-1916.
11. Lucas, M.L., Blair, J.A., Cooper, B.T. and Cooke, W.T. (1976) Biochem. Soc. Trans., 4, 154-156.
12. Swanston, S.K., Blair, J.A., Matty, A.J., Cooper, B.T. and Cooke, W.T. (1977) Biochem. Soc. Trans. 5, 152.

THE EFFECT OF AN IMPLANTED NOVIKOFF HEPATOMA ON THE METABOLISM OF FOLIC ACID IN THE RAT

ANNE E. PHEASANT and JOHN A. BLAIR
Department of Chemistry, University of Aston in Birmingham, UK.

ABSTRACT

(i) A number of folates and scission products have been identified in rat urine following the administration of ^{14}C and ^{3}H folic acid. (ii) Rats bearing an implanted Novikoff hepatoma produced an additional metabolite (iii) More ^{14}C than ^{3}H was recovered in faeces and intact folates only were detected in bile therefore it is suggested that scission takes place in the gut. (iv) A comparison of liver and tumour folates was made.

INTRODUCTION

Barford and Blair[1] reported that the presence of a Walker 256 carcinoma altered urinary folates in the rat. The current study was performed to ascertain whether another tumour type would have a similar effect.

METHODS

Normal rats and rats bearing an implanted Novikoff hepatoma received oral doses of 2-$[^{14}$C$]$, 3', 5', 9-$[^{3}$H$]$ folic acid (100µg/kg body weight). Urine samples were collected 6, 24 and 48h after dosing and faeces after 48h. The animals were then killed and the livers and tumours extracted in (i) boiling phosphate buffer containing ascorbate[2] (ii) cold phosphate buffer containing ascorbate followed by precipitation of the protein with TCA (iii) 0.25M sucrose, pH 7.0, containing ascorbate followed by centrifugation at 100,000g for 1h. Bile cannulations were performed as described[3]. Urine and bile samples were sequentially chromatographed on DEAE-cellulose and Sephadex G15[2]. The Novikoff hepatoma was implanted as s.c. injections of 5x10^{7} (group 1) or 10x10^{7} (group 2) ascitic tumour cells and allowed to grow for 6 or 10 days respectively.

RESULTS AND DISCUSSION

There was an uneven excretion of the two labels between urine and faeces. The normal rats excreted a total of 27.7% ^{14}C, 37.4% ^{3}H in the urine and 21.0% ^{14}C, 11.0% ^{3}H in the faeces. The corresponding values for the tumour-bearing animals were 30.5% ^{14}C, 41.5% ^{3}H in the urine and 26.2% ^{14}C, 15.3% ^{3}H in the faeces. Both groups of animals retained about 11% of the dose in the liver and 1% was present in the tumour. Chromatography of the urine samples showed the presence of at least nine radioactive components including folic acid, 5-methyltetrahydrofolate (5MeTHF), 10-formylfolate, 10-formyltetra-hydrofolate (10CHOTHF), tritiated water, p-acetamidobenzoate urea[4], an unindentified dual-labelled compound (folate A), p-aminobenzoyl-L-glutamate or its acetamido derivative and the oxidisable pterin also found following the administration of 10-formylfolate (see previous communication). Small quantities of $^{14}CO_2$ were detected in the expired air of both groups of rats. The distribution of these metabolites varied with time giving larger percentages of the scission products in the later urine samples.

The tumour-bearing rats of group 2 also excreted another unidentified urinary metabolite B. This was dual-labelled, eluted from DEAE-cellulose at a higher ionic strength than 5MeTHF and represented 25% of the radioactivity in the 6-24h urine sample. It was present in smaller amounts in the other urine samples collected from these rats and completely absent from the urine of normal animals. Folic acid was metabolised more readily by the tumour-bearing animals, less being excreted unchanged over 48h (6.9% of the urinary radioactivity compared to 11.4% in the control animals). The ratio of 10-formyl-folates to folate A was reduced compared to normal rats falling from 2 7:1 for the control animals in the 6-24h urine sample to 0.6:1 in the presence of the tumour. This shift was more evident when less metabolite B was produced. Metabolite B was moderately stable but on lengthy handling broke down to a product eluting from DEAE-cellulose in the same position as folate A, suggesting that the two observed effects of the implanted Novikoff hepatoma are linked.

The overall recoveries indicated that a principally ^{14}C labelled fragment was present in faeces. Experiments performed on control animals with cannulated bile ducts showed that up to 10h after an

oral dose of folic acid, intact folates only were present in bile.
At all time intervals studied, 10CHOTHF, 10-formylfolate and 5MeTHF
were detected representing, on average, 19%, 13% and 52% of the
biliary radioactivity respectively.   Only trace amounts of folic
acid were found.   This is consistent with other reports of a number
of folate species appearing rapidly in bile[5,6].   Since no evidence
for the biliary excretion of scission products was obtained at a time
when scission products appear in the urine, it is probable that
cleavage of the folate molecule takes place in the gut either chemically or due to the gut microflora.   This could be followed by the
reabsorption of the ^{3}H metabolites and their subsequent excretion in
urine;   the ^{14}C scission product being poorly absorbed and the majority
excreted in the faeces.

Sephadex-G15 chromatography of tissue extracts prepared by methods
(i) and (ii) showed the major radioactive species to be a folate
polyglutamate in the control liver, host liver and tumour.   However
differences were observed between cytosol fractions prepared by method
(iii).   In the control liver 56% of the radioactivity was bound to
protein, in the host liver 39% was protein-bound and in the Novikoff
tumour no such binding could be demonstrated.   In the latter case,
10CHOTHF and 5MeTHF were present in a 2:1 ratio, presumably released
by the action of conjugase and other folate metabolising enzymes.
However in the control and host livers 5MeTHF was the dominant
monoglutamate seen.   The significance of the lack of protein binding
is not known and may indicate a change in either the folate binding
proteins or the form of the folate in the tumour tissue.

REFERENCES
1. Barford, P.A. and Blair, J.A. (1975) in Chem.& Biol. of Pteridines.
   ed. W. PFleiderer, Walter de Gruyter.   Berlin N.Y. pp413-427.
2. Barford, P.A., et al. (1977).   Biochem.J. 164 601-605.
3. James, S.P., et al.   (1968).Biochem.J. 109 727-736.
4. Connor, M.J., et al. (1977).   Biochem.Soc.Trans. 5 1319-1320.
5. Lavoie, A. and Cooper, B.A. (1974) Clin.Sci.Mol.Med. 46 729-741.
6. Hillman, R.S., et al. (1977). Trans.Assoc.Am.Phys. 90
   145-156.

IMMUNOREACTIVE HETEROGENEITY OF FOLATE-BINDING PROTEINS FROM HUMAN TISSUES

SHELDON ROTHENBERG, MARIA DA COSTA, CRAIG FISCHER, JEFFREY COHEN

Division of Hematology/Oncology, New York Medical College, 1249 Fifth Avenue,

New York, New York 10029

INTRODUCTION

Proteins which bind several folate analogues have now been identified in extracts

of various human and animal tissues and biologic fluids.[1] The folate-binding pro-

teins (FBP) from milk[2] and chronic myelogenous leukemia (CML) cells[3] have been

purified and their properties characterized. Some of these proteins have similar

binding affinities for folate analogues, the oxidized folate pteroylglutamic acid

(PGA), being bound with greater affinity than N^5-methyltetrahydrofolate (methyl-

FH_4), the naturally-occurring reduced folate in mammalian cells and plasma,

while there is minimal affinity for N^5-formyltetrahydrofolate (formylFH_4).

There are differences, however, in some of the physical properties of these pro-

teins. The FBP from CML cells[4] and human plasma[5] show heterogeneity of ionic

charge by anion exchange chromatography. Also, the molecular size of the FBP in

human milk[2] is smaller than the binding protein in CML cells[4] and plasma[6]. This

report will demonstrate that the folate-binding protein in extracts of several

normal and neoplastic human tissue are also immunologically heterogeneous.

MATERIALS AND METHODS

Human tissues were obtained from surgical specimens. Preliminary studies to

determine the optimum salt solution and method of extraction demonstrated that

homogenization of the tissue in three volumes of 0.05 M sodium citrate, pH 7.2,

using a Virtis homogenizer resulted in the highest yield of the FBP. Following

homogenization, the insoluble debris was separated by centrifugation at 30,000 xg for 30 min, and the supernatant solution was analyzed for its protein concentration, unsaturated folate-binding capacity using [^{3}H]PGA[7] and immunoreactive FBP by double immunodiffusion against guinea pig antiserum to the FBP purified from CML cells. The concentration of FBP was determined by radioimmunoassay (RIA) using the FBP prepared from CML cells as the standard, and rabbit antiserum to this FBP as the immune binding determinant.[8]

RESULTS

Table 1 lists the results only for those samples where neoplastic and adjacent normal tissue could be simultaneously analyzed. All the samples contained FBP by RIA, but unsaturated FBP was not found in all of these tissues.

TABLE 1

FBP MEASURED BY RIA AND FOLATE-BINDING CAPACITY MEASURED BY THE BINDING OF [^{3}H]PGA IN NORMAL AND NEOPLASTIC TISSUE EXTRACTS

Tissue	Normal tissue		Neoplastic tissue	
	FBP by RIA pg/mg protein	Unsaturated folate binding pg/mg protein	FBP by RIA pg/mg protein	Unsaturated folate binding pg/mg protein
Colon				
D.D.	260	0	310	0
R.C.	430	0	440	0
I.K.	310	0	320	0
F.S.	410	4.7	420	3.7
D.P.	340	6.4	380	14
Lung				
P.F.	70,000	24	108,000	25
R.R.	990	35	560	13
Stomach				
J.B.	340	0	250	0
Breast				
A.B.	1,300	0	650	0

By double immunodiffusion in agar against guinea pig antiserum to FBP(Figure

1, A and B), purified from CML lysates, extracts of a spleen from a patient with my-

elofibrosis (A-7) and extracts of lung tumor (B-2), and colon cancer (B-8) gave pre-

cipitin lines. This result was not observed with all tissue extracts even though

immunoreactive FBP was identified by RIA.

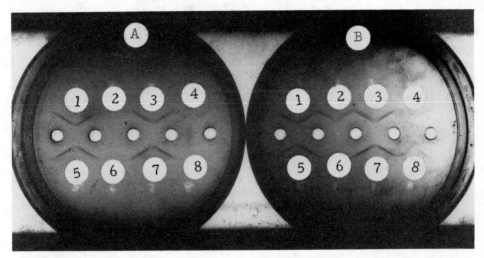

Fig.1. Double immunodiffusion in agar of some tissue extracts against guinea pig
antiserum to the FBP purified from CML cells. The center wells contain the antiserum and outer wells the tissue extracts. A: Wells 1, 3, 5 = CML lysate; 2 = colon
cancer; 4 = normal colon; 6 = gastric cancer; 7 = myelofibrosis spleen; 8 = normal
stomach. B: 1, 3, 5, 7 = CML lysate; 2 = lung cancer; 4 = normal lung; 6 = normal
breast; 8 = colon cancer.

The quantitative results of the RIA for the FBP in extracts of colon tumor, a my-

elofibrotic spleen and lung tumor are shown in Figure 2 and demonstrate the lack of

complete identity with the FBP prepared from CML cells which was used for the

standard dose-response curve because the smaller the volume of extract used, the

higher the concentration of FBP measured, indicating that the protein has lower

immunoreactivity for this rabbit antiserum than the CML-binding protein. In con-

trast, when two volumes of human serum were similarly assayed by RIA, the concen-

tration measured was the same, indicating that the protein measured in the serum is

immunologically the same as the FBP used for the standard curve (Figure 3).

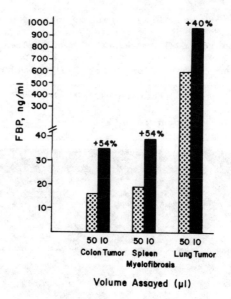

Fig. 2. Nonstoichiometric recovery of FBP in these tissue extracts when measured by RIA using a rabbit antiserum raised against the FBP from CML cells. The standards for this assay were the CML-binding protein.

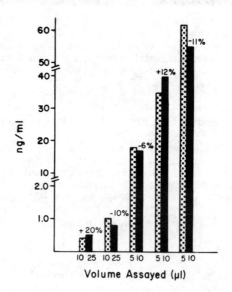

Fig. 3. Stoichiometric recovery of FBP in human serum when measured by this same RIA.

DISCUSSION

It has been previously reported that some serums from patients with a variety of disease processes characterized by cell injury or increased cell turnover contain a significantly higher concentration of FBP than serum from normal subjects when measured by RIA.[8] These studies now demonstrate that a FBP can also be identified in a variety of normal and neoplastic tissue extracts by the same RIA, but there appears to be immunologic differences between these proteins.

One of the basic requirements to assure the validity of any RIA is the proportional recovery of immunoreactive protein upon dilution of the sample being assayed.[9] If the concentration of the protein appears to increase when less sample is assayed, it indicates that the protein being measured is less immunoreactive than the standard FBP with the reagent antiserum, and is probably due to the recognition of slight structural differences by the immune mechanism of this rabbit. Other antiserums may not distinguish similar structural differences, and that may explain the distinct lines of identity with the CML binder observed for some of these tissues by immuno-diffusion against antiserum raised in a guinea pig using the same FBP purified from CML cells.

The significance of these findings is two-fold. Firstly, the concentration of the FBP in tissue extracts measured by this RIA will be underestimated. To determine the true concentration, it will be necessary to establish the dose-response curve with an immunologically-identical binding protein or use an antiserum which does not distinguish between the structural differences of these proteins. Secondly, it is potentially possible to exploit these slight differences in the structure of these pro-teins and develop a RIA which could specifically measure each of these binders. For this purpose, it will be necessary to raise specific antiserum by immunizing animals with FBP obtained from these tissues.

ACKNOWLEDGEMENTS

This work is supported by grants #CA-08976 and #AM-16220 from the National

Institutes of Health.

REFERENCES

1. da Costa, M. and Rothenberg, S. P. (1977) in The Year In Haematology 1977, Gordon, A. S., Silber, R. and Loboue, J. eds., Plenum Publishing Corp., pp 131-151.

2. Waxman, S. and Schreiber, C. (1975) Biochemistry, 14, 5422-5428.

3. Fischer, C., da Costa, M. and Rothenberg, S. P. (1978) Biochim. Biophys. Acta, in press.

4. Fischer, C., da Costa, M. and Rothenberg, S. P. (1975) Blood, 46, 855-867.

5. Colman, N., Pfeffer, D. and Herbert, V. (1977) Blood, 50 (Suppl 1), 91.

6. Colman, N. and Herbert, V. (1976) Blood, 48, 911-922.

7. Rothenberg, S. P. (1970) Proc. Soc. Exp. Biol. Med., 133, 428-432.

8. da Costa, M., Rothenberg, S. P., Fischer, C. and Rosenberg, Z. (1978) J. Lab. Clin. Med., 91, 901-910.

9. Yalow, S. R. and Berson, S. A. (1968) in Principles of Radioimmunassay In Radioisotopes In Medicine In Vitro Studies, Hayes, R. L., Goswitz, F. A. and Murphy, B. P. eds., U.S. Atomic Energy Commission, pp 7-41.

FOLATE METABOLISM IN LECTIN ACTIVATED
HUMAN PERIPHERAL BLOOD LYMPHOCYTES

PETER B. ROWE, EDITH TRIPP AND G.C. CRAIG
Department of Child Health, University of Sydney, N.S.W. AUSTRALIA 2006

ABSTRACT

The exposure of human peripheral blood lymphocytes to phytohemagg-
lutin (PHA) results in blastic transformation which occurs over the
time period 40-72 hours. The massive increase in protein and nucleic
acid synthesis coincides with the uptake of folic acid, aminoacids,
purines and pyrimidines from the incubation medium. There is an associated increase in both the total and specific activities of many
enzyme activities including those of the folate pathway enzymes. Transformation in folate-free medium indicated that certain folate-dependent
enzymatic reactions were preserved while others were considerably
impaired.

INTRODUCTION

The use of lectin-activated lymphocytes as a tool for the study of
mammalian biochemical pathways in general and the biochemistry of the
immune response in particular has gained widespread acceptance in
recent years[1]. Although observations have been made confirming the increase in many metabolic parameters in blastic cells including (i) the
synthesis of nucleic acids and their purine and pyrimidine precursors
(ii) the rate of glycolysis and Krebs cycle activity and (iii) the rate
of amino acid uptake and protein synthesis[2] only recently have more
detailed studies been made on the mechanisms whereby these occur.

While it has been known for many years that folic acid is an essential ingredient of media for mammalian cell culture and that transforming
lymphocytes rapidly accumulate folic acid derivatives, no detailed
systematic study has been made of the role of folate in the lectin-
activated human lymphocyte. In these studies we report our findings
with respect to the timing of cellular folate uptake in relation to (i)
the uptake of other metabolites and (ii) the increase in many different
enzymatic activities including those of the folate pathway. This report
is also concerned with the nature of the intracellular folates and with
the effects of cellular transformation in folate-free media.

MATERIALS AND METHODS

Human peripheral blood lymphocytes were isolated from buffy coats by
the Ficoll-Hypaque technique. These were cultured at a concentration
of 10^6 per ml in RPM1 1640 medium containing 10% fetal calf serum and

0.5μg per ml PHA. The detailed methodology for cell handling, enzyme extraction and isotope pulse studies will be discussed in detail else-where[3]. Metabolite analysis was performed by both thin layer and high pressure liquid chromatography.

RESULTS

Timing of Transformation - linked Metabolic Changes. As shown on Fig.1 the incorporation of glycine - 1 - ^{14}C into the lymphocytes only became significant after 40 hours exposure to PHA. Uptake curves for thymidine, deoxyuridine, hypoxanthine, formate, folate and serine were almost identical in terms of time of onset. Both the total and specific activities of a number of the folate pathway enzymes increased dramatically with blastic transformation (Table 1), the timing of this increase coinciding with the increased metabolite uptake. With specific activity levels there was a three to five-fold increase in the protein content of transformed cells. The changes in total activity of individual folate pathway enzymes was quite variable

Fig.1. The incorporation of glycine-1-^{14}C into (i) the acid soluble amino acid pool (●) and purine nucleotides (O) (ii) proteins (▲) (iii) nucleic acid (△) as a function of time of exposure of cells to PHA.

ranging from 140-fold for thymidylate synthetase to 9-fold for cyclohydrolase. The increases were generally of the order of 10 to 30-fold. A similar increase was observed for the activity of the de novo purine biosynthetic pathway while there was little alteration in the levels of the purine salvage enzymes HGPRTase and APRTase.

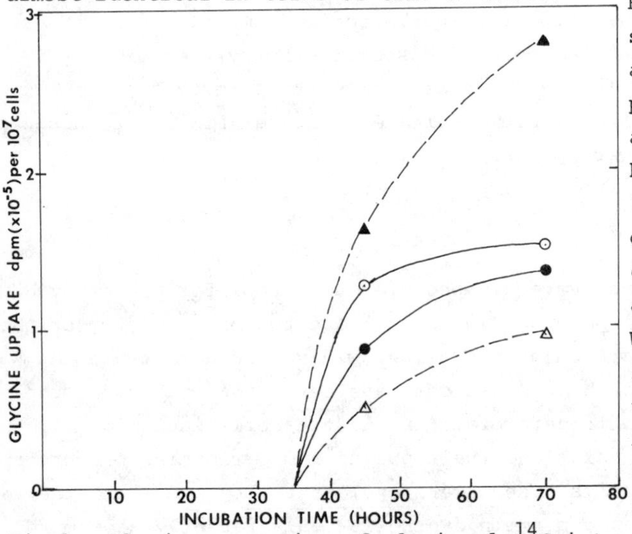

The kinetic parameters of two of the folate pathway enzymes were un-altered by blastic transformation of the cells. Serine transhydro-methylase exhibited Km's for serine and for FH$_4$* of 1.8mM and 0.1mM respectively while 10-formyl FH$_4$ synthetase had Km's for formate and

---

* The abbreviation FH$_4$ designates tetrahydrofolate.

FH_4 of 5.0mM and 0.18mM respectively. The activity of mixtures of enzymes extracted from resting and transformed cells was additive.

TABLE 1

TRANSFORMATION-LINKED CHANGES IN ENZYMATIC ACTIVITY.

ENZYME	ACTIVITY			
	Resting cells		Transformed Cells	
	Total [a]	Specific [a]	Total	Specific
10-FormylFH_4 synthetase	15.00	105.00	356.0	1263.0
MethyleneFH_4 dehydrogenase	9.60	66.20	197.0	699.0
Cyclohydrolase	51.00	352.00	450.0	1596.0
Serine transhydroxymethylase	17.40	120.00	192.0	681.0
Dihydrofolate reductase	2.40	16.50	68.0	241.0
FH_4methyltransferase	0.05	0.34	0.5	1.9
Thymidylate synthetase	0.09	0.62	12.5	44.3
Conjugase	0.55	2.75	6.1	10.2
Denovo purine synthetis	0.29	3.42	5.9	14.8
HGPRTase	80.00	234.00	190.0	130.0
APRTase	149.00	435.00	406.0	278.0

[a] Total activity is expressed as nmoles per hour per 10^7 cells while specific activity is nmoles per hour per mg protein.

Folate Uptake. The uptake of folate essentially paralleled the glycine uptake. Analysis of the radiolabelled folates after the addition of $3',5',7,9-^3$H-folate to the medium over the period 42-66 hours showed that the label was incorporated predominantly into heptaglutamate derivatives.

The effects of Cell Transformation in Folate-free medium. Cell viability and the extent of transformation in folate-free medium was generally less than that seen in complete medium. In addition a variable number of larger transformed cells was seen. There was little difference observed in the uptake of either folate or 5-methylFH_4 under conditions of folate deficiency.

A number of significant differences were noted in pulsed uptake studies of a series of different metabolites (Table 2). The most noticeable changes occurred with serine, leucine and deoxyuridine. There was a 75% reduction of incorporation of the 3-carbon of serine into acid soluble purine and pyrimidine nucleotides and into nucleic acid and a 45% reduction of incorporation of serine into proteins. The

TABLE 2

THE EFFECT OF FOLATE-FREE MEDIUM ON THE INCORPORATION OF RADIOLABELLED
METABOLITES

Cultures of 10^7 cells were pulsed with 10μCi of (i) glycine-1-^{14}C, 0.18
mM (ii) serine-3-^{14}C, 0.3mM (iii) ^{14}C-formate, 0.18mM (iv) leucine-1-
^{14}C 0.38mM (v) 6-^{3}H-deoxyuridine, 0.16μM (vi) methyl-^{3}H-thymidine 5μM
for the 64-68 hour time period of exposure to PHA.

| Metabolite | Medium[a] | Radioactivity incorporated into Cell Fractions[b] | | | |
		Free metabolites	Nucleotides	Nucleic Acid	Protein
Glycine	+	363,311	192,500	158,889	1,161,111
	−	306,472	146,667	152,778	977,778
Serine	+	54,083	1,747,778	4,381,667	1,347,500
	−	116,111	409,444	1,234,444	724,167
Formate	+	−	287,222	467,500	−
	−	−	271,944	281,111	−
Leucine	+	122,222	−	−	2,435,278
	−	116,111	−	−	1,283,383
Deoxyuridine	+	−	244,450	4,412,222	−
	−	−	296,389	1,955,556	−
Thymidine	+	−	70,278	1,347,590	−
	−	−	67,222	1,222,000	−

[a] Medium designation + or − indicates presence or absence of folate.
[b] Expressed as dpm per 10^7 viable transformed cells.

incorporation of leucine into protein was reduced to the same extent.
While the incorporation of deoxyuridine into acid-soluble pyrimidine
nucleotides was usually unaltered, 67% of the deoxyuridine was in the
form of dUMP in folate-deficient cells while control cells contained
almost entirely thymine nucleotides. Deoxyuridine incorporation into
nucleic acid was reduced by 56% in folate-free medium. The incorporation of thymidine into PCA soluble and nucleic acid fractions was
slightly but consistently reduced, of the order of 5% and 10% respectively. The glycine-1-^{14}C incorporation data showed a 16% reduction in
uptake into the free glycine pool and an equivalent drop in incorporation into protein. Despite a 24% decrease in glycine label in purine
nucleotides there was only a 4% decrease in nucleic acid label. The
differences in cell viability, morphology, and biochemical parameters
disappeared if folate were added after 40 hours.

The Effect of Folate-free Medium on Individual Enzymatic Activity. The amino acid uptake studies indicated that protein synthesis was decreased in cells in folate-free medium. The cell protein content was reduced by 20-25%. While the total activities of 10-formylFH$_4$ synthetase methyleneFH$_4$ dehydrogenase, serine transhydroxymethylase and FH$_4$ methyltransferase were reduced, cyclohydrolase, dihydrofolate reductase and thymidylate synthetase were relatively unaffected.

DISCUSSION

It would appear that additional folate was not required for the initial priming events in the transformation process but was essential for an optimal response after this. Whether this folate was required for optimal function of individual T or B cell populations demands further study. The reason for the additional folate requirement is not clear. As the transformed lymphocyte increases some 3 to 5 fold in volume, the uptake may represent an adaptive mechanism for maintaining physiological intracellular folate derivative concentrations. Alternatively, there may be increased folate cofactor breakdown under the stress of increased pathway cycling. The folate uptake studies indicated that the conversion to polyglutamates occured quite rapidly as the heptaglutamate derivative of FH$_4$ appeared to be the dominant compound. Despite this we have only had limited success synthesizing only diglutamate and triglutamate derivatives in in-vitro assay systems. The accumulation of FH$_4$ would be logical as the accumulation of 5-methylFH$_4$ would not be to the advantage of a cell with low FH$_4$ methyltransferase activity. Furthermore there was an absolute requirement for methionine in the medium for both cell viability and transformation.

The increase in both total and specific activity of the folate pathway enzymes was indicative of the pleiotropic effect of the lectin transformation mechanism on DNA transcription. This of course presumes that the increased activity was due to true induction and as yet we have no real proof of this. The activation mechanism was clearly quite variable and not only amongst the individual folate pathway enzymes. Furthermore the increase in enzyme activity could not be suppressed by the addition of product. Added thymidine, had no effect on the massive increase in thymidylate synthetase activity. The transformation-linked increase in activity of the enzymes 10-formylFH$_4$ synthetase, cyclohydrolase and methyleneFH$_4$ dehydrogenase was not the same despite the assignment of these activities to a single polypeptide chain in some mammalian species[4,5].

The uptake studies with serine showed that its major role was the donation of the 3-carbon atom for de novo purine synthesis and for the synthesis of TMP from dUMP. Despite the considerably decreased incorporation in folate-free medium, the radiolabel distribution between purines and pyrimidines remained the same, suggesting that the function of the enzyme common to both pathways was affected, serine transhydroxymethylase. While folate cofactor deficiency might be the underlying reason for this, the equivalent reduction in incorporation of leucine and serine into proteins would suggest that the transport mechanism for these aminoacids was affected.

In comparison there was relatively little effect on any parameter of glycine incorporation indicating that the glycine transport system was not disturbed unduly and that the folate-dependent reactions of the purine synthetic pathway were relatively normal.

The failure of methylation of dUMP in folate-free cells, together with the insignificant effect on the increased thymidylate synthetase under these conditions indicated that folate cofactor deficiency was responsible for the decreased incorporation of medium deoxyuridine into nucleic acid. The nucleic acid synthetic system appeared to be intact on the basis of the thymidine incorporation data.

SUMMARY

1. The lectin-induced transformation of human lymphocytes was associated with a massive increase in a wide range of metabolic parameters which were temporally very closely associated.
2. Transformation of the cells in folate-free medium demonstrated that, while folate was not required for the early events, it was clearly necessary later for the optimum response.
3. Transformation in folate-free medium highlighted (i) the differences in handling of different aminoacids and (ii) the relative sensitivity of thymidylate synthetase to folate deficiency.

REFERENCES.

1. Bernheim, J.L. and Mendelsohn, J. (1977) in Regulatory Mechanism in Lymphocyte Activation, Lucas, D.O. ed., Academic, New York pp 479-505.
2. O'Brien, R.L., Parker, J.W. and Dixon, J.F.P. (1978) in Progress in Molecular and Subcellular Biology, Hahn, F.E., Kersten, H., Kersten, W. and Szybalski, W. eds., Springer-Verlag, Berlin, pp 201-270.
3. Rowe, P.B. MS in preparation.
4. Paukert, J.L., Strauss, L.D. and Rabinowitz, J.C. (1976) J. Biol. Chem., 251, 5104-5111.
5. Tan, L.U., Drury, E.J. and MacKenzie, R.E. (1977) J. Biol. Chem. 252, 1117-1122.

FOLATE BINDING ACTIVITY IN EPITHELIAL BRUSH BORDER MEMBRANES. A SYSTEM FOR
INVESTIGATING MEMBRANE ASSOCIATED FOLATE BINDING PROTEINS *

JACOB SELHUB, ANNA C. GAY, AND IRWIN H. ROSENBERG
University of Chicago, Department of Medicine, 950 East 59th Street, Chicago,
Illinois   60637, U.S.A.

ABSTRACT

The subcellular distribution and properties of folate binding protein (FBP) in
homogenates of rat kidney and intestine were determined with a newly developed
assay for FBP in subcellular particulate fractions, based on selective trapping
of bound folates to cellulose-nitrate filters[1,2]. In both homogenates FBP is
present mostly in particulate fractions with highest enrichment in brush border
(BB) membranes. At pH 7.4 binding constants for PteGlu by folate-free BB membranes from intestine and kidney were 0.035 and 0.042 nM, respectively, whereas
affinities for 5-methylH_4PteGlu and methotrexate were lower under these conditions.
A novel feature of membrane-associated FBP is the observation that anions, particularly chloride ions, enhance the binding of PteGlu; this enhancement is most
pronounced at pH 6.0.

INTRODUCTION

The first description of FBP in membranes employed isolated villous cells from
rat intestine[3]. These cells were found capable of binding, but not transporting,
radioactive folic acid with radioactivity concentrated in the brush border membrane fraction[3]. Other demonstrations of membrane associated FBP include studies
of KB cells[4], L1210 cells[5], rat liver plasma membranes[6], and Lactobacillus casei
cells[7]. A FBP that may also be associated with plasma membranes was reported in
the particulate fraction of rabbit choroid plexus homogenates[8].

In none of these studies, however, was the determination of folate binding
carried out with isolated membranes. No binding of folates could be demonstrated
with isolated brush border membranes from villous cells.

The present study uses cellulose nitrate filters to analyze the distribution
and properties of FBP in brush border membranes of rat kidney and intestine[1,2],
two organs involved in folate transport and conservation.

MATERIALS AND METHODS

Kidneys and intestinal mucosal scrapings from Sprague-Dawley rats were each

*This work is supported by U.S. Public Health Service (National Institute of
Health) Grant AM-15351.

homogenized with 50 mM mannitol, treated with $CaCl_2$ and centrifuged at low speed
to remove cell debris ($Pellet_1$) then at higher speed to separate soluble fraction
(Supernate) from a second pellet ($Pellet_2$) which is enriched with brush border
membranes[1,9]. Pellets were resuspended in mannitol and the various fractions
were analyzed for protein[10], maltase as the BB membrane marker enzyme[11] and FBP
activity. The latter was determined after removing endogenous bound folate by
acidification to pH below 4.0 and centrifugation either as such (for pellet fractions) or after addition of albumin coated charcoal[1]. A sample (20-100 μg protein)
of these preparations was incubated with excess [³H]PteGlu (Amersham-Searle) in
0.05 M potassium phosphate buffer pH 7.2 for 30 min. at room temperature. Bound
radioactivity in insoluble fractions was determined after filtration through a
0.45 μ cellulose-nitrate filter (Schleicher and Schull) followed by washing the
filter with 10 ml of 0.025 M phosphate buffer. The filter was then dried and
assayed for radioactivity in toluene based scintillation fluid. For supernatant
fractions bound radioactivity was determined after treatment with coated charcoal
or after separation on Biogel P-10 columns[1].

RESULTS

Both homogenates of kidney and intestine contain folate binding activity which
is present mostly in the particulate fractions with highest enrichment in the
respective BB membrane fractions (Table 1). The amount and degree of enrichment
of FBP in the BB membrane fractions relative to the original homogenates closely
resembles the pattern of maltase, the BB membrane marker, indicating that the
binding protein is associated with these membranes

TABLE 1

FOLATE BINDING AND MALTASE ACTIVITY IN RAT KIDNEY AND INTESTINE HOMOGENATES
BEFORE AND AFTER FRACTIONATION

Fraction	Kidney			Intestine		
	Folate Binding[a]	Maltase[b]	Protein[c]	Folate Binding[a]	Maltase[b]	Protein[c]
Homogenate	5.4	0.12	140	0.084	0.12	106
$Pellet_1$	7.5	0.15	60	0.103	0.10	55
$Supernate_2$	0.8	0.02	68	0.029	0.03	36
BB Membranes	45	1.10	5.3	0.560	1.38	3.4

[a] pmoles bound/mg protein.
[b] μmoles/min/mg protein.
[c] Total mg protein from 1 g tissue.

For acid-treated BB membranes from kidney and intestine, the binding of [^{3}H]PteGlu is saturable with K_b equal to 0.035 and 0.04 nM, respectively (Fig. 1). The affinities for 5-methyl1H$_4$PteGlu and methotrexate as determined by competition studies with [^{3}H]PteGlu at neutral pH are 3-5 and 30 fold, respectively, lower than for PteGlu[1,2].

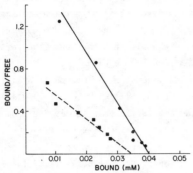

Fig. 1. Scatchard plots of [^{3}H]PteGlu binding by acid-treated BB membranes from kidney (solid line) and intestine (broken line).

Recent studies in this laboratory indicate that FBP's in the BB membranes possess an additional site with affinity for anions, particularly chloride ions, which regulates the binding of folates. For PteGlu this regulation is seen as enhanced binding in the presence of chloride ions and as shifts of peak activities to lower pH optima (pH optima shifted from 7.6 for the kidney FBP to 6.75, and from 7.2 and 7.7 for the intestine FBP to 6.2 and 7.3, respectively). In both kidney and intestine the maximum effect of chloride ions is observed at pH 6.0.

DISCUSSION

The methodology used here allows direct study of FBP in isolated membranes. In both kidney and intestine the properties of the BB membrane associated FBP are similar to the high affinity folate binders found in milk, plasma, and other tissues[8,13]. This is in contrast to the studies with isolated villous cells[3] mentioned above where the binding constant for PteGlu is reported to be in the order of 10^{-5}M, rather than the 10^{-11}M as determined with isolated BB membranes.

This discrepancy in binding constants could reflect the existence of low and high affinity FBP. However, in light of the stability of the FBP-folate complex, obtained from villous cells preincubated with folates, particularly in regard to SDS treatment[3], it is likely that the same FBP is responsible for the demonstrated folate binding by cells and isolated membranes. Differences in binding constants could derive from lower accessibility of folates to FBP in cells due to saturation with endogenous folates, damage during hyaluronidase treatment,

596

lower pH (acid microclimate) at the membrane surface[14], or to a combination of
these factors.

Since they lack any known enzymatic or structural function, and in view of
their location in the brush border membrane fraction, these FBP's are likely candidates for a role in the folate transporting system. The observed regulation of
folate binding by anions may provide the link between binding and transport.
Both anion effects and transport by the intestine are maximum at pH 6.0 (Fig. 2
and Ref. 15, 16) and decrease sharply at higher pH. The participation of anions
in folate transport has been recently suggested by Goldman[17] who showed that
influx of 5-methylH_4PteGlu and methotrexate into Ehrlich ascite tumor cells is
inhibited when chloride ions are partially or totally replaced by other anions.
Oscillation between high and low affinity states of FBP from BB membranes as
indicated here, is analogous to the folate transporting system and membrane
associated-FBP in L. casei cells where the two states are regulated by an oxidoreduction step (instead of anions)[18]. This possibility is now being considered
in our laboratory.

REFERENCES

1. Selhub, J. and Rosenberg, I.H. (1978) Proc. Nat. Acad. Sci., 75, 3090-3093.

2. Selhub, J., Gay, A.C. and Rosenberg I.H. (1978) Gastroenterology, 74, 1144.

3. Leslie, G.I. and Rowe, P.B. (1972) Biochemistry, 11, 1696-1703.

4. McHugh, M.M. and Cheng, Y. (1977) Fed. Proc., 36, 992.

5. McCormick, J.I., Rader, J.I. and Freisheim, J.H. (1977) Fed. Proc. 36, 804.

6. Zamierowski, M.M. and Wagner, C. (1977) J. Biol. Chem., 252, 933-938.

7. Henderson, G.B., Zevely, E.M. and Huennekens, F.M. (1977) J. Biol. Chem,
    252, 3760-3765.

8. Spector, R. (1977) J. Biol. Chem., 252, 3364-3370.

9. Schmitz, J., Preiser, H., Maestracci, O., Gosh, B.K., Cerda, J. and Crane,
    R.K. (1973) Biochim. Biophys. Acta, 323, 98-112.

10. Lowry, O.H., Rosebrough, N.J., Farr, A.L. and Randall, R.J. (1951) J. Biol.
    Chem., 193, 265-275.

11. Dhalqvist, A. (1964) Anal. Biochem., 7, 18-25.

12. Documenta Geigy, Scientific Tables (1973) Diem, K., and Lentner, C. eds.,
    Ciba-Geigy Lim, Basel, Switzerland, pp. 280-283.

13. Rothenberg, S.P. and da Costa, M. (1976) Clinics in Haematology, 5, 569-587.

14. Lucas, M.L. and Blair, J.A. (1978) Proc. R. Soc. Lond., A 200, 27-41.

15. Russell, R.M., Dhar, G.J., Dutta, S.K. and Rosenberg, I.H., J. Lab. Clin.
    Med. (In press).

16. Strum, W.B. (1977) J. Pharmacol. Exp. Therap. 203, 640-645.

17. Goldman, I.D. (1977), in Membrane Toxicity, Miller, M.W. and Shamos, A.E.
    eds., Plenum Press, New York, pp. 85-113.

18. Huennekens, F.M. and Henderson, G.B. (1976) in Chemistry and Biology of
    Pteridines, Pfleiderer, W., ed., Walter de Gruyter, Berlin, pp. 179-196.

STRUCTURAL SPECIFICITY OF FOLATE ANALOG TRANSPORT AND BINDING TO
DIHYDROFOLATE REDUCTASE IN MURINE TUMOR AND NORMAL CELLS: RELEVANCE
TO THERAPEUTIC EFFICACY

F.M. SIROTNAK, P.L. CHELLO, J.R. PIPER, J.A. MONTGOMERY AND J.I. DEGRAW
Memorial Sloan-Kettering Cancer Center, New York, NY 10021, Southern
Research Institute, Birmingham, AL 35205, and Stanford Research
Institute, Menlo Park, CA 94025 (U.S.A.)

ABSTRACT

Structure-activity relationships for transport and dihydrofolate reductase inhibition in murine tumor and intestinal epithelial cells for
a group of folates and analogs are presented. Positions 1, 3, 4, 5 and
8 and the α-carboxyl group are specified for enzyme binding, but position 10 and the γ-carboxyl group are not; positions 4, 5, 8 and 10 and
both α- and γ-carboxyl groups are specified for influx, but not positions 1 and 3; positions 5 and 8 and the γ-carboxyl group are specified
for efflux, but not position 4 or 10 (positions 1 and 3 and the α-
carboxyl group were not evaluated). Differences in specificity between
normal and tumor cells for the 10 position involving transport, but not
enzyme inhibition, are revealed, which appear to explain differences in
selective antitumor action among analogs.

INTRODUCTION

For anticancer agents requiring carrier-mediation for effective penetration into cells, there are at least two separate structural requirements which must be satisfied before a cytotoxic effect is obtained -
one for the carrier and one for an intracellular binding site. In the
case of folate analogs, the latter is the target enzyme, dihydrofolate
reductase. The specificity of the carrier transport system and the intracellular target site may be distinctly different. For folate analogs, some differences have already been well documented in murine tumor tissues[1-3]. Since differences in the specificity of membrane

transport between tumor and normal proliferative tissues appear to account[1-3] for the selective antitumor effects observed with specific analogs, our initial evaluation of the relative structural-specificity for transport and dihydrofolate reductase inhibition has been expanded.

MATERIALS AND METHODS

The source and preparation of the murine ascites tumor cells and intestinal epithelial cells used for transport experiments and dihydrofolate reductase isolation and inhibition assays have been described[1-4]. Kinetic analysis of drug transport and competition by structural analogs was performed[2] following unidirectional influx and efflux measurements carried out at 37°C in a buffered salts solution (pH 7.4). Drug content of cells was assayed by radioactive counting of labeled drug or directly by enzyme assay[4].

RESULTS AND DISCUSSION

Two features of the folate molecule are of crucial importance to enzyme binding and transport in L1210 cells (Tables 1-4): the type of substituent at position 4 of the pteridine ring and the number or location of free carboxyl groups on the glutamyl moiety. Substitution of an amino for the OXO group at position 4 increases enzyme binding 6 orders of magnitude. Also, only a free α-carboxyl group is necessary for effective binding. The same substitution increases influx by the transport system by 2 orders of magnitude, but influx is decreased if there is only one free carboxyl group. Specificities for the primary ring system (Table 1) are in the order quinazoline (qn) > pteridine (ptr) ≃ pyrimidine (pyr) >> purine (pur) for enzyme inhibition; ptr > qn >> pyr ≃ pur for influx; and ptr > pyr >> qn for efflux.

Some 2,4-diamino folates are compared in Table 2. N → C replacement at positions 1 and 3 decreased enzyme binding, but at position 8 increased binding and at position 10 had no effect. Alkyl substitution at position 10 or halogenation (positions 3' and 5') of the benzene ring (data not shown) had no effect on binding. Substitution at the

TABLE 1

STRUCTURE-ACTIVITY RELATIONSHIPS FOR L1210 CELL DIHYDROFOLATE REDUCTASE
INHIBITION AND MEMBRANE TRANSPORT INVOLVING 2,4-DIAMINO FOLATE ANALOGS

Primary ring system	FAH_2 reductase inhibition[a] K_i (nM)	influx[b] K_m (μM)	K_i[c] (μM)	efflux k (min^{-1})
pteridine	0.0032	1.22	1.41	0.249
quinazoline	0.0006	5.65	4.86	0.034
pyrimidine	0.0041	102.00	78.21	0.147
purine	10,100.0	–	132.83	–

[a]Method of Henderson (Biochem. J., 135:101-107, 1973) for titration inhibitors otherwise from Lineweaver-Burk or Dixon plots). SD $\leq$ 33% (n = 3-5).
[b]Values for V_{max} are identical since these are competing analogs. For the same reason $K_m \simeq K_i$. SD $\leq$ 22% (n = 3-5).
[c]K_i determined from Lineweaver-Burk or Dixon plots during measurements of competitive inhibition of [^{3}H]methotrexate uptake.

TABLE 2

STRUCTURE-ACTIVITY RELATIONSHIPS FOR L1210 CELL DIHYDROFOLATE REDUCTASE
INHIBITION AND MEMBRANE TRANSPORT INVOLVING PTERIDINE FOLATE ANALOGS

R_1 (4)	R_2 (1)	R_3 (3)	R_4 (8)	R_5 (10)	R_6 (10')	R_7 α	R_8 γ	FAH_2 reductase inhibition[a] K_i (nM)	influx[b] K_m (μM)	K_i[c] (μM)	efflux k (min^{-1})
OH	N	N	N	N	H	OH	OH	1982.0	–	228.0	–
OH	N	N	CH	N	H	OH	OH	1207.30	–	51.9	–
NH_2	N	N	N	N	H	OH	OH	0.0032	1.2	1.4	0.24
NH_2	N	N	N	N	CH_3	OH	OH	0.0043	3.3	3.5	0.23
NH_2	N	N	N	N	C_2H_5	OH	OH	0.0039	3.8	–	0.25
NH_2	CH	N	N	N	CH_3	OH	OH	338.50	–	1.9	–
NH_2	N	CH	N	N	CH_3	OH	OH	31.10	–	3.5	0.21
NH_2	N	N	N	CH	H	OH	OH	0.0021	1.9	1.6	0.21
NH_2	N	N	N	O	–	OH	OH	–[d]	3.28	3.5	0.23

(continued)

NH$_2$	N	N	N	N	H	OH	glu	0.0041	18.9	–	0.24
NH$_2$	N	N	N	N	CH$_3$	OH	glu	0.0037	49.3	–	0.22
NH$_2$	N	N	N	N	CH$_3$	OH	NH$_2$	0.0027	9.4	8.4	0.15
NH$_2$	N	N	N	N	CH$_3$	OH	NHCH$_3$	0.0027	27.6	–	0.21
NH$_2$	N	N	N	N	CH$_3$	OH	NH(CH$_3$)$_2$	0.0039	48.4	–	0.26
NH$_2$	N	N	N	N	CH$_3$	OH	NH(C$_5$H$_{11}$)	0.0035	16.9	16.8	0.26
NH$_2$	N	N	N	N	CH$_3$	OH	NHCH$_2\phi$	0.0036	3.6	3.8	0.19
NH$_2$	N	N	N	N	CH$_3$	OH	asp	0.0028	>300.0	–	–
NH$_2$	N	N	N	N	CH$_3$	OH	gly	0.0029	3.9	–	2.1
NH$_2$	N	N	N	N	CH$_3$	glu	OH	170.1	–	61.0	–
NH$_2$	N	N	N	N	CH$_3$	asp	OH	208.4	–	146.2	–
NH$_2$	N	N	N	N	CH$_3$	gly	OH	208.2	–	66.6	–

a,b,cSee footnotes in Table 1.   d= methotrexate (estimated from intracellular binding).

α-carboxyl group reduced binding ~200-fold. There was little effect by a N → C replacement at positions 1, 3 or 10, by an N → O replacement at position 10 or halogenation of the benzene ring (data not shown). However, influx was increased by a N → C replacement at position 8 and decreased by alkyl substitution at position 10. Substitution at either time the α- or γ-carboxyl group reduced influx in a substituent specific manner. Efflux was unaffected by N → C or O replacements, alkyl substitution at position 10, or halogenation at positions 3' and 5'. With the exception of the γ-amine derivative, none of the other amide or peptide derivatives evaluated had an altered efflux. Influx and, to a smaller extent, efflux of folate analogs were less (Table 3) in intestinal epithelium than in Ll210 cells. In addition, the effect on influx by N → C replacement, or alkyl substitution at position 10 was greater. The latter observation serves to explain[1,3] the selective action of these agents in murine tumor models. In addition, the influx of natural folates is also less in these normal cells. Influx of 5-substituted-reduced derivatives was 50- to 100-fold greater than folate in Ll210 cells, but only 5-fold greater in epithelial cells. Influx of these natural folates into other murine tumor cells was similar[2] to that seen in L1210 cells, although the influx of methotrexate into these cells was quite different[2].

TABLE 3

STRUCTURE-ACTIVITY RELATIONSHIPS FOR DIHYDROFOLATE REDUCTASE INHIBITION AND MEMBRANE TRANSPORT IN L1210 CELLS AND MURINE INTESTINAL EPITHELIAL CELLS INVOLVING FOLATES AND PTERIDINE FOLATE ANALOGS

				L1210 Cells				Epithelial Cells			
				FAH_2 reductase inhibition[a]	transport			FAH_2 reductase inhibition[a]	influx[b,d]		efflux
R_1	R_2	R_3	R_4	K_i (nM)	influx[b,d] K_m (μM)	K_i^c (μM)	efflux k (min^{-1})	K_i (nM)	K_m (μM)	K_i^c (μM)	k (min^{-1})
OH	–	N	H	1920.0	–	228.0	–	>100.0	–	1769	–
OH	CH_3[e]	N	H	2400.0	–	1.7	–	>100.0	–	318	–
OH	CHO[e]	N	H	2100.0	–	4.4	–	>100.0	–	328	–
NH_2	–	N	H	0.0031	1.2	1.4	0.24	0.0021	7.2	–	0.09
NH_2	–	N	CH_3	0.0043	3.3	3.5	0.23	0.0029	87.1	–	0.08
NH_2	–	N	C_2H_5	0.0039	3.8	–	0.23	0.0024	123.8	–	0.07
NH_2	–	CH	H	0.0036	1.8	1.8	0.22	0.0022	35.2	–	0.08

a,b,cSee footnotes in Table 1. dValues for V_{max} are similar for each cell type. eReduced derivatives with H atoms at position 6, 7 and 8 (racemic mixture, d $\simeq$ ℓ form).

Some quinazoline analogs of aminopterin are compared in Table 4. The 2-amino-4-oxy derivative is a poor inhibitor of dihydrofolate reductase and is poorly transported as is folate itself. Substitution of the L-glutamyl moiety by L-aspartate, D-glutamate or D-aspartate reduces binding to the enzyme. However, substitution of methyl or chlorine at position 5 increases binding, particularly for the L-aspartyl derivative. Influx by L1210 cells of the aspartyl derivatives is markedly reduced compared to the glutamyl derivative, but in both series influx is increased by methyl or chlorine substitution at position 5. Influx of the D-glutamyl derivative is slower than the L-glutamyl derivative, but the reverse is true for the D- and L-aspartyl derivatives. Efflux of the D-glutamyl and D-aspartyl derivatives was more rapid than the corresponding L forms. However, efflux was slower for the 5-substituted *versus* the unsubstituted derivatives.

TABLE 4

STRUCTURE-ACTIVITY RELATIONSHIPS FOR L1210 CELL DIHYDROFOLATE REDUCTASE INHIBITION AND MEMBRANE TRANSPORT INVOLVING QUINAZOLINE FOLATE ANALOGS

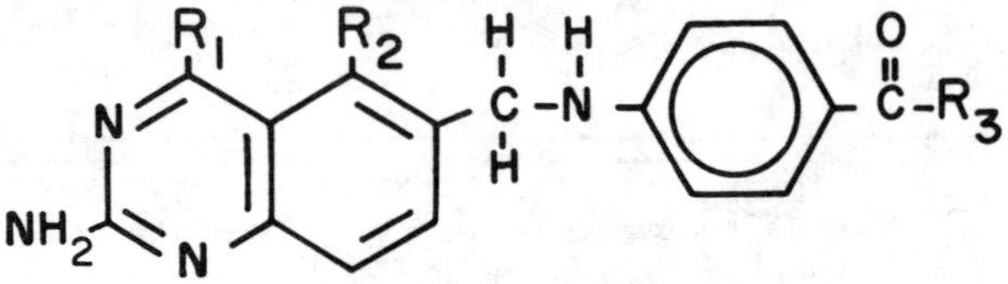

R_1	R_2	R_3	FAH_2 reductase inhibition[a] K_i (nM)	transport: influx[b] K_m (μM)	transport: influx[b] K_i[c] (μM)	transport: efflux k (min^{-1})
OH	H	L-glu	>100.0	-	>20.0	-
NH_2	H	L-glu	0.0006	5.65	4.8	0.034
NH_2	CH_3	L-glu	0.0004	4.76	-	0.027
NH_2	Cl	L-glu	0.0001	2.23	-	0.011
NH_2	H	D-glu	0.0314	45.70	-	0.047
NH_2	H	L-asp	0.0132	30.70	-	0.019
NH_2	CH_3	L-asp	0.0009	21.82	23.9	0.017
NH_2	Cl	L-asp	0.0003	18.74	-	0.018
NH_2	H	D-asp	0.0423	6.13	-	0.053

[a,b,c]See footnotes in Table 1.

ACKNOWLEDGEMENTS

Supported in part by NCI grants CA 08748, CA 18856 and CA 22764 and ACS grant CH26.

REFERENCES

1. Sirotnak, F.M. and Donsbach, R.C. (1975) Cancer Res., 35, 1737-1744.
2. Sirotnak, F.M. and Donsbach, R.C. (1976) Cancer Res., 36, 1151-1158.
3. Chello, P.L., Sirotnak, F.M., Dorick, D.M. and Donsbach, R.C. (1977) Cancer Res., 37, 4297-4303.
4. Sirotnak, F.M. and Donsbach, R.C. (1972) Cancer Res., 32, 2120-2126.

THE EFFECTS OF THYROXINE ON FOLATE AND HISTIDINE METABOLISM

E.L.R. STOKSTAD, MARGARET MAY-SHENG CHAN AND J.E. BLOOMER[*]
Department of Nutritional Sciences, 119 Morgan Hall, University of
California, Berkeley, California 94720 (USA)

ABSTRACT

The effects of thyroxine in producing a pseudo-vitamin B_{12}
deficiency and increasing FIGlu excretion were studied. Rats maintained
on a soy protein diet low in methionine and supplemented with
vitamin B_{12} excreted a moderate amount of FIGlu. This was increased by
giving high levels of thyroxine. Thyroidectomy markedly reduced FIGlu
excretion and also increased the oxidation of $2\text{-}^{14}C$-histidine to $^{14}CO_2$.
Thyroidectomy increased the proportion of tetrahydrofolates in the
liver with a corresponding decrease in the methyltetrahydrofolates.
Thyroidectomy decreased methylenetetrahydrofolic acid reductase in the
liver and addition of thyroid powder to the intact rat increased this
enzyme to higher than normal levels.

INTRODUCTION

The feeding of thyroid powder is known to increase the requirement
for vitamin B_{12}[1,2,3], and to increase the excretion of formimino-
glutamic acid (FIGlu)[4,5,6]. The latter can be restored to normal by
the feeding of methionine[4]. The experiments described here deal with
a study of the effects of hypothyroidism (produced by thyroidectomy)
and hyperthyroidism on the metabolism of folic acid and folate-
dependent enzymes.

MATERIALS AND METHODS

Thyroidectomized and intact albino male weanling rats of the
Sprague-Dawley strain weighing about 50 g were individually caged and
three assigned to each of the six experimental groups which are
described in Table 1. A low-methionine (0.2%) basal diet[6] based on
20% soy assay protein was used which was supplemented with 50 µg
vitamin B_{12} and 5 mg folic acid per kg, together with adequate amounts
of the other known vitamins. Thyroxine (T_4) was administered as
indicated by injection every other day to give an average daily dose
of 2.5 µg/day. This would correspond to the euthyroid state.

[*] Deceased.

In group 6, hyperthyroidism was produced by injecting the equivalent of 100 µg/day. At 20 days, the treatment of half of the groups was changed, and thyroxine administration was either discontinued or initiated as indicated in Table 1.

TABLE 1

DIETARY REGIMENS AND EFFECTS OF THYROXINE (T_4) ON FOLIC ACID METABOLISM

	Thyroidectomized				Intact	
	Grp 1	Grp 2	Grp 3	Grp 4	Grp 5	Grp 6
Days 1-20	−	−	+[a]	+[a]	−	−
Days 21-41	−	+[a]	+[a]	−	−	+++[b]
Body wt. (Day 38), g	88	93	165	125	202	205
% Hepatic uptake of ip ^{3}H-PteGlu	33	16	24	25	29	17
% H$_4$PteGlu[c]	56	38	38	46	37	32

[a] T_4 at 2.5 µg/day.   [b] T_4 at 100 µg/day.

[c] % H$_4$PteGlu = (H$_4$PteGlu/5-CH$_3$-H$_4$PteGlu + H$_4$PteGlu) x 100.

Urine samples were collected and FIGlu measured by the method of Tabor and Wyngarden[7]. Histidine oxidation was measured by injecting 1 µCi 2-^{14}C-histidine per animal, together with 1 µmol of cold histidine per g body weight, and placing the animal in a small respiration chamber. The expired $^{14}CO_2$ was trapped in a 1:1 mixture of ethanolamine and ethyleneglycolmonomethyl ether for two 1.5-hour periods and the radioactivity counted using the scintillating fluid described by Jeffay and Alvarez[8]. All animals were given an ip injection of 25 µCi of a purified ^{3}H-PteGlu (0.5 nmol) 24 hours before they were sacrificed on day 41. The livers were homogenized in 5% ascorbate solution (pH 4.2) and polyglutamate forms of folate were hydrolyzed by autolysis at 37°C for 3 hours. Tritium was measured in the supernatant of the liver homogenate to estimate the hepatic uptake of the ^{3}H-PteGlu dose. Distribution of the single-carbon substituent forms of folic acid in the autolyzed liver was carried out using QAE-Sephadex A25 column chromatography. Hepatic 5,10-methylene-H$_4$PteGlu reductase activity was measured using the method of Kutzbach and Stokstad[9].

RESULTS AND DISCUSSION

The results of the various treatments on FIGlu excretion are shown in Figure 1. Intact control rats were found to excrete approx. 320 μmol of FIGlu/day/kg body weight (Fig. 1, group 5). Thyroidectomy (group 1) reduced FIGlu excretion to very low levels (< 10 μmol/kg/day). Addition of a replacement level of thyroxine to the thyroidectomized animals from the beginning of the experiment (group 3) increased FIGlu excretion to ca. 200 μmol/kg/day which is 60% of that of the intact rat. Addition of thyroxine to the thyroidectomized animal at 20 days (group 2) slowly increased FIGlu excretion so that by 33 days it equalled the group which had received thyroxine for the entire period (group 3). Addition of 100 μg thyroxine to the intact animals (at 20 days) increased FIGlu excretion to 1300 μmol at 28 days. This high value decreased to 900 μmol at 33 days.

The effect of thyroxine on histidine oxidation to respiratory CO_2 (Fig. 2) demonstrated an opposite picture to that of urinary FIGlu. The $^{14}CO_2$ expired in 3 hours from an injected dose of histidine increased from 7% in intact controls at 20 days (group 5) to 46% three weeks after thyroidectomy (group 1). Intact animals given excess thyroxine at 100 μg/rat/day from day 20 showed a marked decrease in $^{14}CO_2$ production to 2% by day 35 (group 6). Thyroxine replacement at 2.5 μg/rat/day beginning at day 0 prevented the elevation in $^{14}CO_2$ production (group 3), and administration of thyroxine at the same dosage three weeks after thyroidectomy led to a reduction in ^{14}C-histidine oxidation from 46% to 19% within 3 days (group 2). Discontinuation of thyroxine administration in group 4 on day 20 resulted in a gradual rise in $^{14}CO_2$ production from 17% to 33% within 2 weeks while the $^{14}CO_2$ level remained at the high level of 45% in the untreated thyroidectomized rats (group 1).

These results show that thyroidectomy increases the oxidation of histidine to CO_2 and decreases its excretion as FIGlu. This is similar to the effect of methionine in reducing FIGlu excretion when added to a methionine-low diet[5,10].

The proportion of $H_4PteGlu$ to total folates was determined, as this would provide a measure of the folate forms capable of functioning in the folate-dependent enzymes involved in the degradation of FIGlu. When liver is autolyzed to hydrolyze folic acid polyglutamates, and the folates separated on QAE-Sephadex, two major peaks are obtained. The first is predominantly $CH_3-H_4PteGlu$ and the second is $H_4PteGlu$.

606

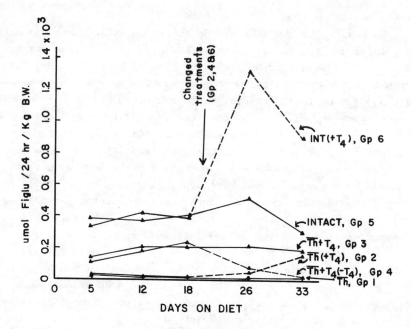

Fig. 1. Effect of thyroxine (T_4) on urinary FIGlu excretion expressed as µmol/day/kg body weight.

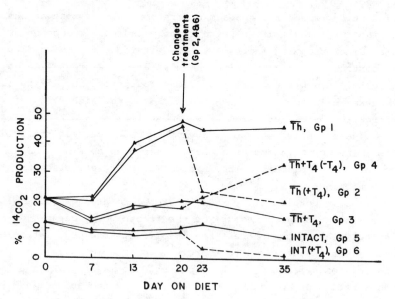

Fig. 2. Effect of thyroxine (T_4) on percent oxidation of injected 2-^{14}C-histidine to respiratory [14]CO_2 in 3 hours.

The results of this analysis, shown in Table 1, are expressed as the percentage of H_4PteGlu to total folates (H_4PteGlu + CH_3-H_4PteGlu). In the intact rat (group 5), H_4PteGlu constitutes 37% of the total folate. Thyroidectomy increases the proportion of H_4PteGlu to 56%. This increase in the proportion of H_4PteGlu is consistent with the observed increase in the rate of oxidation of 2-C of histidine to CO_2 and the decreased excretion of FIGlu. Addition of thyroxine at 20 days reduces the H_4PteGlu level to 38%, which is the same as that for the intact animal (37%). Addition of 100 µg of thyroxine which induces hyperthyroidism reduces the H_4PteGlu level to 32% which was accompanied by a marked increase in FIGlu excretion (Fig. 1, group 6). This reduced level of H_4PteGlu in hyperthyroidism is consistent with the observed increase in FIGlu excretion produced by feeding thyroid powder. This increase in H_4PteGlu level with a corresponding increase in histidine oxidation is similar to the effect of methionine in the perfused liver in increasing the proportion of H_4PteGlu and increasing the oxidation of 2-^{14}C-histidine to $^{14}CO_2$ (Buehring et al.)[11].

Methylenetetrahydrofolic acid reductase activity (Table 2) was reduced by thyroidectomy (group 1) to 38% of the level in intact rats (group 5). Administration of a replacement level (2.5 µg) of thyroxine to the thyroidectomized animals (group 2) raised the enzyme level to normal. Addition of 3 g thyroid powder to the diet of the normal rat, which induces hyperthyroidism, produces a 55% increase in enzyme level.

TABLE 2

EFFECT OF THYROXINE (T_4) ON METHYLENETETRAHYDROFOLATE REDUCTASE

	Thyroidectomized		Intact	
	−	T_4[a]	−	TP[b]
Body wt. (Day 33), g	93	138	158	117
FIGlu (Day 26)[c]	3	255	487	1670
Liver MR (Day 33)[d]	380	990	1010	1560

[a] T_4 at 2.5 µg/day.   [b] Thyroid powder (TP) at 3 g/kg diet.

[c] µmol FIGlu/24 hr/kg body wt.

[d] MR (5,10-methylene-H_4PteGlu reductase) activity as nmol H^{14}CHO formed/hr/g liver wet weight.

608

The reduction in methylenetetrahydrofolic acid reductase provides a metabolic basis for the effect of thyroidectomy in reducing FIGlu excretion and increasing the oxidation of histidine. A reduced activity of this enzyme would decrease the formation of $CH_3-H_4PteGlu$ and thereby increase the proportion of $H_4PteGlu$. This is in accord with the observed increased proportion of $H_4PteGlu$ as shown in Table 1. This effect is similar to the action of methionine in increasing histidine oxidation[6,7,10,11] and can be accounted for by its conversion to S-adenosylmethionine which inhibits methylenetetrahydrofolic acid reductase[9].

Similarly, the effect of thyroid powder in increasing the level of this enzyme to higher than normal is consistent with its effect in increasing FIGlu excretion. Vitamin B_{12} could counter this effect by promoting the synthesis of methionine which after conversion to S-adenosylmethionine would inhibit methylenetetrahydrofolic acid reductase. These observations provide a partial explanation for the observed relationship between thyroxine, vitamin B_{12}, and methionine.

ACKNOWLEDGEMENT

This work was supported in part by USPHS grant no. AM08171 from the National Institutes of Health.

REFERENCES

1. Betheil, J.J. and Lardy, H.A. (1949) J. Nutr., 37, 495-509.

2. Register, U.D., Ruegamer, W.R. and Elvehjem, C.A. (1949) J. Biol. Chem., 177, 129-134.

3. Lewis, U.J., Tappan, D.V., Register, U.D. and Elvehjem, C.A. (1950) Proc. Soc. Exp. Biol. Med., 74, 568-571.

4. Stokstad, E.L.R., Webb, R.S. and Shah, E. (1966) Proc. Soc. Exp. Biol. Med., 123, 752-754.

5. Odell, Amy and Stokstad, E.L.R. (1967) J. Nutr., 92, 127-132.

6. Batra, K.K., Buehring, U. and Stokstad, E.L.R. (1974) Proc. Soc. Exp. Biol. Med., 147, 72-79.

7. Tabor, H. and Wyngarden, L. (1958) J. Clin. Invest., 37, 824-828.

8. Jeffay, H. and Alvarez, J. (1961) Anal. Chem., 33, 12-15.

9. Kutzbach, Carl and Stokstad, E.L.R. (1967) Biochim. Biophys. Acta, 139, 217-220.

10. Brown, D.D., Silva, O.L., Gardiner, R.C. and Silverman, M. (1960) J. Biol. Chem., 235, 2058-2062.

11. Buehring, K.U., Batra, K.K., and Stokstad, E.L.R. (1972) Biochim. Biophys. Acta, 279, 498-512.

ENTEROHEPATIC CIRCULATION OF FOLATES:

I. pH-DEPENDENT INTESTINAL TRANSPORT

WILLIAMSON B. STRUM

Scripps Clinic and Research Foundation, 10666 North Torrey Pines Road,
La Jolla, California 92037

ABSTRACT

The proximal small intestine of the rat can transport folate and
amethopterin against a concentration gradient, apparently by a common
transport system that is pH-dependent, energy-dependent, saturable,
sensitive to temperature, Na^+-dependent, and probably regulated by the
cyclic nucleotide system. The recognition of a marked pH-sensitivity
of the transport system permits further studies to be accomplished
under optimum conditions. An understanding of the details of the
transport system will hopefully lead to methods that will prevent
intestinal toxicity from antifolate cancer chemotherapy.

INTRODUCTION

The mechanism of intestinal transport of folate compounds has been
clarified in recent years by the demonstration of a pH-dependent,
carrier-mediated transport process in rat proximal intestine[1,2,3].
Much of the current interest in intestinal transport of folates is a
reflection of the toxicity to intestinal cells which often results
from antifolate chemotherapy. The folate antagonists, of which amethopterin (methotrexate) is the best known example, block cell replication and are especially toxic to the rapidly dividing non-malignant
intestinal cells. Animal studies have shown that amethopterin accumulates in intestinal mucosa[4] and that the toxicity appears to be related
to the duration of inhibition of DNA synthesis which reflects the persistence of exchangeable drug levels in tissue adequate for complete
inhibition of its target enzyme dihydrofolate reductase[5]. If interaction of amethopterin with dihydrofolate reductase in intestinal
mucosa could be minimized or if the delivery of the drug to these cells
could be manipulated selectively, intestinal toxicity might be controlled. The transport system which determines entry of amethopterin
and other folate compounds into intestinal cells provides a target for
regulatory processes which can control the flow of folate compounds
into these cells to the advantage of the host.

The work from this laboratory has been directed toward determining ways to alleviate intestinal toxicity from antifolate chemotherapy by exploiting the transport system. The studies were carried out with everted sacs of rat intestine using amethopterin as the substrate. In some instances corollary information has been obtained using folate.

GENERAL CHARACTERISTICS

The mucosa-to-serosa transport of amethopterin and folate in rat jejunum is markedly pH-dependent[1,2,3]. Representative data showing the effect of pH on the time-dependent rate of amethopterin transport are shown in Figure 1. The rate of transport for both amethopterin and folate increases sharply with decreasing pH and the maximal rate of transport is observed at pH 6.0. Transport at pH 6.0 is saturable (K_m values for amethopterin ≈ 2.8 μM and folate ≈ 4.4 μM), concentrative, and temperature-dependent; whereas at pH 7.0 and higher these effects are absent or less apparent. These findings are of particular interest since direct measurement of jejunal pH at the absorptive surface is 5.7-6.5 in both human and rat intestine[6].

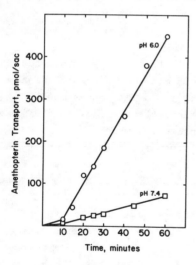

Fig. 1. Time-dependent appearance of amethopterin from the mucosal medium to the serosal compartment of everted sacs of rat jejunum. Each sac was suspended in 5 ml of sodium phosphate buffer at the desired pH containing {³H} amethopterin, 0.5 μM; the serosal solution contained 1 ml of buffer. The sacs were incubated at 37° and removed at the indicated times for recovery of the serosal solution, which was assayed for radioactivity. After an initial lag of approximately 10 minutes the rate was linear for at least 50 minutes. (From ref. 3).

EFFECT ON INHIBITORS

Inhibitors of anaerobic and aerobic metabolism, such as fluoride, hydrozylamine, azide, iodoacetate and p-chloromercuriphenylsulfonate, produce a suppressive effect on amethopterin and folate transport at pH 6.0, but not at higher pH (Table 1). These effects are in contrast to L1210 murine leukemia and Erhlich ascites tumor cells where iodoacetate, azide and other metabolic inhibitors exert an enhancing effect on amethopterin uptake[7,8]. The discovery of an agent which selectively enhances amethopterin or folate transport in the intestine might provide a useful tool for further probing the mechanism of the transport process.

Table 1. Effect of Metabolic Inhibitors on Amethopterin and Folate Transport Across Everted Intestinal Sacs

Condition	Concentration	Amethopterin[a] Transport		Folate Transport	
		pH 6.0	pH 7.4	pH 6.0	pH 7.0
	mM				
No addition		100	100	100	100
Anaerobic		64	93[a]	19	100
Azide	10	47	113[a]	29	111
Iodoacetate	1	31[a]	87	37	85
pCMS[b]	0.1	24	85[a]	21	92
Ouabain	10	32	92	36	100

Transport of folate was measured at pH 6.0 and pH 7.0 or 7.4 at 37° using the standard assay technique (3). Results are expressed as a percentage of a control containing no inhibitor. Initial amethopterin and folate concentrations, 0.1 µM.
[a]From reference 3.   [b]p-Chloromercuriphenylsulfonate.

Amethopterin and folate transport are inhibited competitively by other folate compounds including 5-methyltetrahydrofolate, 5-formyltetrahydrofolate, and 10-formylfolate, as well as by each other. The inhibitory process is markedly pH-dependent, and for amethopterin the inhibition constants of these analogs approximate the K_m for amethopterin transport while for folate the inhibition constants are slightly higher than the K_m for folate transport.

NA-DEPENDENT TRANSPORT

Na^+ has been implicated in the intestinal transport of a wide variety of electrolytes (e.g., calcium, phosphate, sulfate) and organic solutes (e.g., sugars, amino acids, ascorbate)[9]; folates are no exception. Some examples of the effects of cation substitution for Na^+ on amethopterin and folate transport are shown in Table 2. A remarkable feature of this and other Na^+-dependent intestinal transport processes is the unusual degree of specificity for Na^{+}[9]. A variety of inorganic cations have been substituted for Na^+ in the extracellular medium, yet none of these is capable of effectively mimicking the action of Na^+. The addition of ouabain, a Na^+-K^+-ATPase inhibitor, to the serosal medium leads to a profound decrease in the transport of amethopterin and folate at pH 6.0, while only a negligible effect is seen at higher pH (cf. Table 1). Na^+-dependence appears to be restricted to processes capable of transporting certain solutes against an electrochemical gradient[9]; and in the absence of Na^+ accumulation of amethopterin or folate against a chemical gradient is not observed. A novel finding is the inhibitory effect of removal of Na^+ from the extracellular medium on amethopterin transport at both pH 6.0 and 7.5 (cf. Table 2). The observations that Na-dependence occurs at pH 7.5, even though saturation kinetics, concentration against a gradient, and metabolic inhibition are not demonstrable at this pH, support the speculation that the intestinal folate transport system at alkaline pH may be an active transport system which is operating at a low affinity[3].

Table 2. Effect of Cations on Amethopterin Transport Across Everted Intestinal Sacs

Cation Concentration	Amethopterin Transport		Folate Transport	
	pH 6.0	pH 7.5	pH 6.0	pH 7.5
154 mM Na^+	100	100	100	100
154 mM K^+	5	13	3	60
154 mM NH_4^+	14	42	23	52

Standard assay conditions (3) were used and transport was measured at pH 6.0 and 7.5 at $37^\circ C$. Total anion concentration remained constant. Transport is expressed as a percentage of a control containing 154 mM Na^+. Initial amethopterin and folate concentrations, 0.1 μM.

These observations demonstrate the Na^+-dependence of intestinal folate transport, but they do not provide information about the more complex questions regarding the nature of the Na^+ effect, whether Na^+ and folates are co-transported, and whether the energy source for folate transport is the Na^+ concentration gradient across the mucosal brush border membrane. Further studies are needed in this regard.

REGULATION BY CYCLIC NUCLEOTIDES

Transport of folate compounds into L1210 murine leukemia and Erhlich ascites tumor cells[10] appear to be regulated by cyclic nucleotides. In order to determine the effect of cAMP on intestinal amethopterin and folate transport, a study was undertaken to test various phosphodiesterase inhibitors and adenylate cyclase stimulators for their effects on the transport process. Representative results are shown in Table 3. The inhibitory effects seen at pH 6.0 are not demonstrable at pH 7.5. Of the phosphodiesterase inhibitors tested, papaverine is the most effective in suppressing amethopterin and folate transport. Among the compounds known to stimulate various adenylate cyclases, hydrocortisone is the most potent inhibitor of amethopterin and folate transport. The effect of a phosphodiesterase inhibitor and an adenylate cyclase stimulator is illustrated in Table 3 by the combination of papaverine and hydrocortisone.

Table 3. Effect of Phosphodiesterase Inhibitors and Adenyl Cyclase Stimulators on Amethopterin and Folate Transport Across Everted Intestinal Sacs

Compound	Concentration (mM)	Amethopterin Transport		Folate Transport	
		pH 6.0	pH 7.5	pH 6.0	pH 7.5
Phosphodiesterase Inhibitors					
Papaverine	0.5	21	95	16	111
1-Methyl-3-isobutyl-xanthine	5.0	25	100	30	88
Adenylate Cyclase Stimulators					
Hydrocortisone	1.0	23	109	33	108
Histamine	5.0	80	106	102	101
Combination					
Papaverine and Hydrocortisone	0.05 and 0.25	35	89	70	84

Standard assay conditions were used (3) and transport was measured at pH 6.0 and 7.5 at 37°C. Transport is expressed as percent of control containing no inhibitor. Initial amethopterin and folate concentrations, 0.1 µM.

Exogenous cyclic nucleotides are also able to exert an inhibitory effect on amethopterin transport. At concentrations of 5 mM, cAMP produced only slight inhibition of transport (ca. 15%) while cGMP produced substantial inhibition of transport (ca. 45%). The modest effect of cAMP may be referable to poor penetration of this compound into the intestinal mucosal membrane since the dibutyryl derivative of cAMP (5 mM) led to 30% inhibition. The dibutyryl derivative of cGMP (5 mM) had an effect almost identical to that of the parent compound.

Although the mechanism by which cyclic nucleotides regulate folate transport is not yet known, these results suggest that the cyclic nucleotide system may have an important role in controlling the intestinal membrane transport of folate compounds.

ACKNOWLEDGEMENTS

This work was supported by Research Grant No. CA-17809 from the National Cancer Institute, National Institutes of Health. Ann Gauger and Susan Iben provided valuable technical assistance.

REFERENCES

1. Smith, M.E., Matty, A.J. and Blair, J.A. (1970) Biochim. Biophys. Acta 219, 37-46.

2. Blair, J.A., Johnson, I.T. and Matty, A.J. (1976) J. Physiol. 256, 197-208.

3. Strum, W.B. (1977) J. Pharmacol. Exp. Ther. 203, 640-645.

4. Sirotnak, F.M., Donsbach, R.C., Dorick, D.M. and Moccio, D.M. (1976) Cancer Res. 36, 4672-4678.

5. Chabner, B.A. and Young, R.C. (1973) J. Clin. Invest. 52, 1804-1811.

6. Lucas, M.L., Blair, J.A., Cooper, B.T. and Cooke, W.T. (1976) Biochem. Soc. Transact. 4, 154-156.

7. Goldman, I.D. (1969) J. Biol. Chem. 244, 3779-3785.

8. Rader, J.I., Niethammer, D. and Huennekens, F.M. (1974) Biochem. Pharmacol. 23, 2057-2060.

9. Schultz, S.G. and Curran, P.F. (1970) Physiol. Rev. 50, 637-718.

10. Henderson, G.B., Zevely, E.M. and Huennekens, F.M. (1978) Cancer Res. 38, 859-861.

ENTEROHEPATIC CIRCULATION OF FOLATES: II. HEPATIC UPTAKE, INTRACELLULAR ACCUMULATION, AND BILIARY EXCRETION

W.B. STRUM, H.H. LIEM and U. MULLER-EBERHARD
Scripps Clinic and Research Foundation, 10666 North Torrey Pines Road, La Jolla, California   92037

ABSTRACT

Hepatic transport of amethopterin, 5-methyltetrahydrofolate, and folate was studied in the isolated perfused rat liver. The uptake of amethopterin is more rapid than that for 5-methyltetrahydrofolate and folate. The uptake processes for amethopterin and 5-methyltetrahydrofolate are both saturable, and uptake of all three folate compounds is suppressed by metabolic inhibitors and structural analogs. Intracellularly, amethopterin is bound to dihydrofolate reductase. Neither amethopterin nor 5-methyltetrahydrofolate was shown to be appreciably metabolized, but folate is extensively reduced, methylated and/or formylated. All three compounds are excreted into bile against concentration gradients, which are remarkably high for amethopterin. Hepatic uptake and bile excretion systems for amethopterin, 5-methyltetrahydrofolate and folate are energy-dependent and carrier-mediated.

INTRODUCTION

Hepatic transport of the folate analog, amethopterin (methotrexate), occurs via a saturable, energy-dependent, low affinity ($K_m \simeq 1.3$-2.4 mM) uptake system[1,2] and an excretory process in which the drug is excreted into bile against a high concentration gradient[2]. If intestinal toxicity from amethopterin occurs from exposure of the cells to amethopterin from the luminal side (mucosal surface) rather than the circulation (serosal surface), then amethopterin excreted in bile may be critical in producing intestinal injury.

Studies from this laboratory have utilized the in vitro isolated perfused rat liver system for the study of transport of folate compounds from plasma to bile. These studies have been designed to demonstrate the potential influence of hepatic uptake and bile excretion of amethopterin on intestinal toxicity in order to devise ways to offset these effects. This report describes the transport of amethopterin by the isolated perfused liver and compares it to the transport of folate and 5-methyltetrahydrofolate ($meFH_4$) in this system and to transport of folate compounds in isolated hepatocytes.

GENERAL FEATURES OF HEPATIC UPTAKE

The time-dependent uptake of amethopterin, meFH$_4$ and folate is shown
in Fig. 1. At an initial concentration of 1 μM, amethopterin uptake
occurs at a rate of 11.4 nmol/hr/g liver; uptake of meFH$_4$ and folate
occurs at a slower rate of 1.9 and 1.5 nmol/hr/g liver, respectively.
The uptake processes for amethopterin and meFH$_4$ are saturable with a
K$_m$ of 1.3 mM and 0.45 mM, respectively. The effect of concentration
on folate uptake is not yet clear. When metabolic inhibitors, such
as azide, dinitrophenol, iodoacetate and ouabain, or folate analogs
are added to the perfusion medium marked suppression of uptake (50-80%)
is noted for all three compounds.

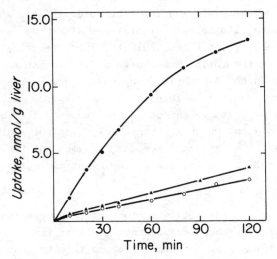

Fig. 1. Hepatic uptake of amethopterin (⊙), meFH$_4$ (Δ), and folate (o)
during perfusion of isolated rat liver. Uptake was determined from
the disappearance of the folate compound from the perfusion medium.
Initial concentrations of folate compound, 1.0 μM. Perfusion procedure as described in reference 2.

INTRACELLULAR EVENTS

Amethopterin is bound to a soluble protein identified as dihydrofolate reductase[2]. Probably as a result of this specific protein binding intracellular accumulation of the drug is concentration-dependent;
e.g., at an initial concentration of 1 μM amethopterin in the perfusion
medium, tissue-to-medium (T/M) ratios of 3-6 are observed after a 2 hr
perfusion and at 0.1 μM amethopterin these ratios rise to 25-50. The
T/M ratios for meFH$_4$ are considerably less than those for amethopterin
with values of 0.5-1.5 being observed with initial meFH$_4$ concentrations

of 0.1-10 μM in the perfusion medium.

Metabolic alteration of amethopterin, meFH$_4$ and folate was studied using ion exchange chromatography of bile. Amethopterin and meFH$_4$ in bile show no conjugation or metabolism; folate is extensively metabolized to meFH$_4$ and probably to 10-formyl folate derivatives.

BILE EXCRETION

The majority of amethopterin which is taken up by the liver is excreted into bile (ca. 70-80%) within a 5 hr perfusion[2]. The drug is concentrated in bile 70-120 fold above that of the initial concentration in the perfusion medium and 450-600 fold above that of the final concentration. Compared to amethopterin, less meFH$_4$ taken up by the liver is excreted into bile (ca. 30-40%) during a 5 hr perfusion. Bile meFH$_4$ concentration reaches values of 8-15 fold above that of the initial concentration in the perfusion medium and 10-24 fold above that of the final concentration. The bile excretion of folate (and its metabolites) closely resembles that of meFH$_4$ regarding the quantity excreted and concentration gradients obtained. After bile excretion amethopterin and meFH$_4$ reach the intestinal mucosal surface and are available for intestinal absorption and reentry into the enterohepatic circulation[2,4].

DISCUSSION

These results for amethopterin transport in the isolated perfused liver are in general agreement with those of Horne, Briggs and Wagner[1] using isolated hepatocytes, who found a K_m of 2.4 mM and an apparent V_{max} of 282 nmol/min/g for amethopterin uptake. Their system required Na$^+$ ions and was sensitive to ouabain and metabolic inhibitors; folate, but not folinate, was slightly inhibitory. Amethopterin concentrated in the isolated hepatic cells with a T/M ratio of 7.3 and 5.8, including and excluding the bound amethopterin fraction, respectively. No metabolism of the drug was observed.

The present studies with meFH$_4$ transport in the isolated perfused liver are also consonant with those of Horne et al. in isolated hepatocytes[3]. Both techniques showed saturation kinetics, energy-dependence, and inhibition by structural analogs. However, both saturation of uptake and inhibition of uptake by analogs were observed only at low concentrations (<5μM) in isolated hepatocytes. The explanation for these differences is not known. Evidence that meFH$_4$ uptake is dependent on the presence of disulfide bonds and that efflux is inhibited by azide has been obtained in the isolated hepatocytes.

Neither the isolated perfused liver nor isolated hepatocytes showed metabolism of $meFH_4$. Extensive metabolism of folate has been observed by both techniques and the formation of 10-formylfolate from folate by rat liver slices has also been described[5].

The similarity in the results obtained for the hepatic transport of amethopterin and $meFH_4$ by the _in vitro_ liver perfusion and isolated hepatocyte techniques is striking. These similarities are noted in spite of the major physiological difference of having both the polarity of the cells and the bile excretion mechanism intact during the _in vitro_ liver perfusion and disorganized in the isolated hepatocyte system.

ACKNOWLEDGEMENTS

This work was supported by Research Grants CA-17809 from the National Cancer Institute (to W.B.S.) and AM-18329 from the Institute of Arthritis, Metabolism, and Digestive Diseases (to U.M.E.), National Institutes of Health.

REFERENCES

1. Horne, D.W., Briggs, W.T. and Wagner, C. (1976) Biochem. Biophys. Res. Commun. 68, 70-76.

2. Strum, W.B. and Liem, H.H. (1977) Biochem. Pharmacol. 26, 1235-1240.

3. Horne, D.W., Briggs, W.T. and Wagner, C. (1978) J. Biol. Chem. 253, 3529-3535.

4. Strum, W.B. and Hanstein, W.G. (1978) Res. Commun. Chem. Path. Pharmacol. 20, 449-456.

5. d'Urso-Scott, M., Uhoch, J. and Bertino, J.R. (1974) Proc. Nat. Acad. Sci. 71, 2736-2739.

STUDIES ON THE ORIGIN OF SERUM FOLATE BINDING PROTEIN

SAMUEL WAXMAN

Department of Medicine, Mount Sinai School of Medicine, New York, New
York   10029

INTRODUCTION

There is now evidence for circulating high affinity, specific
folate binding proteins that are saturated or partially saturated with
folate in normal serum. These folate binding proteins have been characterized in various sera and appear to be of two types. The most
usual folate binding protein (small folate binding protein [S-FABP])
has a molecular weight of approximately 37,000 and is thought to be
derived mainly from the leukocyte[1-3]. In addition, a folate binding
protein with a molecular weight of greater than 200,000 (large folate
binding protein [L-FABP]) is found in the sera from patients with
alcoholism, liver disease and various malignancies[4]. Preliminary data
suggest that the L-FABP may in some way be liver derived. The purpose
of this report is to give further data to support the concept that the
S-FABP protein originates from the granulocyte, is localized in the
specific granule and may be released during phagocytosis while the
L-FABP is distinctly different and may result from abnormalities associated with the liver.

MATERIALS AND METHODS

[3]HPteGlu (40 Ci/mmol-Amersham/Searle Corp.) with a purity which
varies from 90-95% as determined by descending chromatography in 0.1M
phosphate buffer (pH 7.4) was used for these studies. Homogeneous
goat milk folate binding protein and rabbit anti-goat folate binding
protein were prepared as previously reported[5]. Fluorescein conjugated
goat anti-rabbit IgG was purchased from Miles Laboratories. Phorbol
myristate acetate (PMA) was obtained from Consolidated Midland Corpor-

ation, Brewster, New York and dissolved in acetone to give a stock solution of 2 mg/ml and immediately prior to use an aliquot was diluted to the desired concentration (20 ng/ml) with Hank's balanced salt solution (HBSS).

Patient material. The study population consisted of normal subjects and patients with various forms of myeloproliferative disorders and liver disorders. Informed consent was obtained for blood collection.

Preparation of granulocyte-rich fractions. Human granulocytes were obtained from venous blood anticoagulated with EDTA. Granulocytes were separated in a ficoll-hypaque gradient and the red cells sedimented with an equal volume of 3% Dextran T500[6]. The granulocyte fraction was washed twice with HBSS and found to contain greater than 95% granulocytes with a viability greater than 98%, as judged by their ability to exclude trypan blue dye.

PMA release of folate binding protein. Incubations were carried out at 37°C in 5% CO_2 in plastic tubes containing 3×10^{-7} granulocytes with or without PMA in a final volume of 2 ml as previously described[7]. The release of cell contents was calculated by dividing the concentration of the folate binding protein present in the medium by the total amount recovered from the medium and cell lysate and multiplying by 100.

Biochemical assays. Molecular weights of the folate binding proteins were estimated using a 2.2x85 cm column of Sephadex G-200 equilibrated with 0.1M phosphate buffer containing .15M NaCl and 0.02% sodium azide at pH 7.2[2]. DEAE-cellulose chromatography to characterize the various folate binding proteins was done as previously described[2]. Folate binding protein was measured by the binding of exogenous [3]HPteGlu as previously described[2].

Immunofluorescence assay for localization of folate binding proteins. For determination of surface folate binding protein viable cells were obtained from peripheral blood of normals and patients with acute leukemia by Ficoll-hypaque gradient and dextran sedimentation. These viable cells were placed in HBSS and studied for the presence of surface FABP. For the measurement of intracellular FABP cells were placed on glass slides, fixed with ethanol and assayed. For immuno-fluorescence assay the cells were incubated with equal volumes of mono-specific rabbit anti-goat FABP for 60 minutes and fluorescein conju-gated goat anti-rabbit IgG (1:40) for 60 minutes at 37°C. Studies were run with appropriate controls including pre-immune rabbit serum, rabbit anti-goat FABP adsorbed three times with goat FABP, and with and with-out the addition of homogenous goat milk FABP.

RESULTS AND DISCUSSION

Relationship of serum FABP to granulocyte FABP. S-FABP closely resembles the FABP in the granulocyte (Table 1). S-FABP is increased in the serum of some patients with leukocytosis and increases as the leukocyte count rises. The amount of S-FABP decreases when the blood is collected in EDTA-fluoride which is known to diminish the release of certain granulocyte products such as the R-type B_{12} binding protein. PMA simulates the initial events of phagocytosis inducing external degranulation of the specific granule. PMA produced dose related re-lease of intracellular FABP from granulocytes into the medium while preserving cell viability. Incubation with 20 ng/ml resulted in a net release of 60-85% of the intracellular FABP in normal granulocytes. Specific granule products such as B_{12} binding protein and lysozyme are released but not primary granule and cytoplasmic proteins. PMA-re-leased granulocyte FABP is similar to serum S-FABP as measured by G-200 Sephadex column chromatography and DEAE cellulose elution pro-files. In contrast, L-FABP does not appear to be related to the granulocyte released FABP. It does not increase in serum obtained from patients with leukocytosis, is not reduced in EDTA-fluoride plasma as compared to serum and is not found in the media obtained from granulo-cytes incubated with PMA.

TABLE 1

RELATIONSHIP OF SERUM FABP TO GRANULOCYTE FABP

| | Serum | | Granulocyte | |
	L-FABP	S-FABP	Intracellular FABP	PMA-Released FABP (%)
G-200 Sephadex	>200,000	37,000	37,000	37,000
DEAE-cellulose elution	0.2M	0.04M	0.04M	0.04M
% Total serum FABP	10-25	75-90	--	--
Less in EDTA-fluoride plasma	No	Yes	--	--
Increased in leukocytosis	No	Yes	--	--
Increased in liver disease	Yes	No	--	--
% Total granulocyte FABP	--	--	--	60-85

Immunofluorescence localization of cellular FABP. Surface
fluorescence was noted in myeloid precursors, leukemic blasts and proliferating HeLa cells in culture (Table 2). Pre-incubation of the
cells with homogenous FABP goat milk followed by rabbit anti-FABP resulted in a marked increase in the amount of surface immunofluorescence. Surface FABP was not present in viable granulocytes, monocytes,
lymphocytes and red cells. It is suggested, but not proven, that
surface FABP may be part of the membrane carrier transport system involved in the active transport of folic acid.

Intracellular FABP, as determined by immunofluorescence of fixed
preparations, was present in granulocytes, monocytes, myeloid precursors, leukemic blasts and HeLa cells, but less in unstimulated
lymphocytes. No intracellular fluorescence was noted in red blood
cells. Pre-immune rabbit serum or FABP adsorbed anti-FABP serum gave
negative reactions and there was minimal background fluorescence.
Surface-associated FABP occurs in cells that are proliferating and
capable of transporting folic acid and is absent in non-proliferating
cells. In contrast, there is an intracellular FABP present in almost
all cells measured by this immunofluorescence assay with the exception
of the red blood cell.

TABLE 2

IMMUNOFLUORESCENCE LOCALIZATION OF CELLULAR FABP

Cell type	Surface	Intracellular
Granulocytes	-	4+
Monocytes	-	3+
Lymphocytes	-	0-1+
Red blood cells	-	-
Myeloid precursors	+	4+
Leukemic blasts	+	3-4+
HeLa cells	+	3-4+
Pre-incubation with FABP	↑↑	↑or-
Pre-immune rabbit serum	-	-
FABP adsorbed antiserum	-	-

SUMMARY

The FABP released by PMA from human granulocytes is similar to the small molecular weight FABP circulating in the serum and is derived from the specific granule of the granulocyte. A specific immuno-fluorescence assay for FABP reveals the presence of surface FABP in most proliferating cells capable of transporting folic acid while intracellular FABP is present in many cells that do not take up folate or proliferate.

ACKNOWLEDGEMENTS

The author would like to thank Ms. Carol Schreiber for skillful technical assistance and Dr. Harriet Gilbert for providing some of the PMA-treated human granulocytes.

This work was supported by NIH grant AM16690-04, The Chemotherapy Foundation, Inc., and The Gar Reichman Foundation.

REFERENCES

1. Rothenberg, S.P., and daCosta, M. (1971) J. Clin. Invest., 50, 719-727.

2. Waxman, S., and Schreiber, C. (1973) Blood, 42, 291.

3. Colman, N., and Herbert, V. (1976) Blood, 48, 911-918.

4. Waxman, S. (1975) Br. J. Haematol., 29, 23-29.

5. Rubinoff, M., Schreiber, C., and Waxman, S. (1975) FEBS Lett., 75, 244-248.

6. Boyum, P. (1968) Scandinavian J. of Clin. and Lab. Invest., 21, 77-89.

7. Gilbert, H.S., and Waxman, S. (1978) Clin. Research, 26, 581.

LACK OF STEREOSPECIFICITY AT CARBON 6 OF METHYLTETRAHYDROFOLATE TRANSPORT: POSSIBLE
RELEVANCE TO RESCUE REGIMENS WITH METHOTREXATE AND LEUCOVORIN

J. C. White and I. D. Goldman

Medical College of Virginia, Virginia Commonwealth University, Richmond, Virginia

ABSTRACT

Both diastereoisomers of 5-methyltetrahydrofolate (CH_3-H_4folate) are substrates
for the membrane carrier for tetrahydrofolate cofactors and methotrexate (MTX) in
Ehrlich ascites tumor cells. Through interaction at the cell membrane, both isomers
can reduce the level of intracellular MTX and decrease its inhibition of deoxyuridylate incorporation into DNA.

INTRODUCTION

Reduction of H_2folate introduces an asymmetric center at carbon 6. Only the natu-

rally occurring isomer of H_4folate produced by enzymatic reduction can serve as sub-

strate for H_4folate-dependent reactions. Chemical reduction produces a mixture of

diastereoisomers. Specificity of the carrier-mediated membrane transport system for

the diastereoisomers of H_4folate coenzymes has not previously been evaluated in mamma-

lian cells in vitro.

RESULTS AND DISCUSSION

Natural, metabolically active (+) CH_3-H_4folate and unnatural inactive (-) CH_3-H_4

folate were isolated (1) after separation of the isomers of ($\pm$) CH_2-H_4folate on TEAE

cellulose and reduction with borohydride. Stereospecificity of the CH_2-H_4folate was

assayed enzymatically with thymidylate synthetase. Both isomers inhibited influx of

enzymically synthesized (+) $[CH_3-^{14}C]H_4$folate, $[^3H]$MTX, and $[^3H]$aminopterin into

Ehrlich ascites tumor cells (Figure 1). Uptake of radiolabeled stereoisomers of CH_3-

H_4folate was saturable and each diastereoisomer was a competitive inhibitor of the

other (data not shown). Both isomers appear to be transported by the same carrier

though the affinity for the natural (+) isomer (K_m = 2.5) is somewhat greater than

for the unnatural form (K_m = 3.5). When cells brought to a steady state with $[^3H]$

MTX (Figure 2) or $[^3H]$aminopterin (not shown) are exposed to (+) or (-) CH_3-H_4

folate, there is a net efflux of antifolate. If the concentration of CH_3-H_4folate

is sufficiently high, there is a net efflux of antifolates to levels approaching the

component tightly bound to dihydrofolate reductase (1). Perterbation of net

626

Figure 1. Effect of (-) or (+) CH₃-H₄folate on influx of (+) [CH₃-¹⁴C]H₄folate, [³H]MTX, or [³H]aminopterin. At zero time, cells were exposed to substrate at 1 µM concentration alone (●) or simultaneously with 12.3 µM (-) or (+) CH₃-H₄folate (o,□, respectively). A, effects of each isomer on the time course of [³H]MTX uptake. B, composite which evaluates effects of these isomers on influx of (+) CH₃-H₄folate, MTX, or aminopterin. Bars indicate (±) S.E.

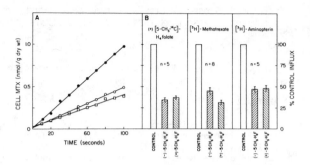

Figure 2. Effect of (-) or (+) CH₃-H₄folate on free intracellular MTX. Cells were exposed to 1.0 µM [³H]MTX and the time course of uptake was measured (●). After 33 min (arrow), portions of the cell suspension were exposed to 27 µM (-) or (+) CH₃-H₄folate (■,□, respectively) and net efflux of [³H]MTX was monitored. Another portion of the cell suspension was separated from the media by centrifugation, washed twice with 0° buffer, and resuspended in MTX-free medium to determine the level of nonexchangeable intracellular MTX (o).

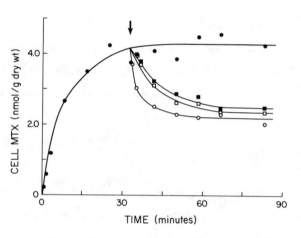

transport of these antifolates by each diastereoisomer further suggests a common transport carrier.

Interaction between MTX and CH₃-H₄folate at the cell membrane may be important in chemotherapy protocols which use high doses of MTX followed by rescue with reduced folate. If the mechanism of rescue is due solely to circumvention of the block in H₄folate synthesis imposed by MTX by providing an exogenous source of H₄folate for intracellular metabolism, then only the natural isomer would be effective. However, since free intracellular MTX is a critical factor in the inhibition of H₂-folate reduction (3) and since both isomers are capable of reducing this intracellular fraction of cell MTX (Figure 2), the unnatural form could also play a role in rescue due to extrusion of free MTX (4). This is seen in Figure 3. Cells were loaded to a steady-state with MTX then (+) or (-) CH₃-H₄folate was added and the incubation

Figure 3. Reversal of MTX inhibition of deoxyuridine incorporation into DNA by (−) or (+) CH_3-H_4folate. Cells were incubated in control media (□) or media containing 1 µM MTX. After 30 min, (+) or (−) CH_3-H_4 folate (●, ○, respectively) was added to achieve a final concentration of 10 µM or 0.3 µM (+) CH_3-H_4folate (▲) or no addition was made (■). After 45 min, during which time a new steady state for MTX was achieved, [^{3}H]deoxyuridine was added and its incorporation into the TCA precipitate was monitored. From enzymic assay during the preparation of (−) CH_3-H_4folate, it was estimated that 3% of the total CH_3-H_4folate is active (+) isomer. Cells exposed to the 0.3 µM (+) CH_3-H_4folate indicated the extent to which this level of the active isomer which accompanies 10 µM (−) CH_3-H_4folate would reverse the MTX block.

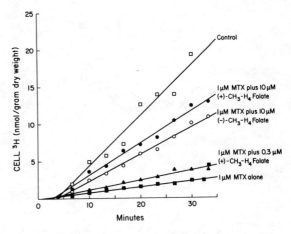

continued until a new steady state for MTX was achieved. Radiolabeled deoxyuridine was then added and its incorporation into DNA was monitored. Both isomers are capable of decreasing MTX inhibition of DNA synthesis. This could not be accounted for on the basis of trace amounts of (+) CH_3-H_4folate present with the (−) diastereoisomer (see the legend to Figure 3). Thus, under these experimental conditions, the unnatural isomer was capable of partial rescue of MTX inhibition of deoxyuridine incorporation into DNA through a membrane transport interaction alone, since this isomer cannot provide substrate for H_4folate-dependent reactions.

REFERENCES

1. White, J.C., Bailey, B.D., Goldman, I.D. (1978), J. Biol. Chem. 253, 247-255.
2. Goldman, I.D. (1969), J. Biol. Chem. 244, 3779-3785.
3. White, J.C., Goldman, I.D. (1976), Mol. Pharmacol. 12, 711-719.
4. Goldman, I.D. (1975), Cancer Chemother. Rep. 6, 63-72.

HIGH-DOSE METHOTREXATE-CARBOXYPEPTIDASE G_1 - A SELECTIVE APPROACH
TO THE THERAPY OF CENTRAL NERVOUS SYSTEM TUMORS

HERBERT T. ABELSON, WILLIAM ENSMINGER, DONALD KUFE, ANDRE ROSOWSKY, AND JACK UREN

Harvard Medical School, Children's Hospital Medical Center, and the Sidney Farber

Cancer Institute, Boston, Massachusetts 02115

ABSTRACT

The identification of dihydrofolate reductase in normal brain and brain tumors has
provided biochemical rationale for antifolate therapy of central nervous system (CNS)
tumors. This report suggests that CNS therapy with classical antifolates can be made
more selective by utilizing carboxypeptidase G_1 ($CPDG_1$) rather than leucovorin (LV)
as a rescue agent.

INTRODUCTION

Biochemical rationale for the treatment of CNS tumors with antifolates was unclear until dihydrofolate reductase (DHFR) was identified in normal rabbit brain[1-3]
and in human brain tumors[4]. The partially characterized enzyme from normal rabbit
brain was similar to that found in liver[1,5]. The brain tumors contained relatively
small amounts of enzyme compared to normal rabbit brain. However, the presence of
DHFR suggested that antifolates might be used for CNS tumors. The rationale behind
this approach is that S phase specific drugs like methotrexate (MTX) do not exhibit
cytotoxicity towards the majority of brain G_0 cells[6]. As MTX-mediated cytotoxicity
is limited to S phase, it is essential that cytotoxic MTX levels[7] be maintained for
as long as possible. Consequently, the concept of concentration x time (C x T) with
respect to MTX is being incorporated into modern treatment protocols[8]. A rescue agent
that would be excluded from certain regions of the body would enhance C x T in those
areas. This kind of selectivity with respect to the CNS can be achieved with $CPDG_1$,
a large polypeptide molecule excluded from the cerebrospinal fluid (CSF) by the blood
brain barrier[9-12].

MATERIALS AND METHODS

Patients. Eight patients with various brain and meningeal tumors have been
treated with between 1 and 5 courses of MTX-$CPDG_1$ in a Phase I study.

Drugs, Treatment Schedule, and Laboratory Studies. MTX was obtained from the
National Cancer Institute. $CPDG_1$ was prepared by the Tufts New England Medical
Center. The pyrogen-free enzyme was supplied in 50 mM Tris-HCl, pH 7.4 containing
10^{-5}M $ZnCl_2$ and had a specific activity of greater than 800 units/mg protein. Most
patients were supplemented with Zn_2SO_4 220 mg/day orally beginning the day before
MTX and continuing until after the last dose of $CPDG_1$. MTX was generally

administered at doses of 10-12 gm/m^2. If MTX was given by continuous infusion over
24 hours, 1/10 of the total dose was given over the first hour and the remainder
over 23 hours. Alternatively, MTX was given over six hours by continuous infusion
with no loading dose. Early in the study, CPDG$_1$ administration was delayed until
36 hours after the initiation of MTX therapy, but now, all patients receive their
first dose of CPDG$_1$ at 24 hours after the start of MTX treatment. CPDG$_1$ (50 IU/kg)
is then given every 12 hours for a total of four doses. Complete blood counts,
serum creatinine, BUN, and liver function tests were obtained, before each course
of treatment, daily during treatment, and for 48 hours after the last CPDG$_1$ dose.
MTX levels were monitored by radioimmunoassay (RIA)[13] and by high-pressure liquid
chromatography (HPLC).

A Waters HPLC Model ALC202 equipped with a U6K injector, dual Model 6000 pumps,
Model 660 solvent programmer, and 280 nm ultraviolet absorbance detector was employed. The analysis was performed on a Waters Bondapak CN column (3.9 mm ID x
30 cm). Folic acid was added to the deproteinated serum specimen or CSF to give
a final concentration of 1 x 10^{-5}M. The initial experiments were carried out with
an eluting buffer containing 0.005 M ammonium acetate, 0.005 M dodecyltrimethyl-
ammonium chloride, and 0.02 M tetraethylammonium chloride in 25% ethanol. Subsequently, superior results with less corrosion of the stainless steel fittings in the
instrument were obtained by using a buffer containing 0.005 M ammonium acetate and
0.008 M tetrabutylammonium hydroxide in 10% ethanol (adjusted to pH 7.6 with acetic
acid). All reagents were of U.S.P. quality, and buffers were prepared daily in
water that had been: (a) deionized by passage through an ion-exchanger (Filterite
Corporation, Timonium, MD), (b) degassed by boiling, and (c) filtered through a
0.2 μm cellulose membrane (Gelman Metricel Type CA-8).

In order to obtain a calibration curve for the assay, standard solutions containing mixtures of MTX (0.2, 0.4, 1.0, 2.0, and 4.0 x 10^{-5}M), 4-amino-4-deoxy-N^{10}-
methylpteroic acid (APA) (0.2, 0.4, 1.0, 2.0, and 4.0 x 10^{-5}M), and folic acid
(1 x 10^{-5}M) were made up in serum previously deproteinated by heat treatment or
addition of perchloric acid or methanol. Each standard solution was injected nine
times, and the peak height ratios (MTX/folic acid, APA/folic acid) were processed
with the aid of a programmable calculator (Texas Instruments Model 59) to obtain a
least-squares linear regression equation of the form $y = b + mx$, with additional
constraints: y intercept $< |0.01|$ and correlation > 0.98. For the analysis of
patient samples, the calculator was programmed to utilize the constants b and m to
convert observed peak height ratios directly into molar concentrations of MTX and
APA. CPDG$_1$ activity was measured spectrophotometrically[9].

RESULTS

CPDG$_1$ hydrolyzes MTX to its cleavage product APA as shown schematically in
Figure 1. We were unable to monitor the decrease in serum MTX by RIA since our

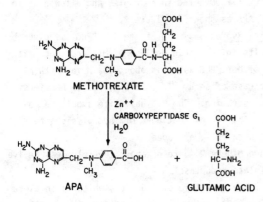

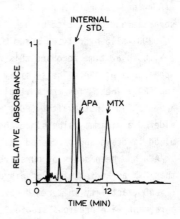

Fig. 1. CPDG₁ hydrolyzes the C-terminal glutamate from MTX producing APA and glutamic acid.

Fig. 2. Separation of MTX and APA by HPLC after MTX and APA were mixed in equimolar amounts (2.5×10^{-5}M) with human serum that had been previously deproteinized.

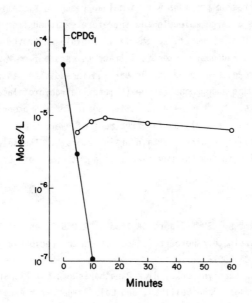

Fig. 3. Initial disappearance of serum MTX and appearance of APA as determined by HPLC after CPDG₁ was given at time zero.

● MTX
O APA

RIA recognizes both MTX and APA. HPLC circumvented this problem and allowed us to separate and quantitate both MTX and APA as shown in Figure 2.

$CPDG_1$ also hydrolyzes serum MTX _in vivo_ as shown in Figure 3. $CPDG_1$ is given by I.V. push at time zero and this results in the rapid decline of MTX and concomitant appearance of APA. The sensitivity of our HPLC assay is about $10^{-7}\underline{M}$ for both MTX and APA. The $t\frac{1}{2}$ for the initial decrease of serum MTX is 3-5 minutes. APA first appears 2-5 minutes after $CPDG_1$ administration. The MTX half-life should be considered a minimum value since the possibility of continued MTX hydrolysis after blood is drawn and processed has not been fully excluded.

APA has been shown by ourselves and others[12,14] to be about 100-fold less active than MTX as an inhibitor of dihydrofolate reductase.

$CPDG_1$ activity in serum decayed with a half-life of 4-6 hours which is in close agreement with previous studies[12]. No $CPDG_1$ activity was identified in the CSF from any patients, and CSF MTX was conserved while serum MTX was destroyed. In fact, egress of MTX from CSF may be slower after $CPDG_1$ than after conventional LV rescue[15]. After LV, CSF MTX decays with a $t\frac{1}{2}$ of about 7 hours; whereas, after $CPDG_1$ rescue, it was prolonged - in one patient, to an average of 20 hours[15].

DISCUSSION

MTX with $CPDG_1$ rescue provides a regional approach to systemic chemotherapy. By virtue of it being a large molecule and therefore excluded from the CSF, $CPDG_1$ cannot hydrolyze CSF MTX. However, serum MTX is rapidly destroyed by the enzyme allowing the bone marrow and gastrointestinal tract to escape from MTX toxicity. C x T for MTX is, therefore, prolonged in the CSF and in addition, there is no exogenous rescue agent (LV) and endogenous rescue (5-methyltetrahydrofolate) is also minimized by $CPDG_1$ hydrolysis. MTX has been an active agent for CNS prophylaxis in acute lymphocytic leukemia[16] as well as for treatment of overt meningeal leukemia[8]. MTX has also shown activity against certain brain tumors[17]. The selective prolongation of MTX concentration in the CNS may make this agent even more useful in CNS therapy in the future.

ACKNOWLEDGEMENTS

Supported in part by USPHS Grants CA 18662, CA 06516, and CA 17979 from the National Cancer Institute. Herbert T. Abelson is the recipient of Research Career Development Award CA 00075.

We wish to thank Carolyn Gorka, Nick Papathanasopoulos, Richard Ragin, Michael Egan, Madison Thompson, John Sullivan, and Lala Sargent for excellent technical assistance. Drs. Emil Frei III, George Canellos, Edward Modest, and David G. Nathan provided advice and encouragement.

REFERENCES

1. Spector, R., Levy, P. and Abelson, H.T. (1977) Biochem. Pharmacol. 26, 1507-1511.

2. Spector, R., Levy, P. and Abelson, H.T. (1977) J. Neurochem. 29, 919-921.

3. Spector, R., Fosburg, M., Levy, P. and Abelson, H.T. (1977) J. Neurochem. 30, 899-901.

4. Abelson, H.T., Gorka, C., Fosburg, M. and Kornblith, P. (1978) Lancet I, 184-185.

5. Pollack, R.J. and Kaufman, S. (1977) J. Neurochem. 30, 253-256.

6. Johnson, L.F., Fuhrman, C.L. and Abelson, H.T. (1978) Cancer Res. 38, 2408-2412.

7. Chabner, B.A. and Young, R.C. (1973) J. Clin. Invest. 52, 1804-1811.

8. Bleyer, W.A., Poplack, D.G., Simon, R.M. (1978) Blood 51, 835-842.

9. McCullough, J.L., Chabner, B.A. and Bertino, J.R. (1971) J. Biol. Chem. 246, 7207-7213.

10. Chabner, B.A., Johns, D.G. and Bertino, J.R. (1972) Nature 239, 395-397.

11. Chabner, B.A., Chello, P.L. and Bertino, J.R. (1972) Cancer Res. 32:2114-2119.

12. Howell, S.B., Blair, H.E., Uren, J. and Frei, E. III (1978) European J. Cancer 14, 787-792.

13. Raso, V. and Schreiber, R. (1975) Cancer Res. 35, 1407-1410.

14. Valerino, D.M., Johns, D.G., Zaharko, D.S., et al. (1972) Biochem. Pharmacol. 21, 821-831.

15. Abelson, H.T., Ensminger, W., Rosowsky, A. and Uren, J. (In press) Cancer Treat. Rep.

16. Sallan, S.E., Camitta, B.M., Cassady, J.R., Nathan, D.G. and Frei, E. III (1978) Blood 51, 425-433.

17. Rosen, G., Ghavimi, F., Nirenberg, A., Mosende, C. and Mehta, B.M. (1977) Cancer Treat. Rep. 61, 681-690.

635

METABOLIC REGULATION OF METHYLENETETRAHYDROFOLATE REDUCTASE

ALBERTA M. ALBRECHT

Sloan-Kettering Institute, 145 Boston Post Rd., Rye, N.Y. 10580

ABSTRACT

Methylenetetrahydrofolate reductase levels were elevated in livers
of Walker tumor-bearing rats provided chow or amino acid-defined diets
ad libitum. Dietary deprivation of folic acid or methionine increased
enzyme levels in normal rats and slightly increased the specific activity values for the liver enzyme in tumor-bearing rats. Reductase levels
rose in tumor-bearing rats also after administration of methotrexate.
Data are discussed in terms of enzyme regulation by folate-dependent
metabolites.

INTRODUCTION

The predominant plasma and storage folate is 5-methyltetrahydrofolate
($meFH_4$)[1]. After its transport across cell membranes, interconversion of
$meFH_4$ to other tetrahydrofolate (FH_4) coenzymes depends primarily upon
the biosynthesis of methionine[2]. The $meFH_4$-dependent methylation of
homocysteine by methionine synthetase provides cells with FH_4 for activation to non-methylated coenzymes. A current hypothesis[3] views the
methylenetetrahydrofolate reductase reaction, previously considered a
uni-directional reduction of methylenetetrahydrofolate (methyleneFH_4)
to $meFH_4$[4], as reversible, thus providing another pathway to FH_4 coenzymes from $meFH_4$. This report on folic acid (FA) metabolism in a
tumor system presents indirect evidence for regulated synthesis of the
latter enzyme and supports the idea that under the stress arising from
administration of methotrexate (MTX), the reductase reaction proceeds
towards methyleneFH_4.

MATERIALS AND METHODS

Rat-tumor system. This was the Walker carcinosarcoma (W-256) in female Fischer rats. Rats were provided *ad libitum* chow or modifications of Teklad Amino Acid-Defined Diet #170010. The diets differed in FA content/g: chow contained 6 µg of FA equivalents and the test diets, 0.5 µg of supplemental FA. Test diets contained 0.5% succinyl sulfathiazole, and were devoid of methionine or FA as required. MTX (100 mg/kg) was administered i.p. 12 days after tumor implant.

Analytical samples. Rats were exsanguinated, dissected and blood (plasma and extracts) was processed according to Bird *et al.*[5]. Organs were washed thoroughly with cold saline and stored (-20°C). Later, tissues were homogenized in 3 parts of 0.25 M sucrose (for enzyme extracts) or 10 mM potassium phosphate buffer (KPB), pH 7.4. Portions of each homogenate in KPB were treated appropriately for subsequent assays. They were (1) centrifuged (4°C, 28,000xg, 40 min.) to yield enzyme extracts or (2) mixed with equal parts of 2% K ascorbate, pH 6.0. The mixtures were heated (95°C), centrifuged and supernatant extracts were treated with hog kidney conjugase[5] and assayed for folates.

Assays. Protein and enzyme activities were determined by methods based upon previously described procedures[4,6]. One enzyme unit was that amount which catalyzed per min. the reduction of 1 nmole of dihydrofolate (dihydrofolate reductase) or the release of 1 nmole of formaldehyde (methylenetetrahydrofolate reductase). Tissue folates were assayed with *Lactobacillus casei*, and with MTX-resistant mutant strains of *L. casei*[7] and *Pediococcus cerevisiae*[8] when samples contained MTX. FA or meFH$_4$ and calcium leucovorin were the reference folates, respectively.

RESULTS AND DISCUSSION

Studies with the W-256 system have provided clues to the controlled synthesis of the methylenetetrahydrofolate reductase in mammalian cells.

This mode of regulation was detected during investigation of the tumor system under different dietary conditions.

Methylenetetrahydrofolate reductase levels were essentially identical in livers of control rats fed chow or the complete test diet, and were elevated equally in tumor-bearing rats on both diets (Table 1). Dietary deprivation of methionine also caused higher enzyme levels in control rats. Limiting total protein synthesis, the substitution of homocystine for methionine did not prevent the tumor effect and, in fact, increased the relative amount (specific activity) of the reductase. Restriction of FA also increased enzyme levels in normal rats and contributed cumulatively to the tumor effect.

TABLE 1

EFFECTS OF TUMOR AND DIETARY DEPRIVATION ON LIVER LEVELS OF METHYLENE-TETRAHYDROFOLATE REDUCTASE

Test diets were initiated with 6-week old rats and W-256 was implanted 5 weeks later. Total test diet period: 9 weeks; liver extracts, in sucrose.

Diets	Protein (mg/g)		Reductase (units/g)[a]	
	N[b]	W[c]	N[b]	W[c]
Chow	110	91	24	42
Test diets				
Complete	110	94	24	45
-Methionine[d]	75	78	34	43
-Folic acid	111	107	31	54

[a] Activity/g of tissue.
[b] N, normal liver.
[c] W, liver of rats 4 weeks after tumor implant.
[d] Homocystine-supplemented.

Values for blood and liver folates indicate that enzyme levels were not directly affected by folate levels (Table 2). Collectively, the data summarized in Tables 1 and 2 imply that the elevations in methylenetetrahydrofolate reductase reflected decreased levels of one or more

TABLE 2

FOLATES OF NORMAL AND TUMOR-BEARING RATS[a]

Diet	Blood[b] (ng/ml)		Liver[c] (µg/g)	
	N	W	N	W
Chow	200	120	14.1	17.1
Test diets				
Complete	65	45	6.0	3.6
-Methionine	115	125	2.5	2.2
-Folic acid	38	35	2.4	1.6

[a] Descriptive details as presented in Table 1.
[b] Before conjugase, as ℓ-meFH$_4$.
[c] Total folates, as ℓ-meFH$_4$.

repressor substances, probably end-products of FA metabolism. The possibility that derivatives of methionine are repressors is suggested by the pattern of enzyme levels observed in the rats fed folic acid- or methionine-free diets. In effect, the nutritional dependence of the tumor on its host simulated dietary deprivation.

Increased levels of methylenetetrahydrofolate reductase were found also after the administration of MTX to tumor-bearing rats. Results of a survey of specific MTX-dependent events (Fig. 1) show that the shift to higher liver levels occurred at the time after MTX when plasma folate was the lowest (A), liver folates were decreased by 25% (B) and apparently 90% of the dihydrofolate reductase was inhibited (D). Increase of the enzyme level at that point was presumably a response to the physiologic stress caused by the drug blockade. Evidently, methylated folates had decreased with the increased demands for meFH$_4$ of other organs and the tumor. Methylated folates also possibly contributed to the non-methylated coenzyme pool. With the overall decrease in FH$_4$ coenzymes, a resultant decline of FH$_4$-dependent metabolites to sub-repressible levels could have sparked the apparent derepression. The speculation that methylenetetrahydrofolate reductase might mediate the formation of methyleneFH$_4$ from meFH$_4$ gains support from the events in the small intestine (Fig. 1, C and E). Despite the marked inhibition of intestinal dihydrofolate reductase (E), the level of non-methylated coenzymes was maintained above the 25% level (C).

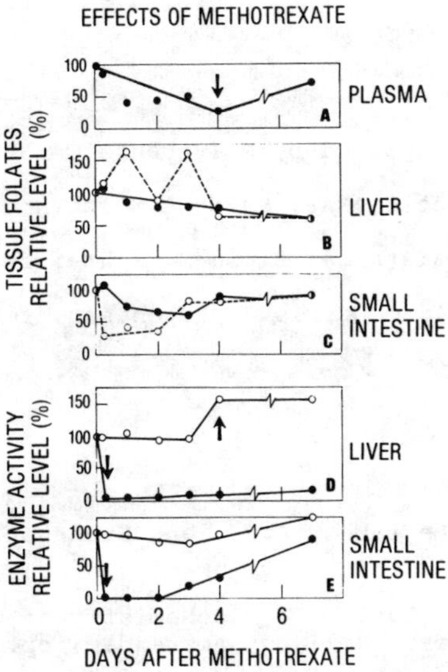

EFFECTS OF METHOTREXATE

DAYS AFTER METHOTREXATE

Fig. 1. Biochemical events following the administration of a single injection of MTX (day 0). Plasma folate (A): reference values (100%), 108 ng of ℓ-meFH$_4$/ml (day 0 to day 4) and 75 ng/ml (day 7); folates of liver (B) and small intestine (C): 100% represents 15.3 µg (B) and 1.2 µg (C) of methylated folates (—●—●—) and 2.3 µg (B) and 0.2 µg (C) of non-methylated (--O--O--) folates/g of tissue of untreated rats; enzyme levels of liver (D) and small intestine (E): 100% represents 1020 units (D) and 140 units (E) of dihydrofolate reductase at pH 6.5 (—●—●—) and 35 units (D) and 12 units (E) of methylenetetrahydro-folate reductase (—O—O—)/g of tissue of untreated rats. Symbols: ↓(frame A) and ↑(frame D) mark the coincidence of the lowest plasma folate level and the shift to higher levels of methylenetetrahydro-folate reductase; ↓(frames D and E) marks the inhibition of dihydro-folate reductase.

640

SUMMARY

This study produced information regarding the possibility of regulated synthesis of methylenetetrahydrofolate reductase. Regulatory metabolites might be derivatives of methionine. Additionally, other data prompt the speculation that the methylenetetrahydrofolate reductase reaction is reversible during the physiologically stressed condition caused by MTX.

ACKNOWLEDGMENTS

This work was supported by NCI grants CA 08748 and CA 17839. The author thanks Eva Boldizsar, Suzanne Zorzo and Margaret Kennedy for their technical assistance; Bipin M. Mehta, for the bio-assays of MTX-containing plasma; and Dorris J. Hutchison, for her interest and support.

REFERENCES

1. Herbert, V., Larrabee, A.R., and Buchanan, J.M. (1962) J. Clin. Invest. 41, 1134-1138.

2. Blakley, R.L. (1969) The Biochemistry of Folic Acid and Related Pteridines, North Holland, Amsterdam, pp. 188-218; 332-351.

3. Thorndike, J. and Beck, W.S. (1977) Cancer Res. 37, 1125-1132.

4. Kutzbach, C. and Stokstad, E.L.R. (1971) Biochim. Biophys. Acta, 250, 459-477.

5. Bird, O.D., McGlohon, V.M. and Vaitkus, J.W. (1965) Anal. Biochem., 12, 18-35.

6. Albrecht, A.M., Biedler, J.L. and Hutchison, D.J. (1972) Cancer Res. 32, 1539-1546.

7. Mehta, B.M. and Hutchison, D.J. (1977) Cancer Treat. Rep. 61, 1657-1663.

8. Mehta, B.M. and Hutchison, D.J. (1975) Cancer Chemother. Rep. 59, 935-937.

FLUOROPYRIMIDINE ANTAGONISM TO METHOTREXATE-SUPPRESSION OF [14C]FORMATE
INCORPORATION INTO NUCLEIC ACIDS AND PROTEIN

DONNELL BOWEN AND ECKARD FÖLSCH
The Genesee Hospital--University of Rochester Cancer Center
Rochester, New York 14607

ABSTRACT

The inhibitory effect of MTX* on [14C]formate incorporation into nucleic acids and
protein of Ehrlich ascites tumor cells is decreased by pretreatment with fluoropyrimidines. Inhibition of formate incorporation into DNA, RNA, and protein in the
presence of MTX only, was 91%, 82%, and 75%, respectively; whereas in the presence
of FUdR plus MTX, formate incorporation in DNA, RNA, and protein was inhibited by
85%, 67%, and 66%. A comparison of the THF/DHF ratio from the soluble fraction of
cells that were incubated with [3H]DHF was 25% greater in the presence of FUdR and
MTX than MTX alone. When MTX alone suppressed formate incorporation by 79% into RNA,
the effect of 0.01, 0.1, and 1μM FUdR plus MTX reduced MTX inhibitory action by 72%,
57%, and 40%, respectively. These data support the concept that fluoropyrimidine-
antagonism to MTX is related, in part, to increased levels of reduced folates available for purine and protein biosynthesis.

INTRODUCTION

The extensive use of MTX and the fluoropyrimidine, FU, in cancer chemotherapy[1-5]
and conflicting evidence as to whether this combination is additive[6-9], less than
additive or antagonistic[8-10], stimulated a series of investigations into the biochemical effects of the MTX-FU combination. Previous studies have attributed antagonism to fluoropyrimidines induced by MTX as a result of (a) a MTX-induced depletion
of $5,10-CH_2THF$[11], the cofactor essential for the covalent association of the fluoropyrimidine, FdUMP, to thymidylate synthetase, and (b) a MTX-induced increase in intracellular dUMP which competes with FdUMP and limits the interaction between FdUMP
and thymidylate synthetase[10]. A diminished MTX effect induced by fluoropyrimidines
has been attributed to (a) fluoropyrimidine protection of cells from the antipurine
effect of MTX on deoxypurine nucleotides[10], and (b) the decreased inhibition of UdR
incorporation into DNA as the basal rate of this reaction was inhibited by FUdR or
FU[12]. A basis for antagonism to MTX induced by fluoropyrimidines on RNA and protein synthesis in contrast to DNA synthesis has not been clarified. In view of the
apparent role of exchangeable intracellular MTX in the inhibition of thymidylate,

---

*Abbreviations: MTX, methotrexate; FUdR, 5-fluorodeoxyuridine; FU, 5-fluorouracil;
DHF, dihydrofolate; THF, tetrahydrofolate; $5,10-CH_2THF$, 5,10-methylene THF; DHFR,DHF
reductase; UdR, deoxyuridine; FdUMP, FUdR monophosphate; dUMP, UdR monophosphate.

purine, and protein synthesis[13,14], studies were undertaken to contrast the effects of fluoropyrimidine-antagonism to free-MTX on nucleic acids and protein synthesis by reducing the rate of thymidylate synthesis with FUdR.

MATERIALS AND METHODS

Ehrlich ascites tumor cells were grown intraperitoneally in CFl mice 6-12 days and prepared for experimentation as described previously[15,16]. The experimental buffer consisted of a modified Eagle's medium[14] without folates, serum and methionine, with the following electrolyte composition: 135mM NaCl, 16mM NaHCO$_3$, 1.1mM Na$_2$HPO$_4$, 4.4mM KCl, 1.9mM CaCl$_2$ and lmM MgCl$_2$. The pH was adjusted to, and maintained at, 7.4 in the presence of 95%O$_2$/5%CO$_2$. The cell suspension was stirred continuously with a motor-driven Teflon paddle as reported previously[16]. All experiments were performed at 37°. [^{14}C]Formate, the sodium salt, and [^{3}H]UdR were supplied by New England Nuclear Corporation (Boston, Mass.). [^{3}H]DHF was prepared from (3', 5', 9-^{3}H) folic acid according to the method of Blakely[17] and purified by DEAE cellulose column chromatography as described previously[18]. The radiochemical purity of [^{3}H] DHF exceeded 90%. Unlabeled FUdR and MTX were obtained from Sigma Chemical Co. (St. Louis, Mo.) and Lederle Laboratories, respectively. All incubations employing DHF were performed in the dark. Incorporation of [^{14}C]formate into DNA, RNA, and protein, as well as [^{3}H]UdR into DNA, was determined from a perchlorate precipitate as described previously[14]. Data are expressed as the mean ± S.E. The MTX concentration was 50μM. The final formate concentration was 100μM.

RESULTS AND DISCUSSION

The Effects of MTX on the Rates of [^{14}C]Formate Incorporation into RNA, DNA, and Protein After Pretreatment with FUdR. Ehrlich ascites tumor cells were exposed to 0.05μM FUdR for 15 min to inhibit thymidylate synthesis and alter the levels of reduced folates utilized for nucleic acids and protein synthesis. The cells were then separated by centrifugation, washed twice, and resuspended into fresh media without FUdR but in the presence and absence of MTX. Thirty min later, when free intracellular MTX was at a steady-state with extracellular MTX, [^{14}C]formate incorporation into DNA, RNA, and protein was monitored over an interval when the rate of incorporation was constant. Cells neither exposed to FUdR or MTX were treated similarly. A representative experiment is illustrated in Fig. 1. In four or more separate experiments, ^{14}C incorporation into DNA, RNA, and protein, in the presence of MTX alone, was 91.1 ± 1.7%, 82.2 ± 3.4%, and 75.0 ± 5.8%, respectively; however, in the presence of FUdR and MTX, formate incorporation into DNA, RNA, and protein was inhibited by 85.5 ± 1.9%, 67.1 ± 5.6%, and 65.8% ± 1.2%.

These data are compatible with the concept that fluoropyrimidines should reduce the inhibitory effect of MTX by diminishing depletion of intracellular THF or reduced folates available for [^{14}C]formate incorporation into DNA, RNA, and protein, which

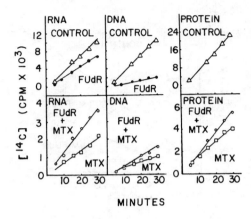

Fig. 1 The effects of FUdR on MTX-suppression of ^{14}C incorporation into RNA, DNA, and protein.

occurs from the insertion of the formate carbon via tetrahydrofolates into purine nucleotides at C-2 and C-8 as well as into thymidine, methionine, and serine[19]. The observation that a greater difference exists in the antagonism of MTX-suppression to [^{14}C]formate incorporation into RNA as compared to DNA and protein suggests that the rate of THF utilization for RNA exceeds that for DNA and protein. The low sensitivity of [^{14}C]formate incorporation into DNA to fluoropyrimidine-antagonism is consistent with the formulation of an irreversible binding of fluoropyrimidines to thymidylate synthetase,

which, mostly, results in a sustained inhibition of thymidine synthesis. Fluoropyrimidine-antagonism to [^{14}C]formate incorporation into protein may be a result of interconversion enzymes sustaining 5-methyl THF levels[20], the principal folate within the mammalian cell[21]. The relative flux of folate coenzymes through the pathways for thymidylate synthesis and methionine synthesis can significantly affect the rate at which folate coenzymes are utilized for protein and RNA synthesis. When thymidylate synthesis is reduced by fluoropyrimidines, that portion of 5,10-CH$_2$THF which is not part of the FdUMP-5,10-CH$_2$THF-thymidylate synthetase ternary complex[22] should be converted to 5-methyl THF, which in the presence of methyl THF:homocysteine methyl transferase synthesizes a molecule of methionine and THF. Thus, for every molecule of methionine that is synthesized and utilized, in part or completely, for protein synthesis, a molecule of THF is available and could be used for purine synthesis. This is consistent with data from five experiments obtained similarly to data in Fig. 1, which indicated that the suppression of ^{14}C incorporation into protein and RNA in the presence of FUdR plus MTX was 66% and 67%, respectively. Hence, ^{14}C incorporation into protein should be least sensitive to (a) depletion of THF by MTX^{14} (Fig.1), and (b) fluoropyrimidine-antagonism because the specific coenzymes necessary to sustain this reaction are less dependent upon the sustained regeneration of THF from DHF.

The Effect of FUdR Dose on MTX-Suppression of [^{14}C]Formate Incorporation into RNA. The relationship between the rates of dTMP synthesis induced by FUdR and antagonism to MTX-suppression of [^{14}C]formate incorporation was assessed by exposing cells to varying concentrations of FUdR (0.01, 0.1, and 1µM) for 15 min to achieve increasing suppression of dTMP synthesis[12]. The cells were then resuspended into a FUdR-free media but in the presence of MTX. A 15 min exposure to 0.01, 0.1, and 1µM FUdR de-

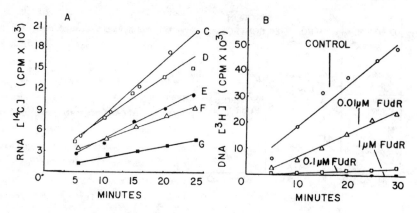

Fig. 2   The effects of FUdR concentration on MTX-suppression of [14C]formate incorporation into RNA (C, Control; D, 1μM FUdR + MTX; E, 0.1μM FUdR + MTX; F, 0.01μM
FUdR + MTX; and G, MTX), and [3H]UdR incorporation into DNA.

creased the rate of [3H]UdR incorporation by 53%, 93%, and 99%, respectively (Fig.2B).
Figure 2A illustrates the effects of FUdR on MTX-suppression of [14C]formate incorporation into RNA. In four experiments, MTX alone suppressed [14C]formate incorporation into RNA by 79.2 ± 2.4%; 0.01, 0.1, and 1μM FUdR plus MTX decreased the rate of
[14C]formate incorporation by 71.8 ± 2.2%, 57.0 ± 7.7%, and 39.6 ± 13.6%, respectively.

The enhancement of [14C]formate incorporation into RNA in the presence of a constant concentration of MTX and increasing concentrations of FUdR further supports the
formulation that fluoropyrimidines cause an increase in reduced folates and diminish
the effect of MTX. Since three of the substrates (dATP, dGTP, and dCTP) for DNA
polymerase are obtained by direct reduction of the corresponding ribonucleotides, the
rate at which 14C appears in purines (adenine and guanine) for RNA should exceed
those for DNA because of fluoropyrimidines limiting the availability of dTMP for
polymerization into DNA. Although dTMP can also arise from thymidine, this reaction
is probably used as a salvage pathway for dTMP formed from thymidylate synthetase.

Metabolism of [3H]DHF in the Presence of FUdR and MTX. The critical role of free-
MTX in suppression of THF synthesis was examined in contrast to conditions in which
cells were exposed to FUdR, MTX, and FUdR plus MTX. In the absence of FUdR and MTX,
Ehrlich tumor cells converted DHF to THF (Fig. 3A). Cells exposed only to FUdR also
converted DHF to THF (Fig. 3B). In the presence of free-MTX alone (Fig. 3C), DHF
reached its maximum level in the cell; this was accompanied with the suppression of
THF production. A similar response to DHF metabolism occurred in the presence of
FUdR plus MTX (Fig. 3D); however, the ratio of THF to DHF was greater in the presence
of FUdR and MTX than MTX alone. In seven experiments, the THF/DHF ratio was 24 ± 6%

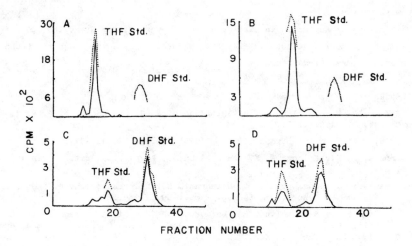

Fig. 3 The effects of FUdR and MTX on [^{3}H]DHF metabolism.

greater in the presence of FUdR and MTX than MTX alone (p<0.05). The presence of THF
in cells treated only with MTX may be a result of competition between a high concentration of DHF extracellularly and increasing intracellular levels of DHF and MTX for
DHFR. When the cells are exposed to MTX and the drug enters the intracellular compartment, the following sequence of events would be expected to occur. Association
of MTX with DHFR which results in a small transient reduction in the rate of THF synthesis with a subsequent increase in the DHF level. Eventually, as MTX binds to the
major portion of DHFR, the rate of THF synthesis will decrease. Since the interaction between DHFR and MTX is not stoichiometric at physiological pH[23], and because
cellular DHF has risen to high levels from MTX binding to DHFR and a high extracellular DHF concentration, DHF can compete with MTX for the few remaining DHFR binding
sites and maintain residual THF synthesis. Similar conditions, therefore, should
exist when cells are exposed to FUdR and MTX. However, the THF level should be less
in cells treated only with MTX because of continual production of DHF from the metabolism of 5,10-CH$_2$THF. This was reflected in the THF/DHF ratio being less in cells
treated with MTX than FUdR and MTX.

SUMMARY

Antagonism to MTX-suppression of formate incorporation into nucleic acids and protein occurs when Ehrlich ascites cells are pretreated with fluoropyrimidines. This
antagonism is related, at least in part, to increased levels of reduced folates
available for purine and protein synthesis.

ACKNOWLEDGEMENTS

This study was supported in part by a Young Investigators Grant (to D.B.) from the National Cancer Institute (CA-24192). We gratefully acknowledge the technical assistance of Mrs. Linda Guernsey.

REFERENCES

1. Creech, R. H., Catalano, R. B., Mastragelo, M. J. and Engstrom, P. R. (1975) Cancer, 35, 1101-1175.

2. Otis, P. T. and Armentrout, S. A. (1975) Cancer, 36, 311-317.

3. Rubens, R. D., Knight, R. K. and Hayward, J. L. (1975) Brit. J. Cancer, 32, 730-736.

4. Umsawasdi, T., Chainuvati, T., Hitannant, S., Nilprabhassorn, P. and Viranovat-ti, V. (1975) Cancer Chemotherapy Rept., 59, 1167-1169.

5. Bonadonna, G., Brusamolino, E., Valagussa, P., Rossi, A., Brugnatelli, L., Brambilla, C., DeLena, M., Tancini, G., Bajetta, E., Musumeci, R. and Veronesi, U. (1976) New Engl. J. Med., 294, 737-744.

6. Kline, I., Venditti, J. M., Mead, J. A. R., Tyrer, D. P. and Goldin, A. (1966) Cancer Res., 26, 848-852.

7. Baribjanian, B. T., Johnson, R. K., Kline, I., Vadlamudi, S., Gang, M., Vendit-ti, J. M. and Goldin, A. (1976) Cancer Treat. Rept., 60, 1347-1361.

8. Bertino, J. R., Sawicki, W. L., Lindquist, C. A. and Gupta, V. S. (1977) Cancer Res., 37, 327-328.

9. Heppner, G. H. and Calabresi, P. C. (1977) Clin. Res., 25, 407A.

10. Tattersall, M. H. N., Jackson, R. C., Connors, T. A. and Harrap, K. R. (1973) European J. Cancer, 9, 733-739.

11. Ullman, B., Lee, M., Martin, D. W. and Santi, D. V. (1978) Proc. Natl. Acad. Sci. U. S. A., 75, 980-983.

12. Bowen, D., White, J. C. and Goldman, I. D. (1978) Cancer Res., 38, 219-222.

13. Goldman, I. D. (1974) Mol. Pharmacol., 10, 257-274.

14. White, J. C., Loftfield, S. and Goldman, I. D. (1975) Mol. Pharmacol., 11, 287-297.

15. Goldman, I. D., Lichtenstein, N. S. and Oliverio, V. T. (1968) J. Biol. Chem., 243, 5007-5017.

16. Bowen, D. and Goldman, I. D. (1975) Cancer Res., 35, 3054-3060.

17. Blakely, R. L. (1960) Nature, 188, 231-232.

18. White, J. C. and Goldman, I. D. (1976) Mol. Pharmacol., 12, 711-719.

19. Stokstad, E. L. R. and Koch, J. (1967) Physiol. Rev., 47, 83-116.

20. Nixon, P. F., Slutsky, G., Nahas, A. and Bertino, J. R. (1973) J. Biol. Chem., 248, 5932-5936.

21. Herbert, V. and Zalusky, R. (1962) J. Clin. Invest., 41, 1263-1276.

22. Santi, D. V., McHenry, C. S. and Sommer, H. (1974) Biochemistry, 13, 471-480.

23. Bertino, J. R., Booth, B. A., Bieber, A. L., Cashmore, A. and Sartorelli, A. C. (1964) J. Biol. Chem., 239, 479-485.

CHEMOTHERAPY WITH ALBUMIN-BOUND METHOTREXATE

BARBARA C. F. CHU and JOHN M. WHITELEY
Scripps Clinic and Research Foundation, La Jolla, California 92037

Methotrexate (MTX) linked to three proteins, bovine serum albumin (BSA), α-chymo-trypsinogen and bovine IgG, has been found to be as effective as MTX alone in pro-longing the survival time of BDF_1 mice bearing the L1210 ascites tumor when injected in a single dose one day after tumor transplant. In contrast, MTX linked to dextrans of varying molecular weights was ineffective (Table 1), which suggests that proteins in general make effective carriers for MTX in drug therapy, whereas dextrans do not. In addition, when MTX-BSA was injected into BDF_1 mice transplanted with the Lewis Lung Carcinoma 1, 5, 9 and 13 days after tumor transplant the derivative decreased the rate of growth of the primary tumor by 40% and reduced by 75% the number of metastatic nodules found on the lungs (Fig. 1), whereas at comparable dose levels MTX alone gave rise to a lesser response. When animals bearing 14-day-old Lewis lung tumors were injected with a single dose of ^{3}[H]MTX or ^{3}[H]MTX-BSA no difference in radioactivity was found in the tumors after 1 h; however, after 8 and 24 h the drug levels in the tumors of the MTX-BSA-treated mice were double those of the MTX-treated tumors (Table 2).

TABLE 1   PROTEINS MAKE EFFECTIVE DRUG CARRIERS:
           DEXTRANS ARE INEFFECTIVE [A]

DRUG	% INCREASE IN SURVIVAL TIME
CONTROL	0
MTX	95
MTX-BSA	92
MTX-CHYMOTRYPSINOGEN	103
MTX-BOVINE IgG	108
MTX-DEXTRAN T70	5
FOLATE-BSA	0

[A] COMPOUNDS INJECTED AT A DOSE LEVEL OF 15 mg/Kg MTX.

TABLE 2

RADIOACTIVITY AT THE PRIMARY TUMOR SITE AFTER TREATMENT OF MICE
CARRYING THE LEWIS LUNG CARCINOMA WITH EITHER MTX OR MTX-BSA [A]

DRUG	MTX, μg/g OF TUMOR [B]		
	1 HR	8 HR	24 HR
^{3}[H]MTX	1.03 ± 0.35	0.72 ± 0.13	0.59 ± 0.13
^{3}[H]MTX-BSA	1.07 ± 0.24	1.60 ± 0.54	1.10 ± 0.34

[A] MEASUREMENTS OF RADIOACTIVITY WERE MADE AT THE INDICATED TIMES AFTER INJECTION OF THE
RADIOLABELED DRUG (12 mg/Kg) INTO MICE CARRYING 12-14 DAY-OLD TUMORS.

[B] RESULTS ARE EXPRESSED AS THE MEAN ± SD OF 6 MICE.

To examine in more detail the interaction of carrier-bound MTX with cells, several *in vitro* experiments with murine L1210 cells were carried out. When the cells were grown with varying concentrations of MTX, MTX-BSA or MTX-Dextran T70 in RPMI 1640 medium, it was found that whereas MTX completely inhibited cell growth at extracellular concentrations of 10^{-7} M, growth was not inhibited with MTX-albumin or dextran until concentrations reached 10^{-6} or 10^{-5} M respectively (Fig. 2). This differing cytotoxic effect of the carrier-bound drugs appears to be proportional to their ability to deliver MTX to the cell. After 1 h at 37°, equal concentrations of L1210 cells incubated with equal dose levels of ^{3}[H]MTX, ^{3}[H]MTX-BSA or ^{3}[H]MTX-

Dextran T70 contained 2.2, 1.12 and 0.42 nmoles MTX/10^9 cells respectively. In each
instance the major part of the label (80-95%) was found in the cell lysate rather
than in the membrane fraction. When the experiment was repeated with MTX-^{125}[I]
BSA and MTX-^{3}[H]Dextran-T70 the concentration of BSA associated with the cells was
8 times greater than that of the Dextran T70, which suggests that one reason for the
poor drug delivery potential of MTX-dextrans may be an inability of the carrier to
bind to the cell wall.

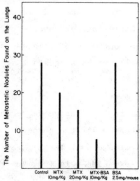

Fig. 1. Number of metastatic nodules found
on the lungs of BDF$_1$ mice carrying the
Lewis Lung Carcinoma after treatment with
MTX, MTX-BSA and BSA. Mice were treated
every fourth day for a total of four doses
at the levels indicated beginning on day 1
after transplant.

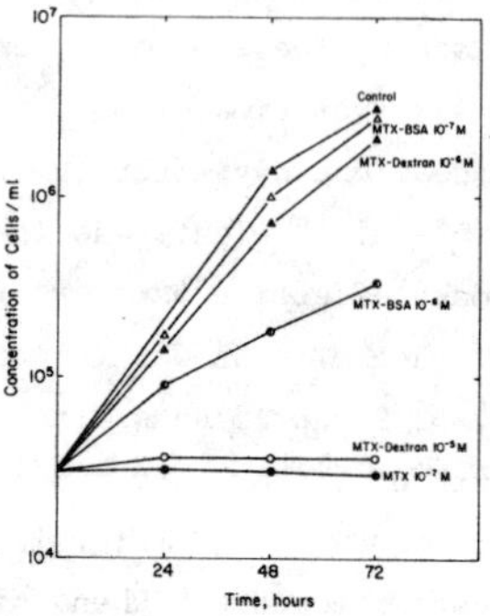

Fig. 2. The comparative inhibition of
growth of L1210 cells in RPMI 1640 medium which occurred in the presence of
MTX, MTX-BSA and MTX-Dextran T70 at the
concentrations indicated.

The entry of MTX-^{125}[I]BSA into L1210 cells was found to be less temperature dependent than that of MTX. At 0° and pH 7.5, MTX transport was >95% inhibited,
whereas that of MTX-BSA was reduced only 50%. At 35° in the presence of p-chloro-
mercurybenzoylsulfonate, a sulfhydryl inhibitor which inhibits MTX transport,[1] the
intracellular drug concentration of MTX-incubated cells dropped an average of 65%,
whereas MTX-BSA transport was reduced only 33%. Similarly the addition of excess 5-
formyl-tetrahydrofolate, which shares the same carrier mechanism as MTX,[2] also
inhibited MTX transport an average of 55%, but reduced MTX-BSA levels only 22%
(Fig. 3). These results suggest that MTX-BSA may gain entry into L1210 cells by an
alternate pathway to that of free MTX.

In order to determine whether the drug-carrier complex enters the cell as one
entity or is degraded on the external membrane surface, the cells were lysed after
they had been incubated at 37° with MTX-^{125}[I]BSA. Aliquots of the membrane, lysate
and extracellular supernatant fractions were then dialyzed to determine the percentage of total radioactivity in each fraction which corresponded to low MW fragments.
Further portions were analyzed by SDS polyacrylamide electrophoresis to determine
the approximate MW of the protein fragments present in each fraction. As is shown

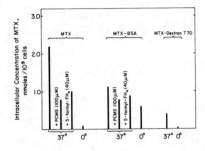

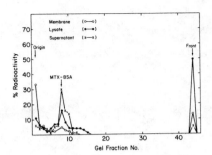

Fig. 3. Intracellular concentrations of MTX observed when L1210 cells grown *in vitro* are treated with MTX and MTX-carrier at 0° and 37°, and in the presence of the indicated levels of *p*-chloromercurybenzoylsulfonate (PCMS) and 5-formyltetrahydrofolate (5-formyl-FH$_4$).

Fig. 4. Radioactive profile obtained by SDS polyacrylamide gel electrophoresis of the cell supernatant (x——x), membrane (o——o) and lysate (●——●) fractions obtained from L1210 cells grown *in vitro* in the presence of MTX-[125][I]BSA.

in Fig. 4, 50% of the carrier in the lysate fraction has been degraded to small MW fragments, the rest remaining as undegraded carrier. With the cell membrane fraction most of the radioactivity remained at the top of the gel suggesting little of the membrane bound carrier had been degraded. The extracellular supernatant fraction was primarily unchanged MTX-[125][I]BSA.

The combined results of the transport experiments suggest that the MTX-BSA complex, and perhaps other drug-protein complexes, are not degraded on the cell surface but bind non-specifically and then enter the cell as one entity, possibly by pinocytosis, where the drug-carrier complex is degraded within the lysosomes causing release of the free drug into the cytoplasm.

ACKNOWLEDGEMENTS

This investigation was supported by USPHS Grant No. CA-11778. John M. Whiteley is the recipient of a USPHS Research Career Development Award (CA-00106) from the National Cancer Institute.

REFERENCES

1. Rader, J.L., Neithammer, D. and Huennekens, F.M. (1974) Biochem. Pharmacol. 23, 2057-2059.

2. Nahas, A., Nixon, P.F. and Bertino, J.R. (1972) Cancer Res., 32, 1416-1421.

651

THE CONCEPT OF METHOTREXATE AS A VERY RAPIDLY REVERSIBLE INHIBITOR OF DIHYDROFOLATE
REDUCTASE WITHIN CELLS: RAMIFICATIONS WITH RESPECT TO MTX-FLUOROPYRIMIDINE
INTERACTIONS AND HIGH DOSE MTX-LEUCOVORIN PROTOCOLS

I. D. GOLDMAN, J. C. WHITE, AND R. C. JACKSON

Medical College of Virginia, Richmond, Virginia, 23298, and Indiana University,
Indianapolis, Indiana, 46202

ABSTRACT

Much greater levels of free intracellular methotrexate (MTX) are required to abolish tetrahydrofolate (THF) synthesis and THF-dependent reactions within cells than
is expected on the basis of MTX-dihydrofolate reductase (DHFR) interactions at physiological pH in cell-free systems. This paper reviews the basis for the observations that in intact mammalian cells, the interaction between MTX and DHFR is a
reversible process which is apparently competitive with dihydrofolate (DHF). The
ramifications of this interaction in terms of (i) clinical applications of high-dose
MTX protocols with leucovorin rescue, (ii) MTX interactions with fluoropyrimidines
and vinca alkaloids, and (iii) the polyglutamation of MTX are described.

INTRODUCTION

Few inhibitors have as high an affinity for their target enzyme as does MTX for

DHFR. With folic acid as substrate, MTX is a stoichiometric inhibitor of this

enzyme. Even at physiological pH, where some competitive behavior with DHF is evi-

dent in cell-free systems, the MTX K_i is very low (1). It was initially assumed that

because of this high affinity for its target enzyme, inhibition of THF synthesis by

MTX in the intact cell required only intracellular drug levels at near molar equiv-

alence with DHFR - that the drug is a stoichiometric inhibitor of DHFR within the

cell. However, it is clear from *in vitro* and *in vivo* studies that the effects of

MTX on the intact cell are rapidly reversible and that free intracellular drug is

required to suppress and abolish THF synthesis and THF-dependent reactions. (This

is reviewed in Reference 2). Studies from the laboratories of the authors have

clarified the basis for these observations and have explored the ramifications of

this functionally reversible interaction between MTX and DHFR within the cell (2-5).

THE ROLE FOR FREE INTRACELLULAR MTX IN THE INHIBITION OF THF SYNTHESIS

When cells are loaded with MTX to an intracellular level above the DHFR binding

capacity and orders of magnitude greater than the MTX K_i, ^{3}H-deoxyuridine incorpor-

ation into DNA, ^{14}C-formate incorporation into RNA, DNA, and protein, and reduction

of ^{3}H-DHF to ^{3}H-THF are abolished (3, 6-8). If these cells, containing high levels

of MTX, are transferred to MTX-free medium, as free intracellular MTX levels decline these biosynthetic reactions rapidly return to near normal rates. This occurs despite the observation that after exchangeable MTX leaves the cells, a fraction of intracellular drug indistinguishable from the DHFR binding capacity remains irreversibly bound within the cell (6, 7, 9). To achieve suppression and abolition of these processes requires the continuous presence of free intracellular MTX orders of magnitude above the MTX K_i (3, 6, 8). Thus MTX which has a high affinity for its target enzyme and appears to be bound irreversibly to DHFR, behaves as a rapidly reversible inhibitor of enzyme function within the cell.

BASIS FOR THE ROLE FOR FREE INTRACELLULAR MTX IN THE INHIBITION OF THF SYNTHESIS

DHFR activity in the cell is far in excess of the cell's capacity to generate DHF in the synthesis of thymidylate from deoxyuridylate. DHF is reduced to THF as rapidly as it is formed and normal cellular DHF concentrations are very low - orders of magnitude below the DHFR K_m for its substrate (2-5, 10). When cells are first exposed to MTX, as drug enters the cell, it is rapidly bound to DHFR and virtually no free drug is present since influx is rate-limiting to binding. Association of MTX with DHFR under these conditions is essentially stoichiometric and results in a reduction of the number of enzyme sites, a reduction in the rate of THF synthesis, and an increase in the DHF level. Since initially, the DHF level is so low compared to the K_m ($\sim 10^{-6}$ M), the reaction kinetics between DHF and DHFR are first order. The increase in intracellular DHF results in a proportional increase in the reaction rate at those enzyme sites unassociated with MTX. THF synthesis is thus maintained at near normal rates until a major portion of DHFR sites are associated with MTX. Eventually, the intracellular DHF concentration approaches its K_m for DHFR and the rate of THF synthesis can no longer increase in proportion to the increase in DHF. At this point, THF synthesis decreases and the rate of THF-dependent reactions falls. Further, because DHF has risen to high levels when free intracellular MTX is very low, DHF competes with MTX for the few remaining sites so that to fully saturate DHFR with MTX and completely suppress THF synthesis requires high levels of free intracellular MTX. The rapid reversibility of the MTX effect is predictable from these considerations. As MTX leaves the cells when the DHF level is high (presumably intracellular DHF is present as a polyglutamate which does not penetrate the cell membrane), DHF will compete with the reduced level of MTX for a few critical enzyme sites. Once a small portion of bound MTX is displaced and has left the cell, resumption of THF synthesis mediated by these few enzyme molecules results in a fall in cellular DHF to usual low levels which cannot compete with MTX for enzyme. This leaves a level of intracellular MTX which is irreversibly bound but is less than, though indistinguishable from, the DHFR binding capacity. It was estimated that 95% of cellular DHFR could be inhibited in log-phase L1210 leukemia cells before DHF reduction becomes rate-limiting to DNA synthesis and the growth rate is appreciably reduced (4). In *in vitro* systems in which DNA synthesis is much lower, the enzyme fraction required to sustain cellular THF levels would be even lower (3, 6, 8). Thus, because the intracellular DHF level can vary in the cell by orders of magnitude, the interaction between MTX and its target enzyme is functionally heterogeneous although the kinetics of the interaction can be explained on the basis of a single enzyme species. This does not preclude the possibility that there may be multiple forms of DHFR within the cell, some of which may have a reduced affinity for MTX. Such enzyme forms if present would further accentuate the reversibility of the MTX effect. Rather, the model indicates that a low affinity form of the enzyme is not required to account for reversal of MTX inhibition of DHFR activity in the cell.

CYTOTOXIC DETERMINANTS OF MTX

According to this model, some of the factors which determine MTX cytotoxicity and cellular resistance are: (1) *Membrane transport* - Since free intracellular MTX must be generated to achieve a pharmacologic effect, the membrane transport system which influences the level of free intracellular drug and its persistance within the cell will be a critical determinant of cytotoxicity (2, 11, 12). Tumor cell resistance to MTX has been associated with a high influx K_m (12, 13). Recently, resistance to MTX was attributed to a marked decrease in the numbers of MTX transport carriers in MTX-resistant L5178Y leukemia cells (14). (2) *The DHFR level* - The higher the enzyme level, the smaller the fraction of total enzyme necessary to sustain cellular demands for THF, the greater the degree of saturation of enzyme that must be achieved by MTX to suppress this critical enzyme fraction and the greater the requirement for free intracellular MTX. Since the capacity of mammalian cells to generate free intracellular MTX is limited due to electrostatic forces, energy metabolism which decreases MTX accumulation, and a saturable influx but first-order efflux mechanism which predicts a finite free drug level generated by the carrier system, increases in cellular DHFR can markedly decrease the pharmacologic effect of MTX (9, 32,22). (3) *The DHFR K_i for MTX* - Obviously, the higher the MTX K_i, the poorer the ability of MTX to interact with DHFR, the more potent the competitive effect of DHF, and the greater the level of free drug required to suppress THF synthesis. (4) *The basal rate of thymidylate synthesis from deoxyuridylate* is an important factor in determining the pharmacologic effect of MTX on THF synthesis. The lower the rate of thymidylate synthesis from deoxyuridylate, the lower the rate of DHF generation, the smaller the fraction of DHFR necessary to sustain THF synthesis, the greater the degree of saturation of enzyme by MTX that will be required, the higher the free level of MTX that will be necessary to achieve this degree of enzyme inhibition and the more refractory the cells will be to any given dose of MTX. Conversely, cells synthesizing DNA at a high rate (i.e., S-phase cells) which utilize a higher fraction of DHFR to sustain THF synthesis would be subject to the greatest pharmacologic effect of MTX at any given MTX dose. (5) *The polyglutamation of MTX* - Another element of MTX pharmacology that is currently emerging is based on the observation that this agent is polyglutamated in a variety of mammalian cells (15-19, 31). Conjugation of MTX with glutamic acid to form long-chain polyglutamate derivatives which presumably do not, or slowly, penetrate the cell membrane, but are fully active as inhibitors of DHFR (20) may have critical ramifications in terms of MTX selectivity and cytotoxicity. Intracellular synthesis of these derivatives of MTX to levels in excess of the DHFR binding capacity would result in the retention of an inhibitor of DHFR after extracellular MTX is removed *in vitro* or cleared from the plasma *in vivo*. This persistence of "free inhibitor" - drug in excess of the DHFR binding capacity thus converts MTX from a reversible to an irreversible inhibitor of the enzyme - irreversible to the extent to which MTX polyglutamates are stable and not hydrolyzed back to shorter-chain polyglutamates or the monoglutamate of MTX and irreversible to the extent to which polyglutamates are not able to penetrate the cell membrane. The differential generation of MTX polyglutamates in host vs. tumor cells may be an element in selectivity. Tissues that generate high levels of MTX polyglutamates would be subject to greater toxicity than those that generate MTX polyglutamates more slowly. The extent to which MTX polyglutamates are produced in tumor cells may be one basis for the efficacy of high-dose MTX regimens. The generation of high levels of free MTX within the cell may favor polyglutamate synthesis in the tumor which may not be reversed by leucovorin or may produce lethal effects before initiation of the rescue.

MTX INTERACTIONS WITH OTHER AGENTS

(1) *Fluoropyrimidines*. As indicated above, the basal rate of thymidylate synthesis from deoxyuridylate controls the generation of DHF in the cell and the fraction of DHFR activity required to sustain cellular THF cofactor pools. Fluoropyrimidines inhibit the generation of thymidylate and lower the rate of DHF production. Accordingly, it would be expected that the pretreatment of cells with fluoropyrimidines would reduce the pharmacologic effects of MTX. This was shown to be the case *in vitro* (21) and correlated well with the demonstration of antagonism between fluorouracil and MTX when the former is administered before or concurrently with MTX *in vivo* (22, 23). Antagonistic interactions between these agents is also expected on the basis of fluoropyrimidine-sparing cellular THF cofactors required for purine biosynthesis (24). MTX inhibition of purine synthesis as well as inhibition of thymidylate synthesis may play an important role in cytotoxicity (25, 26).

(2) *Vinca alkaloid interactions*. Vinca alkaloids slow the exit of MTX from the cell and raise the intracellular MTX concentration in excess of the fraction bound to DHFR (27, 28). This effect is probably mediated through the ability of these agents to inhibit energy-dependent uphill transport of α-aminoisobutyric acid (29). Vinca alkaloid augmentation of intracellular MTX enhances MTX inhibition of deoxyuridine incorporation into DNA (7). Recently, it has been shown that administration of vincristine before, concurrently, or shortly after MTX does not prolong the survival of L1210 leukemia-bearing animals (30). However, administration of vincristine long after MTX results in synergism between the agents (30). The basis for this interaction is uncertain, vincristine-induced changes in the intracellular MTX level could not be detected. It is possible that this interaction occurs at a time when the free

intracellular MTX level has declined to a point where THF synthesis is about to resume – when these cells would be most susceptible to a retardation in the further e-
gress of free intracellular MTX. However, because at low extracellular MTX levels
exchangeable intracellular MTX in the L1210 leukemia system is so low in comparison
to the DHFR binding capacity, changes in exchangeable intracellular drug may be undetectable. A correlation between vinca synergism and a delay in the resumption of
deoxyuridine incorporation into DNA, a parameter that is closely related to the decline in the exchangeable intracellular MTX level, would be an additional way of
assessing whether the vinca-MTX interaction under these conditions *in vivo* is related
to an alteration in MTX transport.

A RATIONALE FOR HIGH-DOSE MTX REGIMENS BASED ON THE REVERSIBLE NATURE
OF THE INTERACTION BETWEEN MTX AND DHFR WITHIN CELLS

The basis for the efficacy of high-dose MTX regimens with leucovorin rescue has
not, as yet, been clearly established and the application of such regimens has preceded a definitive rationale for its use. However, current concepts on the mechanism
of action of MTX provide some scientific basis for this approach. High-dose regimens
with MTX offer a number of pharmacologic advantages. They produce very high extracellular MTX concentrations which permit diffusion of drug into pharmacologic hide-
outs. Because of the marked limitation in the ability of mammalian cells to generate
free intracellular MTX, achievement of high drug levels within the cell requires very
high extracellular drug concentrations – the concentration difference across the cell
membrane may represent a gradient of more than one order of magnitude. Achievement
of high intracellular drug concentrations could deal with many of the factors which
limit the pharmacologic effects of MTX such as impaired membrane transport, DHFR levels, low DHFR K_i for MTX and a low tumor cell basal rate of thymidylate synthesis.
Further, as suggested above, high free intracellular MTX levels might favor the generation of polyglutamates within tumor cells which will have important ramifications
on the extent and duration of the pharmacologic effect produced by MTX. High free
levels of MTX within the cell offers the possibility of inhibiting THF synthesis not
only in S-phase cells, but in cells in other phases of their replicative cycle which
are making thymidylate for DNA repair and for mitochondrial replication – cells in

which thymidylate synthesis is so slow and generation of DHF is so low that only extremely high concentrations of MTX would block THF synthesis in these cells.

REFERENCES

1. Bertino, J.R., Booth, B. A., Bieber, A.L., et al. (1964), J. Biol. Chem. 239, 479-485.
2. Goldman, I.D. (1977), Cancer Treatment Rep. 61, 549-558.
3. White, J.C. and Goldman, I.D. (1976), Mol. Pharmacol. 12, 711-720.
4. Jackson, R.C. and Harrap, K.R. (1973), Arch. Biochem. Biophys. 158, 827-841.
5. Jackson, R.C., Niethammer, D., and Hart, L.I. (1977), Arch. Biochem. Biophys. 182, 646-656.
6. Goldman, I.D. (1974), Mol. Pharmacol. 10, 257-274.
7. Goldman, I.D. and Fyfe, M.J. (1974), Mol. Pharmacol. 10, 275-282.
8. White, J.C., Loftfield, S., and Goldman, I.D. (1975), Mol. Pharmacol. 11, 287-297.
9. Goldman, I.D., Lichtenstein, N.S., Oliverio, V.T. (1968), J. Biol. Chem. 243, 5007-5017.
10. Moran, R.J., Werkheiser, W.C. and Zakrzewski, S.F. (1976), J. Biol. Chem. 251, 3569-3578.
11. Sirotnak, F.M. and Donsbach, R.C. (1974), Cancer Res. 34, 3332-3340.
12. Sirotnak, F.M. and Donsbach, R.C. (1976), Cancer Res. 36, 1151-1158.
13. Jackson, R.C., Niethammer, D., and Huennekens, F.M. (1975), Cancer Biochem. Biophys. 1, 151, 1975.
14. Hill, B.T., Bailey, B.D., Goldman, I.D. (1978), Proc. Am. Assoc. Cancer Res. 19, 49.
15. Baugh, C.M., Krumdieck, C.L., and Nair, M.G. (1973), Biochem. Biophys. Res. Commun. 52, 27.
16. Brown, J.P., Davidson, G.E., Weir, D.G., and Scott, J.M. (1974), Int. J. Biochem. 5, 727.
17. Whitehead, V.M. (1977), Cancer Res. 37, 408-412.
18. Whitehead, V.M., Perrault, M.M., and Stelcner, S. (1975), Cancer Res. 35, 2985.
19. Rosenblatt, D.S., Whitehead, V.M., DuPont, M.M., Vohich, M.-J., and Vera, N. (1978), Mol. Pharmacol. 14, 210.
20. Jacobs, S.A., Adamson, R.H., Chabner, B.A., Derr, C.I., and Johns, D.G. (1975), Biochem. Biophys. Res. Commun. 63, 692.
21. Bowen, D., White, J.C., and Goldman, I.D. (1978), Cancer Res. 38, 219.
22. Bertino, J. R., Sawicki, W.L., Lindquist, C.A., and Gupta, V.S. (1977), Cancer Res. 37, 327.
23. Heppner, G. H. and Calabresi, P. (1977), Cancer Res. 37, 4580.
24. Tattersall, M.H.N., Jackson, R.C., Connors, T.A., and Harrap, K.R. (1973), Euro. J. Cancer 9, 733-739.
25. Grindey, G., and Moran, R.D. (1975), Cancer Res. 35, 1702-1705.
26. Hryniuk, W.M. (1975), Cancer Res. 35, 1085-1092.
27. Zager, R.D., Frisby, S.A., and Oliverio, B.T. (1973), Cancer Res. 33, 1670-1676.
28. Fyfe, M.J. and Goldman, I.D. (1973), J. Biol. Chem. 248, 5067-5073.
29. Fyfe, M.J., Loftfield, S., and Goldman, I.D. (1975), J. Cell. Physiol. 86, 201.
30. Chello, P.L., Sirotnak, F.M., Dorick, D.M., Moccio, D.M., and Gura, T. (1978), Proc. Am. Assoc. Cancer Res. 19, 113.
31. Gewirtz, D.A., White, J.C., and Goldman, I.D. (1978), Fed. Proc. 37, 1346.
32. Goldman, I.D. (1973), Uptake of drugs and resistance. In Drug Resistance and Selectivity, Biochemical and Cellular Basis. New York, Academic Press, 229-358.
33. Goldman, I.D. (1971), Ann. N.Y. Acad. Sci. 186, 400-422.

METABOLISM OF METHOTREXATE AND FOLIC ACID IN CRITHIDIA FASCICULATA

KAZUO IWAI, HIDEO OE AND MASAHIRO KOBASHI
Research Institute for Food Science, Kyoto University, Uji, Kyoto
611 (Japan)

ABSTRACT

Crithidia fasciculata utilized methotrexate for its growth at the
same level as folic acid. Methotrexate was metabolized mainly to 4-
amino-4-deoxy-10-methylpteroic acid. The hydrolyzing activity for
methotrexate was found in cell-free extracts. The enzyme was isolated
in a highly purified state, and appeared as a single band on a polyacrylamide gel electrophoresis. The molecular weight of the enzyme was
about 200,000 and that of the SDS-treated enzyme was 51,000. The optimum pH was found to be 7.0. The enzyme, tentatively named the folate-
hydrolyzing enzyme, catalyzed the cleaving reaction of the amide linkage of folic acid, methotrexate, aminopterin and other folate compounds,
except pteroyltriglutamate. The Km values for folic acid, methotrexate
and aminopterin were 0.13, 0.46 and 0.40 mM, respectively. The purified enzyme also hydrolyzed significantly various N-benzyloxycarbonyl
(Cbz) dipeptides with an aromatic amino acid and Cbz-amino acids, but
not Cbz-Gly-Phe-NH$_2$ and various dipeptides. The enzyme was inhibited
by divalent cations such as Hg^{2+}, Cu^{2+}, Cd^{2+}, Pb^{2+}, and Zn^{2+} at 10^{-4}M and
by chelating agents at 10^{-4}M. Only the addition of Co^{2+} partially recovered the activity of the enzyme which had been previously treated
with a chelating agent, bathophenanthroline. From these results, the
folate-hydrolyzing enzyme in C. fasciculata is assumed to be a new type
of carboxypeptidase. A possible function of this enzyme in the protozoa is also discussed.

INTRODUCTION

The trypanosomid flagellate, Crithidia fasciculata ATCC 12857, a
parasite of mosquitoes, requires unusually high levels of folic acid
for its growth[1-4]. But in the presence of a small amount of 6-alkyl-
pterin such as biopterin, its requirement for folic acid is satisfied
at lower levels.

During the study on the metabolism of folate compounds in the protozoa, we found that anti-folates such as methotrexate and aminopterin
promoted the growth of C. fasciculata at the same level as folic acid.
On the other hand, in vitro, these anti-folates at 0.1 to 1 nM inhibi-

ted strongly the dihydrofolate reductase of this protozoa. The growth-promoting effect of anti-folates stimulated us to clarify the metabolism of methotrexate and folic acid in C. fasciculata.

This paper deals with the identification of a metabolite of methotrexate, and with the occurrence, purification and some properties of an enzyme catalyzing the hydrolysis of methotrexate and folate in C. fasciculata. The metabolism of folic acid in C. fasciculata is also discussed.

MATERIALS AND METHODS

Materials. $[2-^{14}C]$ Folic acid potassium salt (58.2 mCi/mM) and $[3', 5', 9(n)-^3H]$ methotrexate sodium salt (6 Ci/mM) were obtained from the Radiochemical Centre (Amersham). The N-benzyloxycarbonyl (Cbz) dipeptides and Cbz-amino acids used were gifts from Drs. R. Hayashi and T. Matoba, Kyoto university. Pepstatin A and phenylmethylsulfonylfluoride were also from Dr. R. Hayashi. Cbz-Glu and Cbz-Gly-Phe-NH$_2$ were obtained from the Protein Research Foundation (Osaka). Crystalline carboxypeptidase A from bovine pancreas was purchased from Sigma Chemical Co. Other chemicals were acquired from Nakarai Chemicals Ltd.

Media for C. fasciculata. A chemically defined medium[1] was used to investigate the metabolism of methotrexate. The culture medium[5] was used to purify an enzyme catalyzing the hydrolysis of folate compounds. The Crithidia cells were harvested at its logarithmic phase grown at 25 °C.

Standard assay condition for an enzyme catalyzing the hydrolysis of folate compounds. The activity of the enzyme was measured by a radioassay as follows: After incubating the enzyme with 2 μmoles of $[2-^{14}C]$ folic acid (50 nCi) in 0.1 M Tris-HCl buffer, pH 7.0, at 37°C for 1 hour, the $[2-^{14}C]$ pteroic acid formed was separated by thin-layer chromatography on the Avicel cellulose plate. The zone corresponding to pteroic acid was scraped off and its radioactivity was counted[6].

Preparation of 4-amino-4-deoxy-10-methylpteroic acid (AMPte). AMPte was prepared from methotrexate by the folate-hydrolyzing enzyme of C. fasciculata, and separated by thin-layer chromatography on Avicel cellulose plates developed with 0.1 M phosphate buffer at pH 7.0. The zone corresponding to AMPte was scraped off and eluted with water. The eluate was desalted by chromatography on a Sephadex G-10 column and lyophilized. The infrared and UV absorption spectra of the isolated compound coincided with the data established[7].

RESULTS AND DISCUSSION

Metabolism of methotrexate. Methotrexate promoted the growth of C. fasciculata at the same level as folic acid. The amounts of methotrexate and folic acid corresponding to the level of growth at 0.11 nM of biopterin were 9.2 and 12.4 nM, respectively. During the growth of C. fasciculata, methotrexate was found to be metabolized to some compounds. C. fasciculata was cultured at 25°C for 4.5 days in a chemically defined medium containing 0.1 μM of [^{3}H]methotrexate (0.13 μCi), the cells were harvested and sonicated in 3 ml of 10 mM Tris-HCl buffer at pH 7.0 containing 100 mM 2-mercaptoethanol, and the extracts were subjected to a DEAE-cellulose column (1.4 x 7 cm). The cultured medium of 10 ml was subjected to a column of the same size. The elution was performed with a linear gradient of each 60 ml of 10 mM Tris-HCl and 1 M Tris-HCl buffers at pH 7.0, containing 100 mM 2-mercaptoethanol. Figure 1 shows the elution profile of the metabolites. The major metabolite (peak II in Fig. 1) was identified as AMPte by co-chromatography with an authentic compound on Avicel cellulose plates. Upon incubation at 37°C for 1 hr with cell-free extracts of the Crithidia in 50 mM Tris-HCl buffer at pH 7.0, [^{3}H]methotrexate was converted to [^{3}H]AMPte. The extracts also converted folic acid to pteroic acid. Although methotrexate has been reported to be metabolized mainly to its 7-hydroxy compound[8,9] or its poly-γ-glutamyl compounds[10-12] in mammalian tissues, it may be hydrolyzed at the initial metabolic step in C. fasciculata, as in bacteria.[7,10,13-15]

Purification of the folate-hydrolyzing enzyme. In order to investigate its properties, the enzyme was purified from 450 g (wet weight) of the Crithidia cells. Since ammonium sulfate inhibited the enzyme activity, heat treatment (60°C for 5 min), chromatography on DEAE-cellulose and Sephadex G-200 columns, and preparative electrophoresis on polyacrylamide gel[16] were performed. Summary of the purification is shown in Table I. The purified enzyme appeared as a single band on polyacrylamide gel electrophoresis.

Properties of the folate-hydrolyzing enzyme. The molecular weight of the enzyme was estimated to be about 200,000 by gel filtration on a Sephadex G-200 column. The SDS-treated enzyme appeared as a single band whose molecular weight was about 51,000. Optimum pH was 7.0 as shown in Fig. 2. Phosphate buffer was inhibitory at pH 7.0. The enzyme was unstable at alkaline pH over 8.5. The reaction products from folic acid were identified as pteroic acid and L-glutamic acid. Stoichiometry of the reaction was 1/1/1. Methotrexate and aminopterin were hydrolyzed as substrates further than folic acid, as shown in Table II. The reaction products of methotrexate were identified as AMPte and L-glutamic acid. Figure 3 shows an infrared spectrum of the AMPte produced. Cbz-dipeptides with an aromatic amino acid were hydrolyzed 10 times or more than folic acid, but Cbz-dipeptides without aromatic amino acids were less or not as active as the substrate. The enzyme also hydrolyzed Cbz-amino acids significantly, as compared with carboxypeptidase A. Cbz-dipeptide amides, dipeptides such as Gly-Tyr, and γ-peptide such as pteroyltriglutamate were inactive. The Km values of the enzyme for folic acid, methotrexate and aminopterin, were 0.13, 0.46, and 0.40 mM, respectively. Divalent cations such as Hg^{2+}, Cu^{2+}, Cd^{2+}, Pb^{2+} and Zn^{2+} strongly inhibited the reaction at 10^{-4}M. Chelating agents also inhibited the reaction. The activity of the enzyme treated with a chelating

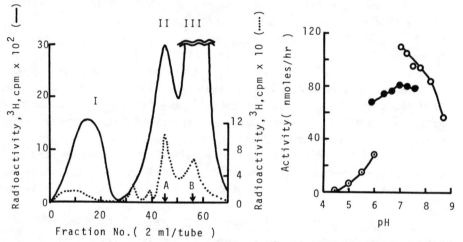

Fig. 1. The elution profile of radio-activity in the cultured medium (—) and cell-free extracts (····) of C. fasciculata after culturing with 0.1 μM of [^{3}H]-methotrexate (0.13 μCi). See the text for details. A, AMPte; B, methotrexate.

Fig. 2. Effect of pH and buffers on the folate-hydrolyzing enzyme Enzyme activity was measured under the standard assay condition. Tris-HCl buffer, ○—○; Tris-maleate, ●—●; sodium citrate, ◉—◉; at 0.1 M.

TABLE I   SUMMARY OF PURIFICATION OF THE FOLATE-HYDROLYZING ENZYME FROM CRITHIDIA FASCICULATA

Step	Protein (mg)	Activity* (nmoles/hr)	Specific activity (nmoles/hr/mg)	Yield (%)
Crude extract	35,853	109,071	3.1	100.0
Heat treatment	20,179	109,030	5.4	100.0
1st DEAE-Sephadex	2,016	60,598	30.1	55.6
2nd DEAE-Sephadex	506	21,526	42.5	19.7
Sephadex G-200	98	10,384	106.1	9.5
Electrophoresis	5.2	1,640	315.4	1.5

* The enzyme activity was estimated as amounts of pteroic acid formed under the standard assay condition.

agent was partially recovered only by the addition of Co^{2+}, as shown in Table III. The enzyme was inhibited completely by p-chloromercuribenzoate at 10^{-4}M, but neither by phenylmethylsulfonylfluoride nor by pepstatin A. The folate-hydrolyzing enzyme has been found in some bacteria and it has been reported that it is inducible and a Zn^{2+}-requiring enzyme, and it specifically hydrolyzes glutamate or aspartate-terminal peptides.[7,13-15] On the other hand, the properties of the enzyme isolated from C. fasciculata differed extremely from those of the bacterial

TABLE II   SUBSTRATE SPECIFICITY OF THE FOLATE-HYDROLYZING ENZYME

Substrate (1 mM)	Activity*	Relative activity	Substrate (1 mM)	Activity*	Relative activity
Pteroylglutamate	0.014	1.0	Cbz-Gly-Leu	0	0
Pteroyl-triglutamate	0	0	Cbz-Gly-Arg	0	0
			Cbz-Gly-Tyr	0.487	34.8
Methotrexate	0.039	2.8	Cbz-Gly-Phe	0.302	21.6
Aminopterin	0.042	3.0	Cbz-Gly-Phe-NH$_2$	0	0
p-Aminobenzoyl-glutamate	0.017	1.2	Cbz-Glu	0.018	1.3
			Cbz-Tyr	0.059	4.2
Cbz-Glu-Glu	0.073	5.2	Cbz-Phe	0.047	3.4
Cbz-Phe-Glu	0.140	10.0	Gly-Tyr	0	0
Cbz-Phe-Ala	0.443	31.6			

* The enzyme activity was assayed by the ninhydrin method[17] and Δ optical density of 0.014 was equivalent to 2.2 nmoles of amino acid released.

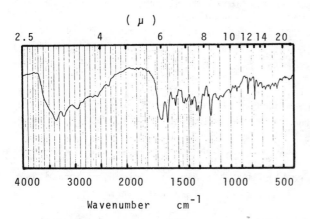

Fig. 3. Infrared spectrum of a compound (AMPte) produced from methotrexate by the folate-hydrolyzing enzyme.
Spectrum was taken in a KBr pellet by a Hitachi Model 285 infrared spectrometer.

TABLE III

EFFECT OF CATIONS ON THE FOLATE-HYDROLYZING ENZYME TREATED WITH BATHOPHENANTHROLINE (BP)

Cation added (0.2mM)	Activity (%)
Control (untreated enzyme)	100.0
None (BP-enzyme*)	19.4
Fe^{2+}	20.3
Fe^{3+}	25.0
Mg^{2+}	20.1
Ca^{2+}	21.7
Co^{2+}	43.6

* The enzyme was preincubated with 0.8 mM of BP at 37°C for 30 min. and dialyzed against 5 mM Tris-HCl buffer at pH 7 for 6 hr, and used for BP-enzyme. The BP-enzyme was incubated with cations as indicated at 37°C for 1 hr.

enzyme. The protozoal enzyme is constitutive, activated by Co^{2+} but inhibited by Zn^{2+}, and hydrolyzes various synthetic peptides and folate compounds, as shown in Table II. Since some of the enzymic properties rather resemble with those of carboxypeptidase A, the substrate specificity of carboxypeptidase A was compared with that of the protozoal enzyme. The results indicated that carboxypeptidase A did not hydrolyze folic acid, methotrexate and p-aminobenzoylglutamic acid at all, while it hydrolyzed Cbz-amino acids only slightly.

From these results, the folate-hydrolyzing enzyme in C. fasciculata is assumed to be a new type of carboxypeptidase. It has been suggested that one of the metabolic functions of folic acid in C. fasciculata is a precursor of an independently functioning unconjugated pteridine,[4,18] and this folate-hydrolyzing enzyme may play an important role in initiating the metabolism of folic acid in this protozoa.

REFERENCE

1. Nathan, H.A. and Cowperthwaite, J. (1954) Proc. Soc. Exp. Biol. Med., 85, 117-119.

2. Nathan, H.A., Hutner, S.H. and Levin, H.L. (1956) Nature, 178, 741-742.

3. Kidder, G.W. and Dutta, B.N. (1958) J. Gen. Microbiol., 18, 621-638.

4. Nathan, H.A. and Funk, H.B. (1959) Am. J. Clin. Nutr., 7, 375-384.

5. Guttman, H.N. (1964) in Pteridine Chemistry, Pfleiderer, W. and Taylor, E.C. eds.,Pergamon, London pp. 255-266.

6. Okinaka, O. and Iwai, K. (1969) Anal. Biochem., 31, 174-182.

7. Levy, C.C. and Goldman, P. (1967) J. Biol. Chem., 242, 2933-2938.

8. Johns, D.G. and Valerino, D.M. (1971) Annal. New York Acad. Sci., 186, 378-386.

9. Johns, D.G., Iannotti, A.T., Sartorelli, A.C., Booth, B.A. and Bertino, J.R. (1965) Biochim. Biophys. Acta, 105, 380-382.

10. Shin. Y.S., Buehring, K.U. and Stokstad, E.L.R. (1974) J. Biol. Chem., 249, 5772-5777.

11. Baugh, C.M., Krumdieck, C.L. and Nair, M.G. (1973) Biochem. Biophys. Res. Commun., 52, 27-34.

12. Bühring, K.V. and Fölsch, E.(1976)Biochim. Biophys. Acta,421,22-32.

13. Goldman, P and Levy. C.C. (1967) Proc. Natl. Acad. Sci., 58, 1299-1306.

14. Pratt, A.G., Crawford, E.J. and Friedkin, M. (1968) J. Biol. Chem., 243, 6367-6372.

15. McCullough, J.L., Chabner, B.A. and Bertino, J.R. (1971) J. Biol. Chem., 246, 7207-7213.

16. Davis, B.J. (1964) Annal. New York Acad. Sci., 121, 404-427.

17. Moore, S. (1968) J. Biol. Chem., 243, 6281-6283.

18. Kidder, G.W., Dewey, V.C. and Rembold, H. (1967) Arch. für Mikrobiol., 59, 180-184.

665

FOLATE ENZYMES IN RAT HEPATOMAS: IMPLICATIONS FOR ANTIFOLATE THERAPY

ROBERT C. JACKSON AND DIETRICH NIETHAMMER
Laboratory for Experimental Oncology, Indiana University, Indianapolis,
Indiana 46202 (U.S.A.) and Department of Paediatrics, University of
Ulm (Germany)

ABSTRACT

Activities of eight folate enzymes were measured in rat liver and
a series of rat hepatomas of widely different growth rates. Only thymidylate synthetase had greater activity in the tumours than in normal
liver (up to 123-fold). The folate-dependent enzymes of histidine
catabolism were markedly decreased in the hepatomas (1 - 33% of liver
activity), as was 5,10-methylenetetrahydrofolate dehydrogenase. These
changes make the neoplastic cells more susceptible to the antipurine
effect of dihydrofolate reductase inhibitors. In addition, well differentiated hepatomas have an appreciable capacity for the degradation
of thymidine; in these tumours the combination of thymidine plus hypoxanthine was unable to block the cytotoxicity of amethopterin to cells
in culture. In vivo, amethopterin alone at the highest tolerated dose
gave no significant increase in lifespan of rats bearing Morris hepatoma 8999, but amethopterin (4 mg/kg) accompanied by thymidine (500 mg/
kg twice daily) gave 45% increase in lifespan.

INTRODUCTION

The process of neoplastic transformation in liver is accompanied by
many alterations in enzyme activity. In the area of folate metabolism
Elford et al.[1] reported increased thymidylate synthetase activity in
hepatomas, correlating with the growth rate. Lepage et al.[2] examined
dihydrofolate reductase, serine hydroxymethyltransferase, 5,10-methyl-
enetetrahydrofolate dehydrogenase, 10-formyltetrahydrofolate synthetase,
and formiminotransferase, and found small to moderate decreases in these
activities relative to host liver. It would be desirable to confirm
these results using normal liver as control tissue. Grossman et al.[3]
showed that methionine synthetase was unchanged in six hepatomas. Some
folate enzymes have been examined in regenerating liver: Labow et al.[4]
reported an elevation in thymidylate synthetase, and Newbold[5] showed
an increase in dihydrofolate reductase. The present report describes
further studies on folate enzymes in transplantable rat hepatomas, and

attempts to relate the selectivity of action of amethopterin in different tumour lines to the pattern of activity of the folate enzymes.

MATERIALS AND METHODS

Animals and tumours. Male ACI/N rats of 200g body weight were used for passage of hepatomas 3924A and 3683, and for the regenerating liver studies. For other tumours 200g male Buffalo rats were used. The hepatomas were supplied by Dr H.P. Morris, and their properties have been previously described[6]. Partial hepatectomy was by the standard method[7].

Cell culture. Origins of the cell lines, and the growth conditions used have been discussed previously[8]. Mean log-phase doubling times of cells used in the present studies were: Novikoff, 12 h; 8999R, 36 h.

Enzyme assays. Tumours were dissected free of necrotic and connective material, minced, and homogenized in 0.25 M sucrose buffered to pH 7.4 with 0.05 M Tris.HCl. Homogenates were centrifuged at 105,000g for 60 min, and all enzymes were measured in the cytosol fraction. Assay techniques followed published procedures: dihydrofolate reductase[9]; thymidylate synthetase[10]; 5,10-methylenetetrahydrofolate dehydrogenase[11]; serine hydroxymethyltransferase[12];10-formyltetrahydrofolate synthetase[13], 10-formyltetrahydrofolate dehydrogenase[14]; 5-formiminotransferase[15]; cyclodeaminase[16]. Cytosol protein was measured by the Lowry method[17].

RESULTS AND DISCUSSION

Folate enzymes in hepatomas. Activities of eight folate cofactor metabolizing enzymes in normal rat liver and in several transplantable hepatomas are shown in Table 1. Dihydrofolate reductase activity in three hepatomas was lower than control activity. In regenerating liver, as previously reported[5], an increase was seen, though this did not become apparent until 48 h after partial hepatectomy. Thymidylate synthetase had the lowest baseline activity in normal liver of all the folate enzymes studied; as shown by Elford et al.[1] thymidylate synthetase activity was markedly elevated in the hepatomas. All the other six enzymes studied had lower activity in the tumours than in normal liver; these decreases were most pronounced for the three enzymes concerned in the catabolism of histidine (5-formiminotransferase, cyclodeaminase and 10-formyltetrahydrofolate dehydrogenase). This pathway apparently is a specialized hepatic function that is progressively lost in the process of neoplastic transformation and malignant progression. The occurence of 10-formyltetrahydrofolate dehydrogenase in liver suggests that in some circumstances liver may acquire one-carbon groups in excess of its requirements for biosynthetic purposes. The retention of small but significant

TABLE 1. ACTIVITY OF FOLATE ENZYMES IN RAT LIVER AND HEPATOMAS

Enzyme	Tissue	Transplant interval (months)	Activity nmol/h/mg protein	percent of normal liver
Dihydrofolate reductase (EC 1.5.1.3)	Liver	–	430	100
	Regenerating liver (24 h)	–	412	96
	" (48 h)	–	1010	235
	Hepatomas:			
	44	5.6	230	53
	7777	1.2	200	47
	3683	0.6	77	18
Thymidylate synthetase (EC 2.1.1.46)	Liver	–	0.2	100
	Regenerating liver (24 h)	–	1.3	650
	Hepatomas:			
	8999	4.0	4.2	2,100
	3924A	0.9	13.2	6,600
	Novikoff	0.4	24.6	12,300
5,10-Methylene tetrahydrofolate dehydrogenase (EC 1.5.1.5)	Liver	–	2400	100
	Regenerating liver (24 h)	–	2860	119
	Hepatomas:			
	8999	4.0	408	17
	3924A	0.9	260	11
	Novikoff	0.4	240	10
Serine hydroxy-methyltransferase (EC 2.1.2.1)	Liver	–	1650	100
	Hepatomas:			
	20	12.0	1570	95
	21	9.0	1620	98
	16	8.7	1070	65
	9633	6.0	1140	69
	7787	5.8	1200	73
	7794A	5.4	1320	80
	5123D	1.8	460	28
	7777	1.2	1155	70
	3924A	0.9	380	23
10-Formyltetra-hydrofolate synthetase (EC 6.3.4.3)	Liver	–	160	100
	Hepatomas:			
	20	12.0	57	35
	16	8.7	54	34
	9633	6.0	31	19
	7787	5.8	67	42
	7794A	5.4	39	24
	8999	4.0	34	21
	3924A	0.9	31	19
10-Formyltetra-hydrofolate dehydrogenase (EC: none)	Liver	–	70	100
	Hepatomas:			
	9618A	10.5	23	33
	8999	4.0	6	9
	3924A	0.9	0.7	1
5-Formimino-transferase (EC 2.1.2.5)	Liver	–	2700	100
	Hepatomas:			
	9618A	10.5	190	7
	8999	4.0	28	1
	3924A	0.9	105	4

TABLE 1.   (continued)

Enzyme	Tissue	Transplant interval (months)	Activity nmol/h/mg protein	percent of normal liver
Cyclodeaminase (EC 4.3.1.4)	Liver Hepatomas:	–	330	100
	8999	4.0	34	10
	3924A	0.6	19	6

Activities shown are means for four or more samples. Assay methods used were as described under "Materials and Methods".

amounts of this enzyme in well differentiated hepatomas suggests that leucovorin may give poor rescue of hepatomas after high-dose amethopterin, while allowing effective rescue of gut and bone marrow. Another hepatic function partially retained in well differentiated hepatomas is the catabolism of thymidine[8]. The exploitation of this effect to increase selectivity of antifolate chemotherapy is discussed below.

10-Formyltetrahydrofolate synthetase, although readily detectable in liver and hepatomas, had much lower activity than serine hydroxymethyltransferase. This reaction seems to be a relatively minor supplier of one-carbon groups, and its primary importance may lie in the removal of free formate. Decreased activity of this enzyme in the hepatomas may reflect a lesser degree of formate production in the malignant tissues. The decreased activities of serine hydroxymethyltransferase and 5,10-methylenetetrahydrofolate dehydrogenase in hepatomas are difficult to explain, since these enzymes appear to play a major role in production of activated one-carbon groups and their direction to the biosynthesis of purines. Since purines are readily synthesized by the de novo pathway in hepatomas, it must be concluded that the reduced activities of the folate-interconverting enzymes are still compatible with undiminished purine production. However, as previously discussed[8], the greatly altered ratio of activities of thymidylate synthetase to 5,10-methylene tetrahydrofolate dehydrogenase in hepatomas markedly enhances the antipurine effect of amethopterin.

Membrane transport of folate and antifolates.   Transport of folic acid, 5-methyltetrahydrofolate, and amethopterin were studied in Novikoff and 8999R cultured hepatoma cells by methods previously described[18]. Results with the Novikoff cells closely resembled those previously obtained with human lymphoblasts[18]. Uptake of amethopterin (1 μM) was initially rapid and a steady state was reached by 20 min (Figure 1). Uptake of 5-methyltetrahydrofolate (1 μM) was biphasic; after an initial rapid phase, the rate decreased and from 5 min to 60 min was linear,

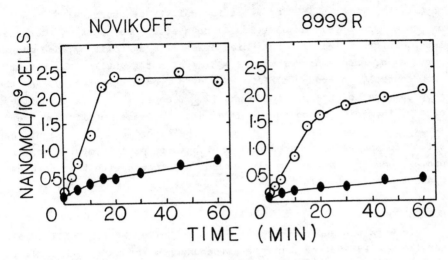

Fig. 1. Transport of amethopterin and folic acid into cultured hepatoma cells. ⊙ amethopterin, 1 μM; ● folic acid, 5 μM.

this second rate probably representing intracellular metabolism of the cofactor. Transport of both amethopterin and 5-methyltetrahydrofolate was completely abolished (< 2% control) following 5 min incubation with 20 μM p-chloromercurisulphonate (pCMS). Folic acid transport (extracellular concentration 5 μM) was much slower (about 20%) than 5-methyltetrahydrofolate, and was unaffected by pCMS. Results with the more slowly growing hepatoma 8999R were generally similar to those obtained with Novikoff cells, except that transport of amethopterin (1 μM) appeared biphasic, with slow linear uptake observed after the rapid initial rate obtained in the first 20 min (Figure 1).

Experimental chemotherapy of hepatomas with antifolates. Malignant hepatomas are notoriously refractory to chemotherapy. However, because of the relatively active catabolism of thymidine in some of these tumours we postulated that the combination of high-dose amethopterin followed by thymidine rescue might have some antihepatoma selectivity[8], since the thymidine would confer some protection upon bone marrow and intestinal mucosa, but much less upon a well differentiated hepatoma that degrades thymidine. This protocol was tested using Morris hepatoma 8999. Five weeks after inoculation (subcutaneously, in the flank) the tumours had reached a diameter of about 1 cm. Animals were divided into groups of 10, and received (a) no treatment; (b) 5 daily i.p. doses of amethopterin, 1 mg/kg/day; (c) 5 daily doses of amethopterin, 4 mg/kg/

day, with thymidine (500 mg/kg) twice daily. Mean survival of the untreated group (a) was 53 ($\pm$S.D.4) days after the start of the experiment. In group (b) 4/10 rats died of early drug toxicity, and mean survival of the remainder was 59 $\pm$ 5 days, not significantly better than control. In group (c) 1/10 rats died from drug toxicity, and the mean survival of the remainder was 77 $\pm$ 7 days, an increase in lifespan of 46%. Thymidine alone (group d) gave no increase in lifespan (mean survival 49 $\pm$3days after the start of the experiment). The significant effect in the group treated with amethopterin plus thymidine confirms and extends the earlier *in vitro* results obtained with this combination against hepatoma cells[8].

ACKNOWLEDGEMENTS

This work was supported by grants from United States Public Health Service (CA 18129) and Deutsche Forschungsgemeinschaft (SFB 112). The authors thank L. Soliven for skilled technical assistance.

REFERENCES

1. Elford,H.L.,Freese,M.,Passamani,E. and Morris,H.P. (1970) J.Biol. Chem. 245:5228-5233.
2. Lepage,R.,Poirier,L.A.,Poirier,M.C. and Morris,H.P. (1972) Cancer Res. 32: 1099-1103.
3. Grossman,M.R.,Finkelstein,J.D.,Kyle,W.E. and Morris,H.P. (1974) Cancer Res. 34: 794-800.
4. Labow,R.,Maley,G.F. and Maley,F. (1968) Cancer Res. 29: 366-372.
5. Newbold,P.C.H. (1973) Brit.J.Dermatol. 89: 343-349.
6. Morris,H.P. and Wagner,B.P.(1968)Methods in Cancer Res.4:125-152.
7. Higgins,G.M. and Anderson,R.M. (1931) Archs.Pathol. 12: 186-202.
8. Jackson,R.C. and Weber,G. (1976) Biochem.Pharmacol. 25: 2613-2618.
9. Mathews,C.K. and Huennekens,F.M.(1963)J.Biol.Chem.238: 3436-3442.
10. Lomax,M.I.S. and Greenberg,G.R.(1967) J.Biol.Chem. 242: 109-113.
11. Ramasastri,B.V. and Blakley,R.L.(1962)J.Biol.Chem. 237: 1982-1988.
12. Scrimgeour,K.G. and Huennekens,F.M.(1962)Meth.in Enzymol.5: 838-843.
13. Rabinowitz,J.C. and Pricer,W.E. (1963) Meth. in Enzymol. 6: 375-379.
14. Kutzbach,C. and Stokstad,E.L.R.(1971) Meth. in Enzymol.18B: 793-798.
15. Tabor,H. (1962) Meth. in Enzymol. 5: 784-789.
16. Uyeda,K. and Rabinowitz,J.C.(1963) Meth. in Enzymol. 6: 380-383.
17. Lowry,O.H.,Rosebrough,N.J.,Farr,A.L. and Randall,R.J. (1951) J. Biol.Chem. 193: 265-275.
18. Niethammer,D. and Jackson,R.C. (1975) in Chemistry and Biology of Pteridines, W.Pfleiderer,ed., deGruyter,Berlin, pp. 197-207.

STUDIES OF THE EFFECTS OF FOLIC ACID ANTAGONISTS ON THYMIDYLATE SYNTHETASE ACTIVITY
IN INTACT MAMMALIAN CELLS

THOMAS I. KALMAN AND JACK C. YALOWICH
State University of New York at Buffalo, Departments of Medicinal Chemistry and
Biochemical Pharmacology, Amherst, New York 14260 (U.S.A.)

INTRODUCTION

The cytotoxicity of antifolates is due to their ability to interfere with DNA
synthesis through the inhibition of two major metabolic pathways: *de novo* thymidylate (dTMP) and purine biosynthesis. The relative extent to which the inhibition of
these pathways contribute to the overall effects of antifolates may depend on a
number of factors[1] and was found to vary among different cell types.

The primary target of 4-deoxy-4-amino derivatives of folic acid, such as the drug
Methotrexate (MTX), is the enzyme dihydrofolate(H_2folate) reductase. Its inhibition
prevents the essential reformation of tetrahydrofolate (H_4folate) from H_2folate and
results in a depletion of H_4folate cofactor pools. Intracellular levels of MTX or
other structurally related drugs exceeding the level of H_2folate reductase may also
block directly the action of certain folate cofactor dependent enzymes[2], such as
dTMP synthetase[2-4].

We have recently developed a rapid method for the measurement of dTMP synthetase
activity in intact mammalian cells[5]. The assay is based on the obligatory displacement of a tritium atom from the labelled substrate 5-^{3}H-deoxyuridylate (dUMP) during
the enzyme catalyzed reaction[6,7]. The assay is performed by incubating the cell
suspension with a properly labelled metabolic precursor of 5-^{3}H-dUMP, such as
5-^{3}H-dUrd, which after uptake and phosphorylation undergoes methylation by dTMP
synthetase with concomitant release of tritium into water:

$$5\text{-}^3\text{H-dUrd} \xrightarrow[\text{membrane}]{\text{cell}} 5\text{-}^3\text{H-dUrd} \xrightarrow[\text{kinase}]{\text{thymidine}} 5\text{-}^3\text{H-dUMP} \xrightarrow[\text{CH}_2\text{H}_4\text{folate}]{\text{dTMP synthetase}} \text{dTMP} + {}^3\text{H-H}_2\text{O}$$

In this report we demonstrate the utility of the tritium release assay for the
evaluation of the effects of antifolates on intracellular dTMP synthetase activity,
as well as their reversal by tetrahydrofolate derivatives and describe the results of
our initial studies[8,9] using leukemia L1210 cells.

EXPERIMENTAL METHODS

Experiments were performed using murine lymphocytic leukemia L1210 cells suspended
in modified Eagle's media (without folate). The L1210 cell line was maintained by
weekly passage of 10^5 cells into DBA/2HA mice.

The standard cellular tritium-release assay of thymidylate synthetase was performed using cells harvested six days after inoculation. In polystyrene tubes,
200 µl aliquots of the tumor cell suspension (2.5×10^7 cells/ml) were mixed with

672

25 µl of various concentrations of antifolate drugs dissolved in Dulbecco's PBS buffer. After 40 min incubation at 37°C, 25 µl of 5-^{3}H-deoxyuridine (dUrd) was added to each tube to achieve a final concentration of 1 µM. All tubes were then incubated at 37°C for 15 min. The reaction was terminated by mixing aliquots of the assay mixture with 10% activated charcoal suspension containing 4% perchloric acid, followed by centrifugation. Portions of the supernate were measured for radioactivity by liquid scintillation counting techniques.

For kinetic studies, cells were mixed with 1 µM 5-^{3}H-dUrd and various antifolates in the absence or presence of tetrahydrofolate derivatives and incubated at 37°C. Aliquots of the reaction mixture were taken at various time intervals for the measurement of tritium release, as described above. Enzyme activity is expressed as percent tritium release relative to the total radioactivity added and the effect of antifolates is expressed as percent inhibition of tritium release relative to that obtained in their absence.

The activity of dTMP synthetase in cell-free extracts of L1210 cells was assayed by the method of Roberts[6] and Lomax and Greenberg[7] using 5-^{3}H-dUMP as substrate, under conditions previously described[10].

RESULTS AND DISCUSSION

The utility of the intact cell tritium release assay of dTMP synthetase for the quantitative evaluation of the effects of antifolates on cellular dTMP formation is demonstrated by the results shown in Figure 1.

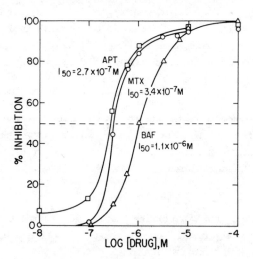

Fig. 1. Inhibition of tritium release by antifolates. BAF (Baker's antifol): triazinate, TZT. L1210 cells were preincubated for 40 min with the drugs before addition of 5-^{3}H-dUrd (see Experimental Methods).

The 50% inhibitory concentrations (I_{50}-values) obtained for MTX, APT and TZT are within a 4-fold range (3.4×10^{-7}M, 2.7×10^{-7}M and 1.1×10^{-6}M, respectively). The similarity between the dose-response profiles of MTX and APT is consistent with their cellular uptake parameters[11] and relative effectiveness as H_2folate reductase inhibitors[12] in the L1210 system. The relatively lower potency of TZT can also be accounted for by its comparative behavior at the level of membrane transport, as well as the inhibition of H_2folate reductase[13].

It was of interest to study the time course of the inhibition of cellular dTMP synthetase activity by the various antifolates. Figure 2 shows the time dependence of the inhibitory effects of various concentrations of MTX without a preincubation period.

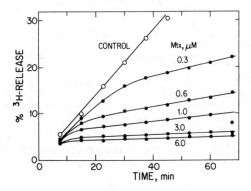

Fig. 2. Effects of MTX on the rate of tritium release.

It is apparent that there is a time requirement for the expression of MTX inhibition. A constant rate of inhibited tritium release is gradually established within 40 min, after an initial lag period. The higher the concentration of MTX the shorter the time required to achieve a linear rate of tritium release. These results are consistent with the notion that before a steady state of free, "exhangable" intracellular drug level is reached, the uptake of MTX and its binding to H_2folate reductase must take place in a time and concentration dependent manner[4,14].

A very similar pattern of time-dependent inhibition of tritium release was obtained with APT. In contrast, in the case of TZT, no lag period was observed and linear plots were obtained at all concentrations tested.

Using the linear portions of the plots such as those shown in Figure 2, the concentration dependence of the inhibition of tritium release by the various antifolates could be evaluated by standard kinetic treatment of the data. Apparent K_i-values of 1.2×10^{-7}M, 5.0×10^{-8}M and 2.4×10^{-6}M for MTX, APT and TZT, respectively were obtained. The corresponding Dixon-plots of the data are shown in Figure 3.

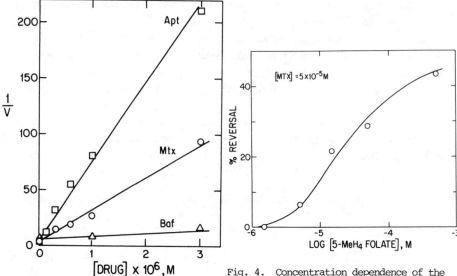

Fig. 3. Dixon-plots of the inhibition of tritium release by antifolates. Baf: triazinate (TZT).

Fig. 4. Concentration dependence of the reversal by 5-methylH$_4$folate of the inhibition of tritium release caused by 50 μM MTX.

The apparent K_i-values are relative indicators of the overall effectiveness of the antifolates as inhibitors of cellular dTMP formation. These inhibitory constants are undoubtedly complex and may reflect differences in the dynamic equilibria of cellular influx-efflux, H$_2$folate reductase binding, H$_4$folate cofactor pool changes and the spectrum and potency of enzyme inhibition. It should be noted that whereas MTX and APT can significantly inhibit dTMP synthetase in cell free extracts of Ll210 cells, no direct effect of TZT on the enzyme could be demonstrated.

In view of the importance of high dose MTX-citrovorum factor rescue treatments in certain types of cancer, we studied the reversal of the inhibitory effects of MTX and TZT by the 5-methyl and 5-formyl derivatives of H$_4$folate, using our cellular dTMP synthetase assay. At 50 μM concentration of MTX and TZT, which is more than sufficient to achieve complete inhibition, the simultaneous addition of equimolar concentrations of 5-methylH$_4$folate (MTHF) or 5-formylH$_4$folate (CF) resulted in a rate of tritium release, which was approximately 30% of that obtained in the absence of the inhibitors and reversing agents.

It was of interest to examine the reversal of antifolate inhibition by H$_4$folate derivatives as a function of the concentrations of the respective agents. Figure 4 shows the pattern of reversal of MTX inhibition by MTHF consistent with a competition for membrane transport between these agents[15]. In contrast, the reversal of TZT inhibition remained constant at a level of ca. 30% throughout a wide range of MTHF concentrations.

The time course of reversals at various antifolate-H$_4$folate combinations are shown in the 4 sets of plots in Figure 5. The pattern of reversal of MTX inhibition is characterized by a significant difference at early times between the effects of

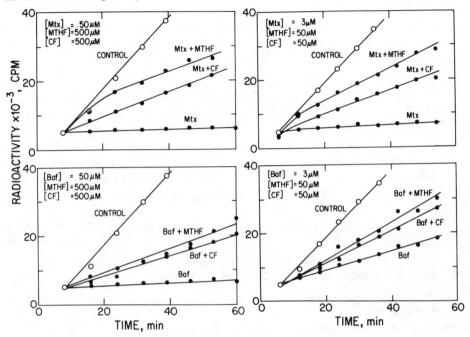

Fig. 5. Kinetics of the reversal of antifolate-inhibition by 5-methylH$_4$folate (MTHF) and 5-formylH$_4$folate (CF). Baf: triazinate (TZT).

MTHF and CF: the former is capable of inducing a lag period, similar to that observed with MTX alone at lower concentrations (see Figure 2). The difference diminishes at latter times and the rate of tritium release becomes very similar in the case of both reversing agents, expecially at 500 μM concentrations. These observations are consistent with the ability of MTHF to effectively compete with MTX for initial transport, due to its higher affinity for the membrane carrier, as indicated by its 5-fold lower K$_t$-value for transport into the cell[15].

In comparison, the reversal of the inhibition of tritium release caused by TZT is immediate, regardless of which H$_4$folate derivative is used. Since, in contrast to MTX, TZT does not share with the reversing agents a common carrier system for transport, the effects of the H$_4$folate derivatives can be fully expressed. At the saturating concentrations employed, a maximal reversal of ca. 30% is obtained, whether tritium release is completely or only partially inhibited by TZT. Thus, dTMP synthetase activity (rate of tritium release) observed under these conditions in L1210 cells may reflect the maximal rate of metabolic conversion of MTHF and CF to 5,10-methyleneH$_4$folate, the cofactor required for this enzyme.

SUMMARY

The effects of antifolates on thymidylate synthetase activity in intact L1210 leukemia cells *in vitro* have been examined utilizing our recently developed tritium release assay.

Preincubation of cells for 40 min at 37°C with methotrexate, aminopterin or triazinate before the addition of 10^{-6} M 5-^{3}H-dUrd resulted in the inhibition of the amount of the tritium released from the substrate, yielding I$_{50}$-values of 3.4×10^{-7} M, 2.7×10^{-7} M and 1.1×10^{-6} M, respectively. Kinetic studies of the inhibitory effects of these antifolates yielded apparent K$_i$-values of 1.2×10^{-7} M, 5×10^{-8} M, and 2.4×10^{-6} M, respectively.

Studies of the reversal of antifolate effects by 5-methyl and 5-formyl tetrahydrofolate revealed characteristic patterns of interactions which could be interpreted in terms of differences in transport properties at the cellular uptake level.

ACKNOWLEDGEMENTS

This work was supported in part by NIH Research Career Development Award GM-34138 and USPHS grant CA-13604.

REFERENCES

1. Goldman, I. D. (1977) Cancer Treat. Rep. 61, 549-558.

2. McBurney, M. W. and Whitmore, G. F. (1975) Cancer Res. 35, 586-590.

3. Borsa, J. and Whitmore, G. F. (1969) Mol. Pharmacol. 5, 318-322.

4. Sirotnak, F. M. and Donsbach, R. C. (1974) Cancer Res. 34, 3332-3340.

5. Kalman, T. I. and Yalowich, J. C. (1977) 174th Amer. Chem. Soc. Meeting, Abstracts, Biol 127.

6. Roberts, D. (1966) Biochemistry 5, 3546-3548.

7. Lomax, M. I. S. and Greenberg G. R. (1967) J. Biol. Chem. 242, 109-113.

8. Kalman, T. I. and Yalowich, J. C. (1978) Proc. Amer. Assoc. Cancer Res. 19, 153.

9. Kalman, T. I. and Yalowich, J. (1978) Fed. Proc. 37, 500.

10. Kalman, T. I., Bloch, A., Szekeres, G. L. and Bardos, T. J. (1973) Biochem. Biophys. Res. Commun. 55, 210-217.

11. Chello, P. L., Sirotnak, F.M., Dorick, D. M. and Donsbach, R. C. (1977) Cancer Res. 37, 4297-4303.

12. Harrap, K. R., Hill, B. T., Furness, M. E. and Hart L. I. (1971) Ann. N. Y. Acad. Sci. 186, 312-324.

13. Skeel, R. T., Sawicki, W. L., Cashmore, A. R. and Bertino, J. R. (1973) Cancer Res. 33, 2972-2976.

14. Goldman, I. D., Lichtenstein and Oliverio, V. T. (1968) J. Biol. Chem. 243, 5007-5017.

15. Goldman, I. D. (1971) Ann. N. Y. Acad. Sci. 186, 400-422.

Kisliuk/Brown, eds. Chemistry and Biology of Pteridines

DISTRIBUTION OF FOLATES FOLLOWING METHOTREXATE-LEUCOVORIN RESCUE REGIMEN IN CANCER PATIENTS

BIPIN M. MEHTA, WILLIAM R. SHAPIRO, GERALD ROSEN AND DORRIS J. HUTCHISON
Memorial Sloan-Kettering Cancer Center, New York, N.Y. 10021

ABSTRACT

Leucovorin is converted to 5-methyltetrahydrofolate in the presence of methotrexate. The determinations of both citrovorum factor and 5-methyltetrahydrofolate along with methotrexate provide new parameters for evaluation of the therapeutic effectiveness of rescue regimen. The relationship of citrovorum factor and 5-methyltetrahydrofolate to the therapeutic and toxic activities of methotrexate has been considered in patients with meningeal carcinomatosis receiving intra-Ommaya methotrexate and intravenous leucovorin and in patients with osteogenic sarcoma receiving high dose methotrexate followed by oral leucovorin rescue.

INTRODUCTION

High dose methotrexate (MTX)-leucovorin rescue regimens have been used extensively for the successful treatment of neoplasms[1-3]. Leucovorin is converted to 5-methyltetrahydrofolate (5-MTHFA)[4], the major serum folate[5].

Patients with meningeal carcinomatosis who received MTX via Ommaya reservoir, were assured of drug entry into both ventricles and the subarachnoid space[6], but persistence of MTX in the systemic circulation could produce bone-marrow depression. A correlation between the cerebrospinal fluid (CSF) levels of MTX and central nervous system toxicity has not been established. In osteogenic sarcoma patients serum levels of MTX proved valuable in predicting toxicity[7].

This report compares the pharmacokinetics of citrovorum factor (CF), 5-MTHFA and MTX in two new protocols, in an attempt to evaluate their therapeutic efficacy and to define the role of leucovorin in rescue.

MATERIALS AND METHODS

Patients. Five patients (40 to 66 years of age) with meningeal carcinomatosis, and ten patients (10 to 25 years of age) with osteogenic sarcoma, were included in the present study.

Drug administration. Meningeal carcinomatosis patients received MTX* at a dose of 6.25 mg/m^2, via Ommaya reservoir[6], and simultaneous intravenous (i.v.) infusion of calcium leucovorin* for 4 1/2-5 hrs.

Osteogenic sarcoma patients were administered MTX[†], 200-500 mg/kg, by i.v. infusion for 4 hrs. and at 24 hrs. leucovorin tablets*, 10-15 mg, were given oral every 6 hrs. x 12 doses.

Samples. From patients with meningeal carcinomatosis, venous blood (5 ml) was drawn at 0, 2, 4, 5, 6, 8, 20, 24 and 48 hrs. into vacu- tainers, and allowed to clot at room temperature then serum was sepa- rated by centrifugation. Ventricular CSF samples were obtained at each time interval[6]. Serum was obtained from osteogenic sarcoma patients as described above at 0, 24, 48 and 72 hrs. Sodium ascorbate (1 mg/ml) was added to all samples prior to storage at -20°C. Samples were assayed within one week.

Assay procedures. Determination of MTX was generally carried out by a microbiological assay method[8]. In samples where CF levels were either higher than or equimolar to MTX, an enzyme titration method[9] was used. CF and 5-MTHFA were measured by microbiological assay[10,11].

RESULTS

Serum and CSF concentrations of MTX, CF and 5-MTHFA of one patient

---

*Lederle Laboratories, Division of American Cyanamid, Pearl River, N.Y.
†Division of Cancer Treatment, National Cancer Institute, Bethesda, Md.

are shown in Figure 1. MTX in CSF persisted above "therapeutic" levels
for about 40 hrs., with serum concentrations less than 50 ng/ml
throughout 48 hrs. CF in the serum peaked at 600 ng/ml at 5 hrs., then
dropped to 3 ng/ml in 24 hrs. Negligible amounts of CF entered the CSF,
and peaked at 4 ng/ml at 2 hrs. 5-MTHFA in the serum peaked at
900 ng/ml at the end of infusion, and dropped close to normal by 48 hrs.
The distribution kinetics of CF and 5-MTHFA following 5 hrs. i.v.
infusion of leucovorin in the absence of MTX are similar.

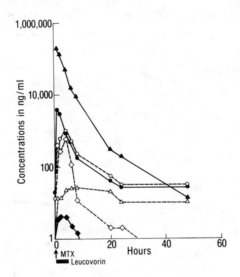

Figure 1. Distribution kinetics following 6.25 mg/m^2 MTX intra-Ommaya
with simultaneous i.v. infusion of Ca-leucovorin (50 mg/m^2) for 5 hrs.
MTX-serum △---△; CSF ▲——▲; 5-MTHFA-serum ○---○; CSF ●——●; CF-serum
◇---◇; CSF ◆——◆.

The half life (t/2) and the areas under the concentration versus time
curves for MTX, CF and 5-MTHFA in both serum and CSF for the five
patients are given in Table 1. The availability of MTX in the CSF was
greater than CF and 5-MTHFA, and the serum concentration of each folate
coenzyme was greater than MTX.

TABLE 1

DISTRIBUTION KINETICS OF MTX, 5-MTHFA AND CF

Half-life (t/2) and the area under the concentration vs. time curve
(CxT) in serum and CSF for MTX, 5-MTHFA and CF in patients receiving
intra-Ommaya MTX (6.25 mg/m^2) with i.v. leucovorin (50 mg/m^2) for 4 1/2-
5 hrs. infusion. Five patients. Mean $\pm$ S.E.

	Serum		CSF	
	t/2	CxT	t/2	CxT
	in hrs.	µg/ml x mins.	in hrs.	µg/ml x mins.
MTX	20.0 $\pm$ 5.4	73.6 $\pm$ 18.8	4.2 $\pm$ 0.2	52,838.0 $\pm$ 15,132.0
5-MTHFA	7.1 $\pm$ 1.4	438.4 $\pm$ 53.6	13.1 $\pm$ 2.9	205.7 $\pm$ 139.1
CF	4.5 $\pm$ 0.6	248.1 $\pm$ 71.0	19.8 $\pm$ 6.7	7.4 $\pm$ 3.0

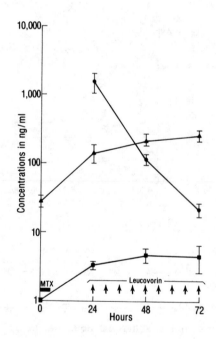

Figure 2. Distribution of MTX ●——●, 5-MTHFA ▲——▲ and CF ■——■ in
patients with osteogenic sarcoma receiving high dose MTX (200-500 mg/kg),
4 hr. i.v. infusion followed 24 hr. later by 10-12 mg leucovorin tablets
every 6 hrs.

Figure 2 represents MTX, CF and 5-MTHFA distribution patterns in 10 patients on high dose MTX-leucovorin rescue protocols. The CF pattern in osteogenic sarcoma patients followed that of normal adults[12]. Serum levels of 5-MTHFA were elevated from 28 ng/ml and persisted at 250 ng/ml during the period of leucovorin administration. On the 7th day following therapy, MTX levels were below 1 ng/ml and 5-MTHFA levels were normal.

DISCUSSION

Our data show that following i.v. infusion of leucovorin in the presence of MTX about 60% of the reduced folates in serum is 5-MTHFA. Nixon and Bertino[4], found that 90 min. after i.v. leucovorin, 40% of the serum folates remained as the administered radiolabeled compound.

The availability of CF and especially 5-MTHFA in the presence of MTX provides the opportunity for differential and selective uptake by host and tumor tissue. Thus, the rescue process associated with therapeutic activity will depend upon differences between the recoverability of normal tissue and the tumors, accordingly it is not expected that all tumors will respond to this type of MTX-leucovorin rescue.

SUMMARY

We suggest that in meningeal carcinomatosis patients, persistently high serum levels of 5-MTHFA, may prevent systemic toxicity, whereas the excess of MTX over 5-MTHFA in the CSF could provide a therapeutic effect. In osteogenic sarcoma patients, high dose MTX maintained higher serum levels than those of 5-MTHFA levels in the serum after leucovorin were higher than MTX, for a prolonged period of time which provide protection from MTX toxicity. The CF levels in serum were never higher than those of MTX or 5-MTHFA.

ACKNOWLEDGMENTS

Supported in part by NCI grants CA 08748, CA 18856; ACS grant CH-39S; Elsa U. Pardee Foundation. We acknowledge the technical assistance of Ann L. Gisolfi.

REFERENCES

1. Djerassi, I., Abir, E., Royer, G., Jr. *et al*. (1966) Clin. Pediat. 5, 502-509.

2. Hryniuk, W.M. and Bertino, J.R. (1969) J. Clin. Invest. 48, 2140-2145.

3. "Proceedings on the Workshop on Antimetabolites and the Central Nervous System", eds. Shapiro, W.R., Mehta, B.M. and Hutchison, D.J. (1977) Cancer Treat. Rep. 61(4), 505-757.

4. Nixon, P.F. and Bertino, J.R. (1972) N. Eng. J. Med. 286, 175-179.

5. Herbert, V., Larrabee, A.R. and Buchanan, J.M. (1962) J. Clin. Invest. 41, 1134-1138.

6. Shapiro, W.R., Young, D.F. and Mehta, B.M. (1975) N. Eng. J. Med. 293, 161-166.

7. Nirenberg, A., Mosende, C., Mehta, B.M. *et al*. (1977) Cancer Treat. Rep. 61, 779-783.

8. Mehta, B.M. and Hutchison, D.J. (1977) Cancer Treat. Rep. 61, 597-601.

9. Sirotnak, F.M. and Donsbach, R.C. (1972) Cancer Res. 32, 2120-2126.

10. Mehta, B.M. and Hutchison, D.J. (1975) Cancer Treat. Rep. 59, 935-937.

11. Mehta, B.M. and Hutchison, D.J. (1977) Cancer Treat. Rep. 61, 1657-1663.

12. Mehta, B.M., Gisolfi, A.L., Hutchison, D.J. *et al*. (1978) Cancer Treat. Rep. 62, 345-350.

According to Fig. 1 MTX by inhibition of the dihydrofolate(FH_2) reductase affects the methylation of deoxiuridine monophosphate (dUMP) to deoxithymidine monophosphate (dTMP). As a consequence of the decreased production of thymidine triphosphate (dTTP) via the de novo pathway the normal feedback inhibition of the thymidine kinase reaction is released. This activation of the thymidine kinase results in an increased production of dTMP and dTTP via the salvage pathway. Thus, both the decrease of the dUR incorporation and the increase of the dTR incorporation into the DNA serve as biochemical parameters of the MTX effect[6,7]. These biochemical effects of MTX can be corrected by the administration of its antidot CF since this activated folate derivative enters directly the pool of the activated one-carbon units[8,9]. Thus, dTMP synthesis and purine de novo synthesis can resume although the FH_2 reductase is still inhibited by MTX. Biochemically the rescue effect of CF is indicated by the normalization of the dUR/dTR-quotient.

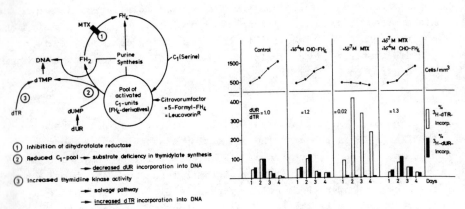

Fig. 1 Biochemical effects of methotrexate(MTX). Abbrev. see text.

Fig. 2 DNA metabolism in cultured human lymphoblasts (LS2). Effects of MTX and CF(=CHO-FH_4).

MATERIALS AND METHODS

The details of the dUR- and dTR-incorporation studies and the estimation of the thymidine kinase activity are described elsewhere[10,11,7]. Serum MTX levels were determined by its inhibition of partially purified dihydrofolate reductase from mammalian liver[12].

RESULTS

The principles of the metabolic changes which are characteristic for the effects of MTX and CF were worked out with the model system of permanent growing lymphoblast cultures (LS2). The results are shown in Fig.2.

BIOCHEMICAL CONTROL OF THE FOLINIC ACID RESCUE EFFECT AFTER HIGH-DOSE
METHOTREXATE (MTX) THERAPY

HANSJÖRG SAUER, ANDREAS SCHALHORN and WOLFGANG WILMANNS
Medical Clinic III, Klinikum Grosshadern, University of Munich and
Institute of Hematology, Department of Clinical Hematology of Gesell-
schaft für Strahlen- und Umweltforschung in Munich (West-Germany)

ABSTRACT

The decrease of the quotient of ^{3}H-deoxiuridine (dUR) and ^{3}H-thymi
dine (dTR) incorporation into the DNA of the cells is a good paramete
for estimating the methotrexate (MTX) effect on rapidly proliferating
cell systems such as lymphoblast cultures and bone marrow. Using this
indicator it could be shown that the usually administered doses of ci
vorum factor (CF) are not sufficient for an effective rescue for the
bone marrow cells as long as the MTX serum concentration is equal or
higher than 10^{-6} M. In critical cases with retarded MTX elimination t
monitoring of DNA metabolism in the bone marrow cells by means of the
dUR/dTR quotient can determine if the used CF dose is enough to promp
the desired rescue effect.

INTRODUCTION

High-dose MTX therapy with following citrovorum factor rescue
(HDMTX/CF)[1,2] is based on the assumption that primary resistant tumor
have an impaired active transport system for folate compounds which i
normally shared by MTX. At very high MTX serum concentrations, howeve
the drug can enter these cells by passive diffusion independent of th
active transport system resulting in cytocidal intracellular MTX conc
trations[3,4,5]. Normal,rapidly proliferating tissues with an intact tr
port system for folates can be protected from death by MTX by the app
cation of relatively small doses of the antidote citrovorum factor (C
5-formyl-tetrahydrofolic acid = $CHO-FH_4$). This is the socalled rescue
effect of CF. Since essentially no CF can enter the cells by passive
diffusion at low serum concentrations, tumor cells lacking the active
transport system do not benefit from the rescue effect.

In this paper the biochemical aspect of the CF rescue in normal bo
marrow cells after HDMTX is described in an attempt to answer two of
most interesting questions:

1) At which time after the MTX infusion does the DNA synthsis re-gain
normal activity?

2) At which MTX serum concentrations is CF really effective when give
in the conventionally recommended doses?

In comparison to the control CF (= CHO-FH$_4$) alone has no significant effect either on the cell growth or on the incorporation rates of ^{3}H-dTR or ^{3}H-dUR. Under normal conditions the incorporation rates of these two nucleosides are nearly equal. The quotient dUR/dTR lies within the normal range of 0.7 to 1.3. As expected from the biochemical mechanism, the dUR incorporation falls almost to zero under MTX whereas the dTR incorporation increases considerably. As a sign of a marked MTX effect the dUR/dTR quotient falls below 0.1. The DNA metabolism of the cells is so much disturbed that the reproduction can no longer occur. After 4 hours preincubation with 10^{-7} M MTX the addition of CF normalizes the incorporation rates. The quotient dUR/dTR raises again to the normal value of 1.3; culture growth is now regular again.

The same parameters as in the model culture were estimated in bone marrow cells of patients under MTX therapy. Fig. 3 shows the results of the dUR/dTR quotient, the thymidine kinase activity(TK) and the corresponding MTX serum levels in a patient with metastatic osteosarcoma who received 3.8 and 14.0 g of MTX respectively. Even 24 hours after the end of the MTX infusion in both cases the DNA metabolism in the bone marrow cells shows a clear MTX effect although up to that time already 7 doses of CF (15 mg each) have been injected. At 24 hours the values of the dUR/dTR quotients are 0.14 and 0.25 and so considerably below the normal range. The thymidine kinase activity is still elevated. Only after 48 hours, when the MTX serum concentrations decreased to the region of 10^{-7} M, have the dUR/dTR quotients (0.81 and 0.90 respectively) and DNA matabolism returned to normal.

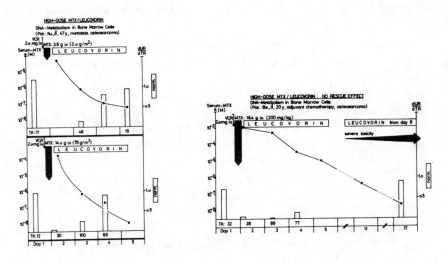

Fig.3 DNA metabolism in bone marrow cells under HDMTX/CF Fig.4
(Leucovorin = CF)

A different course of another patient is demonstrated in Fig. 4.
As expected, the dUR/dTR quotient after MTX application falls to 0.06.
Although CF is given regularly until the 48th hour there is no significant increase in the dUR/dTR quotient. For unknown reasons the MTX
elimination from the patient's serum was considerably retarded. On the
third day after the MTX infusion the MTX concentration in the serum is
still 10^{-5} M and even on the 11th day a pharmacologically effective
level of 2×10^{-7} M is noted. At that time measurement of DNA metabolism
was impossible because of a totally empty bone marrow. On the 17th day
the bone marrow regenerated. Now, under continued CF administration at
a serum concentration of 3×10^{-8} M, the dUR/dTR quotient is again within the normal range. In spite of retake and continuation of CF treatment at the first signs of toxicity (erythema, leucocytopenia, thrombo-
cytopenia) the patient developed a most severe bone marrow depression,
and despite of intensive supportive care (antibiotics, thrombocyte-
and granulocyte-transfusions) he died due to sepsis and renal insuffi-
ciency.
Another 6 patients were treated with 40 courses of HDMTX/CF without
any complications.

DISCUSSION

The decrease of the quotient of ^{3}H-dUR/^{3}H-dTR incorporation
into the DNA of the cells is a good biological parameter for estimating
the MTX effect on rapidly proliferating cell systems as lymphoblast
cultures and bone marrow. The compensation of the MTX effect on the
DNA metabolism by CF leads to the normalization of the dUR/dTR quotient
(= rescue effect of CF).
These parameters were tested in bone marrow cells of patients after high-
dose methotrexate and under citrovorum factor therapy. It could be
shown that the usually administered doses of about 100 mg CF per day
are not sufficient for an effective rescue for the bone marrow cells
as long as the serum MTX concentrations are equal or higher than 10^{-6}M.
At MTX serum concentrations of 10^{-7} M CF is effective in these doses
and leads to the normalization of the dUR/dTR quotient. According to
these results, early CF application before the 24th or 36th hour after
the MTX infusion is not effective and seems to be of no benefit although this is demanded in most of the published schedules for
HDMTX/CF therapy.
In case that MTX elimination is retarded and MTX serum levels remain above 10^{-6} M more than 48 hours, the usually recommended CF doses
are not sufficient to produce a significant rescue effect. In these

patients CF rescue with "normal" doses is ineffective since both MTX and CF enter the cell by the same active transport mechanism and inhibit one another competitively[13]. Thus, high MTX concentrations nearly totally prevent the transport of low CF doses into the cell.

To save these patients from perhaps lethal damage of bone marrow and/or intestinal mucosa, the CF dose must be increased so much that the serum concentration of CF equals that of the MTX. For this purpose several grams of CF per day may be necessary[14]. In critical cases the monitoring of the DNA metabolism in the bone marrow cells by means of the dUR/dTR quotient can determine if the used CF dose is enough to prompt the desired rescue effect.

ACKNOWLEDGEMENTS

This work was supported by the Deutsche Forschungsgemeinschaft.

For skilful technical assistance we thank Mrs. K. Heil, Mrs. R. Sarkar, and Mrs. G. Stupp-Putot.

REFERENCES

1. Jaffe, J. et al.: Weekly high-dose methotrexate-citrovorum factor in in osteogenic sarcoma. Cancer, 39, 45 - 50 (1977).

2. Pratt, C. et al.: Adjuvant multiple drug chemotherapy for osteo-sarcoma of the extremity. Cancer, 39, 51 - 57 (1977).

3. Bleyer, W.A.: Methotrexate: clinical pharmacology, current status and therapeutic guidelines. Cancer Treat. Rev., 4, 87 - 101 (1977).

4. Djerassi, I.: High-dose methotrexate (NSC - 704) and citrovorum factor (NSC - 3590) rescue: bachground and rationale. Cancer Chemoth. Rep., 6, 3 - 6 (1975).

5. Frei, E.: Methotrexate revisited. Med. Ped. Oncol., 2, 227 - 241 (1976).

6. Sauer, H., Wilmanns, W.: Cobalamin dependent methionine synthesis and methyl-folate-trap in human vitamin B12 deficiency. Brit. J. Haematol., 36, 189 - 198 (1977).

7. Wilmanns, W., Kehr, D.: DNS-Synthese in Leukämiezellen unter der Einwirkung von Methotrexat, 5-Fluoro-Uracil und Cytosin-Arabinosid in vitro. Pharmacol. Clin., 2, 161 - 167 (1970).

8. Sauer, H., Jaenicke L.: Zur Aufhebung des zytostatischen Effekts von Amethopterin (Methotrexat[R]) durch Methyl-Tetrahydrofolsäure. Blut, 28, 321 - 326 (1974).

9. Sauer, H., Wilmanns, W.: The activity of the cobalamin dependent methionine-symthetase (5-methyl-5,6,7,8-tetrahydrofolic acid: homocysteine methyltransferase) in rapidly growing human cells and the effect of some folic acid derivatives and analogues. In: Chemistry and Biology of Pteridines, Walter de Gruyter, Berlin-New York, 153 - 163 (1976).

10. Wilmanns, W.: Die Thymidin-Kinase in normalen und leukämischen
    myeloischen Zellen. Klin. Wschr., 45, 501 - 511 (1967).

11. Wilmanns, W.: Dihydrofolat-Reduktase und Thymidin-Kinase im
    Knochenmark unter Einwirkung von Folsäureantagonisten.
    Klin. Wschr., 45, 987 - 994 (1967).

12. Schalhorn, A.: in preparation.

13. Huennekens, F.J. et al.: Folate antagonists: transport and target
    site in leukemic cells. In: Gerlach,E., Moser, K., Deutsch,
    E., Wilmanns, W. (Editors): Erythrocytes, Thrombocytes,
    Leukocytes. Thieme Publishers, Stuttgart, 496 - 503 (1973).

14. Djerassi, I. et al.: New "rescue" with massive dose of citrovorum
    factor for potentially lethal methotrexate toxicity.
    Cancer Treat. Rep., 61, 749 - 750 (1977).

DECREASED SYNTHESIS OF METHOTREXATE POLYGLUTAMATES IN MUTANT HAMSTER CELLS AND
IN FOLINIC ACID-TREATED HUMAN FIBROBLASTS

V. MICHAEL WHITEHEAD AND DAVID S. ROSENBLATT
The Penny Cole Hematology Research Laboratory and the Medical Research Council
Genetics Group, McGill University - Montreal Children's Hospital Research Institute
and Department of Pediatrics, McGill University, Montreal, Quebec, Canada

ABSTRACT

The failure of mutant chinese hamster ovary cells to accumulate methotrexate
polyglutamates was attributed to their lack of folate polyglutamate synthetase
activity. In mutant methotrexate-resistant baby hamster kidney cells, the
failure to accumulate methotrexate polyglutamates was due to competition between
dihydrofolate reductase and the synthetase for methotrexate entering the cell.
Folinic acid caused a depression of polyglutamate synthesis in human fibroblasts
by competing with methotrexate for transport into cells resulting in depletion
of the exchangeable substrate pool of methotrexate and derivatives.

INTRODUCTION

Synthesis of poly-γ-L-glutamyl derivatives of MTX* has been demonstrated by a
number of workers in a variety of tissues[1-11]. Results obtained recently during
study of this metabolism in human fibroblasts[10,11] have substantiated a number
of features of MTX polyglutamate formation which had been suspected from earlier
studies in animals[4,6,8]. Synthesis was found to be dose and time dependent, to
be greatest during logarithmic growth of cells, and to require the continued
presence of MTX in the culture medium. Evidence indicated that MTX and derivatives
in an exchangeable intracellular pool[11] were substrates for polyglutamate synthesis, while MTX and MTX polyglutamates bound to DHFR were not[8]. After synthesis, MTX polyglutamates of longer chain-length displaced those of shorter chain-
length from the non-exchangeable pool. In addition, when fibroblasts were preincubated with MTX for 6 or more hours, and were then transferred into MTX-free
medium they failed to recover their ability to synthesize DNA from deoxyuridine
for a protracted period. This was associated with the presence in these cells
of high levels of polyglutamates in the non-exchangeable pool[11]. Failure of
certain tissues to synthesize MTX polyglutamates has been observed previously[4].
We have studied three instances of decreased polyglutamate synthesis, each of
which was due to a different mechanism.

---

* Abbreviations: MTX, methotrexate, amethopterin; MTX($+G_1$) methotrexate monoglutamate; MTX($+G_n$) MTX polyglutamates longer than MTX($+G_1$); DHFR, dihydrofolate
reductase (EC 1.5.1.3); CHO, chinese hamster ovary; BHK, baby hamster kidney;
PBS, phosphate-buffered saline; GAT, glycine, adenosine and thymidine; folinic
acid, d,l,-5-formyltetrahydrofolate, citrovorum factor.

TABLE I

ACCUMULATION OF NON-EXCHANGEABLE MTX AND DERIVATIVES IN CHO CELLS

Cells were incubated in culture medium containing 10^{-6} M [^{3}H]MTX for 18 h. The non-exchangeable MTX fraction was then examined by gel chromatography as described (see Materials and Methods).

CHO cells	Levels of MTX and derivatives in cells (n moles/g)			
	MTX	MTX(+G_1)	MTX(+G_n)	Total
Wild-type	2.64	0.81	0.31	3.77
GAT$^-$	3.41	0	0.09	3.50

MATERIALS AND METHODS

CHO cells which are auxotrophic for glycine, adenosine and thymidine (GAT$^-$) and which fail to accumulate folate polyglutamates[12] were obtained from Dr. David Hoar. These cells have been shown to lack folate polyglutamate synthetase activity[13]. MTX-resistant BHK cells, A_5, and MTX-sensitive controls, B_1, were obtained from Dr. John Littlefield. A_5 cells contain levels of DHFR two orders of magnitude greater than B_1 cells and can survive in concentrations of MTX 10,000 times greater[14-16].

Cells were incubated in purified [^{3}H]MTX. Labeled MTX and derivatives were separated by Sephadex G-15 gel chromatography[4]. Treatment of the cell extract with hog kidney conjugase[17] caused the MTX(+G_1) and MTX(+G_n) fractions to shift to the position of MTX. Exchangeable and non-exchangeable pools of MTX and derivatives[11] were studied. Results are expressed as nmoles MTX and MTX derivatives per g protein.

RESULTS AND DISCUSSION

MTX polyglutamate synthesis in CHO cells

Compared to wild-type cells, GAT$^-$ cells synthesized little if any MTX polyglutamates (Table I). These results suggested that MTX and folate utilize the same polyglutamate synthetase enzyme. It is of interest that GAT$^-$ and controls accumulated equivalent levels of total non-exchangeable MTX despite the inability of the mutant cells to synthesize polyglutamates.

MTX polyglutamate synthesis in BHK cells

Synthesis of MTX polyglutamates by A_5 and B_1 cells exposed to increasing concentrations of MTX is shown in Table II. At concentration of 10^{-7} and 10^{-6} M MTX, concentrations which are inhibitory to growth of B_1 but not A_5 cells, MTX polyglutamates comprised 80% and 95% respectively of total MTX in B_1 cells. In contrast, polyglutamates comprised 0% and 2% of the total MTX in A_5 cells.

TABLE II

ACCUMULATION OF NON-EXCHANGEABLE MTX AND DERIVATIVES IN BHK CELLS.

Cells were incubated in culture medium containing [^{3}H]MTX for 24 h. The non-exchangeable MTX fraction was then examined by gel chromatography (see Materials and Methods).

[MTX]	Cells	Levels of MTX and derivatives in cells (n moles/g)			
		MTX	MTX($+G_1$)	MTX($+G_n$)	Total
10^{-7} M	B_1	0.38	0.59	1.04	2.01
	A_5	3.27	0	0	3.27
10^{-6} M	B_1	0.53	0.72	8.90	10.15
	A_5	20.34	0.14	0.14	20.62
10^{-5} M	B_1 [a]	1.10	0.25	3.90	5.25
	A_5	106.11	0.54	0.86	107.51
10^{-4} M	B_1	-	-	-	-
	A_5	143.19	7.50	2.90	153.59

[a] B_1 cells were incubated in 10^{-5} M [^{3}H]MTX for 18 h.

Incubation of A_5 cells in greater concentrations of MTX resulted in a further re-markable increase in non-exchangeable cell MTX, and absolute levels of poly-glutamates comparable to those in B_1 cells were obtained. However, polyglutamates never exceeded 7% of the total. A_5 and B_1 cells were incubated in 2.26 μM labeled folic acid. After 3 days, 88% and 86% respectively of the folate in them was present as polyglutamates (analysis performed by Jack Hilton). Thus, A_5 cells were capable of synthesizing both MTX and folate polyglutamates. Clearly, however, polyglutamate synthesis was not the mechanism by which A_5 cells accumulated MTX. We concluded that failure to synthesize MTX polyglutamates in A_5 cells in the face of exceedingly high levels of cell MTX was due to competition between DHFR and folate polyglutamate synthetase for MTX entering the cell, with DHFR possessing the greater affinity. These results provide the most dramatic demonstration that MTX bound to DHFR is not a substrate for polyglutamate synthesis.

Effect of folinic acid on MTX polyglutamate synthesis in human fibroblasts

High-dose MTX therapy with folinic acid "rescue" is widely used to treat patients with leukemia and a variety of other forms of cancer. MTX is given first, usually over several hours, then after an interval folinic acid is given in a series of injections. Folinic acid provides a source of reduced folate to replenish the tetrahydrofolate pool depleted by MTX. In addition, it is known to compete with MTX for transport into cells[18]. The ability of folinic acid to reduce host toxicity with this treatment has been explained in terms of one or another of these mechanisms.

TABLE III

EFFECT OF FOLINIC ACID ON THE ACCUMULATION OF NON-EXCHANGEABLE MTX AND DERIVATIVES IN HUMAN FIBROBLASTS.

Confluent fibroblasts were incubated in culture medium containing 10^{-6} M $[^3H]MTX$ for 1 h. Then folinic acid was added to the culture medium of test cells to achieve a concentration of 10^{-5} M and incubation of test and control cells continued for 24 h. The non-exchangeable MTX fraction was analysed at various times after addition of folinic acid (see Materials and Methods).

Cells	Time	Levels of MTX and derivatives in cells (n moles/g)			
	Hours	MTX	MTX($+G_1$)	MTX($+G_n$)	Total
Control	0^a	0.22	0.30	0.03	0.55
	1	0.11	0.34	0.07	0.52
	2	0.09	0.43	0.14	0.66
	4	0.12	0.62	0.51	1.25
	24	0.18	0.94	4.25	5.37
Folinic acid treated	0^a	0.12	0.21	0.05	0.38
	1	0.14	0.26	0.04	0.44
	2	0.17	0.24	0.03	0.44
	4	0.25	0.24	0.04	0.52
	24	0.99	0.22	0.06	1.27

[a] Time 0 is the time when folinic acid was added to test cells.

TABLE IV

EFFECT OF FOLINIC ACID ON THE ACCUMULATION OF EXCHANGEABLE MTX AND DERIVATIVES IN HUMAN FIBROBLASTS

Results are part of the study described in Table III. At intervals after addition of folinic acid to the culture medium, the exchangeable MTX fraction was analysed (see Materials and Methods).

Cells	Time	Levels of MTX and derivatives in cells (n moles/g)			
	Hours	MTX	MTX($+G_1$)	MTX($+G_n$)	Total
Control	0^a	1.58	0.03	0.03	1.64
	1	0.61	0.04	0.01	0.66
	2	0.51	0.06	0.01	0.59
	4	1.17	0.14	0.06	1.37
	24	1.11	0.21	0.15	1.47
Folinic acid treated	0^a	1.33	0.02	0.01	1.36
	1	0.41	0.01	0.01	0.43
	2	0.37	0.01	0.01	0.39
	4	0.63	0.01	0.01	0.65
	24	0.73	0.01	0.01	0.75

[a] Time 0 is the time when folinic acid was added to test cells.

Table III shows the effect of addition of folinic acid to culture medium containing MTX on subsequent synthesis of MTX polyglutamates by confluent human fibroblasts. In control cells, there was progressive accumulation of non-exchangeable MTX polyglutamates throughout the 25 h of incubation in MTX. In contrast, after folinic acid was added to fibroblasts, there was a marked reduction in the accumulation of total non-exchangeable MTX and MTX polyglutamate synthesis ceased entirely. The effect of folinic acid on the exchangeable MTX pool in these cells is shown in Table IV. Large variations in the level of MTX in this pool were found in both control and folinic acid-treated cells, presumably reflecting MTX associated with or adsorbed on the cell surface[18]. In control cells, there was progressive accumulation of exchangeable MTX polyglutamates. Addition of folinic acid resulted in depletion of exchangeable MTX and MTX polyglutamates, particularly the latter. Thus folinic acid interrupted MTX polyglutamate accumulation by depleting the exchangeable pool of MTX and derivatives, presumably by competing with MTX for transport into the cell[18]. Its effect appears to be the same as would be obtained by removing MTX from the culture medium[10]. These results demonstrate a third mechanism through which folinic acid may "rescue" tissues from MTX toxicity.

SUMMARY

We have shown that an exchangeable pool of MTX and derivatives is the substrate for MTX polyglutamate synthesis. If MTX was removed from the culture medium or if transport of MTX into the cell was blocked by folinic acid, this pool became depleted and polyglutamate synthesis ceased. Competition for intracellular MTX by increased levels of DHFR also deprived the synthetase enzyme of substrate. Absence of folate polyglutamate synthetase activity resulted in failure of synthesis of MTX polyglutamates. The specific role of MTX polyglutamates as distinct from MTX as active compounds is not yet clear. However, it has become apparent that for many cultured cells these polyglutamates are the predominant form of the drug following prolonged exposure or high dosage.

ACKNOWLEDGEMENTS

We thank Mary-Jane Vuchich, Marlene Dupont, Angela Pottier, Nora Matiaszuk and Yolande Guillemot for technical assistance and Claire Pepin and Huguette Ishmael for assistance in the preparation of the manuscript. This work was supported by grants from the Medical Research Council of Canada and the Cancer Research Society to V.M.W. and by a Medical Research Council of Canada Genetics Group grant to D.S.R. Support was also provided by the Lamplighters Leukemia Association and the 1977 and 1978 I.S.C.C. Telethons.

REFERENCES

1. Baugh, C.M., Krumdieck, C.L. and Nair, M.G. (1973) Biochem. Biophys. Res. Commun., 52, 27-34.

694

2. Brown, J.P., Davidson, G.E., Weir, D.G. and Scott, J.M. (1974) Intern. J. Biochem., 5, 727-733.

3. Shin, Y.S., Buehring, K.U. and Stokstad, E.L.R. (1974) J. Biol. Chem., 249, 5772-5777.

4. Whitehead, V.M., Perrault, M.M. and Stelcner, S. (1975) Cancer Res., 35, 2985-2990.

5. Jacobs, S.A., Adamson, R.H., Chabner, B.A., Derr, C.J. and Johns, D.G. (1975) Biochem. Biophys. Res. Commun., 63, 692-698.

6. Whitehead, V.M., Perrault, M.M. and Stelcner, S. (1976) in Chemistry and Biology of Pteridines, Pfleiderer, W. ed., Walter de Gruyter, Berlin, pp. 475-483.

7. Hoffbrand, A.V., Tripp, E. and Lavoie, A. (1976) Clin. Sci. Mol. Med., 50, 61-68.

8. Whitehead, V.M. (1977) Cancer Res., 37, 408-412.

9. Jacobs, S.A., Derr, C.J. and Johns, D.G. (1977) Biochem. Pharmacol., 26, 2310-2313.

10. Rosenblatt, D.S., Whitehead, V.M., Dupont, M.M., Vuchich, M.-J. and Vera, N. (1978) Mol. Pharmacol., 14, 210-214.

11. Rosenblatt, D.S., Whitehead, V.M., Vera, N., Pottier, A., Dupont, M. and Vuchich, M.-J. (1978) Mol. Pharmacol. in press.

12. McBurney, M.W. and Whitmore, G.F. (1974) Cell, 2, 173-182.

13. Taylor, R.T. and Hanna, M.L. (1977) Arch. Biochem. Biophys., 181, 331-344.

14. Nakamura, H. and Littlefield, J.W. (1972) J. Biol. Chem., 247, 179-187.

15. Hanggi, U.J. and Littlefield, J.W. (1974) J. Biol. Chem., 249, 1390-1397.

16. Hanggi, U.J. and Littlefield, J.W. (1976) J. Biol. Chem. 251, 3075-3080.

17. Iwai, K., Luttner, P.M. and Toennies, G. (1964) J. Biol. Chem., 239, 2365-2372.

18. Goldman, I.D., Lichtenstein, N.S. and Oliverio, V.T. (1968) J. Biol. Chem. 243, 5007-5017.

A FLUORESCENT DERIVATIVE OF METHOTREXATE:

AN INTRACELLULAR MARKER FOR DIHYDROFOLATE REDUCTASE

JOHN M. WHITELEY and ANDREA RUSSELL

Scripps Clinic and Research Foundation, La Jolla, California 92037

Dihydrofolate reductase is the principal target enzyme for the folate antagonists used in chemotherapy,[1] yet despite its isolation, ease of purification and character-ization from many sources, little is known of its intracellular properties. To ob-tain information in this area, a fluorescent derivative of the potent dihydrofolate reductase inhibitor methotrexate (MTX) has been synthesized, and its *in vitro* cell-ular uptake properties and intracellular protein binding abilities have been investi-gated.

The fluorescent compound was synthesized by linking fluorescein isothiocyanate (FITC) via a diaminopentyl (DAP) spacer group to MTX. The monoamide product (F-MTX), isolated by chromatography on AE-cellulose and preparative gel electrophoresis,[2] ex-hibited the combined absorbance and fluorescence characteristics of its components (λ_{max} = 365 and 495 nm; fluorescence maximum = 520 nm, pH 7) and was a good inhibitor of dihydrofolate reductase isolated from L1210 murine leukemic leukocytes ($K_i \sim 10^{-7}$M).

At pH 7, the extinction coefficient of F-MTX at 495 nm is 55,000. When irradiated at this wavelength, the emitted fluorescence maximum of 520 nm is identical to that of free fluorescein, however, the intensity is lower which implies that there is an interaction between the fluorescein and pteridine chromophores in aqueous solution. When the polarity of the solvent is decreased by the addition of increasing levels of ethanol, the quantum yield of F-MTX increases towards the level observed with free fluorescein (Table 1).

A similar increase in fluorescence occurs when F-MTX interacts with dihydrofolate reductase from L1210 cells (Fig. 1). This increase was recorded as the enzyme was titrated with increasing quantities of F-MTX, both in the presence (Fig. 1B) and in the absence of NADPH (Fig. 1A). No shift in the peak emission wavelength was ob-served, and maximal fluorescence increments were recorded in both cases at a 1:1 equivalence point. The two double reciprocal plots (Fig. 1C and 1D) afforded K_D values of 3.98 X 10^{-8} M and 3.09 X 10^{-8} M respectively. The nonlinearity of these curves at high concentrations of F-MTX can probably be attributed to the self-quenching of the fluorophore, apparent in the blank rates, rather than an altered binding affinity for the enzyme.

Polyacrylamide gel electrophoresis emphasizes the intimate interaction which occurs between F-MTX and the L1210 dihydrofolate reductase. The homogeneous L1210/R6 reductase (a strain resistant to 10^{-6} M MTX) has a relative mobility of 0.20, where-as the binary complex between enzyme and fluorescent inhibitor forms a new species

TABLE 1

The variation in quantum yield which occurs when the ethanolic content of a 0.1 M potassium phosphate, pH 7, solution of: (a) fluorescein, (b) FITC-DAP and (c) FITC-DAP-MTX (F-MTX) is increased.

Compound	Solvent	Quantum Yield
Fluorescein	0.1 M PO₄, pH 7	0.64
Fluorescein	.../25% EtOH	0.62
FITC-DAP	0.1 M PO₄, pH 7	0.53
FITC-DAP-MTX	0.1 M PO₄, pH 7	0.22
FITC-DAP-MTX	.../25% EtOH	0.42
FITC-DAP-MTX	.../50% EtOH	0.47
FITC-DAP-MTX	.../75% EtOH	0.49

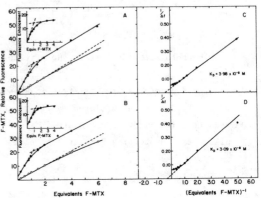

Fig. 1. (*right*) The fluorescence changes observed at 520 nm when the F-MTX concentration is increased from 0 to 6 enzyme equivalents in the presence (●——●) and absence (o——o) of L1210/R8 dihydrofolate reductase: (A) without NADPH, (B) in the presence of 1 equivalent of NADPH. *Inset:* Fluorescence enhancement of F-MTX as a function of concentration. (C) and (D): Double reciprocal plots of changes in relative fluorescence (Δf) vs. F-MTX concentration, again excluding and containing NADPH respectively. Solutions were buffered at pH 7.0 in 0.1 M potassium phosphate.

of relative mobility 0.25. The ternary complex of reductase, NADPH and F-MTX surprisingly occurs as a quartet with relative mobilities of 0.48, 0.55, 0.60 and 0.66. The origin of two of these bands can be attributed to the synthetic route for the preparation of F-MTX which may generate a mixture of α- and λ-linked fluorescent moieties. The band at 0.25 (the binary complex of enzyme and F-MTX) which is broad may also reflect the presence of two unresolved complexes formed between the enzyme and the α- and λ-isomers. The incorporation of NADPH accentuates the separation of the complexes formed by these two isomers, however, and also leads to the appearance of two additional bands which may reflect minor conformational variations in the reductase structure. The bands may be visualized by protein staining,[3,4] or by staining for enzyme activity;[5] in the case of the bands which correspond to complex formation, the latter reactivity is probably due to displacement of the bound inhibitor by dihydrofolate in the activity-staining medium. The enzyme-inhibitor complexes are readily visible (prior to staining) as yellow bands under ordinary light (Fig. 2). In this figure the first gel shows the binary complex of the L1210 enzyme and NADPH, which can be detected as a faint fluorescent band due to the inherent fluorescence of the NADPH which is not affected by binding to the enzyme. In the second gel, the quartet of bands comprising the *ternary* complex of enzyme-NADPH-F-MTX is clearly visible. In contrast, the *binary* complex of enzyme and fluorescent inhibitor shows no fluorescence,

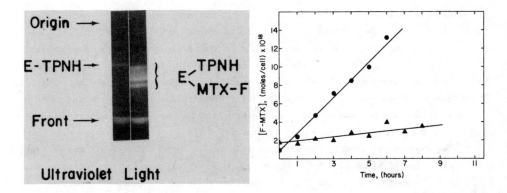

Fig. 2. Polyacrylamide gel electrophoresis of a 0.1 ml solution of L1210/R6
dihydrofolate reductase (∿15μm) in 0.025
M Tris-glycine buffer, pH 8.3 viewed
under UV light: (*left*) after preincubation with excess NADPH, and (*right*)
after preincubation with excess NADPH
plus F-MTX.

Fig. 3. The *in vitro* uptake rate of F-MTX
by MTX-resistant (●——●) and non-resistant
(▲——▲) L1210 cells. F-MTX (7 μm) was
incorporated to log-phase cultures (100 ml)
maintained at 37º. At intervals of 1 h,
10 ml samples were withdrawn and counted.
The fluorescence content of the lysed cells
was then measured at 520 nm and quantitated
by comparison with a standard curve.

suggesting that the fluorescein chromophore is in close contact with the protein or is
compressed close to the pteridine moiety when bound to the active-site. Whatever the
reason, the complex undergoes a major alteration when NADPH is also bound.

The uptake of F-MTX by non-resistant and resistant L1210 cells is illustrated in
Fig. 3. In both cases, F-MTX (∿ 15 μm) was incorporated into early log-phase cultures which were then incubated at 37º. At hourly intervals 10 ml samples were withdrawn, counted, washed with cold phosphate-buffered saline (PBS), centrifuged, and
lysed by sonication after resuspension in phosphate buffer solution, pH 7. The cellular extract after clarification by centrifugation was measured for fluorescence. The
concentration was determined from a calibration curve obtained at 520 nm with differing quantities of F-MTX in the same buffer. It is apparent from Fig. 3 that the resistant cell line demonstrates a more rapid uptake of F-MTX than the non-resistant
line, and that within 30 min the resistant cells contain elevated levels of the
fluorescent inhibitor. After 6 h the resistant cells show a 6-fold increment of
fluorescence compared to the non-resistant line.

The incorporation of F-MTX into L1210 cells has also been examined by Sephadex
G-100 chromatography. A 500 ml culture (8 X 10^8 cells) of L1210/R8 cells (a strain
resistant to 10^{-5} M MTX) was grown, washed repeatedly with PBS, harvested, and disrupted by sonication. The extract, visibly fluorescent when subjected to UV
irradiation and containing an apparent 9.9 units of dihydrofolate reductase activity,
was dialyzed for 12 h against dilute phosphate buffer, pH 7. During dialysis, 93%
of the fluorescence at 520 nm was retained. Chromatography of the dialyzed

solution on a column of Sephadex G-100 led to the emergence of a fluorescent peak which overlapped the peak of dihydrofolate reductase activity. When applied alone to the Sephadex column, F-MTX was retarded to a much greater extent. The movement of the enzyme F-MTX complex down the column and its efflux into the collecting tubes could be monitored visually with a portable UV light source. When the enzymatically active fractions were concentrated by ultrafiltration and subjected to analysis by polyacrylamide electrophoresis, fluorescent bands similar to those described earlier for the purified R6 reductase were observed.

The experiments briefly described in this report suggest that F-MTX may be useful for the visualization of dihydrofolate reductase during purification, and may also provide an approximate measure of the cellular reductase content. The variation in fluorescence intensity observed when F-MTX interacts with the enzyme suggests that the compound may be useful as a solution probe of the active site, which may be sensitive to slight changes in enzyme conformation. In addition, F-MTX may aid the separation of resistant from non-resistant L1210 cells during growth phase, where the primary cause of resistance is an elevated level of dihydrofolate reductase. This observation may be relevant to other cellular systems as has been recently reported for the mouse MTX-resistant AT/300 cell line.[6]

ACKNOWLEDGEMENTS

This investigation was supported by USPHS Grant No. CA-11778. John M. Whiteley is the recipient of a USPHS Research Career Development Award (CA-00106) from the National Cancer Institute.

REFERENCES

1. Blakley, R. L. (1969) The Biochemistry of Folic Acid and Related Pteridines, eds. A. Neuberger and E. L. Tatum, North Holland Publishing Co., p. 489.

2. Gapski, G.R., Whiteley, J. M., Rader, J. F., Cramer, P. L., Henderson, G. B., Neef, V. and Huennekens, F. M. (1975) J. Med. Chem, 18, 526.

3. Ornstein, L. (1964) Ann. N.Y. Acad. Sci., 121, 321.

4. Davis, B. J. (1964) Ann. N.Y. Acad. Sci., 121, 404.

5. Dunlap, R. B., Gunderson, L. E. and Huennekens, F. M. (1971) Biochem. Biophys. Res. Commun., 42, 772.

6. Kaufman, R. J., Bertino, J. R. and Schimke, R. T. (1978) J. Biol. Chem., 253, 5852.

ENZYME DISORDERS IN MOUSE L-CELLS CULTURED
IN THE PRESENCE OF AMETHOPTERIN

ZOFIA M. ZIELINSKA, MALGORZATA BALINSKA, WANDA CHMURZYNSKA, BARBARA
GRZELAKOWSKA-SZTABERT AND MALGORZATA MANTEUFFEL-CYMBOROWSKA
Department of Cellular Biochemistry, Nencki Institute of Experimental
Biology, Polish Academy of Sciences, 02-093 Warsaw (Poland)

ABSTRACT

Activity of dihydrofolate reductase and of some amethopterin
non-target enzymes were assayed in L-cells grown in the media with
this drug at growth-limiting and non-limiting concentrations. Besides
the activity of dihydrofolate reductase, that of lactate dehydrogenase was strongly depressed by amethopterin. The other folate-
related enzymes and folate-unrelated dehydrogenases were affected to
a lesser extent, when examined both in cells at their logarithmic and
stationary phase of growth.

INTRODUCTION

In our study on biochemical aspects of amethopterin inhibition of
growth of mammalian cells in vitro, we have recently focused our
attention on its side effects and followed the activity of some non-
target enzymes.

For mouse L-cells we found the crisis concentration of amethopterin
in the culture medium to be 10^{-8}M. At this concentration, during 48 h
of contact, amethopterin did not interfere with cell survival and only
slightly affected their proliferation rate[1]. However it depressed not
only the activity of dihydrofolate reductase but also (even at concentrations below 10^{-9}M) that of lactate dehydrogenase[2]. The activity
of other folate enzymes was either unaffected, (5,10-methylenetetra-
hydrofolate dehydrogenase and formyltetrahydrofolate synthetase), or
only slightly depressed, (serine hydroxymethyltransferase and
methionine synthetase), even when amethopterin concentrations in the
medium were high enough to suppress cell proliferation. The activity
of isocitrate and glucose-6-phosphate dehydrogenases was only slightly
lowered unless amethopterin concentration was suppressive for L-cell
proliferation.

To gain more insight into enzyme disorders in L-cells cultured
in the presence of amethopterin, we examined the effects of this

drug on the activity of the enzymes in cells at their logarithmic and stationary phases of growth.

MATERIALS AND METHODS

The mouse fibroblast-like L-cells were grown as monolayers in the medium which contained 90% Eagle's MEM plus 10% calf or bovine serum with added antibiotics[3,4]. Approximately 24 h after subculturing (zero time), the standard medium was renewed in the control cultures or changed for that with amethopterin in the experimental ones[1,2]. The cells were then allowed to grow at 37°C for another 24 to 96 hours, than washed out of the medium before processing for enzyme assays[2-4]. In some experiments, the cells were also cultured in the media with amethopterin at a cytocidal concentration for 48 hours in the presence or in the absence of a folate coenzyme at an effective concentration[1].

The activity of the following enzymes was estimated using the commonly used methods listed below: dihydrofolate reductase (1.5.1.4)[3-5], serine hydroxymethyltransferase (2.1.2.1)[5], thymidylate synthetase (2.1.1.b)[6], vitamin B12-dependent methionine synthetase (2.1.1.13)[7], lactate dehydrogenase (1.1.1.27)[8], glucose-6-phosphate dehydrogenase (1.1.1.49)[9], isocitrate dehydrogenase (1.1.1.42)[10].

Protein content was determined by the method of Lowry et al.[11].

RESULTS

In Fig. 1 are presented activity curves of the enzymes in L-cells grown in the control and experimental media with amethopterin at the following concentrations: 2.5×10^{-9}M, at which survival and proliferation rate of the cells were unaffected even after 96 hours of contact; 10^{-8}M, at which survival of the cells was normal but their proliferation rate slightly lowered, and 10^{-6}M, at which cell proliferation fell by 50% already after 24 hours of contact.

The activity of dihydrofolate reductase decreased when the cells passed their logarithmic phase of growth; in the cells from the media with amethopterin, this fall of activity was much sharper and increased with time and with increase in the concentration of the drug. The activity of serine hydroxymethyltransferase was nearly the same as in the control cultures, unless the amethopterin concentration was a growth-limiting one. Methionine synthetase activity fell in the cells of the experimental cultures, parallel to its fall in the control cells. However, a 24 hour-contact of the cells with amethopterin 10^{-6}M resulted in a strong (by 85%) but transient and repeatable depression of the activity of this synthetase, which returned later to the control level. The activity curves for thymidylate synthetase show the maximum between 24 and 48 hours after subculturing. The activity in the cells cultured with amethopterin at the lowest concentration exceeded that of the cells from the control medium, probably because of stabilization of the enzyme molecules by the drug[12].

The activity of isocitrate and that of glucose-6-phosphate dehydrogenases were only slightly lowered by amethopterin at the particular concentration which did not limit the cell proliferation, and decreased by 50% by this drug when applied at the growth-limiting concentration 10^{-6}M. The activity of lactate dehydrogenase, constant in the cells under the control conditions, was strongly lowered in cells cultured in the presence of amethopterin, and this effect increased with time and with increase in the amethopterin concentration.

Addition of folate coenzymes into the medium simultaneously with amethopterin, prevented the effects of the drug on the activity of lactate dehydrogenase and methionine synthetase in L-cells, even at concentrations at which — in the absence of these coenzymes — amethopterin was very toxic for the cells (Table 1). In contrast, none of the folate coenzymes tested could prevent dihydrofolate reductase from inhibiting activity in L-cells.

In summarizing, it is worth noting that amethopterin, even at concentrations not limiting L-cell proliferation, limited the activity of all the enzymes assayed except that of thymidylate synthetase.

Amethopterin - at concentrations far above those in the media we applied - did not inhibit any of the dehydrogenases examined in vitro, and inhibited only slightly the activity of folate-related non-target enzymes. We can conclude therefore, that the observed side effects of the drug are not a consequence of a direct interaction of amethopterin with the enzyme molecules, but rather are secondary effects on some metabolic processes. Our finding that amethopterin decreased significantly the overall protein and DNA synthesis in L-cells (unpublished), is relevant to this point.

We have recently found that the activity of lactate dehydrogenase in L-cells was also strongly depressed by aminopterin and a quinazoline analogue of folate present in the culture medium[13]. Whether

amethopterin and the other drugs influence the isoenzyme pattern
of lactate dehydrogenase and the energy charge in the cells remains
to be assayed.

TABLE 1

ACTIVITY OF DIHYDROFOLATE REDUCTASE (DHFR), VITAMIN B12-DEPENDENT
METHIONINE SYNTHETASE (MS) AND LACTATE DEHYDROGENASE (LDH) IN L-CELLS
CULTURED FOR 48 HOURS IN THE MEDIUM WITH AMETHOPTERIN OR WITH THAT
PLUS A FOLATE COENZYME

Concentrations of amethopterin in the medium were $1.6 \times 10^{-6} M$[a] or
$1.5 \times 10^{-5} M$[b], whereas those of formyl H_4PteGlu and methyl H_4PteGlu
were respectively 24 or 35 times higher than that of the drug. Each
value represents the mean of at least triplicate determinations.

Medium with addition	DHFR[a]		MS[b]		LDH[b]	
	Sp.act.[c]	%	Sp.act.[c]	%	Sp.act.[d]	%
None	93	100	2.0	100	0.90	100
5-formyl-H_4PteGlu	82	88	2.3	115	0.84	93
5-methyl-H_4PteGlu	96	103	2.7	135	0.96	107
Amethopterin	7	7	0.8	40	0.18	20
Amethopterin + 5-formyl-H_4PteGlu	17	18	1.8	90	0.84	93
Amethopterin + 5-methyl-H_4PteGlu	17	18	2.0	100	0.96	107

Sp.act. - specific activity in respective units per mg protein and
per hour: [c]nmole, [d]mmole.

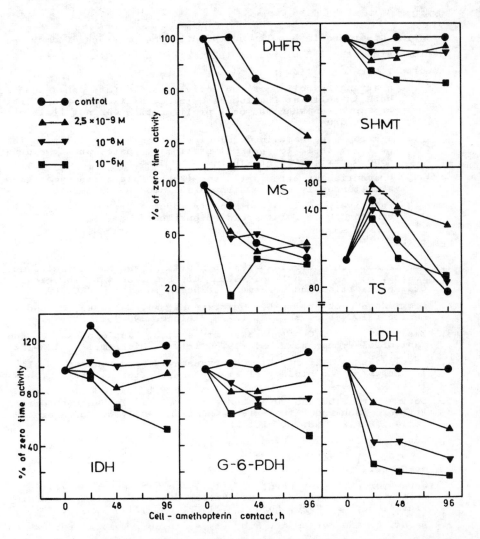

Fig. 1. Activity of dihydrofolate reductase (DHFR), serine hydroxymethyltransferase (SHMT), vitamin B12-dependent methionine synthetase (MS), thymidylate synthetase (TS), isocitrate dehydrogenase
(IDH), glucose-6-phosphate dehydrogenase (G-6-PDH) and lactate dehydrogenase (LDH) in L-cells cultured up to 96 h in the standard
medium, or in the presence of amethopterin at indicated concentrations. The inhibitor was added 24 h after subculturing. The activity
of the enzymes is expressed as a percentage of zero time activity,
whose respective values per mg protein and per hour were for: DHFR 70
nmole, MS 2.5 nmole, TS 0.25 nmole, SHMT 1.5 umole, IDH 60 umole,
G-6-PDH 35 umole, LDH 1.0 mmole. Each value is the mean of the
triplicate estimations in at least three experiments.

SUMMARY

Enzyme disorders in L-cells cultured in the presence of amethopterin besides the inhibition of the target enzyme dihydrofolate
reductase, were as follows:

(1) a strong reduction of the activity of lactate dehydrogenase
    both in cells at the logarithmic and stationary phase of
    growth, even when the cell proliferation was not limited
    by the drug

(2) a strong decrease in methionine synthetase activity in the
    cells at their log but not stationary phase, when the drug
    concentration was growth-limiting

(3) prevention of effects (1) and (2) by folate coenzymes added
    simultaneously with amethopterin into the culture medium

(4) relatively small effects of the drug on the activity of the
    non-log phase folate-related enzymes.

REFERENCES

1. Zielińska, Z.M., Grzelakowska-Sztabert, B. and Manteuffel-Cymborowska, M. (1978) in Proc. VIIth Int. Symp. on the Biological
   Characterization and Treatment of Human Tumors, 4, 294-298.

2. Grzelakowska-Sztabert, B., Chmurzyńska, W., Balińska, M. and
   Manteuffel-Cymborowska, M. (1978) ibidem, 299-302.

3. Zielińska, Z.M., Grzelakowska-Sztabert, B., Koziorowska, J. and
   Manteuffel-Cymborowska, M. (1974) Int. J. Biochem.. 5, 173-182.

4. Grzelakowska-Sztabert, B., Chmurzyńska, W. and Landman, M. (1976)
   in Chemistry and Biology of Pteridines, Walter de Gruyter, New
   York, pp. 143-151.

5. Scrimgeour, K.G. and Huennekens, F.M. (1966) in Handbuch der
   Physiologisch und Pathologisch-Chemische Analyse, Springer
   Verlag, Berlin, 6B, pp. 181-208.

6. Roberts, D.W. (1966) Biochemistry, 5, 3546-3548.

7. Kamely, D., Littlefield, J.W. and Erbe, R.W. (1973) Proc. Natl.
   Acad. Sci., U.S.A., 70, 2585-2589.

8. Bergmeyer, H.U. and Bernt, E. (1974) in Methods of Enzymatic
   Analysis, Bergmeyer H.U. ed., Verlag Chemie Weinheim, Academic
   Press Inc., New York, London, Vol. 2, pp. 574-583.

9. Bernt, E. and Bergmeyer, H.U. (1974) ibidem, Vol. 2, pp. 624-631.

10. Löhr, G.W. and Waller, H.D. (1974) ibidem, Vol. 2, pp. 636-643.

11. Lowry, O.H., Rosebrough, N.J., Farr, A.L. and Randall, K.J.
    (1951) J. Biol. Chem., 193, 265-275.

12. Bonney, R.J., Maley, F. (1975) Cancer Res., 35, 1950-1956.

13. Grzelakowska-Sztabert, B., Balińska, M., Chmurzynska, W. and
    Zielińska, Z.M. (1978) Proc. of the Post-Congress FEBS Symp. on
    Antimetabolites in Biochemistry, Biology and Medicine, in press.

Author Index

Subject Index